Quick Reference to Physical Therapy

Quick Reference to Physical Therapy

SECOND EDITION

Julie A. Pauls, PhD, PT, ICCE

Kathlyn L. Reed, PhD, OTR, FAOTA, MLIS, AHIP

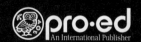

8700 Shoal Creek Boulevard
Austin, Texas 78757-6897
800/897-3202   Fax 800/397-7633
www.proedinc.com

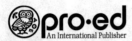
An International Publisher

© 1996, 2004 by PRO-ED, Inc.
8700 Shoal Creek Boulevard
Austin, Texas 78757-6897
800/897-3202 Fax 800/397-7633
www.proedinc.com

NOTICE: The authors have made every effort to ensure the accuracy of the
information herein, particularly with regard to drug selection and dose.
However, appropriate information sources should be consulted, especially
for new or unfamiliar drugs or procedures. It is the responsibility of every
practitioner to evaluate the appropriateness of a particular opinion in the
context of actual clinical situations and with due consideration to new
developments. Authors, editors, and the publisher cannot be held
responsible for any typographical or other errors found in this book.

Library of Congress Cataloging-in-Publication Data

Pauls, Julie A.
    Quick reference to physical therapy/by Julie A. Pauls & Kathlyn L. Reed—
2nd ed.
        p. ; cm.
        Includes bibliographical references and index.
        ISBN 0-89079-961-X
        1. Physical therapy—Handbooks, manuals, etc. I. Reed, Kathlyn L.   II.
        Title.
    [DNLM: 1 Physical Therapy Techniques—Handbooks.   WB 39
P332q2003]
RM701 .P38   2003
615.8′2—dc21

This book is designed in Stone Sans, Lucida Sans and
Lucida Sans Narrow.

Printed in the United States of America

2 3 4 5 6 7 8 9 10   07 06 05 04

This book is dedicated to my family:
Ralph, Lauren, and Mark.

—JP

This book is dedicated to my father,
Herbert C. Reed.

—KR

Contents

Chapter 13
Pulmonary Disorders   587

Acknowledgments

The authors would like to thank the editors of PRO-ED for their expert assistance in producing the second edition of *Quick Reference to Physical Therapy*. In particular, we appreciate the editorial guidance of Senior Editor Peggy Kipping and Permissions Editor Robin Spencer.

Introduction to the First Edition

Purpose

This book provides a synopsis of the diseases, disorders, and dysfunctions referenced in the physical therapy literature. The format used gives all therapists, whether they are students, clinicians, educators, or researchers, quick access to the information needed to assess, educate, and treat clients.

Sources

Most of the references cited were published from 1985 through 1995. Selected older sources supplement the current literature. To qualify for inclusion in the text, one of the authors of the article, chapter, or book had to be identified as a physical therapist. **Publications with no input by a physical therapist were excluded.** Authors who are not physical therapists appear only if the article was published in a physical therapy journal.

Classifications of the disorders were generally derived from the Medical Subject Headings (MeSH) list from the National Library of Medicine (NLM). Using these MeSH classifications, we compiled references from seven computer databases: Allied Alternative Medicine (AMED) from Data-Star, Cumulative Index to Nursing and Allied Health Literature (CINAHL), Current Contents, EMBASE, MEDLINE, NLM Locator, and RNdex. Bibliographies from these references led to a trail of additional references.

The journals researched were:

- *Australian Journal of Physiotherapy*
- *British Journal of Physiotherapy*
- *Clinical Management in Physical Therapy*
- *Clinics in Physical Therapy*
- *Journal of Obstetric and Gynecologic Physical Therapy*
- *Journal of Orthopaedic and Sports Physical Therapy*
- *Journal of Physical Therapy Science*
- *National Association of Physical Therapy*
- *New Zealand Journal of Physiotherapy*
- *Orthopaedic Physical Therapy Clinics of North America*
- *Pediatric Physical Therapy*
- *Physical and Occupational Physical Therapy in Geriatrics*
- *Physical and Occupational Physical Therapy in Pediatrics*
- *Physical Therapy*
- *Physical Therapy Practice*
- *Physiotherapy (South Africa)*
- *Physiotherapy (England)*
- *Physiotherapy Canada*
- *Physiotherapy Theory and Practice*
- *PT Magazine of Physical Therapy*

Titles of the journals are listed in full in the text to facilitate reference location. Physical therapy journals cited should be available through standard library sources.

Format

Each disorder is described according to the same format:

1. *Disorder:* The name of a disorder, followed by any additional names by which the condition is known. Some conditions, such as Raynaud's disease, were omitted because not enough information was found to complete the format. Other conditions, such as balance disorders and vestibular dysfunction, were included as problems of other disorders instead of being listed separately. When it was appropriate, similar conditions were grouped together because their assessment and treatment were the same.
2. *Description:* A brief summary of the disorder, based on the *Merck Manual* or selected references cited at the end of the section.
3. *Cause:* A review of the cause of the disorder, if known, based on the *Merck Manual* or selected references at the end of the section.
4. *Assessment*
   - *Areas:* A list outlining the scope of assessment categories. This list should be adapted to the client's condition. It may *not* be indicated or appropriate to include every area in the initial or subsequent assessments.
   - *Instruments/procedures:* Published tools for evaluation or research, provided under corresponding categories. The tools listed offer a menu of tests, forms, and instrumentation that therapists can use as directed by the client's condition. These instruments were not necessarily invented by a physical therapist but are now cited in the therapeutic literature.
5. *Problems:* Clinical problems or complaints that a client can experience with each disorder.
6. *Treatment/management:* A synopsis of treatment and management options derived from selected references. This section is not intended to be a detailed treatment manual; rather, it is a rapid review of published procedures, protocols, and suggestions for therapeutic care. Therapists are encouraged to refer clients to the support groups listed in the appendices when needed.
7. *Precautions/contraindications:* Notes of caution mentioned by clinicians and researchers. This section is supplemented by a list of contraindications to physical agents and modalities in the appendices.
8. *Desired outcome/prognosis:* The goals of treatment, highlighted by bullets and followed by a mention of expectations found in the physical therapy literature.
9. *References:* A comprehensive list of articles and books, divided into references for assessment and treatment.

Conclusion

This reference guide is based on a survey of physical therapy publications that included contents from seven databases, 23 journal titles, and over 175 texts. It reflects the breadth of current practice and identifies areas in the literature that lack depth. Therapists are encouraged to continue contributions to the literature so as to refine the areas that are well established and to establish the emerging fields.

Introduction to the Second Edition

Positive feedback from clinicians, academics, and students on the first edition of *Quick Reference to Physical Therapy* prompts us to provide an updated, second edition. This new edition continues to offer rapid access to information needed to prevent or treat impairments, disabilities, or other changes in health status due to disease or injury.

The protocol for obtaining references and reviewing information continued, as in the first edition, with the addition of new topics, such as the treatment of vestibular dysfunction. References cited were published primarily between 1991 and 2001 to reflect the physical therapy literature from the past decade. There are also two major changes reflecting new practices: The inclusion of preferred practice patterns recommended in the American Physical Therapy Association's (APTA) *Guide to Physical Therapist Practice* (1998) and an emphasis on tools that promote evidence-based medicine (EBM).

The *Guide to Physical Therapist Practice* was widely distributed in 1997 and used by clinicians, educators, health care administrators, and payers. It is used to promote improved quality of care with a more efficient use of resources.

Physical therapists are also increasingly engaged in evidence-based medicine, also called evidence-based practice. According to Sackett, et al, evidence-based practice is the "conscientious, explicit, and judicious use of current best evidence in making decisions about the care of individual patients." (Sackett DL, et al. *Evidence-based Medicine: How to Practice and Teach EBM*. Edinburgh, Scotland: Churchill Livingstone; 1998:2).

Clinical expertise remains a highly valued ability in identifying each patient's health status, diagnosis, and need for interventions. But, the need for evidence-based practice has emerged in order to cut costs while still giving patients access to the most current therapies. Our new edition seeks to facilitate and expedite this process.

Chapter 1

Conditions in Athletic Injuries

Note: See also Chapter 8, Musculoskeletal Disorders.

Anterior Cruciate Ligament (ACL) Tear

DESCRIPTION

At the onset of injury to the anterior cruciate ligament (ACL), the athlete usually hears a popping noise. This is often followed by rapid swelling and decreased function, including the inability to walk. Other ligaments commonly torn include the posterior cruciate ligament, medial collateral ligament, and lateral collateral ligament. There is also a high incidence of accompanying patellofemoral pain.

CAUSE

In sports that involve jumping, twisting, and pivoting, the ACL is commonly injured through the following forces at the knee joint: valgus stress with external rotation of tibia, varus stress with internal rotation of the tibia, hyperextension, deceleration, or a crossover cut maneuver.

ASSESSMENT

Note: See APTA's Guide to Physical Therapist Practice. 2nd ed. *Physical Therapy.* 2001;81.

Musculoskeletal Preferred Practice Patterns: E, J

AREAS

- History
- Pain
- Gait
- Posture
- Balance
- Joint integrity and structural deviations
- Mobility: active and passive range of motion (ROM) and accessory motion
- Strength
- Neurological: sensation, proprioception, deep tendon reflexes, neural tension
- Skin and soft tissue: temperature, tenderness, tone, edema
- Functional level, including activities of daily living (ADLs)
- Special tests to which the PT may or may not have access

INSTRUMENTS/PROCEDURES

See References for sources.

Balance
- Single-leg standing balance test

Functional Level
- Cincinnati rating system
- Duocondylar rating scale
- Knee society rating scale
- Lysholm knee rating scale
- Modified Lysholm knee score

Joint Integrity and Structural Deviations

Following are orthopedic tests for the knee. Those recommended, especially for this condition, are marked with an asterisk. *Note:* Lachman's test is commonly used for assessing impaired anterial tibial translation.

- A-angle
- Anterolateral Rational Instability (ALRI)
- anterior drawer sign*
- Anteromedial Rotational Instability (AMRI)

- Apley grinding test
- apprehension test*
- bounce home test
- brush or stroke (wipe) test
- Clark sign
- crossover test
- Ely test
- external rotation test*
- flexion rotation drawer test
- fluctuation test*
- gravity drawer test (posterior sag sign)
- hamstring length
- Helfet test
- Hughston plica test
- Hughston posterolateral drawer test
- Hughston test (jerk sign)
- hyperflexion-hyperextension test
- Jakob test (reverse pivot)
- Lachman's test*
- lateral pull test
- limb-length discrepancy
- MacIntosh test (lateral pivot shift)*
- McConnell test
- McMurray-Anderson test*
- Noble's compression test
- Ober's test
- O'Donoghue test
- patellar tap test*
- patellar tilt test
- Perkins test
- plica test
- posterior drawer sign*
- posterior sag sign*
- quadriceps active test
- reverse pivot shift*
- Slocum test
- Steinman's test
- squat test
- tibial displacement test
- valgus stress test
- varus stress test*—at 0 and 30 degrees
- Waldron test
- Wilson test

Mobility
- goniometry
- knee ligament arthrometer
- KT-2000 arthrometer for instrumented laxity testing

Pain
- palpation
- visual analog scale

Skin and Soft Tissue
- temperature, tenderness, tone
- palpation
- edema
- tape measure
- water displacement

Special Tests to Which the Physical Therapist May or May Not Have Access
- arthroscopy

Strength
1. instrumentation
   - cable tensiometers
   - isokinetic dynamometers
   - strain gauge devices
2. manual muscle testing

PROBLEMS

- The athlete with knee instability is usually unable to bear weight normally.
- The athlete may report knee has a history of "giving way."
- There is often weakness at the quadriceps muscle.
- The athlete will often have pain with active movement of the knee.
- There is limited ROM at the knee.

- There may be decreased proprioception.
- There may be an antalgic gait pattern.

- The athlete may have repeated episodes of pain and swelling of the knee.

TREATMENT/MANAGEMENT

ACUTE INJURY

The acronym PRICEMM outlines a general approach for pain and inflammation (see Figure 1.1).

KNEE REHABILITATION

Knee rehabilitation following ACL tears may follow a conservative, nonsurgical course of rehabilitation or, if the client elects surgery, a postsurgical course of rehabilitation. Conservative and postsurgical protocols vary. A therapist should work closely with the athlete's physician during the rehabilitation process.

In general, the phases of knee rehabilitation can be described as follows:

- *Phase 1:* Treat pain, inflammation, and intra-articular swelling. Provide client education.
- *Phase 2:* Regain limited motion and reeducate previously disused tissues. Control swelling and pain.
- *Phase 3:* Retrain function. Tissue realignment should be monitored for proper forces. Reduce risk of reinjury during ADLs.
- *Phase 4:* Begin light activity, progressing toward full functional retraining.
- *Phase 5:* Promote full return to activities and progress maintenance.

The following general suggestions apply to any ACL rehabilitation program:

- Exercise should emphasize hamstring control of anterior tibial translation. Consider the use of closed-chain exercises, including proprioceptive neuromuscular facilitation (PNF), wall slides, leg presses, reclined squats, stair climber, and sta-

---

Protection

Rest: Eliminate aggravating activities

Ice

Compression

Elevation

Medication as prescribed

Modalities: high-voltage electrical stimulation, ultra-sound, ice, heat

---

FIGURE 1.1. PRICEMM acronym outlining general approach for pain and inflammation.

tionary bike. The quadriceps muscle should be exercised in a protected range greater than 45 degrees flexion or with cocontraction. Surgical tubing may be used as an adjunct to exercise.

- Cryotherapy is often used for 15 to 20 minutes after an exercise session.
- Consider the use of transcutaneous electrical nerve stimulation (TENS) for pain.
- Consider the use of a compression pump for swelling.
- The athlete may need an ambulation assistive device using controlled weight bearing.
- Knee immobilizers may be used for a brief period. Assess the need for derotational bracing.
- Electrical stimulation may help with joint effusion and muscular control.
- Consider the incorporation of balance and coordination activities such as a biomechanical ankle platform system (BAPS) board or unsupported single-stance activities.
- Consider using sport-specific activities such as cutting drills, running, and jumping.

Conservative Management of ACL-Deficient Knee

See References for recommended protocols.

Postsurgical Management of the ACL-Reconstructed Knee

Table 1.1 offers a sample postoperative protocol for ACL reconstruction. See References for additional recommended protocols.

PREVENTION

Develop strength and endurance in musculature surrounding the knee to promote stability and injury prevention.

For exercise sequence post anterior cruciate ligament reconstruction and return to sport protocol, see *Clinical Practice Guidelines* by Schunk and Reed.

PRECAUTIONS/CONTRAINDICATIONS

- Conservative and postsurgical protocols vary. A therapist should work closely with the athlete's physician or surgeon during the rehabilitation process.
- All protocols should be tailored to an athlete's individual problems.
- Unnecessary immobilization should be avoided. Consider use of continuous passive motion following surgery.
- The quadriceps should be strengthened with cocontraction or in a protective range (ie, less than 45 degrees flexion).
- Do not progress athletes to the next level of rehabilitation unless they reach success at their current level. Progress depends on the rate of healing.

DESIRED OUTCOME/PROGNOSIS

- The athlete will have diminished or no pain, inflammation, or intra-articular swelling.
- The athlete will be educated in the avoidance of reinjury during ADLs.
- The athlete will not suffer loss of conditioning in uninjured areas of the body.
- The athlete will have full motion and function.
- Postsurgically, the athlete will avoid ligament failure, regain strength, and protect the articular surfaces.

Note: If an athlete's goal is to continue with a sport or stressful work, he or she is usually a candidate for reconstructive surgery instead of conservative treatment.

TABLE 1.1
Accelerated Rehabilitation for Anterior Cruciate Ligament Reconstruction

Rehabilitation Protocol Postoperative Time	Exercise	Activity
0-1 day		Begin gait training and pain control
1-7 days		Monitor wound daily
		Cryo-cuff and PRICE as often as indicated
		Use immobilizer in full extension for sleeping and weight-bearing activities
	Begin weight bearing with crutches as tolerated	
	Use patellofemoral mobilization as tolerated	
	Use wall slide exercise for flexion (< or = 120 degrees as tolerated)	
		Promote full terminal knee extension ASAP
7-14 days	Begin using closed kinematic chain for strengthening	
	Use stationary bike for ROM and strengthening	
	Consider pool exercises if wound is healed	
		Begin incisional mobilization ASAP
	Initiate progressive weight bearing to tolerance	
		Continue PRICE as needed (prn)
	Offer electrical muscle stimulation as needed (prn)	
		Provide proprioceptive balance board activities
2-6 weeks	Progress flexion to full as tolerated	
	Continue weight bearing to full as tolerated	
	Use progressive closed kinematic chain for strengthening	
		Continue PRICE post-exercise
6-12 weeks	Progress to jumping rope, sliding board, lateral shuffles	
	Advance to pool running as tolerated	
	Initiate light jogging	
	Continue using closed kinematic chain for strengthening	
12-24 weeks	Increase closed kinematic chain exercise, agility, and functional activities, such as running, jumping and cutting, as tolerated	
	Consider functional brace for sports or work	

Source: Reprinted with permission from Tomberlin JP, Saunders HD. *Evaluation, Treatment and Prevention of Musculoskeletal Disorders.* The Saunders Group; 1994:2:256.

REFERENCES

Assessment

American Physical Therapy Association. Guide to physical therapist practice. 2nd ed. *Phys Ther*. 2001;81.

Bandy WD, Timm KE. Relationship between peak torque, work, and power for knee flexion and extension in clients with grade I medial compartment sprains of the knee. *J Orthop Sports Phys Ther*. 1992;16:288–292.

Buschbacher RM, ed. *Musculoskeletal Disorders: A Practical Guide for Diagnosis and Rehabilitation*. Boston, Mass: Andover Medical Publishers; 1994.

Ciccotti MG, Kerlan RK, Perry J, et al. An electromyographic analysis of the knee during functional activities: the normal profile. *Am J Sports Med*. 1994;22:645–650.

Clark NC. Functional performance testing following knee ligament injury. *Phys Ther Sport*. 2001;2:91–105.

Daniels L, Worthingham C. *Muscle Testing Techniques of Manual Examination*. 6th ed. Philadelphia, Pa: WB Saunders Co; 1995.

Hall CM, Brody TB. *Therapeutic Exercise: Moving Toward Function*. Philadelphia, Pa: Lippincott Williams and Wilkins; 1999.

Hertling D, Kessler RM. *Management of Common Musculoskeletal Disorders*. 3rd ed. Philadelphia, Pa: JB Lippincott Co; 1996:78, 534.

Itoh H, Ichihashi N, Maruyama T, Kurosaka M, Hirohata K. Weakness of thigh muscles in individuals sustaining anterior cruciate ligament injury. *Kobe J Med Sci*. 1992;38:2:93–107.

Kramer J, Nusca D, Fowler P, Webster-Bogaert S. Knee flexor and extensor strength during concentric and eccentric muscle actions after anterior cruciate ligament reconstruction using the semitendinosus tendon and ligament augmentation device. *Am J Sports Med*. 1993;21:285–291.

Malone TR, McPoil T, Nitz AJ, eds. *Orthopaedic and Sports Physical Therapy*. 3rd ed. St. Louis, Mo: CV Mosby Co; 1997.

McComb FH, Kerr KM. Isokinetic strength of the thigh muscles following the dacron method of reconstruction of the anterior cruciate ligament. *Physiotherapy*. 1992;78:478–483.

Myers RS, ed. *Saunders Manual of Physical Therapy Practice*. Philadelphia, Pa: WB Saunders Co; 1995.

Risberg MA, Ekeland A. Assessment of functional tests after anterior cruciate ligament surgery. *J Orthop Sports Phys Ther*. 1994;19:212–217.

Rothstein JM, Roy SH, Wolf SL. *The Rehabilitation Specialist's Handbook*. 2nd ed. Philadelphia, Pa: FA Davis Co; 1998.

Saidoff DC, McDonough AL. *Critical Pathways in Therapeutic Intervention*. Philadelphia, Pa: CV Mosby Co; 2002.

Schunk C, Reed K. *Clinical Practice Guidelines*. Gaithersburg, Md: Aspen Publishers; 2000.

Snyder-Mackler L, Binder-Macleod SA, Williams PR. Fatiguability of human quadriceps femoris muscle following anterior cruciate ligament reconstruction. *Med Sci Sports Exerc*. 1993;25:783–789.

Snyder-Mackler L, Delitto A, Bailey SL, et al. Strength of the quadriceps femoris muscle and functional recovery after reconstruction of the anterior cruciate ligament. *J Bone Joint Surg Am*. 1995;77:1166–1173.

Tomberlin JP, Saunders HD. *Evaluation, Treatment and Prevention of Musculoskeletal Disorders. Vol 2: Extremities*. Chaska, Minn: The Saunders Group; 1994.

Wilk KE, Andrews JR, Clancy WG. Quadriceps muscular strength after removal of the central third patellar tendon for contralateral anterior cruciate ligament reconstruction surgery: a case study. *J Orthop Sports Phys Ther.* 1993;18:692–697.

Treatment

American Physical Therapy Association. *Sports Physical Therapy: Description of Advanced Clinical Practice.* Alexandria, Va: APTA; 1997. APTA.

Beard DJ, Fergusson CM. The conservative management of anterior cruciate ligament deficiency: a nationwide survey of current practice. *Physiotherapy.* 1992;78:181–186.

Bennell KL, Malcom SA, Wark JD, et al. Skeletal effects of menstrual disturbances in athletes. *Scandinavian J Med Sci Sports.* 1997;7:261–273.

Beynnon BD, Fleming BC, Johnson RJ, et al. Anterior cruciate ligament strain behaviour during rehabilitation exercises in vivo. *Am J Sports Med.* 1995;23:24.

Brewer BW, Van Raalte JL, Petitpas AJ, et al. Preliminary psychometric evaluation of a measure of adherence to clinic-based sport injury rehabilitation. *Phys Ther Sport.* 2000; 1:68–74.

Brownstein B, Bronner S. Patella fractures associated with accelerated ACL rehabilitation in patients with autogenous patella tendon reconstructions. *J Orthop Sports Phys Ther.* 1997;26:168–172.

Buss DD, Warren RF, Wickiewicz TL, Galinat BJ, Panariello R. Arthroscopically assisted reconstruction of the anterior cruciate ligament with use of autogenous patellar-ligament grafts: results after twenty-four to forty-two months. *J Bone Joint Surg.* 1993; 75A:1346–1355.

Chaitow L. *Muscle Energy Techniques.* New York, NY: Churchill Livingstone; 1997.

Corrigan JP, Cashmen WF, Brady MP. Proprioception in the cruciate deficient knee. *J Bone Joint Surg Br.* 1992;74:247–250.

Currier DP, Ray JM, Nyland J, Rooney JG, Noteboom JT, Kellogg R. Effects of electrical and electromagnetic stimulation after anterior cruciate ligament reconstruction. *J Orthop Sports Phys Ther.* 1993;17:177–184.

Dakin A. Management of anterior cruciate ligament deficient patients: group education and exercise. *Physiotherapy.* 2000;86:348–356.

De Bie RA, Verhagen AP, Lenssen AF, et al. Efficacy of 904 nm laser therapy in the management of musculoskeletal disorders: a systematic review. *Phys Ther Rev.* 1998;3: 59–72.

DeCarlo MS, Shelbourne KD, McCarroll JR, Rettig AC. Traditional versus accelerated rehabilitation following ACL reconstruction: a one-year follow-up. *J Orthop Sports Phys Ther.* 1992;15:309–316.

Delitto A. Lower extremity: knee. In: Myers RS, ed. *Saunders Manual of Physical Therapy Practice.* Philadelphia, Pa: WB Saunders Co; 1995:1011.

DeVita P, Hortobagyi T, Barrier J. Gait biomechanics are not normal after anterior cruciate ligament reconstruction and accelerated rehabilitation. *Med Sci Sports Exerc.* In press.

Einhorn AR, Sawyer M, Tovin B. Rehabilitation of intra-articular reconstructions. In: Greenfield BH, ed. *Rehabilitation of the Knee: A Problem-Solving Approach.* Philadelphia, Pa: FA Davis Co; 1993:288–303.

Eyestone ED, Fellinghav G, George J, Fisher AG. Effect of water running and cycling on maximum oxygen consumption and 2-mile run performance. *Am J Sports Med.* 1993; 21:41–44.

Fields J, Murhey M, Horodyski MB, Stopka C. Factors associated with adherence to sport injury rehabilitation in college-age recreational athletes. *J Sport Rehabil.* 1995;9:172–180.

Fitzgibbons RE, Shelbourne KD. "Aggressive" non-treatment of lateral meniscal tears seen during anterior cruciate ligament reconstruction. *Am J Sports Med.* 1995;23:156–165.

Fu FH, Woo SL, Irrgang JJ. Current concepts for rehabilitation following anterior cruciate ligament reconstruction. *J Orthop Sports Phys Ther.* 1992;15:270–278.

Gross MT, Tyson AD, Burns CB. Effect of knee angle and ligament insufficiency on anterior tibial translation during quadriceps muscle contraction: a preliminary report. *J Orthop Sports Phys Ther.* 1993;17:133–143.

Gryzlo SM, Patek RM, Pink M, Perry M. Electromyographic evaluation of closed and open kinetic chain knee rehabilitation exercises. *J Orthop Sports Phys Ther.* 1994;20:36–43.

Guskiewicz KM, Perrin DH. Research and clinical applications of assessing balance. *J Sport Rehabil.* 1996;5:45–63.

Hall CM, Brody TB. *Therapeutic Exercise: Moving Toward Function.* Philadelphia, Pa: Lippincott Williams and Wilkins; 1999.

Harrison EL, Duenkel N, Dunlop R, Russell G. Evaluation of single-leg standing following anterior cruciate ligament surgery and rehabilitation. *Phys Ther.* 1994;74:245–252.

Hutchinson MR, Ireland ML. Knee injuries in female athletes. *Sports Med.* 1995;19:222–236.

Irrgang JJ. *Closed Kinetic Chain Exercises for the Lower Extremity: Theory and Application.* LaCrosse, Wis: Sports Physical Therapy Home Study Course, Sports Physical Therapy Section of the American Physical Therapy Association; 1994.

Jobe C, Jobe FW, Pink M. The sports medicine rehabilitation center. In: Nickel VL, Botte MJ, eds. *Orthopaedic Rehabilitation.* 2nd ed. New York, NY: Churchill Livingstone; 1992: 207–221.

Johnson MI. Acupuncture-like transcutaneous electrical nerve stimulation (AL-TENS) in the management of pain. *Phys Ther Rev* 1998;3:73–93.

Kibbler WB, Herring SA, Press JM, eds. *Functional Rehabilitation of Sports and Musculoskeletal Injuries.* Gaithersburg, Md: Aspen Publishers; 1998.

Lephart SC, Perrin DH, Fu FH, Gieck JH, McCue FC III, Irrgang JJ. Relationship between selected physical characteristics and functional capacity in the anterior cruciate ligament-insufficient athlete. *J Orthop Sports Phys Ther.* 1992;16:174–181.

Lephart SM, Pinccivero DM, Jorge LG, et al. The role of proprioception in the management and rehabilitation of athletic injuries. *Am J Sports Med.* 1997;25:130–137.

Lewis T. Anterior cruciate ligament injury in female athletes: why are women so vulnerable? A Literature Review. *Physiotherapy.* 2000;86:464–472.

Loudon JK. The relationship between static posture and ACL injury in female athletes. *J Orthop Sports Phys Ther.* 1996;24:91–97.

Magee D. *Orthopedic Physical Assessment.* 3rd ed. Philadelphia, Pa: WB Saunders Co; 1997.

Malone TR, McPoil T, Nitz AJ, eds. *Orthopaedic and Sports Physical Therapy.* 3rd ed. St. Louis, Mo: CV Mosby Co; 1997.

Mangine RE, Kremcheck TE. Evaluation-based protocol of the anterior cruciate ligament. *J Sport Rehabil.* 1997;6:157–181.

Mangine RE, Noyes FR. Rehabilitation of the allograft reconstruction. *J Orthop Sports Phys Ther.* 1992;15:294–302.

Mangine RE, Noyes FR, DeMaio M. Minimal protection program: advanced weight bearing and range of motion after ACL reconstruction-weeks 1 to 5. *Orthop.* 1992;15:504–515.

McCarthy MR, Yates CK, Anderson MA, Yates-McCarthy JL. The effects of immediate continuous passive motion on pain during the inflammatory phase of soft tissue healing following anterior cruciate ligament reconstruction. *J Orthop Sports Phys Ther.* 1993: 17:96–101.

Mohr KJ, Pink MM, Elsner C, et al. Electromyographic investigation of stretching: the effect of warm-up. *Clin J Sports Med.* 1998;8:215–220.

Muneta T, Sekiya I, Ogiuchi T, et al. Effects of aggressive early rehabilitation on the outcome of anterior cruciate ligament reconstruction with multi-strand semitendinosus tendon. *Int Orthop.* 1998;22:352–356.

Ninedek A, Kolt GS. Sport physiotherapists' perceptions of psychological strategies in sport injury rehabilitation. *J Sport Rehabil.* 2000;9:191–206.

Norris CM. *Sports Injuries: Diagnosis and Management for Physiotherapists.* Boston, Mass: Butterworth Heinemann; 1993.

Osteras H, Augestad LB, Tondel S. Isokinetic muscle strength after anterior cruciate ligament reconstruction. *Scand J Med Sci Sports.* 1998;8:279–282.

Overend T, Lee W, Speechley M. Anterior cruciate ligament injuries in intercollegiate basketball players: a survey of gender difference. *Physiotherapy Can.* 1999;51:22–26.

Panariello RA, Backus SI, Parker JW. The effect of squat exercise on anterior-posterior knee translation in professional football players. *Am J Sports Med.* 1994;22:768–773.

Parker MG. Biomechanical and histological concepts in the rehabilitation of patients with anterior cruciate ligament reconstructions. *J Orthop Sports Phys Ther.* 1994;20(1):44–50.

Petsche TS, Hutchinson MR. Loss of extension after reconstruction of the anterior cruciate ligament. *J Am Acad Orthop Surg.* 1999;7:119–127.

Prins J, Cutner D. Aquatic therapy in the rehabilitation of athletic injuries. *Clin Sports Med.* 1999;18:447–461.

Rankin AE, Kramer JF, Fowler PJ, et al. Survey of knee brace usage following anterior cruciate ligament reconstruction. *Physiotherapy Can.* 2000;52:215–224.

Roebroeck ME, Dekker J, Oostendorp RA. The use of therapeutic ultrasound by physical therapists in Dutch primary health care. *Phys Ther.* 1998;78:470–478.

St. Clair Gibson A, Lamber MI, Myburgh KH, et al. The relationship between functional capacity, muscle size and strength in chronic ACL deficient and ACL reconstructed individuals. *S Afr J Physiotherapy.* 2000;56:12–18.

Schmidt G. Latest technique in ACL surgery and rehabilitation. *J Orthop Sports Phys Ther.* 1992;15:256–322.

Seto JL, Brewster CE, Lombardo SJ, Tibone JE. Rehabilitation of the knee after anterior cruciate ligament reconstruction. *J Orthop Sports Phys Ther.* 1989;11:8–18.

Shelbourne KD, Davis TJ. Evaluation of knee stability before and after participation in a functional sports agility program during rehabilitation after anterior cruciate ligament reconstruction. *Am J Sports Med.* 1999;27:156–161.

Shelbourne KD, Klootwyk TE, DeCarlo MS. Update on accelerated rehabilitation after anterior cruciate ligament reconstruction. *J Orthop Sports Phys Ther.* 1992;15:303–308.

Shelbourne KD, Nitz P. Accelerated rehabilitation after anterior cruciate ligament reconstruction. *J Orthop Sports Phys Ther.* 1992;15:256–264.

Shrier I. Stretching before exercise does not reduce the risk of local muscle injury: a critical review of the clinical and basic science literature. *Clin J Sports Med.* 1999;9:221–227.

Snyder-Mackler L. Scientific rationale and physiological basis for the use of closed kinetic chain exercise in the lower extremity. *J Sports Rehabil.* 1996;5:2–12.

Sole G, Lambert M, Juritz J. The role of physiotherapy in sports medicine: perceptions of orthopaedic surgeons, sports physicians, biokineticists and physiotherapists. *S Afr J Physiotherapy.* 2000;56:29–35.

Staron RS, Karapondo DL, Kraemenr WJ, et al. Skeletal muscle adaptations during early phase of heavy-resistance training in men and women. *J Appl Physiol.* 1994;76:1247–1255.

Sullivan PE, Markos PD. *Clinical Decision Making in Therapeutic Exercise*. Norwalk, Conn: Appleton & Lange; 1994.

Swanik CB, Lephart SM, Guannantonio FP, Fu F. Reestablishing proprioception and neuro-muscular control in the ACL-injured athlete. *J Sport Rehabil*. 1997;2:182–206.

Swenson C, Sward L, Karlsson J. Cryotherapy in sports medicine. *Scand J Med Sci Sports*. 1996;6:193–200.

ter Haar G. Therapeutic ultrasound. *Eur J Ultrasound*. 1999;9:3–9.

Timm KE. A new model for functional outcomes measurement in sports physical therapy; determination on return to competition. *J Rehabil Outcomes Meas*. 1997;1:35–44.

Tomberlin JP, Saunders HD. *Evaluation, Treatment and Prevention of Musculoskeletal Disorders. Vol 2: Extremities*. Chaska, Minn: The Saunders Group; 1994:245.

Tovin BJ, Tovin TS, Tovin M. Surgical and biomechanical considerations in rehabilitation of patients with intra-articular ACL reconstructions. *J Orthop Sports Phys Ther*. 1992;15:317–322.

Tyler TF, McHugh MP. Neuromuscular rehabilitation of a female Olympic ice hockey player following anterior cruciate ligament reconstruction. *J Orthop Sports Phys Ther*. 2001;31:577–587.

Voight ML, Cook G. Clinical application of closed kinetic chain exercise. *J Sport Rehabil*. 1996;5:25–44.

Weir JP, Housh DJ, Housh TJ, et al. The effect of unilateral concentric weight training and de-training on joint angle specificity, cross-training, and the bilateral deficit. *J Orthop Sports Phys Ther*. 1997;25:264–270.

Weir JP, Housh DJ, Housh TJ, et al. The effect of unilateral eccentric weight training and de-training on joint angle specificity, cross-training, and the bilateral deficit. *J Orthop Sports Phys Ther*. 1995;22:207–215.

Wilk KE, Andrews JR. Current concepts in the treatment of anterior cruciate ligament disruption. *J Orthop Sports Phys Ther*. 1992;15:279–293.

Wilk KE, Arrigo C, Andrews JR, et al. Rehabilitation after all reconstruction in the female athlete. *J Athletic Training*. 1999;34:177–193.

Wilk KE, Naiquan Z, Glenn SF, et al. Kinetic chain exercise: implications for the anterior cruciate ligament patient. *J Sport Rehabil*. 1997;6:125–140.

Worrell TW, Borchert B, Erner K, Fritz J, Leerar P. Effect of a lateral step-up exercise protocol on quadriceps and lower extremity performance. *J Orthop Sports Phys Ther*. 1993; 18:646–653.

Wu GK, NG GY, Mak AF. Effects of knee bracing on the functional performance of patients with anterior cruciate ligament reconstruction. *Arch Phys Med Rehabil*. 2001;82:282–285.

Yack HJ. Anterior tibial translation during progressive loading of the ACL-deficient knee during weight bearing and non-weight bearing exercise. *Am J Sports Med*. 1993; 21:49.

Yack HJ, Collins CE, Whieldon TJ. Comparison of closed and open kinetic chain exercise in the anterior cruciate ligament-deficient knee. *Am J Sports Med*. 1993;21:49–54.

Yeung SS, Yeung EW, Wong TW. Provision of physiotherapy at the Tsing Ma Bridge International Marathon and 10 km Race in Hong Kong. *Br J Sports Med*. 1998;32:336–337.

Zachazewski JE, ed, Magee DJ, Quillen WS. *Athletic Injuries and Rehabilitation*. Philadelphia, Pa: WB Saunders Co; 1996.

Zakaria D, Hartsell H. Efficacy of electrical muscle stimulation during protected immobilization following anterior cruciate ligament surgery. *Physiotherapy Can*. 1993;45: 2:89–93.

Zuluaga M, Briggs C, Carlisle J, et al. *Sports Physiotherapy: Applied Science and Practice*. Melbourne, Australia: Churchill Livingstone, 1995.

Biceps Tendon Strain

DESCRIPTION

The biceps tendon can be strained or ruptured during athletic activity. Strain and rupture of the biceps tendon is linked with an extremely strong elbow flexion force or a hyperextension force leading to elongation and stretch. Strains are graded as first, second, or third degree (ie mild, moderate, or severe).

- *First-degree strain* involves injury and irritation without any structural damage.
- *Second-degree strain* involves a certain degree of damage and functional loss, but the muscle-tendon unit is still intact.
- *Third-degree strain* involves a loss of function due to a complete tear. The onset can be sudden. If the biceps tendon is ruptured, resisted elbow flexion and forearm supination will be weak and painless. It is more common in athletes 50 years or older.

CAUSE

Typically, a hyperextension force causes the biceps tendon to elongate. Anterior and posterior joint capsule impingement may also occur with a hyperextension injury of the elbow. With a biceps tendon rupture, there may be a history of repeated corticosteroid injections.

ASSESSMENT

Note: See APTA's Guide to Physical Therapist Practice. 2nd ed. *Physical Therapy.* 2001;81.

Musculoskeletal Preferred Practice Patterns: D, I

AREAS

- History
- Pain
- Posture
- Joint integrity and structural deviations
- Mobility: active and passive range of motion (ROM) and accessory motion
- Strength: any muscle weakness and/or biomechanical abnormality in the rest of upper extremity that may be contributing to condition
- Neurological
- Skin and soft tissue: temperature, tenderness, tone, and edema
- Functional level

INSTRUMENTS/PROCEDURES

See References for sources.

Joint Integrity and Structural Deviations

The following areas are orthopedic tests for the elbow:
- golfer's elbow test
- ligamentous instability tests
- varus stress and valgus stress

Neurological
- elbow flexion test
- pinch test
- pronator teres syndrome
- Tinel's test

Mobility
- goniometry

Pain
- Nirschl Pain Phase Scale

Skin and Soft Tissue
- palpation for temperature, tone, and tenderness

Strength
1. instrumentation
   - grip test dynamometer
   - isokinetic testing
2. manual muscle testing

PROBLEMS
- The athlete may or may not complain of pain. With a strain, there is usually pain and tenderness.
- If the biceps tendon ruptures, the athlete will usually have weakness in elbow flexion and forearm supination, but no pain.

TREATMENT/MANAGEMENT
- Use ice and compression immediately.
- A compression sleeve and taping can help limit elbow extension and promote healing in a shortened position.
- After healing, use passive stretching to work toward full extension.
- Protective splinting can be discontinued if symptoms are gone.
- Initially, provide strengthening exercises with multiangle isometric work for biceps and supinators, and progress to isotonic and isokinetic muscular work. Eccentric biceps work should use an isotonic and isokinetic mode. Progress to coordination exercises and sport-specific training activities.
- Consider use of electrotherapy and hydrotherapy to increase circulation.
- To prevent further problems, instruct client in a stretching routine and use of taping before athletic activity.

PRECAUTIONS/CONTRAINDICATIONS
- Premature stress on tendon is contraindicated. Avoid massage or heat modalities to area during the early stages of treatment.
- Avoid hyperextension of the elbow.

DESIRED OUTCOME/PROGNOSIS
- The athlete will show no evidence of soft tissue inflammation, swelling, or ecchymosis.
- The athlete will have pain-free, normal joint mobility, and return of strength.
- Muscles are highly vascularized and resilient. Unlike tendons, muscles rarely undergo fatigue degeneration. The decision as to when the athlete can return to competition should be made in conjunction with the attending physician.

REFERENCES

Assessment

American Physical Therapy Association. Guide to physical therapist practice. 2nd ed. *Phys Ther*. 2001;81.

Buschbacher RM, ed. *Musculoskeletal Disorders: A Practical Guide for Diagnosis and Rehabilitation*. Boston, Mass: Andover Medical Publishers; 1994.

Daniels L, Worthingham C. *Muscle Testing Techniques of Manual Examination.* 6th ed. Philadelphia, Pa: WB Saunders Co; 1995.

Hall CM, Brody TB. *Therapeutic Exercise: Moving Toward Function.* Philadelphia, Pa: Lippincott Williams and Wilkins; 1999.

Hertling D, Kessler RM. *Management of Common Musculoskeletal Disorders.* 3rd ed. Philadelphia, Pa: JB Lippincott Co; 1996:78, 534.

Malone TR, McPoil T, Nitz AJ, eds. Orthopaedic and Sports Physical Therapy. 3rd ed. St. Louis, Mo: CV Mosby Co; 1997.

Myers RS, ed. Saunders Manual of Physical Therapy Practice. Philadelphia, Pa: WB Saunders Co; 1995.

Rothstein JM, Roy SH, Wolf SL. *The Rehabilitation Specialist's Handbook.* 2nd ed. Philadelphia, Pa: FA Davis Co; 1998.

Saidoff DC, McDonough AL. *Critical Pathways in Therapeutic Intervention.* Philadelphia, Pa: CV Mosby Co; 2002.

Schunk C, Reed K. *Clinical Practice Guidelines.* Gaithersburg, Md: Aspen Publishers; 2000.

Tomberlin JP, Saunders HD. *Evaluation, Treatment and Prevention of Musculoskeletal Disorders. Vol 2: Extremities.* Chaska, Minn: The Saunders Group; 1994.

Treatment

American Physical Therapy Association. *Sports Physical Therapy: Description of Advanced Clinical Practice.* Alexandria, Va: APTA; 1997.

Andrews JR, Whiteside JA. Common elbow problems in the athlete. *J Orthop Sports Phys Ther.* 1993;17:289–295.

Andrews JR, Wilk KE, Satterwhite YE, Tedder JL. Physical examination of the thrower's elbow. *J Orthop Sports Phys Ther.* 1993;17:296–304.

Bennell KL, Malcom SA, Wark JD, et al. Skeletal effects of menstrual disturbances in athletes. *Scand J Med Sci Sports.* 1997;7:261–273.

Brewer BW, Van Raalte JL, Petitpas AJ, et al. Preliminary psychometric evaluation of a measure of adherence to clinic-based sport injury rehabilitation. *Phys Ther Sport.* 2000; 1:68–74.

Buschbacher RM, ed. *Musculoskeletal Disorders: A Practical Guide for Diagnosis and Rehabilitation.* Boston, Mass: Andover Medical Publishers; 1994.

Chaitow L. *Muscle Energy Techniques.* New York, NY: Churchill Livingstone; 1997.

De Bie RA, Verhagen AP, Lenssen AF, et al. Efficacy of 904 nm laser therapy in the management of musculoskeletal disorders: a systematic review. *Phys Ther Rev.* 1998;3: 59–72.

Hertling D, Kessler RM. *Management of Common Musculoskeletal Disorders.* 3rd ed. Philadelphia, Pa: JB Lippincott Co; 1996.

Johnson MI. Acupuncture-like transcutaneous electrical nerve stimulation (AL-TENS) in the management of pain. *Phys Ther Rev.* 1998;3:73–93.

Kibbler WB, Herring SA, Press JM, eds. *Functional Rehabilitation of Sports and Musculoskeletal Injuries.* Gaithersburg, Md: Aspen Publishers; 1998.

Mohr KJ, Pink MM, Elsner C, et al. Electromyographic investigation of stretching: the effect of warm-up. *Clin J Sports Med.* 1998;8:215–220.

Ninedek A, Kolt GS. Sport physiotherapists' perceptions of psychological strategies in sport injury rehabilitation. *J Sport Rehabil.* 2000;9:191–206.

Prins J. Cutner D. Aquatic therapy in the rehabilitation of athletic injuries. *Clin Sports Med.* 1999;18:447–461.

Quarrier NF. Performing arts medicine: the musical athlete. *J Orthop Sports Phys Ther.* 1993;17:90–95.

Shrier I. Stretching before exercise does not reduce the risk of local muscles injury: a critical review of the clinical and basic science literature. *Clin J Sports Med.* 1999;9:221–227.

Sole G, Lambert M, Juritz J. The role of physiotherapy in sports medicine: perceptions of orthopaedic surgeons, sports physicians, biokineticists and physiotherapists. *S Afr J Physiotherapy.* 2000;56:29–35.

Swenson C, Sward L, Karlsson J. Cryotherapy in sports medicine. *Scand J Med Sci Sports.* 1996;6:193–200.

Symth M. After an injury. What next? *Aust Fam Physician.* 1999 Jun:28(6):555–560.

Timm KE. A new model for functional outcomes measurement in sports physical therapy; determination on return to competition. *J Rehabil Outcomes Meas.* 1997;1:35–44.

Tomberlin JP, Saunders HD. *Evaluation, Treatment and Prevention of Musculoskeletal Disorders. Vol. 2: Extremities.* Chaska, Minn: The Saunders Group; 1994.

Werner SL, Fleisig GS, Dillman CJ, Andrews JR. Biomechanics of the elbow during baseball pitching. *J Orthop Sports Phys Ther.* 1993;17:274–278.

Wilk KE, Arrigo C, Andrews JR. Rehabilitation of the elbow in the throwing athlete. *J Orthop Sports Phys Ther.* 1993;17:305–317.

Wilk KE, Voight ML, Keirns MA, Gambetta V, Andrews JR, Dillman CJ. Stretch-shortening drills for the upper extremities: theory and clinical application. *J Orthop Sports Phys Ther.* 1993;17:225–239.

Zachazewski JE, ed, Magee DJ, Quillen WS. *Athletic Injuries and Rehabilitation.* Philadelphia: WB Saunders Co; 1996.

Zuluaga M, Briggs C, Carlisle J, et al. Sports physiotherapy. *Appl Sci Pract.* Melbourne, Australia: Churchill Livingstone; 1995.

Hamstring Muscle Strain

DESCRIPTION

The hamstring muscle (posterior femoral muscle) can be strained, pulled, or ruptured during athletic activity. The hamstring muscle extends the hip and flexes the knee during running and jumping and opposes the quadriceps muscle, which flexes the hip and extends the knee. The quadriceps muscle is stronger, but hamstring muscle strength should be at least 60% of or equal to the strength of the quadriceps muscle.

The strain usually occurs when the muscle is contracted quickly and vigorously. Other muscles prone to strain include the quadriceps, the hip adductors (gracilis, pectineus, and longus, brevis, and magnus adductors), the iliopsoas, the rectus abdominis, and the gluteus medius.

Strains are classified into first, second, or third degree (ie, mild, moderate, or severe).

- *First-degree strain* involves injury and irritation without any structural damage.
- *Second-degree strain* involves a certain degree of damage and functional loss, but the muscle-tendon unit is still intact.
- *Third-degree strain* involves a loss of function due to a complete tear.

CAUSE

Simultaneous contraction of the hamstrings and the quadriceps can lead to a hamstring tear if the hamstrings are too weak. Risk factors for a hamstring strain include poor posture, inflexibility, inadequate warm-up, neurological and muscular fatigue, improper techniques, strength imbalance, and poor neuromuscular control.

ASSESSMENT

Note: See APTA's Guide to Physical Therapist Practice. 2nd ed. *Physical Therapy.* 2001;81.

Musculoskeletal Preferred Practice Patterns: D, I

AREAS
- History
- Pain
- Posture
- Gait, including weight-bearing pattern
- Joint integrity and structural deviations
- Mobility: active and passive range of motion (ROM) and accessory motion
- Strength
- Neurological sensation, proprioception, deep tendon reflexes, and neural tension
- Skin and soft tissue: temperature, tone, tenderness, and edema
- Functional level, including activities of daily living (ADLs)

INSTRUMENTS/PROCEDURES

See References for sources.

Joint Integrity and Structural Deviations

Following are orthopedic tests for the knee and hip:

- Craig's test
- Ely test
- FABER test
- hamstring tightness and muscle length
- iliotibial band length
- leg-length test
- Noble's compression test
- Ober's test
- piriformis test
- Thomas' test
- Trendelenburg's sign

Mobility
- goniometry

Pain
- visual analog scale

Skin and Soft Tissue
- palpation for temperature, tone, tenderness

Strength
- manual muscle testing

PROBLEMS
- The athlete often reports hearing a "popping" sound with the muscle tear.
- Pain and spasm are proportional to the severity of injury.
- There may be tenderness, especially during a hamstring muscle stretch.
- There is often pain with walking and using the stairs.
- The athlete may have ecchymosis, hemorrhage, and a muscle deficit if strain is severe.
- There is often tightness and weakness in the hamstring muscle.

TREATMENT/MANAGEMENT

ACUTE INJURY

- The acronym **RICE** (**R**est, **I**ce, **C**ompression, and **E**levation) is indicated for pain and inflammation.
- Physical agents can include cold whirlpool, high-voltage pulsed monophasic current, acupuncture point stimulation, phonophoresis, and ultrasound to local area. Treatment with pulsed 1 MHz ultrasound at an intensity of 0.5 W/cm^2 or less has been reported useful during the acute phase.
- Active ROM can be performed after the area has stabilized.
- Consider the use of progressive mobilization, friction massage, and stretching.
- Suggest alternative exercise for general fitness that will not stress the injured area.

STABLE INJURY

- Use scar massage with gentle stretching and phonophoresis.
- Consider cross-fiber friction massage.
- Consider mobilization of sacroiliac joint.
- Review athlete's technique to minimize avoidable stress.
- Pad injury site with wrap before activity.
- Emphasize importance of flexibility and instruct athlete in proper stretching techniques.
- Strengthen areas of weakness in a gradual and conservative progression.
- Warm-up exercises should include movements that mimic the actual sporting event.
- Cool-down exercises should reverse movements that mimic the actual sporting event.
- Running can commence when the athlete can move without an antalgic gait.

Note: A more aggressive approach to rehab using early activity is outlined in Bruckner and Khan (2000).

PRECAUTIONS/CONTRAINDICATIONS

- Any attempt to "run off" a hamstring strain can increase the risk of causing a greater strain.
- A minimum wait of 5 to 7 days is recommended before resuming pain-free stretching after a mild second-degree tear. A second-degree tear can take at least 6 weeks to heal before return to full activity is permitted.
- Before returning to full activity, the client needs normal flexibility, strength, endurance, agility, and power. Adjacent muscles should also be checked.

DESIRED OUTCOME/PROGNOSIS

- The athlete will have early injury stabilization.
- The athlete will experience a reduction in pain.
- There will be a reduction of edema and promotion of healing.
- There will be minimal internal scar formation and muscle defect.
- Treatment will lead to improved remodeling of injury, with reduced cross-linking and random fiber alignment as the collagen repairs.
- Rehabilitation will prevent atrophy and maintain fitness.
- The athlete will maintain ROM in the lower extremities.
- The athlete will have minimal time lost from sport.
- Collagen remodeling can take up to 3 weeks, and full strength gain may take even longer.
- Rehabilitation time of 2 to 3 weeks can be expected if injury is mild or 2 to 6 months if the injury is severe.

REFERENCES

Assessment

American Physical Therapy Association. Guide to physical therapist practice. 2nd ed. *Phys Ther*. 2001;81.

Bandy WD, Irion JM, Biggler M. The effect of time and frequency of static stretching on flexibility of the hamstring muscles. *Phys Ther*. 1997;77:1090.

Bennell K, Tully E, Harvey N. Does the toe-touch test predict hamstring injury in Australian Rules footballers? *Aust J Physiotherapy*. 1999;45:103–109.

Brewer BW, Van Raalte JL, Petitpas AJ, et al. Preliminary psychometric evaluation of a measure of adherence to clinic-based sport injury rehabilitation. *Phys Ther Sport*. 2000;1:68–74.

Buschbacher RM, ed. *Musculoskeletal Disorders: A Practical Guide for Diagnosis and Rehabilitation*. Boston, Mass: Andover Medical Publishers; 1994.

Daniels L, Worthingham C. *Muscle Testing Techniques of Manual Examination*. 6th ed. Philadelphia, Pa: WB Saunders Co; 1995.

Gaidosik RL, Rieck MA, Sullivan DK, Wightman SE. Comparison of four clinical tests for assessing hamstring muscle length. *J Orthop Sports Phys Ther*. 1993;18:614–618.

Hall CM, Brody TB. *Therapeutic Exercise: Moving Toward Function*. Philadelphia, PA: Lippincott Williams and Wilkins; 1999.

Hertling D, Kessler RM. *Management of Common Musculoskeletal Disorders*. 3rd ed. Philadelphia, Pa: JB Lippincott Co; 1996:78, 534.

Kendall FP, McCreary EK, Provance PG. *Muscles: Testing and Function*. 4th ed. Baltimore, Md: Williams and Wilkins; 1993.

Malone TR, McPoil T, Nitz AJ, eds. *Orthopaedic and Sports Physical Therapy*. 3rd ed. St. Louis, Mo: CV Mosby Co; 1997.

Melchione WE, Sullivan MS. Reliability of measurements obtained by use of an instrument designed to indirectly measure iliotibial band length. *J Orthop Sports Phys Ther*. 1993;18:511–515.

Myers RS, ed. *Saunders Manual of Physical Therapy Practice*. Philadelphia, Pa: WB Saunders Co; 1995.

Rothstein JM, Roy SH, Wolf SL. *The Rehabilitation Specialist's Handbook*. 2nd ed. Philadelphia, Pa: FA Davis Co; 1998.

Saidoff DC, McDonough AL. *Critical Pathways in Therapeutic Intervention*. Philadelphia, Pa: CV Mosby Co; 2002.

Schunk C, Reed K. *Clinical Practice Guidelines*. Gaithersburg, Md: Aspen Publishers; 2000.

Tomberlin JP, Saunders HD. *Evaluation, Treatment and Prevention of Musculoskeletal Disorders. Vol 2: Extremities*. Chaska, Minn: The Saunders Group; 1994.

Treatment

American Physical Therapy Association. *Sports Physical Therapy: Description of Advanced Clinical Practice*. Alexandria, Va: APTA; 1997.

Bennell KL, Malcom SA, Wark JD, et al. Skeletal effects of menstrual disturbances in athletes. *Scan J Med Sci Sports*. 1997;7:261–273.

Bentley S. Exercise-induced muscle cramp. Proposed mechanisms and management. *Sports Med*. 1996;21:409–420.

Bruckner P, Khan K, eds. *Clinical Sports Medicine*. 2nd edition. New York, NY: The McGraw-Hill Companies, Inc; 2000.

Chaitow L. *Muscle Energy Techniques*. New York, NY: Churchill Livingstone; 1997.

De Bie RA, Verhagen AP, Lenssen AF, et al. Efficacy of 904 nm laser therapy in the management of musculoskeletal disorders: a systematic review. *Phys Ther Rev.* 1998;3: 59–72.

Johnson MI. Acupuncture-like transcutaneous electrical nerve stimulation (AL-TENS) in the management of pain. *Phys Ther Rev.* 1998;3:73–93.

Kibbler WB, Herring SA, Press JM, eds. *Functional Rehabilitation of Sports and Musculoskeletal Injuries*. Gaithersburg, Md: Aspen Publishers; 1998.

Magee DJ, Quillen WS, eds. *Athletic Injuries and Rehabilitation*. Philadelphia, Pa: WB Saunders Co; 1997:71–91.

Malone TR, Garrett WE, Zachazewski JE. Muscle: deformation, injury, repair. In: Zachazewski JE, Mattick AP, Beattie TF, Macnicol MF. Just a pulled hamstring. *J Accident Emerg Med.* 1999;16:457–458.

McCrory P, Bell S. Nerve entrapment syndromes as a cause of pain in the hip, groin and buttock. *Sports Med.* 1999;27:261–274.

Mohr KJ, Pink MM, Elsner C, et al. Electromyographic investigation of stretching: the effect of warm-up. *Clin J Sports Med.* 1998;8:215–220.

Ninedek A, Kolt GS. Sport physiotherapists' perceptions of psychological strategies in sport injury rehabilitation. *J Sport Rehabil.* 2000;9:191–206.

Prins J. Cutner D. Aquatic therapy in the rehabilitation of athletic injuries. *Clin Sports Med.* 1999;18:447–461.

Roebroeck ME, Dekker J, Oostendorp RA. The use of therapeutic ultrasound by physical therapists in Dutch primary health care. *Phys Ther.* 1998;78:470–478.

Satterfield MJ, Yasumura K, Abreu SH. Retro runner with ischial tuberosity enthesopathy. *J Orthop Sports Phys Ther.* 1993;17:191–194.

Shrier I. Stretching before exercise does not reduce the risk of local muscles injury: a critical review of the clinical and basic science literature. *Clin J Sports Med.* 1999;9:221–227.

Sole G, Lambert M, Juritz J. The role of physiotherapy in sports medicine: perceptions of orthopaedic surgeons, sports physicians, biokineticists and physiotherapists. *S Afr J of Physiotherapy.* 2000;56:29–35.

Swenson C, Sward L, Karlsson J. Cryotherapy in sports medicine. *Scand J Med Sci Sports.* 1996;6:193–200.

ter Haar G. Therapeutic ultrasound. *Eur J Ultrasound.* 1999;9:3–9.

Timm KE. A new model for functional outcomes measurement in sports physical therapy; determination on return to competition. *J Rehabil Outcomes Meas.* 1997;1:35–44.

Tomberlin JP, Saunders HD. *Evaluation, Treatment and Prevention of Musculoskeletal Disorders. Vol 2: Extremities*. Chaska, Minn: The Saunders Group; 1994:200.

Tonsolone PA. Chronic adductor tendinitis in a female swimmer. *J Orthop Sports Phys Ther.* 1993;18:629–633.

Worrell TW, Perrin DH. Hamstring muscle injury: the influence of strength, flexibility, warm-up and fatigue. *J Orthop Sports Phys Ther.* 1992;16:12–18.

Yeung SS, Yeung EW, Wong TW. Provision of physiotherapy at the Tsing Ma Bridge International Marathon and 10 km Race in Hong Kong. *Br J Sports Med.* 1998;32:336–337.

Zachazewski JE, ed, Magee DJ, Quillen WS. *Athletic Injuries and Rehabilitation*. Philadelphia, Pa: WB Saunders Co; 1996.

Zuluaga M, Briggs C, Carlisle J, et al. Sports physiotherapy. *Appl Sci Pract.* Melbourne, Australia: Churchill Livingstone; 1995.

Hip Contusion

Also known as a *hip pointer.*

DESCRIPTION

Contusions are defined as direct blows leading to soft tissue trauma. When a blow occurs in the iliac crest region—usually at or near the anterior superior iliac spine—it is often called a hip contusion. Avulsion of the external obliques is a common secondary problem. Other contusions in the hip region include sacroiliac joint contusion, coccygeal contusion, and contusion injuries to the groin.

CAUSE

A direct blow can cause muscle fibers to be crushed and separated, leading to bleeding and swelling.

ASSESSMENT

Note: See APTA's Guide to Physical Therapist Practice. 2nd ed. *Physical Therapy.* 2001;81.

Integumentary Preferred Practice Patterns: B, E

Musculoskeletal Preferred Practice Patterns: D, E, J

AREAS
- History
- Pain
- Posture
- Gait, including weight-bearing pattern
- Joint integrity and structural deviations
- Mobility: active and passive range of motion (ROM) and accessory motion
- Strength
- Neurological: sensation, proprioception, deep tendon reflexes, and neural tension
- Skin and soft tissue: temperature, tone, tenderness, and edema
- Functional level

INSTRUMENTS/PROCEDURES

See References for sources.

Joint Integrity and Structural Deviations

Following are orthopedic tests for the lower extremities:

- Craig's test
- Ely test
- FABER test
- hamstring tightness
- leg-length test
- Noble's compression test
- Ober's test
- piriformis test
- Thomas' test
- torque test
- Trendelenburg's sign

Mobility
- goniometry

Pain
- visual analog scale

Skin and Soft Tissue
- palpation for temperature, tone, and tenderness

Strength
- manual muscle testing

PROBLEMS
- There is often bleeding and edema.
- The athlete often complains of pain with active trunk movement, coughing, sneezing, or laughing.

TREATMENT/MANAGEMENT
- Rest and ice are indicated, especially in early stages (ie, 48 to 72 hours post injury).
- Following a reduction of swelling and inflammation, begin active ROM and a gradual return to functionality.
- Protective padding is often indicated.
- Begin gentle, graded stretching as symptoms subside.
- Consider transcutaneous electrical nerve stimulation (TENS) for pain.

PRECAUTIONS/CONTRAINDICATIONS
- Avoid overly vigorous stretching to prevent aggravating the soft tissue injury.
- Contusions of the ischial tuberosity must be differentiated from avulsion fractures.
- Severe or chronic contusions can progress to myositis ossificans—a mineralization that forms in the hematoma and usually appears within 1 to 2 weeks following a severe contusion. Massage and stretching are generally contraindicated.

DESIRED OUTCOME/PROGNOSIS
- The athlete will experience a reduction in symptoms.
- The athlete will return to pain-free activities.

REFERENCES

Assessment

American Physical Therapy Association. Guide to Physical Therapist Practice. 2nd ed. *Phys Ther*. 2001;81.

Buschbacher RM, ed. *Musculoskeletal Disorders: A Practical Guide for Diagnosis and Rehabilitation*. Boston, Mass: Andover Medical Publishers; 1994.

Daniels L, Worthingham C. *Muscle Testing Techniques of Manual Examination*. 6th ed. Philadelphia, Pa: WB Saunders Co; 1995.

Hall CM, Brody TB. *Therapeutic Exercise: Moving Toward Function*. Philadelphia, Pa: Lippincott Williams and Wilkins; 1999.

Hertling D, Kessler RM. *Management of Common Musculoskeletal Disorders*. 3rd ed. Philadelphia, Pa: JB Lippincott Co; 1996:78,534.

Kendall FP, McCreary EK, Provance PG. *Muscles: Testing and Function*. 4th ed. Baltimore, Md: Williams and Wilkins; 1993.

Malone TR, McPoil T, Nitz AJ, eds. *Orthopaedic and Sports Physical Therapy*. 3rd ed. St. Louis, Mo: CV Mosby Co; 1997.

Myers RS, ed. *Saunders Manual of Physical Therapy Practice*. Philadelphia, Pa: WB Saunders Co; 1995.

Rothstein JM, Roy SH, Wolf SL. *The Rehabilitation Specialist's Handbook*. 2nd ed. Philadelphia, Pa: FA Davis Co; 1998.

Saidoff DC, McDonough AL. *Critical Pathways in Therapeutic Intervention*. Philadelphia, Pa: CV Mosby Co; 2002.

Schunk C, Reed K. *Clinical Practice Guidelines*. Gaithersburg, Md: Aspen Publishers; 2000.

Tomberlin JP, Saunders HD. *Evaluation, Treatment and Prevention of Musculoskeletal Disorders. Vol 2: Extremities*. Chaska, Minn: The Saunders Group; 1994.

Treatment

Boyd KT, Peirce NS, Batt ME. Common hip injuries in sport. *Sports Med*. 1997;24:273–288.

Brewer BW, Van Raalte JL, Petitpas AJ, et al. Preliminary psychometric evaluation of a measure of adherence to clinic-based sport injury rehabilitation. *Phys Ther Sport*. 2000;1: 68–74.

Cibulka MT, Delitto A. A comparison of two different methods to treat hip pain in runners. *J Orthop Sports Phys Ther*. 1993;17:172–176.

Hicklin SP, DePretis MC. Lower extremity: hip. In: Myers RS, ed; *Saunders Manual of Physical Therapy Practice*. Philadelphia, Pa: WB Saunders Co; 1995:962–968.

Prins J. Cutner D. Aquatic therapy in the rehabilitation of athletic injuries. *Clin Sports Med*. 1999;18:447–461.

Quarrier NF, Wightman AB. A ballet dancer with chronic hip pain due to a lesser trochanter bony avulsion: the challenge of a differential diagnosis. *J Sports Phys Ther*. 1998;28: 168–173.

Swenson C, Sward L, Karlsson J. Cryotherapy in sports medicine. *Scand J Med Sci Sports*. 1996;6:193–200.

Tomberlin JP, Saunders HD. *Evaluation, Treatment and Prevention of Musculoskeletal Disorders. Vol 2: Extremities*. Chaska, Minn: The Saunders Group; 1994:200.

Iliotibial Band Friction Syndrome

DESCRIPTION

Iliotibial band (ITB) friction syndrome is an overuse injury affecting two components at the lateral knee: the iliopatellar band and the iliotibial tract. This condition is a frequent source of knee pain in runners.

CAUSE

Due to overuse of the knee, excess friction between the iliotibial band and the lateral femoral condyle lying underneath can be the cause of this problem. Iliotibial band friction syndrome can also be caused by sudden unaccustomed stress to the knee.

People prone to this condition include those with the following conditions: ITB tightness, pes cavus, genu varus, increased femoral rotation under the ITB, and a crossover gait pattern. Cycling or walking with the foot pronated can also affect the tightness of the ITB.

Overuse injuries are frequently influenced by both extrinsic factors and intrinsic factors. Extrinsic factors may include the following: errors in equipment or training, inadequate training surfaces, environmental conditions, nutritional regimens, and psychological factors.

Intrinsic factors may include the following: body type, endocrine factors, gender, genetic factors, leg length differences, metabolic conditions, muscle weakness and/or imbalance, reduced flexibility, and structural malalignment.

ASSESSMENT

Note: See APTA's Guide to Physical Therapist Practice. 2nd ed. *Physical Therapy.* 2001;81.

Musculoskeletal Preferred Practice Patterns: D, E, J

AREAS
- History
- Pain
- Posture
- Gait
- Joint integrity and structural deviations
- Mobility: active and passive range of motion (ROM) and accessory motion
- Strength
- Neurological: sensation, proprioception, deep tendon reflexes, and neural tension tests
- Skin and soft tissue: temperature, tone, tenderness, and edema
- Functional level and any training/performance errors
- Equipment, including footwear

INSTRUMENTS/PROCEDURES

See References for sources.

Joint Integrity and Structural Deviations

Following are orthopedic tests for the knee. Those recommended especially for this condition are indicated with an asterisk:

- A-angle
- Anteromedial Rotational Instability (AMRI)
- Anterolateral Rotational Instability (ALRI)
- Apley grinding test
- apprehension test
- bounce home test
- brush or stroke (wipe) test
- Clarks sign
- crossover test
- Ely test
- external rotation test
- flexion rotation drawer text
- fluctuation test
- gravity drawer test (posterior sag sign)
- hamstring length
- Helfet test
- Hughston plica test
- Hughston posterolateral drawer test
- Hughston test (jerk sign)
- hyperflexion-hyperextension test
- Jakob test (reverse pivot)
- Lachman's test
- lateral pull test
- leg-length discrepancy*
- MacIntosh test (lateral pivot shift)
- McConnell test
- McMurray-Anderson test
- Noble's compression test*
- Ober's test*
- O'Donoghue test
- patellar tap test
- patellar tilt test
- Perkins test
- plica test
- posterior drawer sign
- posterior sag sign
- quadriceps active test
- reverse pivot shift
- Slocum test
- Steinman's test
- step-down test*
- squat test
- Thomas' test*
- valgus stress test
- varus stress test
- Waldron test
- Wilson test

Mobility
- goniometry

Pain
- visual analog scale

Skin and Soft Tissue
- palpation for temperature, tone, tenderness

Strength
- manual muscle testing

PROBLEMS
- The athlete often complains of diffuse aching or tenderness at the lateral knee with activity. Pain may also be felt at the greater trochanter.
- The athlete may have excessive medial rotation compared to lateral rotation, hip anteversion, and limited extension in gait.
- Pain may have insidious onset but may also be triggered by athletic activity.
- The athlete may be unable to run, secondary to pain.
- There is often excessive tightness of the ITB.
- There may be point tenderness at the lateral femoral condyle.
- The athlete may complain of irritation during stair climbing.
- The athlete may be unable to run.
- There is often weakness at the quadriceps and gluteus medius muscles.

TREATMENT/MANAGEMENT
- Encourage rest.
- Physical agents and modalities can include ice, ultrasound, high-voltage pulsed monophasic current, and iontophoresis for symptoms.
- Stretch ITB and tensor fasciae latae tightness as indicated.
- Correct any structural limb-length inequality.
- Balance subtalar motion leading to any femoral internal rotation or genu varus.
- Consider an orthosis for abnormalities in joint mechanics, especially the effect the foot position adds to any lateral stress at knee. Proper footwear is critical.
- Strengthen hip external rotators and address issues of balance and proprioceptive reeducation.
- Consider friction massage and soft tissue mobilization.
- Counsel athlete about avoiding activities or training errors that irritate the ITB. Consider use of periodization of training with the alternation of vigorous training with less vigorous training and plenty of rest.
- Resume normal athletic routine gradually.

PRECAUTIONS/CONTRAINDICATIONS
- Rule out femoral stress fracture, gluteal strain, lateral meniscal tear, piriformis syndrome, and popliteus tendinitis.
- Pain at the lateral knee will likely increase if there is no modification of the repeated stress.
- Runners need to avoid too much sidehill running and unnecessary stair work.

DESIRED OUTCOME/PROGNOSIS
- The athlete will have a decrease in symptoms such as inflammation.
- The athlete will resume pain-free athletic activities and activities of daily living (ADLs).

Note: If the ITB is related to pes cavus, the recovery may take twice as long to resolve.

REFERENCES

Assessment

American Physical Therapy Association. Guide to physical therapist practice. 2nd ed. *Phys Ther.* 2001;81.

Buschbacher RM, ed. *Musculoskeletal Disorders: A Practical Guide for Diagnosis and Rehabilitation.* Boston, Mass: Andover Medical Publishers; 1994.

Daniels L Worthingham C. *Muscle Testing Techniques of Manual Examination.* 6th ed. Philadelphia, Pa: WB Saunders Co; 1995.

Hall CM, Brody TB. *Therapeutic Exercise: Moving Toward Function.* Philadelphia, Pa: Lippincott Williams and Wilkins; 1999.

Hertling D, Kessler RM. *Management of Common Musculoskeletal Disorders.* 3rd ed. Philadelphia, Pa: JB Lippincott Co; 1996:78, 534.

Malone TR, McPoil T, Nitz AJ, eds. *Orthopaedic and Sports Physical Therapy.* 3rd ed. St. Louis, Mo: CV Mosby Co; 1997.

Melchione WE, Sullivan MS. Reliability of measurements obtained by use of an instrument designed to indirectly measure iliotibial band length. *J Orthop Sports Phys Ther.* 1993;18:511–515.

Myers RS, ed. *Saunders Manual of Physical Therapy Practice.* Philadelphia, Pa: WB Saunders Co; 1995.

Rothstein JM, Roy SH, Wolf SL. *The Rehabilitation Specialist's Handbook.* 2nd ed. Philadelphia, Pa: FA Davis Co; 1998.

Saidoff DC, McDonough AL. *Critical Pathways in Therapeutic Intervention.* Philadelphia, Pa: CV Mosby Co; 2002.

Schunk C, Reed K. *Clinical Practice Guidelines.* Gaithersburg, Md: Aspen Publishers; 2000.

Tomberlin JP, Saunders HD. *Evaluation, Treatment and Prevention of Musculoskeletal Disorders. Vol 2: Extremities.* Chaska, Minn. The Saunders Group; 1994.

Treatment

American Physical Therapy Association. *Sports Physical Therapy: Description of Advanced Clinical Practice.* Alexandria, Va: APTA; 1997.

Bennell KL, Malcom SA, Wark JD, et al. Skeletal effects of menstrual disturbances in athletes. *Scand J Med Sci Sports.* 1997;7:261–273.

Brewer BW, Van Raalte JL, Petitpas AJ, et al. Preliminary psychometric evaluation of a measure of adherence to clinic-based sport injury rehabilitation. *Phys Ther Sport.* 2000;1:68–74.

Chaitow L. *Muscle Energy Techniques.* New York, NY: Churchill Livingstone; 1997.

De Bie RA, Verhagen AP, Lenssen AF, et al. Efficacy of 904 nm laser therapy in the management of musculoskeletal disorders: a systematic review. *Phys Ther Rev.* 1998;3:59–72.

Eng JJ, Peirrynowski MR. The effect of soft foot orthotics on three-dimensional lower-limb kinematics during walking and running. *Phys Ther.* 1994;74:836–844.

Hertling D, Kessler RM. *Management of Common Musculoskeletal Disorders.* 3rd ed. Philadelphia, Pa: JB Lippincott Co; 1996:351.

Holmes JC, Pruitt Al, Whalen NJ. Iliotibial band syndrome in cyclists. *Am J Sports Med.* 1993;21:419–424.

Kendall FP, McCreary EK, Provance PG. *Muscles: Testing and Function*. 4th ed. Baltimore, Md: Williams and Wilkins; 1993.

Johnson MI. Acupuncture-like transcutaneous electrical nerve stimulation (AL-TENS) in the management of pain. *Phys Ther Rev*. 1998;3:73–93.

Johnston J, Plancher KD, Hawkins RJ. Elbow injuries to the throwing athlete. *Clin Sports Med*. 1996;15:307–329.

Kibbler WB, Herring SA, Press JM, eds. *Functional Rehabilitation of Sports and Musculo-skeletal Injuries*. Gaithersburg, Md: Aspen Publishers, 1998.

Mohr KJ, Pink MM, Elsner C, et al. Electromyographic investigation of stretching: the effect of warm-up. *Clin J Sports Med*. 1998;8:215–220.

Myers RS, ed. *Saunders Manual of Physical Therapy Practice*. Philadelphia, Pa: WB Saunders Co; 1995:1349.

Ninedek A, Kolt GS. Sport physiotherapists' perceptions of psychological strategies in sport injury rehabilitation. *J Sport Rehabil*. 2000;9:191–206.

Orchard JW, Fricker PA, Abud At, et al. Biomechanics of iliotibial band friction syndrome in runners. *Am J Sports Med*. 1996;24:375–379.

Pease B. Biomechanical assessment of the lower extremity. *Orthop Phys Ther Clin North Am*. 1994;3:291–325.

Prins J. Cutner D. Aquatic therapy in the rehabilitation of athletic injuries. *Clin Sports Med*. 1999;18:447–461.

Roebroeck ME, Dekker J, Oostendorp RA. The use of therapeutic ultrasound by physical therapists in Dutch primary health care. *Phys Ther*. 1998;78:470–478.

Schwellnus MP, Mackintosh L, Mee J. Deep transverse frictions in the treatment of iliotibial band friction syndrome in athletes: a clinical trial. *Physiotherapy*. 1992;78:564–568.

Shrier I. Stretching before exercise does not reduce the risk of local muscles injury: a critical review of the clinical and basic science literature. *Clin J Sports Med*. 1999;9:221–227.

Sole G, Lambert M, Juritz J. The role of physiotherapy in sports medicine: perceptions of orthopaedic surgeons, sports physicians, biokineticists and physiotherapists. *S Afr J Physiotherapy*. 2000;56:29–35.

Swenson C, Sward L, Karlsson J. Cryotherapy in sports medicine. *Scand J Med Sci Sports*. 1996;6:193–200.

ter Haar G. Therapeutic ultrasound. *Eur J Ultrasound*. 1999;9:3–9.

Timm KE. A new model for functional outcomes measurement in sports physical therapy; determination on return to competition. *J Rehabil Outcomes Meas*. 1997;1:35–44.

Tomberlin JP, Saunders HD. *Evaluation, Treatment and Prevention of Musculoskeletal Disorders. Vol 2: Extremities*. Chaska, Minn: The Saunders Group; 1994:233.

Yeung SS, Yeung EW, Wong TW. Provision of physiotherapy at the Tsing Ma Bridge International Marathon and 10 km Race in Hong Kong. *Br J Sports Med*. 1998;32:336–337.

Zachazewski JE, ed, Magee DJ, Quillen WS. *Athletic Injuries and Rehabilitation*. Philadelphia, Pa: WB Saunders Co; 1996.

Zuluaga M, Briggs C, Carlisle J, et al. *Sports Physiotherapy: Applied Science and Practice*. Melbourne, Australia: Churchill Livingstone; 1995.

Medial Collateral Ligament (Elbow) Sprain

DESCRIPTION

The medial collateral ligament of the elbow may be sprained during throwing activities. Injury to the medial collateral ligament accompanied by medial elbow muscle hypertrophy is sometimes called "Little League elbow." In an adolescent whose growth plate has not fused, a repetitive valgus stress can lead to an avulsion injury of the medial epicondyle. Ligamentous injury has 4 stages: edema, scarring and disassociation of fibers, calcification, and ossification.

CAUSE

Throwing can place severe stress on the soft tissues of the elbow, resulting in an overuse injury. The acceleration phase of throwing is the most stressful to the elbow joint due to the valgus stress on the medial joint structures. This repeated valgus extension overload leads to microtraumatic injury. Factors influencing overuse injury risk may be both intrinsic and extrinsic:

- Intrinsic factors include malalignment, muscular imbalance, inflexibility, muscular weakness, and instability.
- Extrinsic factors include training errors, equipment, environment, technique, and sports-imposed deficiencies.

Injury can also be caused by a direct blow or elbow dislocation. A complete ligamentous rupture is usually associated with acute trauma.

ASSESSMENT

Note: See APTA's Guide to Physical Therapist Practice. 2nd ed. *Physical Therapy.* 2001;81.

Integumentary Preferred Practice Pattern: A

Musculoskeletal Preferred Practice Patterns: D, E, J

AREAS
- History
- Pain
- Posture
- Joint integrity and structural deviations
- Mobility: active and passive range of motion (ROM) and accessory motion
- Strength: any muscle weakness and/or biomechanical abnormality in the rest of upper extremity that may be contributing to condition
- Neurological: including sensation, proprioception, deep tendon reflexes, and upper limb tension tests (ie, median nerve, radial nerve, and ulnar nerve dominant)
- Skin and soft tissue: temperature, tone, tenderness, and edema
- Gait
- Functional level

INSTRUMENTS/PROCEDURES

See References for sources.

Joint Integrity and Structural Deviations

Following are orthopedic tests for the elbow. Those recommended especially for this condition are indicated with an asterisk:

- golfer's elbow test
- ligamentous instability tests
- tennis elbow test
- varus stress and valgus stress tests*
- elbow flexion test
- pinch test
- pronator teres syndrome
- Tinel's test

Pain
- Nirschl Pain Phase Scale

Skin and Soft Tissue
- palpation for temperature, tone, and tenderness

Strength
1. instrumentation
    - grip test dynamometer
    - isokinetic testing
2. manual muscle testing

PROBLEMS
- The athlete often has medial instability of the elbow joint with a valgus stress.
- The athlete often has swelling of the elbow at the medial region.
- The athlete may have pain with throwing or pushing motions.
- The involved elbow may be painful to touch over the ulnar collateral ligament.

TREATMENT/MANAGEMENT
- Prescribe rest from stressful activities.
- Immobilization may be indicated if there is evidence of osteochondritis dissecans of the capitulum, if the athlete is post surgery, or if the symptoms are severe.
- Use physical agents and modalities as indicated.
- An exercise program can include a progression from passive exercise, including joint mobilization and stretching, to isometric, isotonic, and isokinetic work. One schedule recommends isokinetic work at 3 times per week for 10 to 30 seconds at 30 degree/second increments with 10 to 12 repetitions.
- Use proprioceptive exercise to prevent reinjury.
- Consider use of preventive taping or bracing.
- Teach proper mechanics of throwing.

PRECAUTIONS/CONTRAINDICATIONS
- During stages of healing, ligamentous rupture can still occur.
- Chronic valgus stress of the ligament, along with hyperextension at the humero-ulnar joint, can lead to the formation of bone spurs and ossific bodies. Surgical removal of these spurs may be necessary for restoration of the function of the elbow.
- Surgical repair or reconstruction may be used with acute instability.
- Communication with surgeon about progression of rehabilitation is important.

DESIRED OUTCOME/PROGNOSIS
- The athlete will show no evidence of soft tissue inflammation or swelling.
- The athlete will have pain-free, normal joint mobility and return of strength.
- The athlete will be able to demonstrate a correct throwing technique.

Note: The decision of when the athlete can return to competition should be made in conjunction with the primary caregiver.

REFERENCES

Assessment

American Physical Therapy Association. Guide to physical therapist practice. 2nd ed. *Phys Ther.* 2001;81.

Buschbacher RM, ed. *Musculoskeletal Disorders: A Practical Guide for Diagnosis and Rehabilitation.* Boston, Mass: Andover Medical Publishers; 1994.

Daniels L, Worthingham C. *Muscle Testing Techniques of Manual Examination.* 6th ed. Philadelphia, Pa: WB Saunders Co; 1995.

Hall CM, Brody TB. *Therapeutic Exercise: Moving Toward Function.* Philadelphia, Pa: Lippincott Williams and Wilkins; 1999.

Hertling D, Kessler RM. *Management of Common Musculoskeletal Disorders.* 3rd ed. Philadelphia, Pa: JB Lippincott Co; 1996:78, 534.

Malone TR, McPoil T, Nitz AJ, eds. *Orthopaedic and Sports Physical Therapy.* 3rd ed. St. Louis, Mo: CV Mosby Co; 1997.

Myers RS, ed. *Saunders Manual of Physical Therapy Practice.* Philadelphia, Pa: WB Saunders Co; 1995.

Rothstein JM, Roy SH, Wolf SL. *The Rehabilitation Specialist's Handbook.* 2nd ed. Philadelphia, Pa: FA Davis Co; 1998.

Saidoff DC, McDonough AL. *Critical Pathways in Therapeutic Intervention.* Philadelphia, Pa: CV Mosby Co; 2002.

Schunk C, Reed K. *Clinical Practice Guidelines.* Gaithersburg, Md: Aspen Publishers; 2000.

Tomberlin JP, Saunders HD. *Evaluation, Treatment and Prevention of Musculoskeletal Disorders. Vol 2: Extremities.* Chaska, Minn: The Saunders Group; 1994.

Treatment

American Physical Therapy Association. *Sports Physical Therapy: Description of Advanced Clinical Practice.* Alexandria, Va: APTA; 1997.

Andrews JR, Whiteside JA. Common elbow problems in the athlete. *J Orthop Sports Phys Ther.* 1993;17:289–295.

Andrews JR, Wilk KE, Grob D. Elbow rehabilitation. In: Brotzman SB, ed. *Handbook of Orthopaedic Rehabilitation.* St. Louis, Mo: Mosby Year Book; 1996.

Andrews JR, Wilk KE, Satterwhite YE, Tedder JL. Physical examination of the thrower's elbow. *J Orthop Sports Phys Ther.* 1993;17:296–304.

Bernhardt-Bainbridge D. Sports injuries in children. In: Campbell SK, ed. *Physical Therapy for Children.* Philadelphia, Pa: WB Saunders Co; 1994:383–422.

Brewer BW, Van Raalte JL, Petitpas AJ, et al. Preliminary psychometric evaluation of a measure of adherence to clinic-based sport injury rehabilitation. *Phys Ther Sport.* 2000; 1:68–74.

Buschbacher RM, ed. *Musculoskeletal Disorders: A Practical Guide for Diagnosis and Rehabilitation.* Boston, Mass: Andover Medical Publishers; 1994.

Chaitow L. *Muscle Energy Techniques.* New York, NY: Churchill Livingstone; 1997.

Conway JE, Jobe FW, Gousman RE, et al. Medial instability of the elbow in throwing athletes. *J Bone Joint Surg.* 1992;74:67–83.

De Bie RA, Verhagen AP, Lenssen AF, et al. Efficacy of 904 nm laser therapy in the management of musculoskeletal disorders: a systematic review. *Phys Ther Rev.* 1998;3: 59–72.

Dilorenzo CE, Parkes JC II, Chemlar RD. The importance of shoulder and cervical dysfunction in the etiology and treatment of athletic elbow injuries. *J Orthop Sports Phys Ther.* 1990;11:398–401.

Fox GM, Jebson PJL, Orwin JF. Overuse injuries of the elbow. *Physician and Sportsmedicine.* 1995;23:58–66.

Kibbler WB, Herring SA, Press JM, eds. *Functional Rehabilitation of Sports and Musculoskeletal Injuries.* Gaithersburg, Md: Aspen Publishers; 1998.

Massie DL, Sager J, Spiker JC. Rehabilitation of the injured elbow. *Orthop Phys Ther Clin North Am.* 1994;3:385–401.

Prins J. Cutner D. Aquatic therapy in the rehabilitation of athletic injuries. *Clin Sports Med.* 1999;18:447–461.

Quarrier NF. Performing arts medicine: the musical athlete. *J Orthop Sports Phys Ther.* 1993;17:90–95.

Roebroeck ME, Dekker J, Oostendorp RA. The use of therapeutic ultrasound by physical therapists in Dutch primary health care. *Phys Ther.* 1998;78:470–478.

Sole G, Lambert M, Juritz J. The role of physiotherapy in sports medicine: perceptions of orthopaedic surgeons, sports physicians, biokineticists and physiotherapists. *S Afr J Physiotherapy.* 2000;56:29–35.

Stroyan M, Wilk KE. The functional anatomy of the elbow complex. *J Orthop Sports Phys Ther.* 1993;17:279–288.

Swenson C, Sward L, Karlsson J. Cryotherapy in sports medicine. *Scand J Med Sci Sports.* 1996;6:193–200.

Syed AA, O'Flanagan J. Simultaneous bilateral elbow dislocation in an international gymnast. *Br J Sports Med.* 1999;33:132–133.

ter Haar G. Therapeutic ultrasound. *Eur J Ultrasound.* 1999;9:3–9.

Timm KE. A new model for functional outcomes measurement in sports physical therapy; determination on return to competition. *J Rehabil Outcomes Meas.* 1997;1:35–44.

Tomberlin JP, Saunders HD. *Evaluation, Treatment and Prevention of Musculoskeletal Disorders. Vol 2: Extremities.* Chaska, Minn: The Saunders Group; 1994.

Werner SL, Fleisig GS, Dillman CJ, Andrews JR. Biomechanics of the elbow during baseball pitching. *J Orthop Sports Phys Ther.* 1993;17:274–278.

Wilder RP, Nirschl PR, Sobel J. Elbow and forearm. In: Buschbacher RM, ed. *Musculoskeletal Disorders: A Practical Guide for Diagnosis and Rehabilitation.* Boston, Mass: Andover Medical Publishers; 1994:153–169.

Wilk KE, Arrigo C, Andrews JR. Rehabilitation of the elbow in the throwing athlete. *J Orthop Sports Phys Ther.* 1993;17:305–317.

Wilk KE, Voight ML, Keirns MA, Gambetta V, Andrews JR, Dillman CJ. Stretch-shortening drills for the upper extremities: theory and clinical application. *J Orthop Sports Phys Ther.* 1993;17:225–239.

Zachazewski JE, ed, Magee DJ, Quillen WS. *Athletic Injuries and Rehabilitation.* Philadelphia, Pa: WB Saunders Co; 1996.

Zuluaga M, Briggs C, Carlisle J, et al. *Sports Physiotherapy: Applied Science and Practice.* Melbourne, Australia: Churchill Livingstone; 1995.

Meniscal Tear

DESCRIPTION

A meniscal tear is common among athletes. The tear may be confined to the periphery or may involve the meniscal body. It is not uncommon to have an anterior cruciate ligament (ACL) injury concurrent with medial meniscal injury. The injury may be preceded by degenerative damage leading to chronic pain.

CAUSE

Injury to the meniscus of the knee can be caused by varus or valgus contact with rotation but is usually triggered by noncontact knee stress. Often a quick change of direction can trigger injury. If the knee is twisted—in hyperflexion or in hyperextension (as in jumping)—it is more vulnerable to injury. Degenerative damage is usually due to repeated stress in a squatting or kneeling position.

ASSESSMENT

Note: See APTA's Guide to Physical Therapist Practice. 2nd ed. *Physical Therapy.* 2001;81.

Musculoskeletal Preferred Practice Patterns: D, H, I

AREAS

- History
- Pain
- Posture
- Gait
- Joint integrity and structural deviation
- Mobility: active and passive range of motion (ROM) and accessory motion
- Strength
- Neurological: sensation, proprioception, deep tendon reflexes, and neural tension
- Skin and soft tissue: temperature and edema
- Functional level
- Equipment, including footwear

INSTRUMENTS/PROCEDURES

See References for sources.

Functional Level
- Modified Lysholm Knee Score

Joint Integrity and Structural Deviations

Following are orthopedic tests for the knee. Those commonly used with this condition are indicated with an asterisk:

- A-angle
- Anteromedial Rotational Instability (AMRI)
- anterior drawer sign
- Anterolateral Rotational Instability (ALRI)
- Apley grinding test*
- apprehension test
- bounce home test
- brush or stroke (wipe) test
- Clark sign
- crossover test
- Ely test
- external rotation test
- flexion rotation drawer test
- fluctuation test
- gravity drawer test (posterior sag sign)
- hamstring length
- Helfet test*
- Hughston plica test
- Hughston posterolateral drawer test
- Hughston test (jerk sign)
- hyperflexion-hyperextension test
- Jakob test (reverse pivot)
- Lachman's test

- lateral pull test
- limb-length discrepancy
- MacIntosh test (lateral pivot shift)
- McConnell test
- McMurray-Anderson test*
- Noble's compression test
- Ober's test
- O'Donoghue test
- patellar tap
- patellar tilt
- Perkins test
- plica test
- posterior drawer sign
- posterior sag sign
- quadriceps active test
- reverse pivot shift
- Slocum test
- Steinman's test
- squat test
- valgus stress test
- varus stress test
- Waldron test
- Wilson test

Mobility
- goniometry

Skin and Soft Tissue
1. temperature, tone, tenderness
   - palpation
2. edema
   - tape measure
   - water displacement

Strength
- manual muscle testing

PROBLEMS
- The athlete may complain of deep pain associated with a feeling of the joint "giving way."
- The athlete may report a feeling of the knee catching or locking.
- There may be pain at the knee joint line and with movement, especially with weight bearing.
- The athlete often has an antalgic gait.
- There may be limited knee flexion.

TREATMENT/MANAGEMENT
- Treatment, in general, is based on the nature of the lesion, extent of degeneration, and residual joint stability.
- Use physical agents and modalities for symptom control.
- Gait activities may indicate the use of an assistive device. Usually, full weight bearing is allowed around 4 to 7 days postoperatively with a partial meniscectomy. Non-weight-bearing status is common for 3 to 6 weeks after meniscal repairs with gradual return to full weight-bearing status.
- Initially, exercise can include open-chain activities and progress to closed-chain activities. Aquatic therapy and proprioceptive training may be useful.

PRECAUTIONS/CONTRAINDICATIONS
- To prevent reinjury, exercise should avoid excessive joint swelling or pain. The process of rehabilitation after surgery should be gradual, avoiding strenuous activity.
- The therapist may be unable to perform McMurray's test if effusion restricts knee flexion or the Helfet test because of incomplete extension.

DESIRED OUTCOME/PROGNOSIS
- The athlete will have decreased or no symptoms.
- The athlete will have pain-free and full ROM with resumption of activities of daily living (ADLs) including athletic activities.

- Nonoperative postmeniscal injury and partial meniscectomy rehabilitation lasts approximately 6 to 12 weeks. Rehab after surgery may take about 3 to 5 weeks but complete recovery after surgical repair may last 6 months. In general, the more conditioned the athlete, the quicker the recovery. Conservative treatment of injury is more likely to be successful if the athlete is able to bear weight and there is minimal swelling and previous history of rapid recovery from a similar injury.

REFERENCES

Assessment

American Physical Therapy Association. Guide to physical therapist practice. 2nd ed. *Phys Ther.* 2001;81.

Brewer BW, Van Raalte JL, Petitpas AJ, et al. Preliminary psychometric evaluation of a measure of adherence to clinic-based sport injury rehabilitation. *Phys Ther Sport.* 2000; 1:68–74.

Buschbacher RM, ed. *Musculoskeletal Disorders: A Practical Guide for Diagnosis and Rehabilitation.* Boston, Mass: Andover Medical Publishers; 1994.

Daniels L, Worthingham C. *Muscle Testing Techniques of Manual Examination.* 6th ed. Philadelphia, Pa: WB Saunders Co; 1995.

Hall CM, Brody TB. *Therapeutic Exercise: Moving Toward Function.* Philadelphia, Pa: Lippincott Williams and Wilkins; 1999.

Hertling D, Kessler RM. *Management of Common Musculoskeletal Disorders.* 3rd ed. Philadelphia, Pa: JB Lippincott Co; 1996:78, 534.

Kendall FP, McCreary EK, Provance PG. *Muscles: Testing and Function.* 4th ed. Baltimore, Md: Williams and Wilkins; 1993.

Malone TR, McPoil T, Nitz AJ, eds. *Orthopaedic and Sports Physical Therapy.* 3rd ed. St. Louis, Mo: CV Mosby Co; 1997.

Myers RS, ed. *Saunders Manual of Physical Therapy Practice.* Philadelphia, Pa: WB Saunders Co; 1995.

Rothstein JM, Roy SH, Wolf SL. *The Rehabilitation Specialist's Handbook.* 2nd ed. Philadelphia, Pa: FA Davis Co; 1998.

Saidoff DC, McDonough AL. *Critical Pathways in Therapeutic Intervention.* Philadelphia, Pa: CV Mosby Co; 2002.

Schunk C, Reed K. *Clinical Practice Guidelines.* Gaithersburg, Md: Aspen Publishers; 2000.

Tomberlin JP, Saunders HD. *Evaluation, Treatment and Prevention of Musculoskeletal Disorders. Vol 2: Extremities.* Chaska, Minn: The Saunders Group; 1994.

Treatment

American Physical Therapy Association. *Sports Physical Therapy: Description of Advanced Clinical Practice.* Alexandria, Va: APTA; 1997.

Buckwalter JA. Articular cartilage: injuries and potential for healing. *J Orthop Sports Phys Ther.* 1998;28:192–202.

Chaitow L. *Muscle Energy Techniques.* New York, NY: Churchill Livingstone; 1997.

De Bie RA, Verhagen AP, Lenssen AF, et al. Efficacy of 904 nm laser therapy in the management of musculoskeletal disorders: a systematic review. *Phys Ther Rev.* 1998;3: 59–72.

Delitto A. Lower extremity: knee. In: Myers RS, ed. *Saunders Manual of Physical Therapy Practice.* Philadelphia, Pa: WB Saunders Co; 1995.

Kibbler WB, Herring SA, Press JM, eds. *Functional Rehabilitation of Sports and Musculoskeletal Injuries.* Gaithersburg, Md: Aspen Publishers; 1998.

Moffet H, Richards CL, Malouin F, et al. Early and intensive physiotherapy accelerates recovery postarthroscopic meniscectomy: results of a randomized controlled study. *Arch Phys Med Rehabil.* 1994;75:415–426.

Mohr KJ, Pink MM, Elsner C, et al. Electromyographic investigation of stretching: the effect of warm-up. *Clin J Sports Med.* 1998;8:215–220.

Ninedek A, Kolt GS. Sport physiotherapists' perceptions of psychological strategies in sport injury rehabilitation. *J Sport Rehabil.* 2000;9:191–206.

Prins J, Cutner D. Aquatic therapy in the rehabilitation of athletic injuries. *Clin Sports Med.* 1999;18:447–461.

Roebroeck ME, Dekker J, Oostendorp RA. The use of therapeutic ultrasound by physical therapists in Dutch primary health care. *Phys Ther.* 1998;78:470–478.

Rothstein JM, Miller PJ, Roetgger RF. Goniometric reliability in a clinical setting: elbow and knee measurements. *Phys Ther.* 1983.

Shrier I. Stretching before exercise does not reduce the risk of local muscles injury: a critical review of the clinical and basic science literature. *Clin J Sports Med.* 1999;9:221–227.

Sole G, Lambert M, Juritz J. The role of physiotherapy in sports medicine: perceptions of orthopaedic surgeons, sports physicians, biokineticists and physiotherapists. *S Afr J Physiotherapy.* 2000;56:29–35.

Swenson C, Sward L, Karlsson J. Cryotherapy in sports medicine. *Scand J Med Sci Sports.* 1996;6:193–200.

ter Haar G. Therapeutic ultrasound. *Eur J Ultrasound.* 1999;9:3–9.

Timm KE. A new model for functional outcomes measurement in sports physical therapy; determination on return to competition. *J Rehabil Outcomes Meas.* 1997;1:35–44.

Tomberlin JP, Saunders HD. *Evaluation, Treatment and Prevention of Musculoskeletal Disorders. Vol 2: Extremities.* Chaska, Minn: The Saunders Group; 1994.

Walker JM. Cartilage of human joints and related structures. Zachazewski JE, Magee DJ, Quillen WS, eds. *Athletic Inj Rehabil.* Philadelphia, Pa: WB Saunders Co; 1996.

Zachazewski JE, ed, Magee DJ, Quillen WS. *Athletic Injuries and Rehabilitation.* Philadelphia, Pa: WB Saunders Co; 1996.

Zuluaga M, Briggs C, Carlisle J, et al. Sports physiotherapy. *Appl Sci Pract.* Melbourne, Australia: Churchill Livingstone, 1995.

Osteitis Pubis

DESCRIPTION

Osteitis pubis is a chronic inflammatory condition of the pubic bone leading to degeneration of the bony articulation. Small avulsion fractures may accompany the inflammation of the ligaments.

CAUSE

Forceful abduction of the legs—as in gymnastics, equestrian events, and water skiing—may stress the anterior aspect of the pelvis at the pubic symphysis joint. A single-leg weight-bearing stance can lead to downward shear forces. Pubic symphysitis may be a precursor to or variation of osteitis pubis.

ASSESSMENT

Note: See APTA's Guide to Physical Therapist Practice. 2nd ed. *Physical Therapy.* 2001;81.

Musculoskeletal Preferred Practice Patterns: A, H, I

AREAS
- History
- Gait
- Joint integrity and structural deviations
- Mobility: including active and passive range of motion (ROM) and accessory motion
- Strength: abdominal, adductor, and lower back musculature
- Neurological
- Pain
- Skin and soft tissue: temperature, tone, tenderness, and edema
- Functional level

INSTRUMENTS/PROCEDURES

See References for sources.

Joint Integrity and Structural Deviation

Following are orthopedic tests for the lower quadrant:

- Craig's test
- Ely test
- FABER test
- hamstring tightness
- leg-length discrepancy
- Noble's compression test
- Ober's test
- piriformis test
- Thomas' test
- Trendelenburg's sign

Strength
- manual muscle testing

PROBLEMS
- The athlete often reports that pain comes on gradually after trauma accumulation.
- There may be joint tenderness and pain with adductor contraction or stretch.
- The athlete tends to ignore the symptoms.

TREATMENT/MANAGEMENT
- Encourage rest.
- Consider using ice followed by heat modalities.
- Begin gentle stretching of adductor muscles to tolerance.
- Swimming can be used as an alternative exercise if the athlete avoids kicks such as whip kicks, which can aggravate the condition.
- Gradually begin a progressive strengthening program following the acute phase.

PRECAUTIONS/CONTRAINDICATIONS
- Pain from osteitis pubis may be confused with referred pain from the viscera or the adductor muscles.
- Avoid cycling, which can aggravate symptoms.

DESIRED OUTCOME/PROGNOSIS

- The athlete will return to a pain-free resumption of activities.

REFERENCES

Assessment

American Physical Therapy Association. Guide to physical therapist practice. 2nd ed. *Phys Ther.* 2001;81.

Brewer BW, Van Raalte JL, Petitpas AJ, et al. Preliminary psychometric evaluation of a measure of adherence to clinic-based sport injury rehabilitation. *Phys Ther Sport.* 2000; 1:68–74.

Buschbacher RM, ed. *Musculoskeletal Disorders: A Practical Guide for Diagnosis and Rehabilitation.* Boston, Mass: Andover Medical Publishers; 1994.

Daniels L, Worthingham C. *Muscle Testing Techniques of Manual Examination.* 6th ed. Philadelphia, Pa: WB Saunders Co; 1995.

Hall CM, Brody TB. *Therapeutic Exercise: Moving Toward Function.* Philadelphia, Pa: Lippincott Williams and Wilkins; 1999.

Hertling D, Kessler RM. *Management of Common Musculoskeletal Disorders.* 3rd ed. Philadelphia, Pa: JB Lippincott Co; 1996:78, 534.

Kendall FP, McCreary EK, Provance PG. *Muscles: Testing and Function.* 4th ed. Baltimore, Md: Williams and Wilkins; 1993.

Malone TR, McPoil T, Nitz AJ, eds. *Orthopaedic and Sports Physical Therapy.* 3rd ed. St. Louis, Mo: CV Mosby Co; 1997.

Myers RS, ed. *Saunders Manual of Physical Therapy Practice.* Philadelphia, Pa: WB Saunders Co; 1995.

Rothstein JM, Roy SH, Wolf SL. *The Rehabilitation Specialist's Handbook.* 2nd ed. Philadelphia, Pa: FA Davis Co; 1998.

Saidoff DC, McDonough AL. *Critical Pathways in Therapeutic Intervention.* Philadelphia, Pa: CV Mosby Co; 2002.

Schunk C, Reed K. *Clinical Practice Guidelines.* Gaithersburg, Md: Aspen Publishers; 2000.

Tomberlin JP, Saunders HD. *Evaluation, Treatment and Prevention of Musculoskeletal Disorders. Vol 2: Extremities.* Chaska, Minn: The Saunders Group; 1994.

Treatment

American Physical Therapy Association. *Sports Physical Therapy: Description of Advanced Clinical Practice.* Alexandria, Va: APTA; 1997.

Chaitow L. *Muscle Energy Techniques.* New York, NY: Churchill Livingstone; 1997.

De Bie RA, Verhagen AP, Lenssen AF, et al. Efficacy of 904 nm laser therapy in the management of musculoskeletal disorders: a systematic review. *Phys Ther Rev.* 1998;3: 59–72.

Johnson MI. Acupuncture-like transcutaneous electrical nerve stimulation (AL-TENS) in the management of pain. *Phys Ther Rev.* 1998;3:73–93.

Kibbler WB, Herring SA, Press JM, eds. *Functional Rehabilitation of Sports and Musculoskeletal Injuries.* Gaithersburg, Md: Aspen Publishers, 1998.

Mohr KJ, Pink MM, Elsner C, et al. Electromyographic investigation of stretching: the effect of warm-up. *Clin J Sports Med.* 1998;8:215–220.

Ninedek A, Kolt GS. Sport physiotherapists' perceptions of psychological strategies in sport injury rehabilitation. *J Sport Rehabil.* 2000;9:191–206.

Prins J, Cutner D. Aquatic therapy in the rehabilitation of athletic injuries. *Clin Sports Med.* 1999;18:447–461.

Shrier I. Stretching before exercise does not reduce the risk of local muscles injury: a critical review of the clinical and basic science literature. *Clin J Sports Med.* 1999;9:221–227.

Sole G, Lambert M, Juritz J. The role of physiotherapy in sports medicine: perceptions of orthopaedic surgeions, sports physicians, biokineticists and physiotherapists. *S Afr J Physiotherapy.* 2000;56:29–35.

Swenson C, Sward L, Karlsson J. Cryotherapy in sports medicine. *Scand J Med Sci Sports.* 1996;6:193–200.

Timm KE. A new model for functional outcomes measurement in sports physical therapy; determination on return to competition. *J Rehabil Outcomes Meas.* 1997;1:35–44.

Tomberlin JP, Saunders HD. *Evaluation, Treatment and Prevention of Musculoskeletal Disorders. Vol 2: Extremities.* Chaska, Minn: The Saunders Group; 1994.

Tonsolone PA. Chronic adductor tendinitis in a female swimmer. *J Orthop Sports Phys Ther.* 1993;18:629–633.

Zachazewski JE, ed, Magee DJ, Quillen WS. *Athletic Injuries and Rehabilitation.* Philadelphia, Pa: WB Saunders Co; 1996.

Zuluaga M, Briggs C, Carlisle J, et al. *Sports Physiotherapy: Applied Science and Practice.* Melbourne, Australia: Churchill Livingstone; 1995.

Rotator Cuff Tendinitis

Also known as *shoulder impingement syndrome, swimmer's shoulder, tennis shoulder*, and *pitcher's shoulder*.

DESCRIPTION

Rotator cuff tendinitis is a tearing and inflammation of the rotator cuff muscle tendons—supraspinatus, infraspinatus, subscapularis, and teres minor—which hold the head of the humerus into the glenoid fossa of the scapula. It is common in sports in which the arm is repeatedly moved forward and overhead. Examples include the forward motion of the arm during freestyle, backstroke, and butterfly swimming strokes; overhead lifting in weight-lifting; the serve in tennis; and the pitching motion in baseball. Rotator cuff tendinitis is the most common shoulder problem in sports medicine.

The disorder can be classified into the following stages:

- *Stage 1 lesion* is simple tendinitis of acute onset. Age of onset is generally under 25 years.
- *Stage 2 lesion* shows fibrosis and tendinitis. Age of onset is generally between 25 and 40 years, but can be any age.
- *Stage 3 lesion* demonstrates bone spurs and tendon rupture.
- *Stage 4 lesion* results in a complete-thickness rotator cuff tear.

CAUSE

Rotator cuff tendinitis is a progressive process, with overuse as the primary etiologic factor. Forward and overhead motion causes the humeral head of the anteriorly flexed shoulder to rub against the acromium and coracoacromial ligament, leading to friction and impingement at the supraspinatus tendon. This mechanical cause of impingement can also affect the adjacent biceps tendon, which may also become impinged.

Structural causes of impingement include congenital abnormalities and/or degenerative alterations in the subacromial arch. Functional causes of impingement include glenohumeral capsular laxity or tightness, cervical spine dysfunction with radiculopathy, postural deviations, and inadequate rotator cuff function with diminished humeral head depression.

If the irritation is chronic, it can lead to subacromial bursitis, inflammation of the tendons, and the rotator cuff tearing by an acute excessive force. If the patient ignores the pain and continues to exercise, the problem can progress to periostitis with avulsion of the tendons at their attachments.

ASSESSMENT

Note: See APTA's Guide to Physical Therapist Practice. 2nd ed. *Physical Therapy.* 2001;81.

Musculoskeletal Preferred Practice Patterns: D, E, I

AREAS
- History
- Pain
- Posture
- Joint integrity and structural deviations
- Mobility: active and passive range of motion (ROM) and accessory motion
- Strength
- Neurological: sensation, proprioception, deep tendon reflexes, and neural tension tests
- Skin and soft tissue: temperature, tone, tenderness, and edema
- Gait
- Functional level

INSTRUMENTS/PROCEDURES

See References for sources.

Functional Level
- Impingement–Instability Classifications
- shoulder pain and disability index

Joint Integrity and Structural Deviations/Neurological Involvement

Following are neurological and orthopedic tests for the upper extremity. Those commonly used with this condition are indicated with an asterisk:

- differentiation tests
- impingement sign
- instability tests*
- lock test*
- neural tension tests
- rotator cuff resistive tests*
- shoulder quadrant test*

Mobility
- goniometry

Skin and Soft Tissue
- palpation for temperature, tone, and tenderness

Special Tests to Which the Physical Therapist May or May Not Have Access
- arthroscopic examination of the throwing shoulder
- electromyograph (EMG) analysis of posterior rotator cuff exercises
- EMG analysis of the upper extremity in pitching
- EMG maximal voluntary isometric contraction (MVIC)
- magnetic resonance imaging (MRI) anatomy of the shoulder

Strength
1. instrumentation
   - cable tensiometry
   - hand-held dynamometry
   - isokinetic assessment
2. manual muscle testing

PROBLEMS

Note: See Description section for definition of stages.

STAGE 1
- The athlete may be unable to sleep on affected side.
- The involved joint may be warm to touch.
- The athlete often has aching pain after a sporting activity.
- There is often point tenderness over the greater tuberosity of the humerus.
- There may be tenderness over the anterior acromion.
- The athlete often demonstrates the classic painful arch between 60 to 120 degrees of flexion.
- There may be involvement of the biceps tendon.

STAGE 2
- The athlete often has biceps tendon involvement.
- Often, symptoms progress to restricted movement and a refraining from any activity that leads to pain.
- There is no relief with avoidance.
- The athlete may have increased tenderness over the acromioclavicular joint.
- The athlete may have pain and weakness with muscle testing, especially with supraspinatus.
- The athlete may complain of a painful catching sensation.

STAGE 3
- There is often increased involvement and frequency of earlier symptoms.
- Pain often limits any athletic activity.

STAGE 4
- The athlete often reports prolonged history of shoulder problems.
- The athlete often demonstrates weakness and atrophy.
- The athlete often has limited ROM, especially during abduction and external rotation.
- There is often difficulty initiating abduction.
- Often, the biceps tendon is involved.

TREATMENT/MANAGEMENT

STAGE 1
- Encourage rest, and consider physical agents and modalities such as microcurrent, pulsed electromagnetic field therapy, iontophoresis, phonophoresis, cryotherapy, and low frequency transcutaneous electrical nerve stimulator (TENS) to decrease inflammation and pain.
- Initiate active-assistive exercises of pendulum activity, pulley motion, and cane exercises with flexion to maintain mobility of glenohumeral, scapulothoracic, acromioclavicular, and sternoclavicular joints.

- Initiate modified isometric exercises. One schedule suggests 3 sets of 12 to 20 repetitions at a submaximal effort and in a slow, rhythmic action to prevent atrophy. Activities include external and internal rotation, abduction, flexion, extension, and scapular motions. Modified aerobic and non-weight-bearing arm activities may be prescribed as needed.
- Educate the patient about activities to avoid, and provide arm protection with support.
- Progress to next stage when athlete reports no pain at rest and no warmth of joint and tolerates Stage 1 activities well.

STAGE 2
- Physical agents and modalities to enhance circulation to the subacromial space may include the following:
  1. ultrasound to supraspinatus fossa
  2. effleurage massage to supraspinatus and infraspinus muscles
  3. ice massage where indicated
  4. transverse friction massage if lesion is superficial
- Initiate abduction movement with rope and pulley and use of cane into external rotation at 90 degrees of abduction to increase ROM and flexibility. Consider use of PNF patterns for glenhumeral motion.
- Consider progressive joint mobilization and self-stretching for shoulder capsule.
- Add total-arm strengthening exercises to promote scapular stabilization, submaximal biceps, tricep, and forearm musculature. One suggested schedule uses light isotonic exercise of 3 sets of 10 repetitions progressing to 20 repetitions as tolerated.
- Progress to Stage 3 if athlete demonstrates normal ROM and is symptom-free with activities of daily living (ADLs), and shows improvement in muscle performance.

STAGE 3
- Use increasingly aggressive joint mobilization to normalize arthokinematics. Client can use active-assisted ROM with cane or T bar in all directions. Teach self-stretches for capsular stretch. Use arm ergometer before and after ROM exercises.
- Use arm ergometry and isotonic dumbbell program to regain shoulder muscle strength. A cable system is preferable if available. May use surgical tubing as an equipment adjunct. Address proximal stability of scapula. Progress to sport-specific training. Consider use of plyometrics to duplicate athletic activity and improve neuromuscular control.
- Progress to Stage 4 if athlete regains full, nonpainful ROM, with no tenderness and with satisfactory strength on clinical examination.

STAGE 4
- Athlete is able to perform functional activities, gradually progressing to full activity. Institute maintenance exercise program for flexibility and strengthening of arm.

PRECAUTIONS/CONTRAINDICATIONS
- Do not perform full ROM initially to avoid undue stress on the musculotendinous junctures.
- Rope and pulley exercises should start with flexion, with palm supinated and humerus externally rotated to avoid impingement. Avoid any discomfort with the movement.
- Grades 1 and 2 (mobilization) may be used in the glenohumeral joint to avoid discomfort from the inflammatory process of the joint.

Note: Progressing too rapidly into Stage 2 is a common fault in unsuccessful rehabilitation.

DESIRED OUTCOME/PROGNOSIS

- The athlete will be free of pain.
- The athlete will have a decrease in the inflammatory response and no swelling.
- The athlete will demonstrate a full range of active and passive motion.
- The athlete will demonstrate maximized shoulder function with coordinated neuromuscular timing.
- The athlete will be able to perform sports with proper technique.
- The athlete will wear properly fitted sporting equipment.
- The athlete will have been instructed in correction or modification of joint abuse and prevention of recurrence.
- Tears of the supraspinatus occur before biceps ruptures in a 7:1 ratio.
- Steroid injections have been reported to weaken a normal tendon for up to 14 days. Athletes should be limited to light work activities for a minimum of 2 weeks post injection.
- An athlete who demonstrates structural changes and is not responding to rehabilitation may require surgery.
- Generally, 70% of athletes fit well into the rehabilitation program, 15% need to be accelerated, and 15% need to go slower.

REFERENCES

Assessment

American Physical Therapy Association. Guide to physical therapist practice. 2nd ed. *Phys Ther.* 2001;81.

Bak KM, Magnusson SP. Shoulder strength and range of motion in symptomatic and pain-free elite swimmers. *Am J Sports Med.* 1997;25:454–459.

Baybar SR. Excessive scapular motion in individuals recovering from painful and stiff shoulders: causes and treatment strategies. *Phys Ther.* 1996;76:226–238.

Beach ML, Whitney SL, Dickoff-Hoffman SA. Relationship of shoulder flexibility, strength, and endurance to shoulder pain in competitive swimmers. *J Orthop Sports Phys Ther.* 1992;16:262–268.

Buschbacher RM, ed. *Musculoskeletal Disorders: A Practical Guide for Diagnosis and Rehabilitation.* Boston, Mass: Andover Medical Publishers; 1994.

Daniels L, Worthingham C. *Muscle Testing Techniques of Manual Examination.* 6th ed. Philadelphia, Pa: WB Saunders Co; 1995.

Davies GJ, Dickoff-Hoffman S. Neuromuscular testing and rehabilitation of the shoulder complex. *J Orthop Sports Phys Ther.* 1993;18:427–432.

Dillman CJ, Fleisig GS, Andrews JR. Biomechanics of pitching with emphasis upon shoulder kinematics. *J Orthop Sports Phys Ther.* 1993;18:402–408.

Ellenbecker TS. Shoulder internal and external rotation strength and range of motion of highly skilled junior tennis players. *Isokinetics Exerc Sci.* 1992;2:1–8.

Ellenbecker TS, Feiring DC, DeHart RL, Rich M. Isokinetic shoulder strength: coronal versus scapular plane testing in upper extremity unilaterally dominant athletes. *Phys Ther.* 1992;72(suppl):580.

Elliott J. Shoulder pain and flexibility in elite water polo players. *Physiotherapy.* 1993;79: 693–697.

Falkel JE, Murphy TC, Murray TF. Prone positioning for testing shoulder internal and external rotation on the Cybex II isokinetic dynamometer. *J Orthop Sports Phys Ther.* 1987;8:368–370.

Glousman R. Electromyographic analysis and its role in the athletic shoulder. *Clin Orthop Related Res.* 1993;288:27–34.

Hall CM, Brody TB. *Therapeutic Exercise: Moving Toward Function.* Philadelphia, Pa: Lippincott Williams and Wilkins; 1999.

Hartsell SD. Postsurgical shoulder strength in the older patient. *J Orthop Sports Phys Ther.* 1993;18:667–672.

Hertling D, Kessler RM. *Management of Common Musculoskeletal Disorders.* 3rd ed. Philadelphia, Pa: JB Lippincott Co; 1996:78, 534.

Jobe FW, Pink M. Classification and treatment of shoulder dysfunction in the overhead athlete. *J Orthop Sports Phys Ther.* 1993;18:427–432.

Kendall FP, McCreary EK, Provance PG. *Muscles: Testing and Function.* 4th ed. Baltimore, Md: Williams and Wilkins; 1993.

Malone TR, McPoil T, Nitz AJ, eds. *Orthopaedic and Sports Physical Therapy.* 3rd ed. St. Louis, Mo: CV Mosby Co; 1997.

Myers RS, ed. *Saunders Manual of Physical Therapy Practice.* Philadelphia, Pa: WB Saunders Co; 1995.

Pellecchia GL, Paolino J, Connell J. Intertester reliability of the Cyriax evaluation in assessing patients with shoulder pain. *J Orthop Sports Phys Ther.* 1996;23:34–38.

Rothstein JM, Roy SH, Wolf SL. *The Rehabilitation Specialist's Handbook.* 2nd ed. Philadelphia, Pa: FA Davis Co; 1998.

Saidoff DC, McDonough AL. *Critical Pathways in Therapeutic Intervention.* Philadelphia, Pa: CV Mosby Co; 2002.

Schunk C, Reed K. *Clinical Practice Guidelines.* Gaithersburg, Md: Aspen Publishers; 2000.

Tomberlin JP, Saunders HD. *Evaluation, Treatment and Prevention of Musculoskeletal Disorders. Vol 2: Extremities.* Chaska, Minn: The Saunders Group; 1994.

Walmsley RP, Hartsell H. Shoulder strength following surgical rotator cuff repair: a comparative analysis using isokinetic testing. *J Orthop Sports Phys Ther.* 1992;15:215–222.

Weir JP, Wagner LL, Housh TJ, Johnson GO. Horizontal abduction and adduction strength at the shoulder of high school wrestlers across age. *J Orthop Sports Phys Ther.* 1992;15:183–186.

Williams JW, Holleman DR, Simel DL. Measuring shoulder function with the shoulder pain and disability index. *J Rheumatol.* 1995;22:727–732.

Wilk KE, Andrews JR, Arrigo CA, et al. The strength characteristics of internal and external rotators in professional baseball pitchers. *Am J Sports Med.* 1993;21:61–66.

Wilk KE, Arrigo CA. Isokinetic exercise and testing for the shoulder. In: Andrews JR, Wilk KE, eds. *The Athlete's Shoulder.* New York, NY: Churchill Livingstone; 1994:523–542.

Worrell TW, Corey BJ, York SL, Santiestaban J. An analysis of supraspinatus EMG activity and shoulder isometric force development. *Med Sci Sports Exerc.* 1992;24:744–748.

Treatment

Allegrucci M, Whitney SL, Irrgang JJ. Clinical implications of secondary impingement of the shoulder in freestyle swimmers. *J Orthop Sports Phys Ther.* 1994;20:307–318.

American Physical Therapy Association. *Sports Physical Therapy: Description of Advanced Clinical Practice.* Alexandria, Va: APTA; 1997.

Andrews JR, Wilk KE, eds. *The Athlete's Shoulder.* New York, NY: Churchill Livingstone; 1994:523–542.

Bertoft ES. Painful shoulder disorders from a physiotherapeutic view: a review of literature. *Crit Rev Phys Rehabil Med.* 1999;11:229–277.

Blevins FT. Rotator cuff pathology in athletes. *Sports Med.* 1997;24:205–220.

Boublik M, Hawkins RJ. Clinical examination of the shoulder complex. *J Orthop Sports Phys Ther.* 1993;18:379–385.

Brewer BW, Van Raalte JL, Petitpas AJ, et al. Preliminary psychometric evaluation of a measure of adherence to clinic-based sport injury rehabilitation. *Phys Ther Sport.* 2000;1:68–74.

Brewster C, Schwab ER. Rehabilitation of the shoulder following rotator cuff injury or surgery. *J Orthop Sports Phys Ther.* 1993;18:422–426.

Bush TA, Mork DO, Sarver KK, et al. The effectiveness of shoulder taping in the inhibition of the upper trapezius as determined by the electromyogram (abstract). *Phys Ther.* 1996;76:S17.

Cavallo RJ, Speer KP. Shoulder instability and impingement in throwing athletes. *Med Sci Sports Exerc.* 1998;30:S18–S25.

Culham E, Peat M. Functional anatomy of the shoulder complex. *J Orthop Sports Phys Ther.* 1993;18:342–350.

Diamond W. Upper extremity: shoulder. In: Myers RS, ed. *Saunders Manual of Physical Therapy Practice.* Philadelphia, Pa: WB Saunders Co; 1995:802–822.

DiGiovine NM, Jobe FW, Pink M, Perry J. An electromyographic analysis of the upper extremity in pitching. *J Shoulder Elbow Surg.* 1992;1:15–25.

Dillman CJ, Murrary TA, Hintermeister RA. Biomechanical differences of open and closed chain exercises with respect to the shoulder. *J Sport Rehabil.* 1994;3:228–238.

Donatelli RA. *Physical Therapy of the Shoulder.* 3rd ed. New York, NY. Churchill Livingstone; 1997.

Ellenbecker TS. Etiology and evaluation of rotator cuff pathology and rehabilitation. In: Donatelli RA. *Phys Ther Shoulder.* 3rd ed. New York, NY. Churchill Livingstone; 1997.

Falkel JE, Murphy TC. Principles of rehabilitation and prehabilitation. In: Falkel JE, Malone TR, eds. *Sports Inj Manage: Shoulder Inj.* Baltimore, Md: Williams and Wilkins; 1988:1:2:42–54.

Herrera-Lasso I, Mobarak L, Fernandez-Dominguez L, et al. Comparative effectiveness of packages of treatment including ultrasound or transcutaneous electrical nerve stimulation in painful shoulder syndrome. *Physiotherapy.* 1993;79:251–253.

Hertling D, Kessler RM. *Management of Common Musculoskeletal Disorders.* 3rd ed. Philadelphia, Pa: JB Lippincott Co; 1996:169–204.

Ho CP. Applied MRI anatomy of the shoulder. *J Orthop Sports Phys Ther.* 1993;18:351–359.

Host HH. Scapular taping in the treatment of anterior shoulder impingement. *Phys Ther.* 1995;75:803–812.

Ingber RS. Shoulder impingement in tennis/racquetball players treated with subscapularis myofascial treatments. *Arch Phys Med Rehabil.* 2000;81:110–122.

Itoi E, Tabata S. Conservative treatment of rotator cuff tears. *Clin Orthop Related Res.* 1992:275:165–173.

Jacobson RP, Benson DJ. Amateur volleyball attackers competing despite shoulder pain: analysis of play habits, anthropometric data, and specific pathologies. *Phys Ther Sport.* 2001;2:112–122.

Jensen C, Nilsen K, Hansen K, et al. Trapezius muscle load as a risk indicator for occupational shoulder-neck complaints. *Intern Arch Occup Environ Health.* 1993;64:415–423.

Jobe C, Jobe FW, Pink M. The sports medicine rehabilitation center. In: Nickel VL, Botte MJ, eds. *Orthop Rehabil.* 2nd ed. New York, NY: Churchill Livingstone; 1992:207–221.

Jobe FW, Pink M. Classification and treatment of shoulder dysfunction in the overhead athlete. *J Orthop Sports Phys Ther.* 1993;18:427–432.

Kamkar A, Irrgang JJ, Whitney SL. Non-operative management of secondary shoulder impingement syndrome. *J Orthop Sports Phys Ther.* 1993;17:212–224.

Kibbler WB, Herring SA, Press JM, eds. *Functional Rehabilitation of Sports and Musculoskeletal Injuries.* Gaithersburg, Md: Aspen Publishers; 1998.

Lake DA. Neuromuscular electrical stimulation: an overview and its application in the treatment of sports injuries. *Sports Med.* 1992;13:320–336.

Leivseth G, Reikeras O. Changes in muscle fiber cross-sectional area and concentrations of Na, K-ATPase in deltoid muscle in patients with impingement syndrome of the shoulder. *J Orthop Sports Phys Ther.* 1994;19:146–149.

Lephart SM, Henry TJ. The physiological basis for open and closed kinetic chain rehabilitation for the upper extremity. *J Sport Rehabil.* 1996;5:71–87.

Litchfield R, Hawkins R, Dillman CJ, Atkins J, Hagerman G. Rehabilitation for the overhead athlete. *J Orthop Sports Phys Ther.* 1993;18:433–441.

Malerba JL, Adam ML, Harris BA, Krebs DE. Reliability of dynamic and isometric testing of shoulder external and internal rotators. *J Orthop Sports Phys Ther.* 1993;18:543–552.

Malone TR. Elements of a standardized shoulder examination. In: Andrews JR, Wilk KE, eds. *The Athlete's Shoulder.* New York, NY: Churchill Livingstone; 1994:39–44.

Matsen FA, Lippett SB, Slidles JA, et al, eds. *Practical Evaluation and Management of the Shoulder.* Philadelphia, Pa: WB Saunders Co; 1993.

McConville OR, Iannotti JP. Partial-thickness Tears of the Rotator Cuff: Evaluation and Management. *J Am Acad Ortho Surg.* 1999;7:32–43.

McDermott DM, Neumann L, Frostick SP, et al. Early results of Bankart repair with a patient-controlled rehabilitation program. *J Shoulder Elbow Surg.* 1999;8:146–150.

McQuade KJ, Wei SH, Smidt GL. Effects of local muscle fatigue on three-dimensional scapulohumeral rhythm (abstract). *Phys Ther.* 1993;73:S109.

Meister K, Andrews JR. Classification and treatment of rotator cuff injuries in the overhand athlete. *J Orthop Sports Phys Ther.* 1993;18:413–421.

Mohr KJ, Pink MM, Elsner C, et al. Electromyographic investigation of stretching: the effect of warm-up. *Clin J Sports Med.* 1998;8:215–220.

Mosely JB, Jobe FW, Pink M, et al. EMG analysis of the scapular muscles during a shoulder rehabilitation program. *Am J Sports Med.* 1992;20:128–134.

Paine RM, Voight M. The role of the scapula. *J Orthop Sports Phys Ther.* 1993;18:386–391.

Pink M, Jobe FW, Perry J. The normal shoulder during the butterfly stroke: an electromyographic and cinematographic analysis of twelve muscles. *Clin Orthop Related Res.* 1993;288:48–59.

Prins J, Cutner D. Aquatic therapy in the rehabilitation of athletic injuries. *Clin Sports Med.* 1999;18:447–461.

Reid DC, Saboe LA, Chepeha JC. Anterior shoulder instability in athletes: comparison of isokinetic resistance exercise and an elecromyographic biofeedback reeducation program: a pilot program. *Physiotherapy Can.* 1996;251–256.

Roebroeck ME, Dekker J, Oostendorp RA. The use of therapeutic ultrasound by physical therapists in Dutch primary health care. *Phys Ther.* 1998;78:470–478.

Savoie FH. Arthroscopic examination of the throwing shoulder. *J Orthop Sports Phys Ther.* 1993;18:409–412.

Shehab D, Adham N. Comparative effectiveness of ultrasound and transcutaneous electrical stimulation in treatment of periarticular shoulder pain. *Physiotherapy Can.* 2000;52:208–214.

Shrier I. Stretching before exercise does not reduce the risk of local muscles injury: a critical review of the clinical and basic science literature. *Clin J Sports Med.* 1999;9:221–227.

Sole G, Lambert M, Juritz J. The role of physiotherapy in sports medicine: perceptions of orthopaedic surgeons, sports physicians, biokineticists and physiotherapists. *S Afr J Physiotherapy.* 2000;56:29–35.

Swenson C, Sward L, Karlsson J. Cryotherapy in sports medicine. *Scand J Med Sci Sports.* 1996;6:193–200.

Tata GE, Ng L, Kramer JF. Shoulder antagonistic strength ratios during concentric and eccentric muscle actions in the scapular plane. *J Orthop Sports Phys Ther.* 1993;18:654–660.

ter Haar G. Therapeutic ultrasound. *Eur J Ultrasound.* 1999;9:3–9.

Timm KE. A new model for functional outcomes measurement in sports physical therapy; determination on return to competition. *J Rehabil Outcomes Meas.* 1997;1:35–44.

Tomberlin JP, Saunders HD. *Evaluation, Treatment and Prevention of Musculoskeletal Disorders. Vol 2: Extremities.* Chaska, Minn: The Saunders Group; 1994;73–112.

Van der Hiejden GJ, Van der Windt DA, de Winter AF. Physiotherapy for patients with soft tissue shoulder disorders: a systematic review of randomized clinical trial. *Br Med J.* 1997;315:25–30.

Veiersted KB, Westgaard RH. Development of traezius myalgia among female workers performing light manual work. *Scand J Work Environ Health.* 1993;19:277–283.

Wilk KE, Andrews JR. Rehabilitation following arthroscopic shoulder subacromial decompression. *Orthop.* 1993;16:349–358.

Wilk KE, Arrigo C. Current concepts in the rehabilitation of the athletic shoulder. *J Orthop Sports Phys Ther.* 1993;18:365–378.

Wilk KE, Arrigo CA. Isokinetic testing and exercises of microtraumatic shoulder injuries. In: Davies GJ, ed. *The Compendium of Isokinetics.* 4th ed. Onalaska, Wis: S & S Publishing; 1992.

Wilk KE, Arrigo CA. Isokinetic testing and exercise. In: Souza TA, ed. *Sports Injuries of the Shoulder.* New York, NY: Churchill Livingstone; 1994:237–256.

Wilk KE, Arrigo CA, Andrews JR. Closed and open kinetic chain exercise for the upper extremity. *J Sport Rehabil.* 1996;5:88–102.

Wilk KE, Arrigo CA, Keirns MA. Shoulder abduction/adduction isokinetic test results: window vs unwindow data collection. *J Orthop Sports Phys Ther.* 1992;15:107–112.

Wilk KE, Voight ML, Keirns MA, Gambetta V, Andrews JR, Dillman CJ. Stretch-shortening drills for the upper extremities: theory and clinical application. *J Orthop Sports Phys Ther.* 1993;17:225–239.

Wooden MJ, Greenfield B, Johanson M, Litzelman L, Mundrane M, Donatelli RA. Effects of strength training on throwing velocity and shoulder muscle performance in teenage baseball players. *J Orthop Sports Phys Ther.* 1992;15:223–228.

Zachazewski JE, ed, Magee DJ, Quillen WS. *Athletic Injuries and Rehabilitation.* Philadelphia, Pa: WB Saunders Co; 1996.

Ankle Sprains

DESCRIPTION

Injury to the ligaments of the ankle is very common. Most ankle sprains (80–90%) involve injury to the lateral ligaments, including the anterior talofibular ligament, the posterior talofibular ligament, and the calcaneal fibular ligament. The anterior talofibular ligament is often injured first (64% injure the ATL only). Less commonly, medial ankle ligaments may also be sprained.

Sprains can be classified by grade (1, 2, or 3), degree (first, second, or third), or description (mild, moderate, or severe).

- In a *grade 1* or *first-degree sprain,* there is some tearing of collagen fibers, and minimal hemorrhaging may occur. The ligament is still intact.
- In a *grade 2* or *second-degree sprain,* part of the ligament or joint capsule is damaged; there is accompanying hemorrhaging and a partial loss of function.
- In a *grade 3* or *third-degree sprain,* the ligament is completely torn, with severe hemorrhaging, edema, and loss of function. There may be capsular disruption as well.

CAUSE

When the lateral ligament is injured, it is usually sprained in a plantar-flexed, inverted position with a twisting motion. Some clients with ligamentous laxity are more vulnerable to inversion injury.

ASSESSMENT

Note: See APTA's Guide to Physical Therapist Practice. 2nd ed. *Physical Therapy.* 2001;81.

Musculoskeletal Preferred Practice Patterns: D, I

AREAS

- History
- Pain
- Posture
- Gait
- Joint integrity and structural deviations: including comparative girth measurements with figure eight technique or malleolar levels
- Mobility: active and passive range of motion (ROM)
- Strength including strength in weight bearing
- Balance: single-limb and double-limb balance using stable and mobile surfaces
- Foot mechanics
- Neurological: sensation, proprioception, deep tendon reflexes, and neural tension
- Skin and soft tissue: temperature, tone, tenderness, and edema
- Functional level
- Equipment, including footwear

INSTRUMENTS/PROCEDURES

See References for sources.

Balance
- Chattecx balance systems

Gait
1. dynamic assessment of foot mechanics
   - dynamic plantar pressure distribution
   - foot pressure EMED system
   - pedabarograph three-dimensional kinematic analysis
2. footprint analysis

Joint Integrity and Structural Deviations

Following are orthopedic tests of the ankle. Those commonly used for this condition are indicated with an asterisk:

- Achilles tendon test
- anterior drawer sign*
- Homan's sign
- inversion stress test
- kinesthetic awareness

- Kleiger test
- talar tilt*
- Thomas' test
- Thompson test

Mobility
- goniometric subtalar and ankle joint measurements
- open and closed kinetic chain subtalar joint neutral positions and navicular drop test
- visual estimates of ankle joint active range of motion

Posture
- postural responses to lateral perturbation
- postural sway following inversion sprain of the ankle

Skin and Soft Tissue
- palpation of temperature, tone, and tenderness

Special Tests
- electromyography (EMG)

Strength
- Biodex dynamometer
- manual muscle testing

PROBLEMS
- The athlete often has ankle edema. Reports of increased circumference greater than 4cm indicate a 70% chance of lignamentous rupture.
- The athlete often has pain, especially with weight bearing.
- The athlete may complain of tenderness over area of injured ligaments.
- The athlete may report a feeling of the joint "giving way."

TREATMENT/MANAGEMENT
In general:
- Control weight bearing as tolerated with assistive devices such as crutches. Progressively increase weight bearing.
- Consider ankle support or bracing. Keep damaged ligament in shortened position when supported.
- Use modalities, such as cryotherapy in combination with electrotherapy, for symptoms.
- Compression pumps or padding or compressive stockings in key areas can decrease edema. Cold and compression can be delivered simultaneously with commerical units. Use elevation to also help control edema.
- Exercises can include proprioceptive exercises and open-chain exercises. Progress with closed-chain exercise as allowed by healing. Consider use of aquatic therapy and/or light effleurage massage (with leg elevated and in a caudocephalad direction) after exercise to assist in venous drainage.
- Stretch gastrocsoleus region and consider use of manual distraction. Stretching can be facilitated with heel cord wedges.

Treatment by degree of sprain is as follows:
- Grade 1
  1. Begin with non-weight-bearing activities, especially for a client with a muscle strength grade of fair or lower.
  2. Use compression such as orthotics or wrap with tape for support.
  3. Consider use of contrast baths or ice and elevation for swelling.

- Grade 2
    1. Wrap with tape for support and apply felt pads over area for extra support.
    2. Consider use of balance board system, such as Biomechanical Ankle Platform System (BAPS) board or KAT system, for proprioceptive training.
- Grade 3
    1. Avoid stretching ligaments in early stages.
    2. Gradually facilitate increase in ROM and strength. Consider use of progressive resistance strengthening exercises with elastic resistance bands. Stress ankle in a controlled manner to return to sport-specific activities. Equipment such as a sliding board, trampoline, and cross-country skiing track—such as Nordic Track—can be used to simulate sport activities. Plyometrics techniques can be applied to the use of this equipment.
    3. Consider use of balance board system—such as Biomechanical Ankle Platform System (BAPS) board—for proprioceptive training.
    4. Consider use of ultrasound or electrotherapeutic modalities if indicated.
    5. Apply manual therapy techniques such as joint mobilization and soft tissue techniques and friction massage.
    6. Home program can emphasize flexibility, strengthening, plyometrics, running progression, edema, and pain control measures.

PRECAUTIONS/CONTRAINDICATIONS
- Subtalar and midtarsal joints should remain in a neutral position during measurement of ankle dorsiflexion.
- Be alert for signs of fracture with acute sprains. Signs of fracture include pain at the distal end of percussion and extreme sensitivity at one particular spot.
- Severe sprains may need surgery. Atypical sprains that may lead to persistent ankle pain include medial ligament sprain, syndesmosis sprain (AITFL), and subtalar joint sprain.

DESIRED OUTCOME/PROGNOSIS
- The athlete will have decreased pain.
- The athlete will have decreased edema.
- The athlete will restore normal ROM.
- The athlete will restore normal strength.
- The athlete will return to full function.

Prolonged ankle instability persists in 10% to 20% of patients with lateral ankle ruptures. Load sensitivity that is atypical could indicate a chondral lesion.

REFERENCES

Assessment

American Physical Therapy Association. Guide to physical therapist practice. 2nd ed. *Phys Ther.* 2001;81.

Buschbacher RM, ed. *Musculoskeletal Disorders: A Practical Guide for Diagnosis and Rehabilitation.* Boston, Mass: Andover Medical Publishers; 1994.

Daniels L, Worthingham C. *Muscle Testing Techniques of Manual Examination.* 6th ed. Philadelphia, Pa: WB Saunders Co; 1995.

Hall CM, Brody TB. *Therapeutic Exercise: Moving Toward Function.* Philadelphia, Pa: Lippincott Williams and Wilkins; 1999.

Hertling D, Kessler RM. *Management of Common Musculoskeletal Disorders.* 3rd ed. Philadelphia, Pa: JB Lippincott Co; 1996:78,534.

Johnson MB, Johnson CL. Electromyographic response of peroneal muscles in surgical and nonsurgical injured ankles during sudden inversion. *J Orthop Sports Phys Ther.* 1993; 18:497–501.

Kendall FP, McCreary EK, Provance PG. *Muscles: Testing and Function.* 4th ed. Baltimore, Md: Williams and Wilkins; 1993.

Malone TR, McPoil T, Nitz AJ, eds. *Orthopaedic and Sports Physical Therapy.* 3rd ed. St. Louis, Mo: CV Mosby Co; 1997.

Myers RS, ed. *Saunders Manual of Physical Therapy Practice.* Philadelphia, Pa: WB Saunders Co; 1995.

Picciano AM, Rowlands MS, Worrell T. Reliability of open and closed kinetic chain subtalar joint neutral positions and navicular drop test. *J Orthop Sports Phys Ther.* 1993;18: 553–558.

Rothstein JM, Roy SH, Wolf SL. *The Rehabilitation Specialist's Handbook.* 2nd ed. Philadelphia, Pa: FA Davis Co; 1998.

Schunk C, Reed K. *Clinical Practice Guidelines.* Gaithersburg, Md: Aspen Publishers; 2000.

Tomberlin JP, Saunders HD. *Evaluation, Treatment and Prevention of Musculoskeletal Disorders. Vol 2: Extremities.* Chaska, Minn: The Saunders Group; 1994.

Youdas JW, Bogard CL, Suman VJ. Reliability of goniometric measurements and visual estimates of ankle joint active range of motion obtained in a clinical setting. *Arch Phys Med Rehabil.* 1993;74:1113–1118.

Treatment

American Physical Therapy Association. *Sports Physical Therapy: Description of Advanced Clinical Practice.* Alexandria, Va: APTA; 1997.

Brewer BW, Van Raalte JL, Petitpas AJ, et al. Preliminary psychometric evaluation of a measure of adherence to clinic-based sport injury rehabilitation. *Phys Ther Sport.* 2000;1: 68–74.

Brunt D, Andersen JC, Huntsman B, et al. Postural responses to lateral perturbation in healthy subjects and ankle sprain patients. *Med Sci Sports Exerc.* 1992;24:2:171–176.

Bullock-Saxton JE. Local sensation changes and altered hip muscle function following severe ankle sprain. *Phys Ther.* 1994;74:17–28.

Bullock-Saxton JE. Local sensation changes and altered hip muscle function following severe ankle sprain. *Phys Ther.* 1994;74:17–28.

Donatelli RA. *The Biomechanics of the Foot and Ankle.* 2nd ed. Philadelphia, Pa: 1996.

Feurerbach JW, Grabiner MD. Effect of the aircast on unilateral postural control: amplitude and frequency variables. *J Orthop Sports Phys Ther.* 1993;17:149–154.

Giallonardo LM. Lower extremity: ankle. In: Myers RS, ed. *Saunders Manual of Physical Therapy Practice.* Philadelphia, Pa: WB Saunders Co; 1995:1031–1053.

Green T, Refshauge K, Crosbie J, et al. A randomized controlled trial of a passive accessory joint mobilization on acute ankle inversion sprains. *Phys Ther.* 2001;81:984–994.

Gross MT, Ballard CL, Mears HG, Watkins EJ. Comparison of DonJoy Ankle Ligament Protector and Aircast Sport-Stirrup orthoses in restricting foot and ankle motion before and after exercise. *J Orthop Sports Phys Ther.* 1992;16:60–67.

Gross MT, Everts JR, Roberson SE, et al. Effect of DonJoy Ankle Ligament Protector and Aircast Sport-Stirrup orthosis on functional performance. *J Orthop Sports Phys Ther.* 1994;19:150–156.

Hanson C, Madras D. Ankle sprain. *Phys Ther Case Rep.* 2000;3:220–225.

Heil B. Lower limb biomechanics related to running injuries. *Physiotherapy.* 1992;78:400–406.

Holme E, Magnusson SP, Becher K, et al. The effect of supervised rehabilitation on strength, postural sway, position sense and re-injury risk after acute ankle ligament sprain. *Scand J Med Sci Sports*. 1999;9:104–109.

Keely G, Sanders B. Ankle injury: the masquerading talar fracture. *Phys Ther Case Rep*. 1998;1:242–249.

Kibbler WB. Diagnosis, treatment and rehabilitation principles in complete tendon rupture in sports. *Scand J Sci Sports*. 1997;7:119–129.

Kibbler WB, Herring SA, Press JM, eds. *Functional Rehabilitation of Sports and Musculoskeletal Injuries*. Gaithersburg, Md: Aspen Publishers;1998.

Lemak KJ, Ellis EA. Acute and chronic ankle sprains: assessment and management. *Sport Med Update*. 1993;8:6–11.

Losito JM, O'Neil J. Rehabilitation of foot and ankle injuries. *Clin Podiatr Med Surg*. 1997;14:533–557.

Lynch SA, Renstrom PA. Treatment of acute lateral ankle ligament rupture in the athlete. Conservative versus surgical treatment. *Sports Med*. 1999;27:61–71.

Mascaro TB, Swanson LE. Rehabilitation of the foot and ankle. *Orthop Clin North Am*. 1994;25:147–160.

McCulloch MU, Brunt D, Vander-Linden D. The effect of foot orthotics and gait velocity on lower limb kinematics and temporal events of stance. *J Orthop Sports Phys Ther*. 1993;17:2–10.

McPoil TG. Footwear. *Phys Ther*. 1988;68:1857–1964.

McPoil TG, Hunt GC. Evaluation and management of foot and ankle disorders: present problems and future directions. *J Orthop Sports Phys Ther*. 1995;21:381–388.

Melham TJ, Sevier TL, Malnofski MJ, Wilsoon JK, et al. Chronic ankle pain and fibrosis successfully treated with a new noninvasive augmented soft tissue mobilization technique (ASTM): a case report. *Med Sci Sports Exerc*. 1998;30:801–804.

Mohr KJ, Pink MM, Elsner C, et al. Electromyographic investigation of stretching: the effect of warm-up. *Clin J Sports Med*. 1998;8:215–220.

Ninedek A, Kolt GS. Sport physiotherapists' perceptions of psychological strategies in sport injury rehabilitation. *J Sport Rehabil*. 2000;9:191–206.

Prins J, Cutner D. Aquatic therapy in the rehabilitation of athletic injuries. *Clin Sports Med*. 1999;18:447–461.

Pugia MK, Middel CJ, Seward SW, et al. Comparison of acute swelling and function in subjects with lateral ankle injury. *J Orthop Sports Phys Ther*. 2001;31:384–388.

Roebroeck ME, Dekker J, Oostendorp RA. The use of therapeutic ultrasound by physical therapists in Dutch primary health care. *Phys Ther*. 1998;78:470–478.

Sammarco GJ. *Rehabilitation of the Foot and Ankle*. St. Louis, Mo: CV Mosby Co; 1995.

Scotece GG, Guthrie MR. Comparison of three treatment approaches for Grade I and II ankle sprains in active duty soldiers. *J Orthop Sports Phys Ther*. 1992;15:19–23.

Shrier I. Stretching before exercise does not reduce the risk of local muscles injury: a critical review of the clinical and basic science literature. *Clin J Sports Med*. 1999;9:221–227.

Sole G, Lambert M, Juritz J. The role of physiotherapy in sports medicine: perceptions of orthopaedic surgeons, sports physicians, biokineticists and physiotherapists. *S Afr J Physiotherapy*. 2000;56:29–35.

Swenson C, Sward L, Karlsson J. Cryotherapy in sports medicine. *Scand J Med Sci Sports*. 1996;6:193–200.

Tatro-Adams D, McGann SF, Carbone W. Reliability of the figure-of-eight method of ankle measurement. *J Orthop Sports Phys Ther*. 1995;22:161–163.

ter Haar G. Therapeutic ultrasound. *Eur J Ultrasound.* 1999;9:3–9.

Timm KE. A new model for functional outcomes measurement in sports physical therapy; determination on return to competition. *J Rehabil Outcomes Meas.* 1997;1:35–44.

Tomberlin JP, Saunders HD. *Evaluation, Treatment and Prevention of Musculoskeletal Disorders. Vol 2: Extremities.* Chaska, Minn: The Saunders Group; 1994:265–302.

Weinstein ML. An ankle protocol for second-degree ankle sprains. *Milit Med.* 1993;158:771–774.

Vandervoort AA, Chesworth BM, Cunningham DA, Rechnitzer PA, Paterson DH, Koval JJ. An outcome measure to quantify passive stiffness of the ankle. *Can J Public Health.* 1992;83: (suppl 2): S19–23.

Wester JU, Jespersen SM, Nielsen KE, et al. Wobble board training after partial sprains of the lateral ligaments of the ankle: a prospective randomized study. *J Orthop Sports Phys Ther.* 1996;23:332–336.

Wilkerson GB, Horn-Kingery HM. Treatment of the inversion ankle sprain: comparison of different modes of compression and cryotherapy. *J Orthop Sports Phys Ther.* 1993;17:240–246.

Yeung SS, Yeung EW, Wong TW. Provision of physiotherapy at the Tsing Ma Bridge International Marathon and 10 km Race in Hong Kong. *Br J Sports Med.* 1998;32:336–337.

Zachazewski JE, ed, Magee DJ, Quillen WS. *Athletic Injuries and Rehabilitation.* Philadelphia, Pa: WB Saunders Co; 1996.

Zuluaga M, Briggs C, Carlisle J, et al. Sports physiotherapy. *Appl Sci Pract.* Melbourne, Australia: Churchill Livingstone; 1995.

Chapter 2
Cardiovascular Conditions

Coronary Artery Disease

DESCRIPTION

Coronary artery disease (CAD) generally results from atherosclerotic lesions that affect the medium and large cardiac arteries. The narrowing and obstruction caused by the atheroma lead to insufficient blood flow to the heart. Other causes may include coronary spasm, drug use, embolus, Kawasaki syndrome, and vasculitis. CAD's primary complications are angina pectoris, myocardial infarction (MI), and sudden cardiac death.

ANGINA PECTORIS

Angina pectoris is due to myocardial ischemia. Angina pectoris may lead to symptoms as slight as an ache or may be characterized by pressure or crushing pain in the mid-chest region and be triggered by exertion and relieved by rest or sublingual nitroglycerin. The pain may also radiate to the teeth, jaw, throat (tickling sensation), posterior neck, shoulder blade areas, or even the abdominal region. Women often have atypical chest pain (see Problems following). There are several types of angina including unstable angina that may not be associated with activity and can occur at rest. Asymptomatic, or "silent" angina can occur without client awareness of an episode.

MYOCARDIAL INFARCTION

Myocardial infarction results in ischemic myocardial necrosis. This leads to reduced cardiac output. It is usually triggered by a sudden decrease in coronary blood flow to a portion of the myocardium. The initial symptoms of an acute attack are usually deep, substernal, visceral pain described as pressure or aching. The pain may radiate into the jaw, left arm, or back. Women often have atypical chest pain (see Problems). Older clients may experience more shortness of breath than ischemic pain.

SUDDEN CARDIAC DEATH

Sudden cardiac death is defined as sudden death within 1 hour of initial symptoms. The contraction of the ventricles is absent or inadequate and results in immediate circulatory failure.

CAUSE

Risk factors associated with CAD are age, gender, family history, cigarette smoking, hypertension, diabetes mellitus, and high serum lipid levels. Other factors may include a lack of physical activity, obesity, elevated homocysteine levels, and infectious agents. The role of personality type as a risk factor is under debate.

ANGINA PECTORIS

Angina pectoris is caused by transient myocardial ischemia without the death of any myocardial cells usually triggered by physical activity.

MYOCARDIAL INFARCTION (MI)

For more than 90% of clients, an acute MI is usually triggered by a thrombus—caused by plaque rupture—that occludes an artery supplying the area that is damaged. The clot is possibly formed by altered platelet function due to endothelial change in the atherosclerotic plaque.

Very rarely, an MI can be caused by arterial embolization. Coronary spasm, which can be triggered by cocaine, can also lead to MI.

SUDDEN CARDIAC DEATH

Sudden cardiac death is often caused by ventricular fibrillation if known factors have been ruled out.

ASSESSMENT

Note: See APTA's Guide to Physical Therapist Practice. 2nd ed. *Physical Therapy.* 2001;81.

Acute MI:

Musculoskeletal Preferred Practice Pattern: C

Cardiovascular/Pulmonary Preferred Practice Patterns: D, E

Atherosclerosis:

Cardiovascular/Pulmonary Preferred Practice Patterns: B, D

Musculoskeletal Preferred Practice Pattern: J

Integumentary Preferred Practice Patterns: A, E

AREAS

- History
- General Appearance
- Equipment, including use of oxygen, humidification, drips, and any chest tubes
- Vital signs, including temperature, resting heart rate, resting BP, resting respiratory rate, and rhythm
- Cardiovascular, including results of exercise testing
- Musculoskeletal, including posture, head and neck musculature, and chest shape
- Skin and soft tissue, including edema and condition of hands, especially nails
- Selected cardiopulmonary tests and measures

CARDIOPULMONARY TESTS AND MEASURES

- aerobic capacity and endurance, including vital signs and palpation of pulses
- auscultation of heart, lungs, and major vessels
- breathing patterns, including thoracoabdominal movements and chest wall mobility
- claudication time tests
- cough/sputum production and airway clearance
- edema assessment
- functional level (see following)
- quality of life measures (see following)
- rating of perceived exertion (RPE) scales
- response to positional changes
- skin coloration, including cyanosis
- size and body fat composition
- ventilatory muscle ability

INSTRUMENTS/PROCEDURES

Functional Level
- Barthel ADL index
- PULSES profile
- Chronic Respiratory Disease Questionnaire (CRQ)
- Classes of Respiratory Impairment
- Functional Independence Measure (FIM)
- Katz Index of ADLs
- Klein Bell Activities Scale
- New York Functional and Therapeutic Classification of Heart Disease
- Pulmonary Functional Status Scale (PFSS)
- Pulmonary Functional Status and Dyspnea Questionnaire (PFSDQ)

- St. George's Respiratory Questionnaire
- visual analog scale for dyspnea and/or pain

Quality of Life Measures for Cardiac Care
- Cardiac Depression Scale (CDS)
- Controlled job simulation
- Ferrans and Powers Quality of Life Index – Cardiac Version (QLI-C)
- Function Status Questionnaire
- Human Activity Profile
- MacNew Quality of Life after Myocardial Infarction (QLI-H-Fp)
- MET activity tables
- Minnesota Living with Heart Failure Questionnaire (MLHFQ)
- New York Heart Association Functional Classification
- Outcomes Institute Angina TyPE Specification (HOI TyPE-A)
- Physical Activity Readiness Questionnaire (PAR-Q)

Physical Activity Measures
- Seattle Angina Questionnaire (SAQ)
- Specific Activity Scale
- The Duke Activity Status Index (DASI)
- 6-minute walk assessment
- 12-minute walk assessment
- Quality of Life after Myocardial Infarction

Exercise Testing Measures
- angina and dyspnea rating scales
- bicycle test
- blood pressure response to exercise
- graded exercise test
- intermittent claudication rating scale
- rating received exertion (Borg scales)
- signs/symptoms
- submaximal exercise test
- symptom-limited maximum tests
- single-staged endurance tests
- telemetry (continuous or intermittent)
- treadmill exercise assessment protocols such as Bruce, Stanford, and Balke
- walk test
- 12-lead ECG
- vital signs

Special Tests to Which the Physical Therapist May or May Not Have Access
- arterial blood gas analysis (ABG)
- bacterial and cytological tests of sputum
- chest x-ray (CXR)
- exercise tests (ie, walk test, cycle test, treadmill tests)
- flexible bronchoscopy
- oximetry
- Ventilation/Perfusion Scan

Pulmonary Function Tests (PFTs)
- airways resistance (Raw)
- alveolar ventilation (VA)
- body plethysmography – lung volumes (TGV)
- diffusion capacity of lungs for carbon monoxide (DL co)
- graded exercise tests (GXT)
- expiratory reserve volume (ERV)
- flow-volume loop (F-V loop)
- forced expiratory volume in 1 second (FEV1)
- forced vital capacity (FVC)
- functional residual capacity (FRC)
- helium dilution method
- inspiratory reserve volume (IRV)

- maximum voluntary ventilation (MVV)
- maximum minute expired volume (VE)
- methacholine provocation test
- nitrogen washout test
- peak expiratory flow rate (PEFR)
- residual volume (RV)
- spirogram
- spirometry
- tidal volume (TV)
- total lung capacity (TLC)
- vital capacity (VC)
- Ventilation/Perfusion Scan

PROBLEMS

ANGINA

- Client reports pressure or crushing pain in the mid-chest region, which is triggered by exertion and relieved by rest.
- The pain may also radiate to the teeth, jaw, throat (tickling sensation), posterior neck, or shoulder blade areas.
- Other symptoms include dyspnea, nausea, indigestion and belching. Women, in particular, may experience variations in symptoms (see following).
- Unstable angina may not be associated with activity and can occur at rest.

Women may have the following variations in symptoms:
- palpitation without chest pain or left chest pain without mid-chest pain
- ache in right biceps
- back pain
- chest pain or heartburn unrelieved by medications
- extreme lethargy
- nocturnal dyspnea

MYOCARDIAL INFARCTION

The client may describe symptoms in the following terms:
- burning/indigestion
- chest tightness or squeezing
- discomfort/angina lasting 30 minutes or greater or unrelieved by rest or medication
- dizziness/feeling faint/weakness
- shortness of breath
- shoulder ache/radiation of pain down arms bilaterally/RSD
- pallor/diaphoresis

Women may have the following variations in symptoms:
- palpitation without chest pain or left chest pain without mid-chest pain
- ache in right biceps
- back pain
- chest pain or heartburn unrelieved by medications
- extreme lethargy
- nocturnal dyspnea

CORONARY ARTERY DISEASE

- exercise-induced myocardial ischemia
- functional capacity at or below 5 metabolic equivalent units (METs)
- impaired aerobic capacity which may include abnormal heart rate and blood pressure responses

TREATMENT/MANAGEMENT

CARDIAC REHABILITATION

Angina, MI, and Coronary Artery Disease

Management of nonacute coronary heart disease includes individually designed care based on the essential component of cardiac rehabilitation. According to the US Department of Health and Human Services (DHSS) 1995 report (see References following), "cardiac rehabilitation services are comprehensive, long-term programs involving medical evaluation, prescribed exercises, cardiac risk factor modification, education, and counseling. Cardiac rehabilitation centers have an increased emphasis on prevention of secondary complications from coronary artery disease."

Cardiac care includes a continuum of care that begins with inpatient and transitional care and continues in a more aggressive mode within an outpatient setting employing risk stratification. Inpatient care generally lasts the first 2 weeks post-hospitalization of cardiac event or procedure. Transitional care generally lasts from 1 to 6 weeks post-hospitalization of cardiac event or procedure and occurs in a subacute facility or at home. Outpatient programs typically last from 1 to 12 weeks post-hospitalization of cardiac event or procedure and occur at a cardiac rehabilitation center. This continuum of care should be extended to a lifelong maintainance program that is home-based or occurs at a community facility.

Initiation of Rehabilitation in the Inpatient or Transitional Period

Conditions for initiating activity include the following:

- Absence of chest pain for 8 hours
- Absence of new signs of uncompensated failure, abnormal cardiac rhythms, or ECG changes for 8 hours

Conditions for progression of rehabilitation include the following:

- HR increase of 5–20 beats above resting rate in response to activity
- Systolic BP rises to within 10–40 mmHg from resting rate in response to activity
- Absence of cardiac symptoms and rhythm or ECG changes

Inpatient Progression of Activity

In the CCU, the client will be on bedrest until stable and progress to sitting up in a chair and using a bedside commode. MET level is in the 1 to 2 METs range. Progression to a Step-Down Unit includes self-care activities, gentle ROM in sitting, and walking in the room. MET level is in the 2 to 3 METs range. The client will then progress to ADLS in the 3 to 4 METs level range for self-care, walking in the hall for 5 to 10 minutes from 2 to 4 times a day, and progressing to stairs or treadmill with supervision.

Cardiac rehabilitation is a multifactorial process but this text will focus on the physical activity component. Before beginning an exercise program, the client's risk status should be assessed followed by an individualized treatment plan for exercise training.

Prescribed exercise training is based on risk level and client goals and will be either supervised or unsupervised with ECG monitoring versus no monitoring. Exercise prescription methodologies may include exercise intensity methods using percentage of peak heart rate, heart rate reserve, MET values, and perception of exertion.

Generally, a minimum goal for physical activity is 30 minutes of activity, 3 to 4 times per week (American Heart Association's Consensus Panel Statement, 1995).

Physical activity prescription consists of the following parameters:

- *Duration:* 30 to 60 minutes
- *Frequency:* 3 to 4 times per week

- *Type:* moderate intensity activities such as walking, jogging, biking, or increased physical activity in ADLs such as stair climbing, household work, and gardening
- *Qualifications:* Moderate- to high-risk patients should be in a medically supervised program.

American Association of Cardiovascular and Pulmonary Rehabilitation (AACVPR) recommends assessment of risk for progression of CAD when determining the parameters of treatment within a secondary prevention program in an outpatient setting. See Table 2.1 for an illustration of the stratification of risk and recommendations for monitoring patients.

Cardiac rehabilitation also applies to clients with coronary insufficiency, which may also be treated with percutaneous transluminal coronary angioplasty (PTCA) or bypass surgery (ie, coronary artery bypass graft [CABG]), and clients with pacemakers, heart valve repair, cardiac transplantation, heart failure, and arrhythmias.

Cardiac rehabilitation is also described in phases beginning with Phase I, the acute or monitoring phase, Phase II, the subacute or conditioning phase, Phase III, training or intensive rehabilitation, and Phase IV, ongoing conditioning (ie, maintenance phase or prevention program).

PRECAUTIONS/CONTRAINDICATIONS

Absolute contraindications to exercise testing include the following:

- Acute cardiopulmonary conditions such as MI, myocarditis, pericarditis, or pulmonary infarction
- Unstable angina, uncontrolled arrhythmias or heart failure, or severe aortic stenosis (symptomatic)

Relative contraindications to exercise testing include:

- Severe symptoms of hypertension or high-degree atrioventricular block
- Coronary stenosis (left main) or moderate stenotic valvular heart disease
- Arrhythmias (tachy or brady cardia) or electrolyte imbalances
- Outflow tract obstruction

Discontinue exercise if the following adverse responses occur:

- Elevated heart rate higher than 130 bpm or an increase of 30 bpm above pre-activity level
- Elevated diastolic blood pressure above 110 mmHG or decrease in systolic blood pressure greater than 10 mmHG
- Arrhythmias or heart block (2nd or 3rd degree)
- Exercise intolerance symptoms of angina pectoris or significant dyspnea
- Management of the client will vary depending on pre-existing conditions such as chronic renal insufficiency or cardiovascular complications such as post-operative bleeding.

DESIRED OUTCOME/PROGNOSIS

OUTCOMES OF CARDIAC REHABILITATION

The most scientifically supported substantial benefits reported by the DHHS (1995) include the following:

- Improvement in exercise tolerance
- Improvement in symptoms
- Improvement in blood lipid levels
- Reduction in cigarette smoking
- Improvement in psychosocial well-being and reduction of stress
- Reduction in mortality

TABLE 2.1

Stratification for Risk of Event (Not Specific Solely to Exercise) and Recommendations for ECG Monitoring and Close Supervision During Exercise

---

Lowest Risk

1. No significant LV dysfunction (EF > 50%)
2. No resting or exercise-induced complex dysrhythmias
3. Uncomplicated MI; CABG; angioplasty; atherectomy, or stent
4. Absence of CHR or signs/symptoms indicating postevent ischemia
5. Normal hemodynamics with exercise or recovery
6. Asymptomatic including absence of angina with exertion or recovery
7. Functional capacity greater or equal to 7.0 METs (if available)
8. Absence of clinical depression

Lowest risk classification is assumed when each of the risk factors in the category is present. Lowest risk patients may be monitored for 6-18 sessions, beginning with continuous ECG monitoring along with close clinical supervision, decreasing the intensity of ECG monitoring to intermittent during sessions 8 through 12. Hemodynamic response to exercise should be normal and progression of the exercise prescription should be regular during those sessions. Close clinical supervision, which may include direct supervision of exercise sessions, should continue for at least 30 days postevent.

Moderate Risk

1. Moderately impaired left ventricular function (EF = 40%-49%)
2. Signs/symptoms including angina at moderate levels of exercise (5-6.9 METs) or in recovery.

Moderate risk is assumed for patients who do not meet the classification of either highest risk or lowest risk. Moderate patients may be monitored for 12-24 sessions initially, with continuous ECG monitoring along with close clinical supervision, decreasing the intensity of ECG monitoring to intermittent during latter sessions. Hemodynamic response to exercise should be normal and progression of the exercise prescription should be regular during those sessions. Close clinical supervision, which may include direct supervision of exercise sessions, may be required for 60 to 90 days postevent.

Highest Risk

1. Decreased LV function (EF < 40%)
2. Survivor of cardiac arrest or sudden death
3. Complex ventricular dysrhythmia at rest or with exercise
4. MI or cardiac surgery complicated by cardiogenic shock, CHF, or signs/symptoms of postprocedure ischemia
5. Abnormal hemodynamics with exercise (especially flat or decreasing systolic blood pressure or chronotropic incompetence with increasing workload)
6. Signs/symptoms including angina pectoris at low levels of exercise (< 5.0 MET) or in recovery
7. Functional capacity < 5.0 MET (if available)
8. Clinically significant depression

Highest risk classification is assumed with the presence of any one of the risk factors included in this category. High-risk patients may be monitored for 18-24 sessions or more initially, with continuous ECG monitoring along with close clinical supervision, decreasing the intensity of ECG monitoring to intermittent during latter sessions. Hemodynamic response to exercise should be normal and progression of the exercise prescription should be regular during those sessions. Close clinical supervision, including direct supervision of exercise sessions, may be required for 90 days or more postevent.

Note. LV = left ventricular; EF = ejection fraction; MI = myocardial infarction; CABG = coronary artery bypass grafts; METs = metabolic equivalents; CHF = congestive heart failure. Reprinted with permission from American Association of Cardiovascular & Pulmonary Rehabilitation, *Guidelines for cardiac rehabilitation and secondary prevention programs*, 3rd ed. Champaign, IL: Human Kinetics; 1999:45.

REFERENCES

Assessment

American Physical Therapy Association. Guide to physical therapist practice. 2nd ed. *Phys Ther*. 2001;81.

Cahalin LP. Auscultation of the heart: a cursory review of basic principles and practice skills. *CardioPulmonary Phys Ther J*. 1997;8:8–12.

Dean E. Preferred practice patterns in cardiopulmonary physical therapy: a guide to physiologic measures. *CardioPulmonary Phys Ther J*. 1999;10:124–134.

Eason JM. Cardiopulmonary assessment. *CardioPulmonary Phys Ther J*. 1999;10:135–142.

Goodman C, Snyder T. *Differential Diagnosis in Physical Therapy*. 3rd ed. Philadelphia, Pa: WB Saunders Co; 2000.

Frownfelter D, Dean E. *Principles and Practice of Cardiopulmonary Physical Therapy*. 3rd ed. New York, NY: CV Mosby Co; 1996.

Hillegass EA, Sadowsky HS. *Essentials of Cardiopulmonary Physical Therapy*. 2nd ed. Philadelphia, Pa: WB Saunders Co; 2001.

Myers RS, ed. *Saunders Manual of Physical Therapy Practice*. Philadelphia, Pa: WB Saunders Co; 1995.

Pashkow FJ, Dafoe WA. *Clinical Cardiac Rehabilitation: A Cardiologist's Guide*. 2nd ed. Baltimore, Md: Williams and Wilkins; 1999.

Paz JC, Panik M. *Acute Care Handbook for Physical Therapists*. Burlington, Mass: Butterworth Heinemann; 1997.

Rothstein JM. *Measurement in Physical Therapy*. 2nd ed. New York, NY: Churchill Livingstone; 1998.

Williams MA. *AACVPR Guidelines for Cardiac Rehabilitation and Secondary Prevention Programs*. 3rd ed. Champaign, IL: Human Kinetics; 1999.

Treatment

Ades PA, Pashkow PF, Nestor JR, Pashkow FJ. Evaluation of outcomes. In: Pashkow FJ, Dafoe WA. *Clinical Cardiac Rehabilitation: A Cardiologist's Guide*. 2nd ed. Baltimore, Md: Williams and Wilkins; 1999:52–64.

Alexander KM, Devine NL, Wintz GS. Using surveys in physical therapy. *CardioPulmonary Phys Ther J*. 1999;10:101–104.

Alexander K, LaPeir TK, Provosty Y, Lahdenpera H, et al. A comparison of automatic finger blood pressure monitoring and sphygmomanometry with auscultation at rest and during progressive exercise. *CardioPulmonary Phys Ther J*. 1997;8:4–9.

Borjesson M, Eriksson P, Dellborg M, Eleasson T, et al. Transcutaneous electrical nerve stimulation in unstable angina pectoris. *Coronary Artery Disease*. 1997;8:543–550.

Brooks B. Cardiac case study: ECG monitoring. *Cardiopulmonary Phys Ther*. 1996;7:16–17.

Cahalin LP. Auscultation of the heart: a cursory review of basic principles and practice skills. *CardioPulmonary Phys Ther J*. 1997;8:8–12.

Cassady LS, Duffy AM, Meier KM, Venteicher JM, et al. *Cardiopulmonary Phys Therapy*. 1996;7:8–12.

Certo C. Cardiovascular system. In: Myers RS, ed. *Saunders Manual of Physical Therapy Practice*. Philadelphia, Pa: WB Saunders Co; 1995:193–251.

Cohen MC, Rohtla KM, Mittleman MA, et al. Meta-analysis of the morning excess of acute myocardial infarction and sudden cardiac death. *Am J Cardiology*. 1997;79:1512–1516.

Dean E. Preferred practice patterns in cardiopulmonary physical therapy: A guide to physiologic measures. *CardioPulmonary Phys Ther J.* 1999;10:124–134.

DeTurk WE, Buck L, Cahalin J, Jewell D, et al. Revalidation of advanced clinical practice in cardiopulmonary physical therapy. *CardioPulmonary Phys Ther J.* 1999;10:105–108.

Eason JM. Cardiopulmonary assessment. *CardioPulmonary Phys Ther J.* 1999;10:135–142.

El-Ansary D, Adams R, Ghandi A. Musculoskeletal and neurological complications following coronary artery bypass graft surgery: a comparison between saphenous vein and internal mammary artery grafting. *Aust J Physiotherapy.* 2000;46:19–25.

Flarey DL, Blancett SS, eds. *Cardiovascular Outcomes: Collaborative, Path-Based Approaches.* Gaithersburg, Md: Aspen Publishers; 1998.

Francis K, Murray D. Walking and running energy expenditure estimated by the Tritrac and indirect calorimetry. *CardioPulmonary Phys Ther J.* 1998;9:6–10.

Goodman C, Synder T. *Differential Diagnosis in Physical Therapy.* 2nd ed. Philadelphia, Pa: WB Saunders Co; 2000.

Grabois M, Garrison SJ, Hart KA, Lehmkuhl LD. *Physical Medicine and Rehabilitation: The Complete Approach.* Malden, Mass: Blackwell Science; 2000.

Hamer P, Slocombe B. The psychophysical and heart rate relationship between treadmill and deep-water running. *Aust J Physiotherapy.* 1997;43:265–271.

Hillegass EA, Sadowsky HS. *Essentials of Cardiopulmonary Physical Therapy.* 2nd ed. Philadelphia, Pa: WB Saunders Co; 2001.

Humphrey E. Exercise physiology in patients with left ventricular assist devices. *J Cardiopulmonary Rehabil.* 1997;17:73–75.

Humphrey R, Bartels MN. Exercise, cardiovascular disease, and chronic heart failure. *Arch Phys Med Rehabil.* 2001;82:S76–81.

Humphrey R, Manetz C, Tolman DE, et al. Exercise training responses in a patient with a left ventricular assist device. *J Cardiopulmonary Rehabil.* 1996;16:5:310.

Keeling B, Weaver J, Murph E. Improving outcomes related to the cooperative cardiovascular project. In: Farey DL, Blancett SS, eds. *Cardiovascular Outcomes.* Gaithersburg, Md: Aspen Publishers; 1998:62–80.

LaPier TK, Cleary KK. Clinical profile. Cardiac rehabilitation after acute myocardial infarction. *Phys Ther Case Reports.* 2000;3:124–131.

LaPier TK, Donovan C. Reliability and validity issues in cardiopulmonary physical therapy. *CardioPulmonary Phys Ther J.* 1999;10:148–152.

Mathes P. Exercise and physical therapy in elderly, more severely incapacitated patients in cardiac rehabilitation. *Coronary Artery Dis.* 1999;10:33–36.

Morrin L, Mayhew A, Reid R, et al. Home vs. supervised exercise programs: do participant characteristics and outcomes differ? *J Cardiopulmonary Rehabil.* 1997;17:354.

Pashkow P, Ades PA, Emery CF, et al. Outcome measurement in cardiac and pulmonary rehabilitation. *J Cardiopulmonary Rehabil.* 1995;15:394–405.

Pashkow P, MacDonald CL. Patient outcomes in cardiac rehabilitation: what, why, and when to measure. In: Wenger NK, Smith LK, Froelicher ES, Comoss PM, eds. *Cardiac Rehabilitation: A Guide to Practice in the 21st Century.* New York, NY: Marcel Dekker, Inc; 1999:423–434.

Pashkow FJ, Pashkow PL. Program models for cardiac rehabilitation. In: Pashkow FJ, Dafoe WA. *Clinical Cardiac Rehabilitation: A Cardiologist's Guide.* 2nd ed. Baltimore, Md: Williams and Wilkins; 1999:453–457.

Petta A, Jenkins S, Allison F. Ventilatory and cardiovascular responses to unsupported low-intensity upper limb exercise in normal subjects. *Aust J Physiotherapy.* 1998;44:123–129.

Ribisl PM, Morrin L, Lefroy S. Program standards and organizational issues. In: Pashkow FJ, Dafoe WA. *Clinical Cardiac Rehabilitation: A Cardiologist's Guide.* 2nd ed. Baltimore, Md: Williams and Wilkins; 1999:418–445.

Scherer S, Cassady SL. Rating of perceived exertion: development and clinical applications for physical therapy exercise testing and prescription. *CardioPulmonary Phys Ther J.* 1999;10:143–147.

Scherer S. Exercise in the patient with claudication pain. *CardioPulmonary Physical Therapy Journal.* 1999;10:45–48.

Schuster NB. Simultaneous implementation of two cardiopulmonary preferred practice patterns across the continuum of care. *Phys Ther Case Rep.* 1999;2:6:241–248.

Shaw DK, Artois JW, McCord AM, et al. Efficacy and telemedicine in the evaluation of patients with cardiopulmonary disease. *Phys Ther Case Rep.* 2000;3:37–39.

Siler WL, Koch NQ, Frese EM. The path utilized affects the distance walked in the 12 minute walk test. *CardioPulmonary Phys Ther J.* 1999;10:84–89.

Sokolski DM, Cahalis LP, Hill J, Johansen J, Pedersen S, LaPier TK. Evaluation of a complicated patient with coronary artery disease: a case study. *CardioPulmonary Phys Ther J.* 1997;8:8–11.

Sparks KE, Shaw DK, Jennings HS III, Quinn LM. Cardiovascular complications of outpatient cardiac rehabilitation programs utilizing transtelephonic exercise monitoring. *CardioPulmonary Phys Ther J.* 1998;9:3–6.

Stewart AV, Eales CJ, DeCharmoy S. The knowledge profile of patients with hypertension. *S Afr J Physiotherapy.* 2001;56:17–21.

Ståhle A, Tollback A. Effects of aerobic group training on exercise capacity, muscular endurance and recovery in elderly patients with recent coronary events: a randomized, controlled study. *Adv Physiotherapy.* 2001;3:29–37.

Vanhees L, Schepers D, Heidbuchel H, et al. Exercise performance and training in patients with implantable cardioverter-defibrillators and coronary heart disease. *Am J Cardiology.* 2001;87:712–715.

Wells CL. Physiological response to upper extremity exercise and the clinical implications. *CardioPulmonary Phys Ther J.* 1998;9:7–9.

Wenger NK, Froelicher ES, Smith LK, Ades PA, Berra K, Blumenthal JA, Certo CME, et al. *Cardiac Rehabilitation: Clinical Practice Guideline No. 17.* Rockville, Md: U.S. Department of Health and Human Services, Public Health Service, Agency for Health Care Policy and Research and the National, Heart, Lung, and Blood Institute; October 1995. AHCPR publication 96-0672.

Williams MA, ed. *AACVPR Guidelines for Cardiac Rehabilitation and Secondary Prevention Programs.* 3rd ed. Champaign, Ill: Human Kinetics; 1999.

Cardiac Surgery

DESCRIPTION

Just as there are a variety of approaches to cardiac surgery, there are a variety of approaches to physical therapy after cardiac surgery. The therapist should work closely with the surgical team and client on treatment decisions. Clients undergoing cardiac surgery are at an increased risk for postoperative complications such as thrombosis or pneumonia. This section applies to the following surgeries:

- atrial septal defect
- complete transposition of the great vessels
- coronary artery bypass grafting (CABG)
- corrective surgery in adults

- pacemakers
- percutaneous transluminal coronary angioplasty (PTCA)
- pulmonary stenosis or aortic stenosis
- repair of ascending aortic aneurysm
- tetralogy of Fallot
- transplantation
- valve repair
- valve replacement
- ventricular aneurysmectomy
- ventricular septal defect
- ventricular tachycardia

CAUSE

Valvular lesions can be caused by complications from rheumatic fever, degenerative changes, congenital defects, or subacute bacterial endocarditis. Pulmonary valve problems are usually caused by congenital defects. Congenital defects are often a result of maternal disease, arrested development in utero, or genetic factors. See also Chapter 12, Pediatric Cardiac Conditions.

Congenital disorders are divided into acyanotic conditions and cyanotic conditions. Acyanotic conditions lead to excessive pulmonary blood flow, and cyanotic conditions lead to inadequate pulmonary blood flow. Acyanotic conditions include valvular stenosis, atrial septal defect, ventricular septal defect, persistent ductus arteriosus, and aortic coarctation. Cyanotic conditions include tetralogy of Fallot and transposition of great vessels.

The need for a pacemaker may be triggered by the following conditions: arrhythmias, heart block, hypersensitive carotid sinus syndrome, Stokes-Adams syndrome, and sick sinus syndrome. Arrhythmias are caused by abnormal conduction patterns.

ASSESSMENT

Note: See APTA's Guide to Physical Therapist Practice. 2nd ed. *Physical Therapy.* 2001;81.

Cardiovascular/Pulmonary Preferred Practice Patterns: C, F

AREAS
- History, including operative notes, type of incision, use of any grafts
- General Appearance
- Equipment, including use of oxygen, humidification, drips, and any chest tubes
- Vital signs, including temperature, resting heart rate, resting BP, resting respiratory rate and rhythm.
- Intake and output, presence of any drainage tubes
- Cardiovascular, including results of exercise testing
- Musculoskeletal, including posture, head and neck musculature, and chest shape
- Skin and soft tissue, including edema and condition of hands, especially nails
- Strength: little or no resistance in upper extremities after sternotomy
- Selected cardiopulmonary tests and measures

CARDIOPULMONARY TESTS AND MEASURES
- aerobic capacity and endurance, including vital signs and palpation of pulses
- auscultation of heart, lungs, and major vessels
- breathing patterns, including thoracoabdominal movements and chest wall mobility
- claudication time tests
- cough/sputum production and airway clearance
- edema assessment
- functional level (see following)
- quality of life measures (see following)
- rating of perceived exertion (RPE) scales
- response to positional changes

- skin coloration including cyanosis
- size and body fat composition
- ventilatory muscle ability

INSTRUMENTS/PROCEDURES

Functional Level
- Barthel ADL index
- PULSES profile
- Chronic Respiratory Disease Questionnaire
- Classes of Respiratory Impairment
- Functional Independence Measures
- Katz Index of ADLs
- Klein Bell Activities Scale
- New York Functional and Therapeutic Classification of Heart Disease
- Pulmonary Functional Status Scale
- Pulmonary Functional Status and Dyspnea Questionnaire
- St. George's Respiratory Questionnaire
- visual analog scale for dyspnea and/or pain

Quality of Life Measures for Cardiac Care
- Cardiac Depression Scale
- Controlled job simulation
- Ferrans and Powers Quality of Life Index–Cardiac Version
- Function Status Questionnaire
- Human Activity Profile
- MacNew Quality of Life after Myocardial Infarction
- MET activity tables
- Minnesota Living with Heart Failure Questionnaire
- New York Heart Association Functional Classification
- Outcomes Institute Angina Type Specification
- Physical Activity Readiness Questionnaire

Physical Activity Measures
- Seattle Angina Questionnaire
- Specific Activity Scale
- The Duke Activity Status Index
- 6-minute walk assessment
- 12-minute walk assessment
- Quality of Life after Myocardial Infarction

Exercise Testing Measures
- angina and dyspnea rating scales
- bicycle test
- blood pressure response to exercise
- graded exercise test
- intermittent claudication rating scale
- rating received exertion (Borg scales)
- signs/symptoms
- submaximal exercise test
- symptom-limited maximum tests
- single-staged endurance tests
- telemetry (continuous or intermittent)
- treadmill exercise assessment protocols such as Bruce, Stanford, and Balke
- walk test
- 12-lead ECG
- vital signs

Special Tests to Which the Physical Therapist May or May Not Have Access
- arterial blood gas analysis (ABG)
- bacterial and cytological tests of sputum
- chest x-ray (CXR)
- exercise tests (ie, walk test, cycle test, and treadmill tests)
- flexible bronchoscopy

- oximetry
- Ventilation/Perfusion Scan

Pulmonary Function Tests (PFTs)
- airway resistance (Raw)
- alveolar ventilation (VA)
- body plethysmography
- diffusion capacity of lungs for carbon monoxide (DL co)
- graded exercise tests (GXT)
- expiratory reserve volume (ERV)
- flow-volume loop (F-V loop)
- forced expiratory volume in 1 second (FEV1)
- forced vital capacity (FVC)
- functional residual capacity (FRC)
- helium dilution method
- inspiratory reserve volume (IRV)
- maximum voluntary ventilation (MVV)
- maximum minute expired volume (VE)
- methacholine provocation test
- nitrogen washout test
- peak expiratory flow rate (PEFR)
- residual volume (RV)
- spirogram
- spirometry
- tidal volume (TV)
- total lung capacity (TLC)
- vital capacity (VC)

PROBLEMS

POSTOPERATIVELY
- The client is usually in pain.
- There may be diminished air entry with dyspnea and impaired respiratory function.
- The client may have an increase in retained secretions with change in baseline breath sounds and chest radiograph.
- The client may have decreased extremity movement and general mobility, especially on the side from which the saphenous vein was donated for CABG.
- There may be brachial plexus injury.
- There may be weakness on one side, or foot drop.
- There may be edema.

POSSIBLE COMPLICATIONS FROM CARDIAC SURGERY
- anemia
- arrythmias
- cardiac arrest
- cerebral infarction
- embolus (peripheral or pulmonary)
- infection
- neurological deficits
- renal failure
- respiratory failure
- unstable sternum

TREATMENT/MANAGEMENT

Note: See APTA's Guide to Physical Therapist Practice. 2nd ed. *Physical Therapy.* 2001;81.

Cardiovascular/Pulmonary Preferred Practice Patterns: C, D

PREOPERATIVELY
- Explain equipment to client.
- Instruct client in range-of-motion (ROM) exercises, posture awareness, breathing exercises, effective cough and huffing techniques, and general mobility.
- Teach support of incision.

POSTOPERATIVELY, IN GENERAL
- Be sure client is adequately medicated before starting treatment.
- Instruct in unilateral and bilateral deep breathing exercises.
- Client may need IPPB.

- Consider unilateral, posterior shaking at base of lungs, huffing, and coughing with accompanying sternal support.
- Client may need percussion after the first 2 days if sputum is viscous.
- Instruct in active exercise (ie, active ankle-pumping) to extremities one at a time.
- Instruct in ADLs for bed mobility and transfers.
- Begin gait activities—with physician approval—a few days after surgery.
- Stimulate progressive increase in mobility, progressing to exercise and stairs.
- Prescribe exercise as indicated. Monitor as per precautions.

The continuum of cardiac rehabilitation, outlined in the previous section "Coronary Artery Disease," applies to clients with coronary insufficiency that may be treated with PTCA or CABG, as well as to clients with pacemakers, heart valve repair, cardiac transplantation, heart failure, and arrhythmias.

See Certo, "Cardiovascular system," in References, for sample protocol for inpatient cardiac rehabilitation program following CABG surgery.

AFTER TRANSPLANTATION SURGERY
- Client may be isolated in room to avoid infection.
- Provide chest physical therapy postoperatively.
- During the first few days postoperatively, initiate transfers, gait training, and dangling feet at side of bed as indicated.
- Postural exercises are usually indicated, especially for weakened back musculature.
- Initiate ROM and strengthening exercises as tolerated by client.
- After sternum has healed, instruct client in activities to stretch anterior chest via scapular exercises.
- Begin aerobic conditioning program, such as walking or cycling, under close supervision.

PRECAUTIONS/CONTRAINDICATIONS

EXERCISE

The American Heart Association recommends monitoring during exercise for the following signs indicating that client is responding abnormally to exercise:

- flat or progressive decrease in systolic blood pressure
- bradycardia or excessive tachycardia
- significant arrhythmias
- angina
- undue shortness of breath
- dizziness
- confusion
- lower extremity claudication
- cyanosis
- pallor
- mottling of skin
- cold sweat
- ataxia
- glassy stare
- abnormal heart sounds

The American Heart Association also lists the following contraindications to exercise:

- acute febrile illness
- uncontrolled, active chronic systemic disease
- anatomical abnormalities
- functional abnormalities, such as third-degree heart block

INTRA-AORTIC BALLOON PUMP
- Any interference of electrodes can interrupt the synchronization of the balloon pump.
- Avoid hyperextending the hip or flexing more than 50 degrees.

PACEMAKERS
- Pacemakers are subject to possible generator failure.
- Diathermy can interfere with pacemaker function.

- Temporary pacemaker wires should be kept dry.
- The physician may have client on limited ROM after pacemaker placement.
- Monitor blood pressure and any electrocardiogram (ECG) abnormalities during exercise for exercise intolerance.
- Use of rate of perceived exertion is helpful for clients with pacemakers.
- Avoid any excessive shortness of breath during exercise.
- Avoid forced coughing.

AFTER TRANSPLANTATION SURGERY
- Client should avoid anyone with infection (ie, a cold).
- Avoid any stress on sternum.
- Consult with physician before initiating use of weights.
- Monitor exercise response using Borg's perceived levels of exertion and Stanford's dyspnea index.

Note: Be aware that a denervated heart may respond with little or no increase in heart rate to low levels of exercise.

DESIRED OUTCOME/PROGNOSIS
- The client will achieve maximum expansion of lungs and prevention of pulmonary complications.
- The client will prevent circulatory complications.
- The client will maintain maximum mobility.
- The client will increase endurance.
- The client will return to full activities of daily living.

Note: Improved normality of heart rate has been reported at 1 year post transplant.

REFERENCES

Assessment

American Physical Therapy Association. Guide to physical therapist practice. 2nd ed. *Phys Ther.* 2001;81.

Cahalin LP. Auscultation of the heart: a cursory review of basic principles and practice skills. *CardioPulmonary Phys Ther J.* 1997;8:8–12.

Dean E. Preferred practice patterns in cardiopulmonary physical therapy: a guide to physiologic measures. *CardioPulmonary Phys Ther J.* 1999;10:124–134.

Eales CJ, Stewart AV. Health and responsibility: self-efficacy, self-care and self-responsibility. *S Afr J Physiotherapy.* 2001;57:20–25.

Eason JM. Cardiopulmonary assessment. *CardioPulmonary Phys Ther J.* 1999;10:135–142.

Frownfelter D, Dean E. *Principles and Practice of Cardiopulmonary Physical Therapy.* 3rd ed. New York, NY: CV Mosby Co; 1996.

Goodman C, Snyder T. *Differential Diagnosis in Physical Therapy.* 3rd ed. Philadelphia, Pa: WB Saunders Co; 2000.

Hillegass EA, Sadowsky HS. *Essentials of Cardiopulmonary Physical Therapy.* 2nd ed. Philadelphia, Pa: WB Saunders Co; 2001.

Myers RS, ed. *Saunders Manual of Physical Therapy Practice.* Philadelphia, Pa: WB Saunders Co; 1995.

Pashkow FJ, Dafoe WA. *Clinical Cardiac Rehabilitation: A Cardiologist's Guide.* 2nd ed. Baltimore, Md: Williams and Wilkins; 1999.

Paz JC, Panik M. *Acute Care Handbook for Physical Therapists*. Burlington, Mass: Butterworth Heinemann; 1997.

Rothstein JM. Measurement in Physical Therapy. 2nd ed. New York, NY: Churchill Livingstone; 1998.

Williams MA. *AACVPR Guidelines for Cardiac Rehabilitation and Secondary Prevention Programs*. 3rd ed. Champaign, Ill: Human Kinetics; 1999

Treatment

Bellet N, Tucker B, Jenkins S. Breathing exercises. *Aust J Physiotherapy*. 1997;43:61–65.

Brooks D, et al. Accuracy and reliability of specialized physical therapists in auscultating tape recorded lung sounds. *Physiotherapy Can*. 1993;45:21–24.

Brooks D, Crowe J, Kelsey CJ, et al. A clinical practice guideline on peri-operative cardiorespiratory physical therapy. *Physiotherapy Canada*. 2001;52:9–25.

Cahalin LP. Exercise training early after cardiac transplantation: a comparative case report. *CardioPulmonary Phys Ther J*. 1996;7:3–8.

Certo C. Cardiovascular system. In: Myers RS, ed. *Saunders Manual of Physical Therapy Practice*. Philadelphia, Pa: WB Saunders Co; 1995:193–251.

Cockram J, Jenkins S, Clugston R. Cardiovascular and respiratory response to early ambulation and stair climbing following coronary artery surgery. *Physiotherapy Theory Pract*. 1999;15:1:3–15.

Crowe JM, et al. The effectiveness of incentive spirometry with physical therapy for high-risk patients after coronary artery bypass surgery. *Phys Ther*. 1997;77:260–268.

De Charmoy S, Eales CJ. The role of prophylactic chest physiotherapy after cardiac valvular surgery: Is there one? *S Afr J Physiotherapy*. 2000;56:24–28.

Deng MC, Wilhelm MJ, Scheld HH. Effects of exercise during long-term support with a left ventricular assist device. *Circ*. 1998;97:1212–1213.

El-Ansary D, Adams R, Toms L, et al. Sternal instability following coronary artery bypass. *Physiotherapy Theory Pract*. 2000;16:35–42.

El-Rahmany HK, et al. Forced-air warming decreases vasodilator requirement after coronary artery bypass surgery. *Anesth Analg*. 2000;90:286–291.

Hardy KA, Anderson BD. Noninvasive clearance of airway secretions. *Respir Care Clin North Am*. 1996;2:323–345.

Henderson K, Marshall G, Sambrook P, Keogh A. Two cases of hip pain in patients with heart transplantation. *Aust J Physiotherapy*. 1997;43:131–133.

Hill J, Johansen J, Pedersen S, LaPier TK. Site of measurement and subject position affect chest excursion measurements. *CardioPulmonary Phys Ther J*. 1997;8:12–17.

Hillegass EA, Sadowsky HS. *Essentials of Cardiopulmonary Physical Therapy*. 2nd ed. Philadelphia, Pa: WB Saunders Co; 2001.

Hodgson C, Carroll S, Denehy L. A survey of manual hyperinflation in Australian hospitals. *Aust J Physiotherapy*. 1999;45:185–193.

Irwin S, Tecklin JS, eds. *Cardiopulmonary Physical Therapy*. 3rd ed. St Louis, Mo: CV Mosby Co; 1995.

Laurikka JO, Toivio I, Tarkka MR. Effects of a novel pneumatic vest on postoperative pain and lung function after coronary artery bypass grafting. *Scand Cardiovascular J*. 1998;32:141–144.

Maiorana AJ, Briffa TG, Goodman C, Hung J. A controlled trial of circuit weight training on aerobic capacity and myocardial oxygen demand in men after coronary artery bypass surgery. *J Cardiopulmonary Rehabil*. 1997;17:239–247.

Noble BJ, Borg GAV, Jacobs I, Ceci R, et al. A category-ratio perceived exertion scale: Relationship to blood and muscle lactates and heart rate. *Med Sci Sports Exerc*. 1983;15: 523–528.

Orfanos P, Ellis E, Johnston C. Effects of deep breathing exercises and ambulation on pattern of ventilation in post-operative patients. *Aust J Physiotherapy*. 1999;45:173–182.

Pashkow P, Ades, PA, Emery CF, et al. Outcome measurement in cardiac and pulmonary rehabilitation. *J Cardiopulmonary Rehabil*. 1995;15:394–405.

Patman S, Jenkins S, Bostock S, Edlin S. Cardiovascular responses to manual hyperinflation in post-operative coronary artery surgery patients. *Physiotherapy Theory Pract*. 1998; 14:1:5–12.

Patman S, Sanderson D, Blackmore M. Physiotherapy following cardiac surgery: is it necessary during the intubation period? *Aust J Physiotherapy*. 2001;47:7–16.

Rothstein JM. *Measurement in Physical Therapy*. 2nd ed. New York, NY: Churchill Livingstone; 1998.

Sadowsky HS. Cardiac transplantation: A review. *Phys Ther*. 1996;76:498.

Schuster NB. Simultaneous implementation of two cardiopulmonary preferred practice patterns across the continuum of care. *Phys Ther Case Rep*. 1999;2:6:241–248.

Tucker D, Jenkins S, Davies K, McGann R, et al. The physiotherapy management of patients undergoing coronary artery surgery: a questionnaire survey. *Aust J Physiotherapy*. 1996;42:129–137.

Wattie J. Incentive spirometry following coronary artery bypass surgery. *Physiotherapy*. 1998;84:508–514.

Heart Failure

Also known as *(chronic) congestive heart failure*.

DESCRIPTION

Heart failure (HF) is a myocardial dysfunction characterized by ineffective pumping of the heart, leading to diminished and inadequate cardiac output. Initially, this syndrome may be symptomatic only during exertion, but in later stages the symptoms of congestion and fatigue appear even when the client is at rest.

CAUSE

Heart failure has multiple etiologies. Two causes are left ventricular failure and right ventricular failure. HF also occurs when plasma volume increases, and the lungs, abdominal organs, and peripheral tissues are filled with fluid.

ASSESSMENT

Note: See APTA's Guide to Physical Therapist Practice. 2nd ed. *Physical Therapy*. 2001;81.

Cardiovascular/Pulmonary Preferred Practice Patterns: B, D

Integumentary Preferred Practice Pattern: A

AREAS
- History
- General Appearance

- Equipment, including use of oxygen, humidification, drips, and any chest tubes
- Vital signs, including temperature, resting heart rate, resting BP, resting respiratory rate, and rhythm
- Cardiovascular, including results of exercise testing
- Musculoskeletal, including posture, head and neck musculature, and chest shape
- Skin and soft tissue, including edema and condition of hands, especially nails
- Selected cardiopulmonary tests and measures

CARDIOPULMONARY TESTS AND MEASURES
- aerobic capacity and endurance, including vital signs and palpation of pulses
- auscultation of heart and lungs and major vessels
- breathing patterns, including thoracoabdominal movements and chest wall mobility
- claudication time tests
- cough/sputum production and airway clearance
- edema assessment
- functional level (see following)
- quality of life measures (see following)
- rating of perceived exertion (RPE) scales
- response to positional changes
- skin coloration including cyanosis
- size and body fat composition
- ventilatory muscle ability

INSTRUMENTS/PROCEDURES

Functional Level
- Barthel ADL index
- PULSES profile
- Chronic Respiratory Disease Questionnaire
- Classes of Respiratory Impairment
- Functional Independence Measure
- Katz Index of ADLs
- Klein Bell Activities Scale
- New York Functional and Therapeutic Classification of Heart Disease
- Pulmonary Functional Status Scale
- Pulmonary Functional Status and Dyspnea Questionnaire
- St. George's Respiratory Questionnaire
- visual analog scale for dyspnea and/or pain

Quality of Life Measures for Cardiac Care
- Cardiac Depression Scale
- Controlled job simulation
- Ferrans and Powers Quality of Life Index–Cardiac Version
- Function Status Questionnaire
- Human Activity Profile
- MacNew Quality of Life after Myocardial Infarction
- MET activity tables
- Minnesota Living with Heart Failure Questionnaire
- New York Heart Association Functional Classification
- Outcomes Institute Angina Type Specification
- Physical Activity Readiness Questionnaire

Physical Activity Measures
- Seattle Angina Questionnaire
- Specific Activity Scale
- The Duke Activity status Index
- 6-minute walk assessment
- 12-minute walk assessment
- Quality of Life after Myocardial Infarction

Exercise Testing Measures
- angina and dyspnea rating scales
- bicycle test
- blood pressure response to exercise
- graded exercise test
- intermittent claudication rating scale
- rating received exertion (Borg scales)
- signs/symptoms
- submaximal exercise test
- symptom-limited maximum tests
- single-staged endurance tests
- telemetry (continuous or intermittent)
- treadmill exercise assessment protocols such as Bruce, Stanford, and Balke
- walk test
- 12-lead ECG
- vital signs

Special Tests to Which the Physical Therapistw May or May Not Have Access
- arterial blood gas analysis (ABG)
- bacterial and cytological tests of sputum
- chest x-ray (CXR)
- exercise tests (ie, walk test, cycle test, treadmill tests)
- flexible bronchoscopy
- oximetry
- Ventilation/Perfusion Scan

Pulmonary Function Tests (PFTs)
- airways resistance (Raw)
- alveolar ventilation (VA)
- body plethysmography
- diffusion capacity of lungs for carbon monoxide (DL co)
- graded exercise tests (GXT)
- expiratory reserve volume (ERV)
- flow-volume loop (F-V loop)
- forced expiratory volume in 1 second (FEV1)
- forced vital capacity (FVC)
- functional residual capacity (FRC)
- helium dilution method
- inspiratory reserve volume (IRV)
- Maximum voluntary ventilation (MVV)
- Maximum minute expired volume (VE)
- methacholine provocation test
- nitrogen washout test
- peak expiratory flow rate (PEFR)
- residual volume (RV)
- spirogram
- spirometry
- tidal volume (TV)
- total lung capacity (TLC)
- vital capacity (VC)
- Ventilation/Perfusion Scan

PROBLEMS

The client may display the following signs and symptoms:

- abdominal pain
- edema, especially ankle/leg swelling
- bloating
- cough (accompanied by rales) producing sputum with blood
- cyanosis
- dyspnea and/or paroxysmal nocturnal dyspnea
- fatigue with orthopnea
- increased heart and respiratory rates
- nausea
- decreased renal function or increased nocturnal urination
- acute pulmonary edema
- LV failure or RV failure
- right-side upper quadrant (RUQ) pain with RV failure

TREATMENT/MANAGEMENT

A comprehensive rehabilitation program for chronic heart failure includes an exercise prescription and a referral for nutritional counseling. Generally, the client needs a functional ability to perform activities at least 3 METs or higher and a left ventricular ejection fraction over 20 percent. Exercise sessions usually begin with a warm-up session and include activities on the low end of functional capacity (40 to 60%), exercising for 2 to 4 minutes and resting for 1 to 2 minutes, for a total of 10 to 15 minutes. This may be extended gradually to reach a total of 40 minutes for a frequency of 3 to 5 times per week. Monitoring of vital signs is critical via BP, ECG, and RPE. Exercise should be stopped if the client shows any signs of deterioration in cardiovascular status.

For an LVAD patient, consider progressive exercise with treadmill and resistance training with elastic bands and hand-held weights (light). Protocol is the same as post-surgery patients.

- Prescribe low-level exercise.
- Instruct in energy conservation techniques during acute phase.
- Progress through continuum of cardiac rehabilitation as tolerated (see section preceding, "Coronary Artery Disease").
- Consider use of oxygen.
- Consider use of chest physical therapy.

PRECAUTIONS/CONTRAINDICATIONS

The following precautions should be observed in exercise testing:

- Elderly persons with stable, uncomplicated medical histories who report fatigue with exertion should be monitored via respiratory rate, heart rate, blood pressure, and electrocardiogram, to closely assess their ability to participate in an exercise program.
- Additional monitoring can include resting and exercise pulmonary function, oxygen saturation, and analysis of expired gas at maximum exercise effort.
- Full 12-lead ECG monitoring is indicated if client has severe cardiac symptoms or specific medical complications (ie, respiratory infection).

Note: See additional precautions in previous section "Coronary Artery Disease."

DESIRED OUTCOME/PROGNOSIS

- Client will improve in cardiac output and performance.

Note: If intervention is directed to specific impairments, there may be productive central and peripheral adaptations that may lead to improved symptoms.

REFERENCES

Assessment

American Physical Therapy Association. Guide to Physical Therapist Practice. 2nd ed. *Phys Ther.* 2001;81.

Cahalin LP. Auscultation of the heart: a cursory review of basic principles and practice skills. *CardioPulmonary Phys Ther J.* 1997;8:8–12.

Dean E. Preferred practice patterns in cardiopulmonary physical therapy: a guide to physiologic measures. *CardioPulmonary Phys Ther J.* 1999;10:124–134.

Eason JM. Cardiopulmonary assessment. *CardioPulmonary Phys Ther J.* 1999;10:135–142.

Goodman C, Snyder T. *Differential Diagnosis in Physical Therapy.* 3rd ed. Philadelphia, Pa: WB Saunders Co; 2000.

Frownfelter D, Dean E. *Principles and Practice of Cardiopulmonary Physical Therapy.* 3rd ed. New York, NY: CV Mosby Co; 1996.

Hillegass EA, Sadowsky HS. *Essentials of Cardiopulmonary Physical Therapy.* 2nd ed. Philadelphia, Pa: WB Saunders Co; 2001.

Myers RS, ed. *Saunders Manual of Physical Therapy Practice.* Philadelphia, Pa: WB Saunders Co; 1995.

Pashkow FJ, Dafoe WA. *Clinical Cardiac Rehabilitation: A Cardiologist's Guide.* 2nd ed. Baltimore, Md: Williams and Wilkins; 1999.

Paz JC, Panik M. *Acute Care Handbook for Physical Therapists.* Burlington, Mass: Butterworth Heinemann; 1997.

Rothstein JM. *Measurement in Physical Therapy.* 2nd ed. New York, NY: Churchill Livingstone; 1998.

Williams MA. *AACVPR Guidelines for Cardiac Rehabilitation and Secondary Prevention Programs.* 3rd ed. Champaign, Ill: Human Kinetics; 1999.

Treatment

American Physical Therapy Association. Guide to physical therapist practice. 2nd ed. *Phys Ther.* 2001;81.

Buck LA. Physical therapy management of three patients following left ventricular assist device implantation: a case report. *Cardiopulmonary Phys Ther.* 1998;9:8–14.

Buck L, Morrone T, Goldsmith R, Humphrey R, et al. Exercise training of patients with left ventricular assist devices: A pilot study of physiologic adaptations. *J Cardiopulmonary Rehabil.* 1997;17:324.

Cahalin LP. Applying the cardiopulmonary practice patterns: heart failure. *Cardiopulmonary Phys Ther J.* 1999;10:90–97.

Cahalin LP. Physiotherapy for the disablement of heart failure. Part I. *Physiotherapy Singapore.* 2000;3:31–38.

Cahalin LP. Physiotherapy for the disablement of heart failure. Part II. *Physiotherapy Singapore.* 2000;3:20–30.

Cahalin LP, Blessey RL, Kummer D, Simard M. The safety of exercise testing performed independently by physical therapists. *J Cardiopulmonary Rehabil.* 1987;7:269–276.

Certo C. Cardiovascular system. In: Myers RS, ed. *Saunders Manual of Physical Therapy Practice.* Philadelphia, Pa: WB Saunders Co; 1995.

Deng MC, Wilhelm MJ, Scheld HH. Effects of exercise during long-term support with a left ventricular assist device. *Circulation.* 1998;97:1212–1213.

Hare DL, Ryan TM, Selig SE, Pellizzer A, et al. Resistance exercise training increases muscle strength, endurance, and blood flow in patients with chronic heart failure. *Am J Cardiol.* 1999;83:1674–1677.

Hillegass EA, Sadowsky HS. *Essentials of Cardiopulmonary Physical Therapy.* 2nd ed. Philadelphia, Pa: WB Saunders Co; 2001.

Humphrey R. Cardiopulmonary exercise response in a patient with a left ventricular assist device: inability of conventional cardiopulmonary exercise testing to identify functional capabilities. *Phys Ther Case Rep.* 1998;1:172–177.

Humphrey R. Exercise physiology in patients with left ventricular assist devices. *J Cardiopulmonary Rehabil.* 1997;17:73–75.

Humphrey R, Buck L, Cahalin L, Morrone T. Physical therapy assessment and intervention for patients with left ventricular assist devices. *CardioPulmonary Phys Ther J.* 1998; 9:3–7.

Humphrey R, Maetz C, Tolman DE, Guerraty A. Exercise training responses in a patient with a left ventricular assist device. *J Cardiopulmonary Rehabil.* 1996;16:310.

Makin F. The vented electric left ventricular assist device: an alternative to cardiac trans-plantation? *Physiotherapy*. 1996;82:295–298.

Morrone TM. The use of mechanical assistance to treat congestive heart failure: a prelimi-nary look at a clinical trial. *CardioPulmonary Phys Ther J*. 1998;9:15.

Morrone TM, Buck LA, Catanese KA, Goldsmith RL, et al. Early progressive mobilization of patients with left ventricular assist devices is safe and optimizes recovery before heart transplantation. *J Heart Lung Transplantation*. 1996;14:423–429.

Overend TJ, Anderson CM, Lucy SD, et al. The effect of incentive spirometry on postopera-tive pulmonary complications: a systematic review. *Chest*. 2001;120:971–978.

Tyni-Lenne R, Gordon A, Jansson E, Bermann G. Skeletal muscle endurance training im-proves peripheral oxidative capacity, exercise tolerance, and health-related quality of life in women with chronic congestive heart failure secondary to either ischemic car-diomyopathy or idiopathic dilated cardiomyopathy. *Am J Cardiol*. 1997;80:1025–1029.

Chapter 3

Connective Tissue Conditions

Ankylosing Spondylitis

DESCRIPTION

Ankylosing spondylitis (AS) is a type of systemic rheumatic arthritis producing symptoms of inflammation primarily in the axial skeleton, leading to complaints of recurrent back pain. Less frequently, the disease begins with pain in the peripheral joints. It is seen 3 times more often in men than women. Onset is usually between the ages of 20 and 40.

CAUSE

Any neurological symptoms are often the result of compression radiculitis or sciatica, cauda equina syndrome, or vertebral subluxation and fractures. Ankylosing spondylitis may also be associated with acute iritis, cardiovascular and pulmonary manifestations, Reiter's syndrome, ulcerative colitis, and Crohn's disease. There appears to be a genetic component to this disorder; AS is 10 to 20 times more common in relatives compared to the general population.

ASSESSMENT

Note: See APTA's Guide to Physical Therapist Practice. 2nd ed. *Physical Therapy.* 2001;81.

Musculoskeletal Preferred Practice Patterns: F, G

AREAS

- History, including height
- Integumentary
- Gait, including asymmetrical gait pattern
- Pain
- Posture
- Cardiovascular, including endurance level
- Pulmonary capacity
- Mobility, including spinal mobility and active range of motion (ROM) in peripheral joints
- Functional level, including activities of daily living (ADLs), ergonomic factors, and sleep posture
- Health status

Special Tests to Which the Physical Therapist May or May Not Have Access
- radiological tests
- sedimentation rate

INSTRUMENTS/PROCEDURES

See References for sources.

Functional Level
- Arthritis Self-Efficacy Scale
- Bath Ankylosing Spondylitis Functional Index (BASFI)
- Dougados Functional Index
- Maximum work capacity by ergometry
- Functional Index (FI)
- Spondylitis Functional Index Instrument (SFI)

Health Status
- Health Assessment Questionnaire for the Spondylarthropathies (HAQ-S)
- Sickness Impact Profile (SIP)

Mobility
- cervical rotation
- chin-to-chest distance
- finger-to-floor distance
- occiput-to-wall distance
- FABER test
- Schober test
- thoracolumbar flexibility

Pain
- visual analog scale

Pulmonary Capacity
- chest expansion (CE)
- vital capacity (VC)

PROBLEMS
- The client often has back pain, especially in the lumbar region.
- There may be tenderness in the sacroiliac region.
- The client often reports stiffness in the morning and after inactivity.
- The spine becomes progressively rigid.
- The client often has postural changes such as forward head, increase in thoracic kyphosis, and loss of lumbar curve.
- There may be a decrease in chest expansion and a sunken chest appearance.
- The client may have flexion contractures at shoulders and hips.
- The client may complain of pain due to achilles tendinitis and plantar fasciitis.

TREATMENT/MANAGEMENT
- Consider use of modalities (eg, heat and hydrotherapy) for pain relief.
- Stretch areas of tightness, especially at hips and shoulders.
- Prescribe land-based or aquatic exercises. Daily exercise should be encouraged. Include the following:
  1. breathing exercises and exercises for chest expansion
  2. spinal rotation, extension, and lateral movements
  3. hip and shoulder exercises
  4. postural exercises, especially extensor muscles
- Instruct in home program to be performed twice a day.
- Consider ergonomic applications to ADLs such as driving, working, and sleeping.
- Provide education about the disorder, refer to support groups, and provide long-term support.
- Reassess at least 1 month post treatment and again yearly.

PRECAUTIONS/CONTRAINDICATIONS
- Diagnosis should be confirmed by x-ray.

DESIRED OUTCOME/PROGNOSIS
- The client will improve posture and prevent deformity.
- The client will increase chest expansion and vital capacity.
- The client will maintain or improve mobility, fitness, functioning, and overall health.

Notes: Outcomes research by Ammer has demonstrated that exercise therapy has beneficial outcomes in cervical mobility, overall health assessment, and patient's perception of disability. In general, given proper treatment, a client with ankylosing spondylitis can expect to live a productive life.

REFERENCES

Assessment

American Physical Therapy Association. Guide to physical therapist practice. 2nd ed. *Phys Ther.* 2001;81.

Cronstedt H, Waldner A, Stenstorim CH. The Swedish version of the Bath ankylosing spondylitis functional index: Reliability and validity. *Scand J Rheumatol Supplement.* 1999;111:1–9.

Heikkila S, Viitanen JV, Kautiainen H, et al. Sensitivity to change of mobility tests; effect of short term intensive physiotherapy and exercise on spinal, hip, and shoulder measurements in spondyloarthropathy. *J Rheumatol.* 2000;27:1251–1256.

Hidding A, van der Linden S, Boers M, et al. Is group physical therapy superior to individualized therapy in ankylosing spondylitis? *Arthritis Care Res.* 1993;6:3:117–125.

Kraag G, Stokes B, Groh J, Helewa A, Goldsmith C. The effects of comprehensive home physiotherapy and supervision of patients with ankylosing spondylitis: a randomized controlled trial. *J Rheumatol.* 1990;17:228–233.

Langely GB, Sheppeard H. The visual analogue scale: its use in pain measurement. *Rheumatol Int.* 1985;5:145–148.

Lomi C, Nordholm LA. Validation of a Swedish version of the Arthritis Self-Efficacy Scale. *Scand J Rheumatol.* 1992;21:231–237.

Lubrano E, Butterworth M, Hesselden A, et al. *Clin Rehabil.* 1998;12:216–220.

Moncur C, Cannon GW, Shaw M, et al. Inter-observer reliability of the Spondylitis Functional Index Instrument for assessing spondylarthropathies. *Arthritis Care Res.* 1996;9:182–188.

Ruof J, Stucki G. Comparison of the Dougados Functional Index and the Bath ankylosing spondylitis Functional Index: A literature review. *J Rheumatol.* 1999;26:955–960.

Van der Heijde D, Calin A, Dougados M, et al. Selection of instruments in the core set for DC-ART, SMARD, physical therapy, and clinical record keeping in ankylosing spondylitis. *J Rheumatol.* 1999;26:951–954.

Vandervoort AA, Chesworth BM, Cunningham DA, et al. An outcome measure to quantify passive stiffness of the ankle. *Can J Public Health.* 1992;83(suppl 2):S19–S23.

Viitanen JV, Suni J, Kautiainen H, et al. Effect of physiotherapy on spinal mobility in ankylosing spondylitis. *Scand J Rheumatol.* 1992;21:38–41.

Treatment

Ammer K. Physiotherapy in seronegative spondylarthropathies—a systematic review. *Eur J Phys Med Rehabil.* 1997;7:114–119.

Bakker C, Hidding A, van der Linden S, et al. Cost effectiveness of group physical therapy compared to individualized therapy for ankylosing spondylitis: a randomized controlled trial. *J Rheumatol.* 1994;21:264–268.

Bakker C, Rutten-van Molken M, Hidding A, et al. Patient utilities in ankylosing spondylitis and the association with other outcome measures. *J Rheumatol.* 1994;21:1298–1304.

Bakker C, van der Linden S, van Santen-Hoeufft M, et al. Problem elicitation to assess patient priorities in ankylosing spondylitis and fibromyalgia. *J Rheumatol.* 1995;22:1304–1310.

Band DA, Jones SD, Kennedy LG, et al. Which patients with ankylosing spondylitis derive most benefit from an inpatient management program? *J Rheumatol.* 1997;24:2381–2384.

Carbon RJ, Macey MG, McCarthy DA, et al. The effect of 30 minute cycle ergometry on ankylosing spondylitis. *Br J Rheumatol.* 1996;35:167–177.

Clarke AK. Effectiveness of rehabilitation in arthritis. *Clin Rehabil.* (suppl) 1999;13:51–62.

Dagfinrud H, Hagen K. Physiotherapy interventions for Ankylosing Spondylitis (Cochrane Review). *Cochrane Database Systematic Rev.* 2001;4:CD002822.

David C, Lloyd J. *Rheumatol Physiotherapy*. London, England: CV Mosby Co;1999.

Dougados M, et al. Spondylarthropathy treatment: progress in medical treatment, physical therapy, and rehabilitation. *Baillieres Clin Rheumatol*. 1998;12:717–736.

Goodman C, Snyder TE. *Differential Diagnosis in Physical Therapy*. 2nd ed. Philadelphia, Pa: WB Saunders Co; 2000.

Grabois M, Garrison SJ, Hart KA, Lehmkuhl LD. *Physical Medicine and Rehabilitation: The Complete Approach*. Malden, Mass: Blackwell Science; 2000.

Heikkila S, Viitanen JV, Kautiainen H, et al. Does improved spinal mobility correlate with functional changes in spondyloarthropathy after short term physical therapy. *J Rheumatol*. 2000;27:2942–2944.

Helliwell PS, Abbott CA, Chamberlain MA. A randomized trial of three different physiotherapy regimes in ankylosing spondylitis. *Physiotherapy*. 1996;82:85–90.

Hidding A, van der Linden S. Factors related to change in global health after group physical therapy in ankylosing spondylitis. *Clin Rheumatol*. 1995;14:347–351.

Hidding A, van der Linden S, deWitts L. Therapeutic effects of individual physical therapy in ankylosing spondylitis related to duration of disease. *Clin Rheumatol*. 1993;12:334–340.

Hidding A, van der Linden S, Gielen X, et al. Continuation of group physical therapy is necessary in ankylosing spondylitis: results of a randomized controlled trial. *Arthritis Care Res*. 1994;7:90–96.

Russell P, Unsworth A, Haslock I. The effect of exercise on ankylosing spondylitis: a preliminary study. *Br J Rheumatol*. 1993;32:498–506.

Ryall NH, Hellowell PS. A critical review of ankylosing spondylitis. *Crit Rev Phys Rehabil Med*. 1998;10:265–301.

Solchaga MR, Castellanos CO, Soro JMG. Influence of physical therapy exercises on the evolution of ankylosing spondylitis. *Rehabil*. 1998;32:316–323.

Stucki G, von-Felten A, Speich R, Michel BA. Ankylosing spondylitis and sarcoidosis—coincidence or association? Case report and review of the literature. *Clin Rheumatol*. 1992;11:436–439.

Van der Heijde D, Bellamy N, Calin A, et al. Preliminary core sets for endpoints in ankylosing spondylitits. Assessments in Ankylosing Spondylitis Working Group. *J Rheumatol*. 1997;24:225–2229.

Viitanen JV, Suni J, Kautiainen H, Liimatainen M, Takala H. Effect of physiotherapy on spinal mobility in ankylosing spondylitis. *Scand J Rheumatol*. 1992;21:38–41.

Fibromyalgia

Also known as *fibrositis, fibromyositis*.

DESCRIPTION

Fibromyalgia is a nonarticular rheumatic condition. With fibromyalgia, there is pain in fibrous tissues such as muscles, ligaments, and tendons. It is characterized by extreme tenderness in a minimum of 11 of 18 specific tender points (see Table 3.1 for classification). The disorder occurs more frequently in females; reportedly 5 to 10 times more frequently. Although there are similarities, myofascial pain syndrome (MPS) is considered a separate disorder from fibromyalgia (see section "Myofascial Pain Syndrome" following). Some clients may have symptoms of both disorders.

CAUSE

The cause of fibromyalgia is still under investigation but may be associated with a viral infection. The etiology has been associated with sleep disturbance, specifically a decrease of stage IV non-REM sleep. Some clients have a psychological component that aggravates the disorder. The disorder has also been linked with irritable bowel syndrome (IBS). In general, clients with fibromyalgia have an increased sensitivity to pain. Other pain triggers include stress, trauma, cold, and systemic disorders.

ASSESSMENT

Note: See APTA's Guide to Physical Therapist Practice. 2nd ed. *Physical Therapy.* 2001;81.

There is no specific preferred practice pattern listed. See reference index as indicated by symptoms.

AREAS
- History, including detailed list of symptoms and results of other specialists' diagnostic tests
- Pain, including nature of pain and influence of motion and position
- Posture
- Joint integrity and structural deviations
- Mobility, including passive and active range of motion (ROM)
- Skin and soft tissue, including trigger points

INSTRUMENTS/PROCEDURES

See References for sources.

Functional Capacity
- Arthritis Impact Measurement Scale (AIMS)
- Fibromyalgia Impact Questionnaire (FIQ)
- Short Form 36 Health Survey (SF-36)

Pain
- body chart
- Multidimensional Pain Inventory – Swedish (MPI-S)
- visual analog scale

TABLE 3.1
American College of Rheumatology 1990 Criteria for the Classification of Fibromyalgia

1. History of widespread pain present for a minimum of 3 months.
2. Pain in at least 11 of 18 total tender point sites—9 bilateral points—on digital palpation
· occiput
· low cervical
· trapezius
· supraspinus
· second rib
· lateral epicondyle
· gluteal area
· greater trochanter
· knee

Source: Reprinted with permission from Wolfe F, et al. The American College of Rheumatology 1990 Criteria for the Classification of Fibromyalgia. *Arthritis and Rheumatology.* JB Lippincott Co; 1990:160–172.

Skin and Soft Tissue
- palpation of trigger points

Special Tests to Which the Physical Therapist May or May Not Have Access
- blood tests
- bone scan
- CT scan
- electrodiagnostic tests
- electromyography (EMG); integrated EMG
- phosphorus magnetic resonance imaging (MRI)
- radiographs

Quality of Life
- Quality of Life Questionnaire (QOLS)

PROBLEMS

The client is tender upon palpation of muscles, with tenderness in at least 11 of 18 tender points (see criteria for classification in Description section previous).

- The client has chronic pain in muscles.
- The pain is often diffuse and often described as stiffness or achiness.
- The client is often fatigued.

- The client may report disturbed sleep.
- The client may report frequent headaches.
- Women may report painful menstrual periods.

TREATMENT/MANAGEMENT

Note: Symptoms usually respond to modalities, moderate activity, and stretching exercise.
- Modalities used to decrease symptoms may include:
  1. heat packs before massage
  2. massage: concentrate on relaxing strokes such as stroking and kneading as client tolerates
  3. ice massage
  4. quick, cold stimulant such as vapocoolant spray or ice combined with stretching for trigger points
  5. electrical stimulation
  6. ultrasound
- Provide a carefully controlled, gradual program of conditioning, cardiovascular activity, flexibility, and posture reeducation. Consider use of PNF techniques, muscle energy techniques, and manual therapies that employ the use of gentle movement. Later phases of treatment may include closed chain eccentric exercise, and resistance work with tubing.
- Instruct in relaxation techniques that may include biofeedback, progressive relaxation, and autogenic deep breathing.
- Teach pacing of activities to alternate work with frequent rest periods.
- Client education is a key component of treatment.
- Restful sleep is a critical component of successful treatment.

PRECAUTIONS/CONTRAINDICATIONS
- Too vigorous an exercise program may worsen symptoms.
- Massage should not increase pain. Client will probably not be able to tolerate deep pressure.
- Contraindications to ice massage include a client who has an aversion or adverse reaction to cold or poor circulation.

- Contraindication to massage can include inflammation due to bacterial infection, signs of myositis ossificans, hematoma, traumatic arthritis, severe rheumatoid arthritis, massage of bursa, nerve entrapment, phlebitis, cellulitis, metastatic cancer, or infectious skin disease.

DESIRED OUTCOME/PROGNOSIS
- The client will experience a decrease in symptoms.
- The client will experience an increase in functional activity.

Notes: Fibromyalgia has a tendency to become chronic. Effective management depends on a client who engages in active self-care with home exercise activities.

REFERENCES

Assessments

American Physical Therapy Association. Guide to physical therapist practice. 2nd ed. *Phys Ther.* 2001;81.

Caldron PH. Screening for rheumatic disease. In: Boissonnault WG, ed. *Examination in Physical Therapy Practice.* 2nd ed. Philadelphia, Pa: Churchill Livingstone; 1995:237–253.

Mannerkorpi K, Svantesson U, Carlsson J, et al. Tests of functional limitations in fibromyalgia syndrome: a reliability study. *Arthritis Care Res.* 1999;12:193–1999.

Marques AP, Rhoden L, de Oliveira Siqueira J, et al. Pain evaluation of patients with fibromyalgia, osteoarthritis, and low back pain. *Rev Hosp Clin Fac Med Sao Paulo.* 2001;56:5–10.

Miller B. Manual therapy treatment of myofascial pain and dysfunction. In: Rachlin ES, ed. *Myofascial Pain and Fibromyalgia.* St Louis, Mo: CV Mosby Co; 1993:455–472.

Roy SH. Combined use of surface electromyography and 31P-NMR spectroscopy for the study of muscle disorders. *Phys Ther.* 1993;73:892–901.

Russell IJ. The reliability of algometry in the assessment of patients with fibromyalgia syndrome. *J Musculoskeletal Pain.* 1998;6:33–45.

Stokes MJ, Colter C, Klestov A, Cooper RG. Normal paraspinal muscle electromyographic fatigue characteristics in patients with primary fibromyalgia. *Br J Rheumatol.* 1993; 32:711–716.

Treatment

Ali HM. Fibromyalgia: case report. *Physiotherapy.* 2001;87:140–145.

Ambrogia N, Cuttiford J, Lineker S. A comparison of three types of neck support in fibromyalgia patients. *Arthritis Care Res.* 1998;11:405–410.

Borenstein D. Prevalence and treatment outcome of primary and secondary fibromyalgia in patients with spinal pain. *Spine.* 1995;20:796.

Buckelew SP, Murray SE, Hewett JE, et al. Self-efficacy, pain, and physical activity among FM subjects. *Arthritis Care Res.* 1995;8:43–50.

Burckhardt CS, Clark SR, Campbell SM, et al. Multidisciplinary treatment of fibromyalgia. *Scand J Rheumatol.* 1992;(S94):51.

Burckhardt CS, Mannerkorpi K, Hendenberg L, et al. A randomized controlled clinical trial of education and physical training for women with fibromyalgia. *J Rheumatol.* 1994; 21:714–720.

Cantu RI, Grodin AJ. *Myofascial Manipulation: Theory and Clinical Application*. 2nd ed. Gaithersburg, Md: Aspen Publishers; 2001.

Clark SR. Prescribing exercise for fibromyalgia patients. *Arthritis Care Res*. 1994;7:221–225.

Essenberg VJ Jr, Tollan M. Etiology and treatment of fibromyalgia syndrome. *Orthop Phys Ther Clin North Am*. 1995;4:443–457.

Fischer AA. Algometry in diagnosis of musculoskeletal pain and evaluation of treatment outcome: an update. *J Musculoskeletal Pain*. 1998;6:5–32.

Fisher AA, ed. *Myofascial Pain: Update in Diagnosis and Treatment*. Philadelphia, Pa: WB Saunders Co; 1997.

Gerwin RD. Myofascial pain and fibromyalgia: diagnosis and treatment. *J Back Musculoskeletal Rehabil*. 1998;11:175–181.

Grabois M, Garrison SJ, Hart KA, Lehmkuhl LD. *Physical Medicine and Rehabilitation: The Complete Approach*. Malden, Mass: Blackwell Science; 2000.

Hanten WP, Olson SL, Butts NL, et al. Effectiveness of home program of ischemic pressure followed by sustained stretch for treatment of myofascial trigger points. *Phys Ther*. 2000;80:997–1003.

Henriksson C, Gundmark I, Bengtsson A, Ek AC. Living with fibromyalgia. *Clin J Pain*. 1992;8:138–144.

Henriksson CM. Living with continuous muscular pain—patient perspectives. *Scand J Caring Sci*. 1995;9:67–76.

Isomeri R, Mikkelsson M, Latikka P. Effects of amitriptyline and cardiovascular fitness training on the pain of fibromyalgia patients. *Scand J Rheumatol*. 1992;(S94):47.

Keel PJ, Bodoky C, et al. Comparison of integrated group therapy and group relaxation training for fibromyalgia. *Clin J Pain*. 1998;14:232–238.

Kruger LR, van der Linden WJ, Cleaton-Jones PE. Transcutaneous electrical nerve stimulation in the treatment of myofascial pain dysfunction. *S Afr J Surg*. 1998;36:35–38.

Krsnich-Shriwise S, Hensley J, Thomson K, et al. Fibromyalgia syndrome. *PT – Magazine Phys Ther*. 1997;56–67.

Leslie M. Fibromyalgia syndrome: a comprehensive approach to identification and management. *Clin Excellence Nurse Pract: Int J NPACE*. 1999;3:165–171.

Lindh M, Johansson G, Hedberg M, et al. Studies on maximal voluntary contraction in patients with fibromyalgia. *Arch Phys Med Rehabil*. 1994;75:1217–1222.

Mannerkorpi K, Burchhardt CS, Bjelle A. Physical performance characteristics of women with FM. *Arthritis Care Res*. 1994;7:123–129.

Mannerkorpi K, Krorksmark T, Ekdahl C. How patients with fibromyalgia experience their symptoms in everyday life. *Physiotherapy Res Int*. 1999;4:110–122.

Martin L, Nutting A, Macintosh BR, et al. An exercise program in the treatment of fibromyalgia. *J Rheumatol*. 1996;23:1050–1053.

Mengshoel AM. Fibromyalgia and responses to exercise. *J Manual Manipulative Ther*. 1998; 6:144–150.

Mengshoel AM, Komnaes HB, Forre O. The effect of 20 weeks of physical fitness training in female patients with fibromyalgia. *Clin Exp Rheumatol*. 1992;10:345–349.

Mengshoel AM, Vollestadt NK, Forre O. Pain and fatigue induced by exercise in fibromyalgia patients and sedentary healthy subjects. *Clin Exp Rheumatol*. 1995;13:477–482.

Nichols DS, Gless TM. Effects of aerobic exercise on pain perception, affect and level of disability in individuals with FM. *Phys Ther*. 1994;74:327–332.

Norregaard J, Lykkegaard JJ, et al. Exercise training in treatment of fibromyalgia. *J Musculoskeletal Pain*. 1997;5(1):71–79.

Offenbacher M, Stucki G. Physical therapy in the treatment of fibromyalgia. *Scand J Rheumatol.* 2000;113:78–85.

Penner B. *Managing Fibromyalgia: A Six-Week Course on Self-Care.* Helena, Mont: Capital Physical Therapy, 1997.

Rachlin I. Therapeutic massage in the treatment of myofascial pain syndromes and fibromyalgia. In: Rachlin ES, ed. *Myofascial Pain and Fibromyalgia.* St. Louis, Mo: CV Mosby Co; 1993:455–472.

Ramsay C, Moreland J, Ho M, et al. An observer-blinded comparison of supervised and unsupervised aerobic exercise regimens in fibromyalgia. *Rheumatol.* 2000;39:501–505.

Rosen NB. Physical medicine and rehabilitation approaches to the management of myofascial pain and fibromyalgia syndromes. *Baillieres Clin Rheumatol.* 1994;8:881–916.

Schutz L. Fibromyalgia and myofascial pain syndrome. In: Buschbacher RM, ed. *Musculoskeletal Disorders: A Practical Guide for Diagnosis and Rehabilitation.* Boston, Mass: Andover Medical Publishers; 1994:239–244.

Simms RW. Controlled trials of therapy in FMS. *Baillieres Clin Rheumatol.* 1994;8:917–934.

Simons DG, Travell JG, et al. *Myofascial Pain and Dysfunction: The Trigger Point Manual.* 2nd ed. Baltimore, Md: Williams and Wilkins; 1999.

Simons LS, Simons DG. Chronic myofascial pain syndrome. In: Tollison CD, ed. *Handbook of Chronic Pain Management.* Baltimore, Md: Williams and Wilkins; 1994:509–529.

Sims J, Adams N. Physical and other non-pharmacological interventions for fibromyalgia. *Baillieres Best Pract Res Clin Rheumatol.* 1999;13:507–23.

Sprott H, Muller W. Functional symptoms in fibromyalgia: monitored by an electronic diary. *Clin Bull Myofascial Ther.* 1998;3:61–67.

Turk DC, Okifuji A. Assessment of patients' reporting of pain: an integrated perspective. *Lancet.* 1999;353:1784–1788.

Turk DC, Okifuji A, Starz TW, et al. Effects of type of symptom onset on psychological distress and disability in fibromyalgia syndrome patients. *Pain.* 1996;68:423–430.

Vecchiet L, Pizzigallo E, et al. Differentiation of sensitivity in different tissues and its clinical significance. *J Musculoskeletal Pain.* 1998;6:33–45.

Worrell LM, Krahn LE, Sletten CD. Treating fibromyalgia with a brief interdisciplinary program: initial outcomes and predictors of response. *Mayo Clin Proc.* 2001;76:384–390.

Zohn DA, Clauw DJ. A comparison of skin rolling and tender points as a diagnostic test for fibromyalgia. *J Musculoskeletal Pain.* 1999;7:127–136.

Myofascial Pain Syndrome

DESCRIPTION

Myofascial pain syndrome (MPS) is muscular pain combined with trigger points and occasionally accompanied by autonomic symptoms. MPS is equally common in men and women.

CAUSE

MPS is thought to be caused by acute or chronic physical stress of muscle due to trauma, overstretching, or overwork fatigue. Mechanical factors such as poor posture or leg-length difference can contribute to or perpetuate the stress. Symptoms may be exacerbated by anxiety, infection, allergy, arthritis, or other underlying disorders.

ASSESSMENT

Note: See APTA's Guide to Physical Therapist Practice. 2nd ed. *Physical Therapy.* 2001;81.

There is no specific preferred practice pattern listed. See reference index as indicated by symptoms.

AREAS
- History, including a detailed list of symptoms
- Pain, including nature of pain and influence of motion and position
- Posture
- Joint integrity and structural deviations
- Mobility, including passive and active range of motion (ROM)
- Skin and soft tissue, including trigger points

INSTRUMENTS/PROCEDURES

See References for sources.

Joint Integrity and Structural Deviations
- leg-length discrepancy

Pain
- body chart
- visual analog scale

Skin
- trigger point palpation

Special Tests to Which the Physical Therapist May or May Not Have Access
- blood tests
- bone scan
- electrodiagnostic tests
- magnetic resonance imaging (MRI)
- radiographs

PROBLEMS
- The client often has complaints of regional muscle pain, but pain may also be localized.
- Muscles are tender during palpation.
- There are often one or more trigger points characterized by a twitch response (ie, involuntary contraction) and radiation of pain to referred zone.
- Trigger points may lead to headache.
- The trigger points may refer pain to arm or leg. Radiculopathy should be ruled out.

TREATMENT/MANAGEMENT
- Educate client about nature of disorder, posture, and body mechanics for activities of daily living (ADLs). Avoid muscle overwork.
- Instruct client in relaxation and stress management techniques.
- Therapeutic exercise may include traditional stretching, strengthening, conditioning exercise, and movement therapy. Alternate voluntary contraction with passive stretch as well as contract-relax techniques. Emphasis is on optimal muscle control and active involvement of client.
- Consider use of manual therapy, including soft tissue mobilization, neurosensorimotor reeducation, and joint mobilization. Soft tissue techniques vary depending on desired effect; they may be sustained or varied in rate and described as compressing or stripping.

- Assistive devices, such as tape, can be used for proper alignment of tissues. Rubber balls, foam, or cardboard rollers or tools may apply therapeutic pressure on tissues.
- Consult with physician on use of injections for trigger points.
- Address mechanical factors that may perpetuate stress, such as structural anatomical variations, postural abnormalities, and vocational factors.
- Massage may be helpful, including techniques of compression (especially useful for trigger points), friction, kneading, stroking, stripping, and digital pressure; also ice massage.
- Possible adjuncts to massage:
  1. vapocoolant sprays or ice combined with stretching
  2. accupressure
  3. ultrasound
  4. transcutaneous electrical nerve stimulation (TENS)
  5. electrical stimulation-generally recommended for electrodes to parallel the shape of tissue being treated
  6. cold laser

PRECAUTIONS/CONTRAINDICATIONS
- Contraindications to soft tissue manual therapies listed include acute infection, inflammation, neoplasm, fever, change in neurological status, instability, and recent injury to tissue. Contraindications are relative to the extent of condition and manner in which therapy is conducted.
- Soreness after treatment can be normal, but if soreness persists longer than 24 hours, it may indicate that treatment was too vigorous.

Note: It is important to address any underlying medical condition contributing to pain.

DESIRED OUTCOME/PROGNOSIS
- The client will have decreased pain.
- The client will regain normal function of myofascial tissue with diminished hardened areas of the muscle.
- The client will have an inhibition of undesired muscle activity.
- The client will have an increased level of function.
- There will be improved efficiency of desired movement.

REFERENCES

Assessment

PAIN

Miller B. Manual therapy treatment of myofascial pain and dysfunction. In: Rachlin ES, ed. *Myofascial Pain and Fibromyalgia.* [Body chart and visual analogue scale] St Louis, Mo: CV Mosby Co; 1993:455–472.

Treatment

American Physical Therapy Association. Guide to physical therapist practice. 2nd ed. *Phys Ther.* 2001;81.

Cantu RI, Grodin AJ. *Myofascial Manipulation: Theory and Clinical Application.* 2nd ed. Gaithersburg, Md: Aspen Publishers; 2001.

Fisher AA, ed. *Myofascial Pain: Update in Diagnosis and Treatment*. Philadelphia, Pa: WB Saunders Co; 1997.

Grabois M, Garrison SJ, Hart KA, Lehmkuhl LD. *Physical Medicine and Rehabilitation: The Complete Approach*. Malden, Mass: Blackwell Science; 2000.

Kahn J. Electrical modalities in the treatment of myofascial conditions. In: Rachlin ES, ed. *Myofascial Pain and Fibromyalgia*. St Louis, Mo: CV Mosby Co; 1993:473–485.

Manheim CJ, Lavett DK. *The Myofascial Release Manual*. 2nd ed. Thorofare, NJ: Slack; 1994.

Miller B. Manual therapy treatment of myofascial pain and dysfunction. In: Rachlin ES, ed. *Myofascial Pain and Fibromyalgia*. St Louis, Mo: CV Mosby Co; 1993:415–454.

Schutz L. Fibromyalgia and myofascial pain syndrome. In: Buschbacher RM, ed. *Musculoskeletal Disorders: A Practical Guide for Diagnosis and Rehabilitation*. Boston, Mass: Andover Medical Publishers; 1994:239–244.

Simons DG, Travell JG, et al. *Myofascial Pain and Dysfunction: The Trigger Point Manual*. 2nd ed. Baltimore, Md: Williams and Wilkins; 1999.

Simons LS, Simons DG. Chronic myofascial pain syndrome. In: Tollison CD, ed. *Handbook of Chronic Pain Management*. Baltimore, Md: Williams and Wilkins; 1994:509–529.

Osteoarthritis

Also known as *degenerative joint disease*.

DESCRIPTION

Osteoarthritis (OA) is the most frequent type of articular disorder. OA leads to the breakdown of hyaline cartilage followed by involvement of the subchondral bone and hypertrophy of surrounding tissues leading to the production of osteophytes. Joints commonly affected include the cervical and lumbar spine, peripheral joints, and knee and hip joints.

CAUSE

The etiology of osteoarthritis is unknown, but factors influencing the course of the disease include aging, congenital joint abnormalities, genetic defects, and acute or chronic trauma to the joint. OA may also appear secondary to other joint diseases such as Legg-Calve-Perthes disease or slipped femoral capital epiphysis; diseases of the hyaline cartilage; or neuropathic, endocrine, metabolic, and infectious diseases.

ASSESSMENT

Note: See APTA's Guide to Physical Therapist Practice. 2nd ed. *Physical Therapy*. 2001;81.

Cardiopulmonary Preferred Practice Pattern: B

Musculoskeletal Preferred Practice Patterns: A, B, C, D, F, G, H, I, J

AREAS
- History, including psychosocial evaluation as indicated
- Posture
- Pain
- Gait
- Joint integrity and structural deviations
- Mobility, including range of motion (ROM), hypermobility, and hypomobility
- Strength

- Neurological: position sense (if damage suggested by weakness or paresthesia)
- Skin and soft tissue: inflammation, temperature, edema
- Functional level, including activities of daily living (ADLs) and activity level
- Equipment, including shoes and any assistive devices

INSTRUMENTS/PROCEDURES

See References for sources.

Functional Level
- Arthritis Self-Efficacy Scale
- Functional Status Index
- Functional Independence Measure (FIM)
- Impact of Rheumatic Diseases on General Health and Lifestyle (IRGL)
- Katz Index of ADLs
- Knee Injury and Osteoarthritis Outcome Score (KOOS)
- Hospital for Special Surgery Knee Rating Scale
- Self-Efficacy Scale
- Outcomes Assessment Measures
- Western Ontario and McMaster Universities Osteoarthritis Index (WOMAC)

Gait
- walking speed
- oxygen cost of walking

Health Status
- Sickness Impact Profile

Joint Integrity and Structural Deviations
- joint circumference as indicated
- leg-length discrepancy as indicated
- palpation for crepitus and laxity
- Patrick's test
- test for hip dislocation

Mobility
- relaxed oscillation test
- Timed Up and Go Test

Skin
- palpation for temperature, tenderness

Special Tests to Which the Physical Therapist May or May Not Have Access
- electromyography (EMG)
- joint surface separation
- knee kinematics
- x-rays

Strength
- angular velocity testing
- dynamometer testing
- muscle endurance testing
- hand-held dynamometry
- isometric and isokinetic torque
- manual muscle testing

PROBLEMS

EARLY STAGES
- The client often reports pain with weight bearing, especially later in the day or with overexertion.
- The client often has mild limitation of ROM, especially into internal rotation, abduction, and extension at the hip.

LATER STAGES

- The client often reports aching, even during sleep.
- There is often morning stiffness.
- There are often muscle spasms.
- There may be joint swelling, which is usually moderate.
- There is often joint crepitus, sometimes audible.
- Hip joint deformity often follows a pattern of adduction, flexion, and lateral rotation.
- Pain at hip joint varies depending upon stage of disease.
- Knee joint deformity often follows a pattern of varus or valgus deformity with flexion.
- The client may have a leg-length discrepancy.
- The client often has a progressive loss of ROM.
- The client may have an antalgic gait pattern.
- The client may need assistive devices.
- The client may report a decrease in balance.
- The client may have decreased independence with ADLs such as dressing or stairs.

TREATMENT/MANAGEMENT

GENERAL

- Select modalities for pain such as heat or ice, ultrasound, interferential, and/or shortwave diathermy.
- Unload or modify excessive force patterns on joint.
- Provide careful prescription of exercise based on degree of joint damage.
- Encourage loss of any excessive weight.

TREATMENT OF THE HIP

Early Stages
- Instruct in active ROM exercises.
- Instruct in postural exercises as indicated.
- Provide joint mobilization for ROM and decrease in pain.
- Consider modalities for pain such as ultrasound and moist heat.
- Instruct in strengthening exercises, especially for hip abductors. Consider use of isometric and isotonic exercise, graduated resistive exercise, proprioceptive neuromuscular facilitation (PNF) patterns, pendular exercise, and aquatic exercise.
- Consider need for weight reduction to decrease stress on joints.

Later Stages
- Consider more vigorous mobilization such as grade 2 level.
- Provide gait training as indicated.
- Prescribe assistive device for weight-bearing activities and adaptive equipment such as raised toilet seat. Prescribe orthotics as indicated. Assess footwear.
- People with hip disease should carry loads bilaterally to reduce force on hip joint.
- The treatment modalities considered most effective for OA of hip include hydrotherapy, home exercises, and individual exercises.

POST HIP REPLACEMENT

- Begin rehabilitation with isometric exercises like quadriceps setting and gluteal isometrics. Add ankle-pumping activity and diaphragmatic breathing as early as in recovery room.
- Initiate bed transfers at day 1 postoperatively.
- Perform gait training as indicated by weight-bearing status and client's response to surgery (e.g. partial weight bearing with noncemented hips and weight bearing as tolerated with cemented hips). Generally clients begin gait activities by using a walker or crutches to protect joint and then progress to cane.

- Instruct in transfers.
- Perform active ROM exercises for lower extremities within acceptable range.

POST TOTAL SHOULDER REPLACEMENT (TSR)
- Protect the surgical repair. Abduction brace may be indicated after rotator cuff repair.
- Prescribe individualized treatment program based on soft tissue constraints of client.
- Begin continuous passive motion if earlier mobilization is desired.
- After adequate healing, pendulum exercise may begin.
- Progress to pulley exercises and passive stretching.
- Mobilization and isometrics may also be included with caution.

PRECAUTIONS/CONTRAINDICATIONS
- Heat from shortwave diathermy may aggravate condition.
- Use traction with caution.
- Consult with surgical team on recommended precautions after joint replacement surgery.
- After total hip replacement surgery, the client should avoid hip flexion (less than 90 degrees), adduction past midline, and internal rotation.
- After constrained total shoulder replacement, motion—particularly external rotation—should not be forced beyond the limits discovered at surgery.

Note: Vigorous or heavy use of shoulder could cause the prosthesis to loosen.

DESIRED OUTCOME/PROGNOSIS
- The client will experience pain relief.
- The client will gain increased mobility.
- The client will experience increased strength.
- The client will increase in functional independence.
- The client will be educated about OA.

Notes: Within 3 months after total hip arthroplasty, the client should be independent in activities of daily living.

Post total shoulder replacement, muscle-strengthening exercise must be continued for the rest of the patient's life. Total Shoulder Replacement (TSR) may relieve pain and increase function, but it may not return the client to normal strength or ROM.

Repaired rotator cuff may need 6 to 12 weeks to heal before resuming active motion.

REFERENCES

Assessment

American Physical Therapy Association. Guide to physical therapist practice. 2nd ed. *Phys Ther.* 2001;81.

Angst F, Aeschlimann A, Steiner W, et al. Responsiveness of the WOMAC osteoarthritis index as compared with the SF-36 inpatients with osteoarthritis of the legs undergoing a comprehensive rehabilitation intervention. *Ann Rheum Dis.* 2001;60:834–840.

Burckardt CS, Moncur C, Minor MA. Exercise tests as outcome measures. *Arthritis Care Res.* 1994;7:4:169–175.

Fisher NM, Gresham GE, Abrams M, Hicks J, Horrigan D, Pendergast DR. Quantitative effects of physical therapy on muscular and functional performance in subjects with osteoarthritis of the knees. *Arch Phys Med Rehab.* 1993;74:840–847.

Fisher NM, Gresham GE, Pendergast DR. Effects of a quantitative progressive rehabilitation program applied unilaterally to the osteoarthritic knee. *Arch Phys Med Rehabil.* 1993; 74:1319–1326.

Hayes KW, Falconer J. Reliability of hand-held dynamometry and its relationship with manual muscle testing in patients with osteoarthritis in the knee. *J Orthop Sports Phys Ther.* 1992;16:145–149.

Holm I, et al. Reliability of goniometric measurements and visual estimates of hip ROM in patients with osteoarthrosis. *Physiotherapy Res Int.* 2000;5:241–248.

Jevsevar DS, Riley PL, Hodge WA, Krebs DE. Knee kinematics and kinetics during locomotor activities of daily living in subjects with knee arthroplasty and in healthy control subjects. *Phys Ther.* 1993;73:229–242.

Lomi C, Nordholm LA. Validation of a Swedish version of the Arthritis Self-Efficacy Scale. *Scand J Rheumatol.* 1992;21:231–237.

Marks R. The effect of isometric quadriceps strength training in mid-range for osteo-arthritis of the knee. *N Z J Physiotherapy.* 1993;21:2:16–19.

Marks R, Ghanagaraja S, Ghassemi M. Ultrasound for osteo-arthritis of the knee: a systematic review. *Arthritis Care Res.* 2000;86:452–463.

Marks R, Quinney AH, Wessel J. Reliability and validity of the measurement of position sense in women with osteoarthritis of the knee. *J Rheumatol.* 1993;20:1919–1924.

Marques AP, Rhoden L, de Oliveira Siqueira J, et al. Pain evaluation of patients with fibromyalgia, osteoarthritis, and low back pain. *Revista Do Hospital Das Clinicas; Faculdade de Medicina da Universidade de Sao Paulo.* 2001;56:5–10.

Meenan RF, Mason JH, Anderson JJ, et al. AIMS2: the content and properties of a revised and expanded Arthritis Impact Measurement Scales health status questionnaire. *Arthritis Rheum.* 1992;35:1–10.

Neumann DA, Cook TM, Sholty RL, Sobush DC. An electromyographic analysis of hip abductor muscle activity when subjects are carrying loads in one or both hands. *Phys Ther.* 1992;72:207–217.

Oatis CA. The use of a mechanical model to describe the stiffness and damping characteristics of the knee joint in healthy adults. *Phys Ther.* 1993;73:740–749.

Roos EM, Roos HP, Lohmander LS. Knee Injury and Osteoarthritis Outcome Score (KOOS) – development of a self-administered outcome measure. *J Orthop Sports Phys Ther.* 1998;28:88–96.

Rothstein JM, Roy SH, Wolf SL. *The Rehabilitation Specialist's Handbook.* 2nd ed. Philadelphia, Pa: FA Davis Co; 1998.

Vandervoort AA, Chesworth BM, Cunningham DA, et al. An outcome measure to quantify passive stiffness of the ankle. *Can J Public Health.* 1992;83(suppl 2):S19–S23.

Vaz MD, Kramer JF, Rorabeck CH, Bourne RB. Isometric hip abductor strength following total hip replacement and its relationship to functional assessments. *J Orthop Sports Phys Ther.* 1993;18:526–531.

Weidenhielm L, Mattsson E, Brostrom L, Wersall-Robertsson E. Effect of preoperative physiotherapy in unicompartmental prosthetic knee replacement. *Scand J Rehabil Med.* 1993;25:33–39.

Treatment

Allen SH, Minor MA, Hillman LS, et al. Effect of exercise on the bone mineral density and bone remodelling indices in women with rheumatoid arthritis. *J Rheumatol.* 1993;20: 1247–1249.

Aubin M, Marks R. The efficacy of short-term treatment with transcutaneous electrical nerve stimulation for osteo-arthritic knee pain. *Physiotherapy.* 1995;81:669–676.

Balint G, Szebenyi B. Non-pharmalogical therapies in osteoarthritis. *Baillieres Clin Rheumatol.* 1997;11:795–815.

Bohannon RW, Cooper J. Total knee arthroplasty: evaluation of an acute care rehabilitation program. *Arch Phys Med Rehabil.* 1993;74:1091–1094.

Borjesson M, Robertson E, Weidenhielm L, et al. Physiotherapy in knee osteoarthrosis: effect on pain and walking. *Physiotherapy Res Int.* 1996;1:89–97.

Brotzman SB, Cameron HU, Boolos M. Rehabiliation after total joint arthroplasty. In: Gratzman SB, ed. *Handbook of Orthopaedic Rehabilitation.* St. Louis, Mo: Mosby Year Book; 1996.

Chiarello CM, Gundersen L, O'Halloran T. The effect of continuous passive motion duration and increment on range of motion in total knee arthroplasty patients. *J Orthop Sports Phys Ther.* 1997;25:119–127.

Clark BM. Rheumatology: 9. Physical and occupational therapy in the management of arthritis. *CMAJ.* 2000;163:999–1005.

Creamer R, Flores R, Hochberg ME. Management of osteoarthritis in older adults. *Clin Geriatr Med.* 1998;14:435–454.

David C, Lloyd J. *Rheumatol Physiotherapy.* London: CV Mosby Co; 1999.

Deyle GD, Henderson NE, Matekel RL, et al. Effectivenes of manual physical therapy and exercise in osteoarthritis of the knee. A randomized, controlled trial. *Ann Intern Med.* 2000;132:173–181.

Dieppe P, Altman R, Lequesne M, et al. Osteoarthritis of the knee: Report of a task force of the international league of associations for rheumatology and the Osteoarthritis Research Society. *J Am Geriatr Soc.* 1997;45:850–852.

D'Lima DD, Colwell DD, Colwell CW, et al. The effect of preoperative exercise on total knee replacement outcomes. *Clin Orthop.* 1996;78:174–182.

Elke R, Meier G, Warnke K, et al. Outcome analysis of total knee replacements in patients with rheumatoid arthritis versus osteoarthritis. *Arch Orthop Trauma Surg.* 1995; 114:330–334.

Enloe L J, Shields RK, Smith K, et al. Total hip and knee replacement treatment programs: A report using consensus. *J Orthop Sports Phys Ther.* 1996;23:3–17.

Ettinger WH Jr, Burs S. A randomized trial comparing aerobic exercise with a health education program in older adults with knee osteoarthritis. *JAMA.* 1997;277:25–31.

Falus A, Lakatos T, Smolen J. Dissimilar biosynthesis of interleukin-6 by different areas of synovial membrane of patients with rheumatoid arthritis and osteoarthritis. *Scand J Rheumatol.* 1992;21:116–119.

Felson DT. Nonmedicinal therapies for osteoarthritis. *Bull Rheum Dis.* 1998;47:5–7.

Fisher NM, Gresham GE, Abrams M, et al. Quantitative effects of physical therapy on muscular and functional performance in subjects with osteoarthritis. *Arch Phys Med Rehabil.* 1993;74:840–847.

Fisher NM, Pendergast DR. Application of quantitative and progressive exercise rehabilitation to patients with osteoarthritis of the knee. *J Back Musculoskeletal Rehabil.* 1995; 5:33–53.

Fisher NM, White SC, Yack HJ, et al. Muscle function and gait in patients with knee osteoarthritis before and after muscle rehabilitation. *Disability Rehabil.* 1997;19:47–55.

Foldes K, Balint P, Gaal M, Buchanan WW, Balint GP. Nocturnal pain correlates with effusions in diseased hips. *J Rheumatol.* 1992;19:1756–1758.

Foldes K, Gaal M, Balint P, et al. Ultrasonography after hip arthroplasty. *Skeletal Radiol.* 1992;21:297–299.

Foster RR, Khalifa S. Total knee replacement rehabilitation. *Sports Med Arthroscopic Rev.* 1996;4:83–91.

Fransen M, Crosbie J, Edmonds J. Physical therapy is effective for patients with osteoarthritis of the knee: a randomized controlled clinical trial. *J Rheumatol.* 2001;28:156–164.

Fransen M, Crosbie J, Edmonds J. Reliability of gait measurements in people with osteoarthritis of the knee. *Phys Ther.* 1997;77:944–953.

Gerber L. Rehabilitation of patients with rheumatic diseases. In: Schumacher HR Jr, ed. *Primer on the Rheumatic Diseases.* 10th ed. Atlanta, Ga: Arthritis Foundation; 1993: 90–95.

Gianini MJ, Protas EJ. Comparison of peak isometric knee extensor torque in children with and without juvenile rheumatoid arthritis. *Arthritis Care Res.* 1993;6:82–88.

Givens-Heiss DL, Krebs DE, Riley PO, Strickland EM. In vivo acetabular contact pressures during rehabilitation: post-acute phase. *Phys Ther.* 1992;72:700–710.

Grabois M, Garrison SJ, Hart KA, Lehmkuhl LD. *Physical Medicine and Rehabilitation: The Complete Approach.* Malden, Mass: Blackwell Science; 2000.

Guccione AA. Arthritis and the process of disablement. *Phys Ther.* 1994;74:408–414.

Hart LE. Combination of manual physical therapy and exercises for osteoartitis of the knee. *Clin J Sports Med.* 2000;10:305.

Holm I, Bolstad B, Lutken T, et al. Reliability of goniometric measurements and visual estimates of hip ROM in patients with osteoarthrosis. *Physiotherapy Res Int.* 2000;5:241–248.

Holpit LA. Preoperative and postoperative physical therapy for the total shoulder, hip, and knee replacement patient. *Orthop Phys Ther Clin North Am.* 1993;2:97–118.

Hopman-Rock M, Westhoff MH. The effects of a health education and exercise program for older adults with osteoarthritis of the hip or knee. *J Rheumatol.* 2000;27:1947–1954.

Hughes K, Kuffner L, Dean B. Effect of weekend physical therapy treatment on postoperative length of stay following total hip and total knee arthroplasty. *Physiotherapy Can.* 1993;45:245–249.

Hurley MV, Newham DJ. The influence of arthrogenous muscle inhibition on quadriceps rehabilitation of patients with early, unilateral osteoarthritic knees. *Br J Rheumatol.* 1993;32:131–137.

Iudica AC. Can a program of manual physical therapy and supervised exercise improve the symptoms of osteoarthritis of the knee? *J Fam Pract.* 2000;49:466–467.

Jansen CM, Windau JE, Bonuttie PM, et al. Treatment of a knee contracture using a knee orthosis incorporating stress-relaxation techniques. *Phys Ther.* 1996;76:182–186.

Jensen GM, Lorish CD. Promoting patient cooperation with exercise programs. *Arthritis Care Res.* 1994;7:181–189.

Jevsevar DS, Riley PO, Hodge WA, Krebs DE. Knee kinematics during locomotor activities of daily living in subjects with knee arthroplasty and in healthy control subjects. *Phys Ther.* 1993;73:229–239.

King L. Case study: physical therapy management of hip osteoarthritis prior to total hip arthroplasty. *J Orthop Sports Phys Ther.* 1997;26:35–38.

Kolisek FR, Gilmore KJ, Peterson EK. Slide and flex, tighten, extend (SAFTE): a safe, convenient, effective, and no-cost approach to rehabilitation after total knee arthroplasty. *J Arthroplasty.* 2000;15:1013–1016.

Kumar PJ, McPherson EJ, Dorr LD. Rehabilitation after total knee arthroplasty: a comparison of 2 rehabilitation techniques. *Clin Orthop.* 1996;89:93–101.

Lane NE, Thompson JM. Management of osteoarthritis in the primary-care setting: an evidence-based approach to treatment. *Am J Med.* 1997;103:25S–30S.

Lechner DE. Rehabilitation of the knee with arthritis. In: Greenfield BH, ed. *Rehabilitation of the Knee: A Problem-Solving Approach.* Philadelphia, Pa: FA Davis Co; 1993:206–241.

Lorig K, Fries JF. *The Arthritis Help Book*. 4th ed. Reading, Mass: Addison-Wesley; 1995:124.

Loudon JK. Case report: manual therapy management of hip osteoarthritis. *J Manual Manipulative Ther*. 1999;7:203–208.

Magee DJ. *Orthopedic Physical Assessment*. 3rd ed. Philadelphia, Pa: WB Saunders Co; 1997.

Marks R. Peripheral articular mechanisms in pain production in osteoarthritis. *Aust J Physiotherapy*. 1992;38:289–298.

Marks R. Muscles as a pathogenic factor in osteoarthritis. *Physiotherapy Can*. 1993; 45:251–259.

Marks R. Quadriceps strength training for osteoarthritis of the knee: a literature review and analysis. *N Z J Physiotherapy*. 1993;21:1:15–20.

Marks R. Symptomatic osteoarthritis of the knee: the efficacy of physiotherapy. *Physiotherapy*. 1997;83:306–312.

Marks R, Ungar M, Ghasemmi M. Electrical muscle stimulation for osteoarthritis of the knee: Biological basis and Systematic Review. *N Z J Physiotherapy*. 2000;28:6–20.

Mayer ME. Physical therapy and exercise in osteoarthritis of the knee. *Ann Int Med*. 2000; 132:923.

Messier SP. Osteoarthritis of the knee and associated factors of age and obesity—effects on gait. *Med Sci Sports Exerc*. 1994;26:1446.

Minor MA. Exercise in the management of osteoarthritis of the knee and hip. *Arthritis Care Res*. 1994;7:4:198–204.

Minor MA, Brown JD. Exercise maintenance of persons with arthritis after participation in a class experience. *Health Educ Q*. 1993;20:1:83–95.

Minor MA, Sanford MK. Physical interventions in the management of pain in arthritis: an overview for research and practice. *Arthritis Care Res*. 1993;6:4:197–206.

Mohomed NN. Manual physical therapy and exercise improved function in osteoarthritis of the knee. *J Bone Joint Surg Am*. 2000;82:1324.

Ogino T, Obata H, Ishii S. Tendon ball interposition arthroplasty for traumatic ankylosis of the MP joint. *J Hand Surg*. 1993;18B:704–707.

Reid JC, Minor MA, Mitchell JA, et al. OA rehab: designing a personalized exercise program for people with osteoarthritis. *J Am Med Inf Assoc*. Vol. 272. 1994; (suppl): S987.

Rice JR, Pisetsky DS. Pain in the rheumatic diseases. Practical aspects of diagnosis and treatment. *Rheumatol Dis Clin North Am*. 1999;25:15–30.

Rijken RP, Dekker J. Clinical experience of rehabilitation therapists with chronic diseases: a quantitative approach. *Clin Rehabil*. 1998;12:143–150.

Rodgers JA, Garvin KL, Walker CW, et al. Preoperative physical therapy in primary total knee arthroplasty. *J Arthroplasty*. 1998;13:414–421.

Scott CM, Gatti L. Physical therapy following total hip and total knee replacement. *Orthop Phys Ther Clin North Am*. 1993;2:161–172.

Sevick MA, Bradham DD, Muender G, et al. Cost-effectiveness of aerobic and resistance exercise in seniors with knee osteoarthritis. *Med Sci Sports Exerc*. 2000;32:1534–1540.

Sharma L, Sinacore J, Daugherty C. Prognostic factors for functional outcome of total knee replacement: a prospective study. *J Gerontol*. 1996;51A:M152–M157.

Shelton S. Rehabilitation following total hip arthroplasty. *Topics I Geriatric Rehabilitation*. 1996;12:9–22.

Shields RK, Enoie LJ, Evans R, et al. Analysis of the reliability of clinical functional tests in total hip replacement patients. *Phys Ther*. 1992;72:S113.

Shish CH, Du YK, Lin YH, Wu CC. Muscular recovery around the hip joint after total hip arthroplasty. *Clin Orthop*. 1994;302:115–120.

Sims K. Assessment and treatment of hip osteoarthritis. *Man Ther.* 1999;136–144.

Sims K. The development of hip osteoarthritis: implication for conservative management. *Man Ther.* 1999;4:127–135.

Stenstrom C. Therapeutic exercise in rheumatoid arthritis. *Arthritis Care Res.* 1994;7:190–197.

Strickland EM, Fares M, Krebs DE, et al. In vivo acetabular contact pressures during rehabilitation: acute phase. *Phys Ther.* 1992;72:691–699, 706–710.

Threikeld JA, Currier D. Osteoarthritis: effects of synovial joint tissues. *Phys Ther.* 1998;68:364–370.

Walker-Bone K, Javaid K, Arden N, et al. Regular review: medical management of osteoarthritis. *BMJ.* 2000;321:936–940.

Wegener L, Kisner C, Nichols D. Static and dynamic balance responses in persons with bilateral knee osteoarthiris. *J Orthop Sports Phys Ther.* 1997;25:13–50.

Weidenhielm L, Mattsson E, Brostrom LA, Wersall-Robertsson E. Effect of preoperative physiotherapy in unicompartmental prosthetic knee replacement. *Scand J Rehabil Med.* 1993;25:33–39.

Welch V, Brosseau L, Peterson J. Therapeutic ultrasound for osteoarthritis of the knee (Cochrane Review). *Cochrane Database Systematic Rev.* 2001;3:CD003132.

Rheumatoid Arthritis

DESCRIPTION

Rheumatoid arthritis (RA) is a chronic disorder that leads to inflammation of the peripheral joints, often progressing to destruction of the articular and periarticular structures of these joints. At the joint there is synovial inflammation, proliferation, thickening, and engorgement. The disease's severity can range from a few joints minimally involved to many joints affected by complete ankylosis. A joint is considered damaged if there is a loss of range of motion (ROM) of 15 degrees or more, ligamentous laxity, gross crepitus, and/or joint deformity. Hands and feet are usually the first areas involved, typically at the second and third metacarpophalangeal (MP) joints and proximal interphalangeal joints (PIP). Women are affected 2 to 3 times more often than men.

CAUSE

The specific cause is unknown, but the immunologic changes that trigger the manifestations of RA are multifactorial.

ASSESSMENT

Note: See APTA's Guide to Physical Therapist Practice. 2nd ed. *Physical Therapy.* 2001;81.

Cardiopulmonary Preferred Practice Pattern: B

Musculoskeletal Preferred Practice Patterns: A, B, C, D, F, G, H, I, J

AREAS

- History, including psychosocial evaluation if indicated
- Inflammation
- Pain
- Posture
- Mobility, including ROM, hypermobility, and hypomobility
- Strength
- Neurological, if indicated by weakness or paresthesia

- Joint integrity, including crepitus and laxity
- Skin and soft tissue: temperature, edema
- Balance
- Gait
- Functional level, including activities of daily living (ADLs)
- Equipment, including shoes and any assistive devices

INSTRUMENTS/PROCEDURES

See References for sources.

Functional Level
- Arthritis Self-Efficacy Scale
- Arthritis Community Research and Evaluation Unit Rheumatoid Arthritis Knowledge Questionnaire (KQ)
- Function Independence Measure
- functional inquiry joint examination by ARA classification system
- Geriatric population tests
  1. Functional Life Scale
  2. Lawton's Instrumental Activities of Daily Living Scale
  3. OARS Multidimensional Functional Assessment Questionnaire
  4. Philadelphia Geriatric Center Multilevel Assessment
- Health Assessment Questionnaire (HAQ)
- Katz Index of ADLs
- MACTAR: Patient Preference Disability Questionnaire
- Nottingham Health Profile (NHP)
- Ritchie Index
- Short-form Arthritis Impact Assessment Questionnaire (HAQ)
- Stanford Arthritis Self-Efficacy Scale (SES)
- Thompson/Kirwan Articular Index
- timed 50-feet walking test

Gait
- videotaped observational gait analysis assessments
- observational gait analysis

Inflammation
- duration of morning stiffness
- erythrocyte sedimentation rate
- number of active joints
- numerical scale for joint inflammation

Mobility
- fingertip-to-floor distances
- goniometry
- relaxed oscillation test
- Timed Up and Go Test
- Romberg test
- heel to shin test
- proprioception
- reflexes
- visual acuity
- mental status exam

Pain
- Numeric Pain Rating Scale (NPRS)
- visual analog scale

Special Tests to Which the Physical Therapist May or May Not Have Access
- modified Larsen's radiological index
- Ritchie's articular index

Strength
- hand-held dynamometer
- maximal isometric contraction

- modified sphygmomanometer
- manual muscle testing

PROBLEMS

GENERAL

- The client often complains of pain with movement.
- The client often complains of stiffness in the morning.
- The joints are inflamed and tender and there may be effusion.
- The client often reports loss of movement.
- There is a tendency to flexion contractures.
- There is often weakness, instability, and altered joint-loading responses.
- Gait patterns are often inefficient.
- The client may also have pulmonary problems of pleural effusions, pleuritis, or diffuse interstitial pneumonitis, leading to shallow breathing and chest pain during inspiration.

HANDS

- There may be dorsal subluxation of the ulnar head and palmar displacement of the extensor carpi ulnaris tendon.
- There may be deformity in radiocarpal joint.
- The client may have fusion of the wrist.
- There may be deviation and subluxation of the finger metacarpophalangeal joints.
- At finger interphalangeal joints or thumb joints (MP and PIP), there may be boutonniere deformity (eg, PIP joint flexion and distal interphalangeal [DIP] joint extension) or swan-neck deformity (eg, PIP joint extension, MP joint, and DIP joint flexion).

LOWER EXTREMITIES

- There is often valgus deformity at the knees and ankles.
- There may be a clawed-toes deformity.
- The metatarsal heads may be callused.
- Rheumatoid nodules may be visible on extensor surface with thinning of skin.

TREATMENT/MANAGEMENT

GENERAL

Acute Phase
1. Encourage rest as indicated.
2. Provide splints as indicated for rest and pain relief, especially at hands, wrists, knees, or ankles.
3. Consider use of ice or other modalities for pain, eg, moist heat or paraffin wax for hands and hydrotherapy for relaxation.
4. Maintain ROM with active and active assistive movement within pain-free range, especially in the neck and shoulder region.
5. Do not move joint beyond limit of pain. Passive ROM is not advised during the acute phase.
6. Consider use of suspension devices for exercise or pendular exercises.
7. Educate the client about RA, including the following topics:
   - pathology
   - importance of rest
   - exercise program
   - protection of joints and energy pacing

Subacute Phase
1. Physical agents and modalities
   - Use cryotherapy, if tolerated.
   - Use moist heat packs.
   - Use paraffin wax.
   - Use transcutaneous electrical nerve stimulation (TENS).
   - Use diathermy.
   - Use galvanic muscle stimulation.
   - Ultrasound may be used on localized soft tissue lesions, trigger points, bursae, and tendon sheaths but is not indicated over acute inflammatory lesions.
   - Use massage, including friction, deep transverse friction, ice massage, and accupressure.
   - Use traction with caution.
2. Exercise
   - Begin with isometric exercise, progressing to active movement and concentrating especially on the postural muscles.
   - Use ROM exercises, and increase repetitions depending on degree of morning stiffness and degree of acute synovitis.
   - Consider use of hydrotherapy or aquatic therapy for relaxation and strengthening.
   - Exercises may include PNF patterns on land or in water.
   - Provide gait activities with weight bearing as tolerated.
3. Education
   - Offer group or individual educational sessions.
   - Encourage adequate rest periods.
   - Offer guidelines for lifestyle choices of recreation.

Chronic Phase
1. Continue to stress ROM activities; do not force areas with passive subluxation. ROM exercises are generally active or active assistive, with low repetition as tolerated by client.
2. Reduce contracture with splinting, mobilization, and gentle stretching. Include spray-and-stretch techniques.
3. Continue strengthening program, with hydrotherapy or isometric contractions. If pain persists for more than 2 hours after exercise, decrease intensity. No resistive exercise through full range if joint is swollen. Aerobic activities may include swimming, bicycling, walking, low-impact aerobics, and aquatics. Start slowly, and gradually increase to 45 minutes. Precede and conclude activity with warm-up exercise. Special adaptations for clients with arthritis include the following: progress number of repetitions slowly, modify equipment as needed, use braces or other devices to protect joints, and avoid excess to avoid joint swelling.
4. Provide client with gait-assistive devices as indicated. Crutches should be used only if client can demonstrate sufficient hand grip strength, wrist dorsiflexion, elbow extensor strength, and latissimus dorsi strength. The client may find a platform crutch or a cane with a pistol grip or modified handle more suitable. Assess for the need of a wheelchair. Consider insoles for footwear or wedge to raise as needed for correction of leg-length discrepancy.
5. Assess home environment for needed changes such as handrails or alterations in furniture.
6. Encourage adequate rest periods. Provide improvements in functional capacity with assistive devices or energy conservation techniques.
7. Encourage weight management.
8. Consider physical agents and modalities for pain such as TENS.

HANDS

Acute Phase
- Fit with splints—which may include cock-up or tripoint splints—for protection and rest.
- Use isometric hand exercises.
- Perform ROM exercises as tolerated.
- Provide modalities for edema and pain.
- Elastic gloves may be used at night to assist with swelling.

Subacute Phase
- Provide modalities for pain.
- Instruct in rest and protection of joints.
- Initiate active-assistive exercises, progressing to isotonic exercises at MP joint, especially into extension.
- Fit with adaptive devices for ADLs as indicated.
- Provide education on RA.

Chronic Phase
- Consider splinting for ROM and prevention of contracture using a spring coil splint.
- Use isotonic exercise with mild resistance.
- Postsurgical protocols for procedures performed on MP joints vary among physicians. One protocol recommends the use of dynamic splints placed on day 3 after surgery and worn for 6 to 8 weeks. Switch to night use only until week 14 post surgery.

Note: See preceding section, "Osteoarthritis," for a discussion of and references to joint arthroplasty.

PRECAUTIONS/CONTRAINDICATIONS

- Avoid overexertion.
- Do not have client engage in resistive exercise through full range when there is gross crepitus or when joint is swollen.
- Do not apply heat when joints are inflamed. Prolonged heat can lead to an increase in edema and discomfort.
- Assess sensation before using ice. Ice should not be applied to the skin directly except when using ice massage. The body part involved should not be placed directly on the pack.
- TENS complications can include skin irritation, cutaneous burns, and electric shock. TENS is not to be used on clients with a demand cardiac pacemaker.
- Ultrasound is contraindicated over the spinal cord and anesthetic areas, areas of malignancy, areas with compromised circulation, and on clients with a demand cardiac pacemaker. Ultrasound may be contraindicated over metallic joint implants.
- Shortwave diathermy and microwave diathermy are contraindicated if client has a pacemaker.
- Splints should be removed at least daily and client tolerance should be monitored closely.
- Manual therapy can be used with arthritis only after careful assessment of joint and recent x-rays. When a joint is in the acute phase, even gentle mobilization can lead to increased pain. Techniques should be used cautiously and modified as indicated.
- Isometric exercise is contraindicated in the rheumatoid hand because it may lead to ulnar subluxation.
- Temperature of water for hydrotherapy is recommended at 98 degrees F. Use hydrotherapy cautiously with clients with high blood pressure or recent myocardial disease. Hydrotherapy is always contraindicated if the client is hydrophobic.

Note: Therapists have a tendency to consider only the physical disabilities and underestimate possible depression and anxiety.

DESIRED OUTCOME/PROGNOSIS
- The client will experience a reduction in pain and swelling.
- Therapy will prevent further deterioration and deformity.
- There will be improvement or restoration and maintenance of normal motion and function.
- Cardiovascular conditioning will increase maximal aerobic power and aerobic capacity.
- The client will have enhanced endurance and fitness.
- The client will increase strength.
- The client may have an enhanced sense of well-being.

Notes: The effectiveness of therapy for RA is closely related to the effectiveness of medications. Randomized controlled trial found 4 hours of community-based PT intervention for 6 weeks led to increased self-efficacy, decreased joint stiffness, and disease management knowledge (Bell, et al).

REFERENCES

Assessment

American Physical Therapy Association. Guide to physical therapist practice. 2nd ed. *Phys Ther.* 2001;81.

DeJong Z, Van der Heijde D, McKenna SP, et al. The reliability and construct validity of the RAQoL: a rheumatoid arthritis specific quality of life instrument. *Br J Rheumatol.* 1997;36:878–883.

Ekdahl C. Postural control, muscle function and psychological factors in rheumatoid arthritis: are there any relations? *Scand J Rheumatol.* 1992;21:297–301.

Ellis JI, Orti M. Rheumatoid arthritis in the general hospital setting. In: Peat M, ed. *Curr Phys Ther.* 103–106.

Helewa A, Smythe HA. Physical therapy in rheumatoid arthritis. In: Wolfe F, Pincus T, eds. *Rheum Arthritis.* New York, NY: Marcel Dekker Inc;1994:419.

Lia IM. The Knee Functional Outcome Score—a retrospetive evaluation of responsiveness. *Physiotherapy Singapore.* 2000;3:10–15.

Lomi C, Nordholm LA. Validation of a Swedish version of the Arthritis Self-Efficacy Scale. *Scand J Rheumatol.* 1992;21:231–237.

Mengshoel AM, Clarke-Jenssen A, Fredriksen B, et al. Clinical examination of balance and stability in rheumatoid arthritis patients. *Physiotherapy.* 2000;86:342–347.

Oatis CA. The use of a mechanical model to describe the stiffness and damping characteristics of the knee joint in healthy adults. *Phys Ther.* 1993;73:740–749.

Stenstrom CH. Radiologically observed progression of joint destruction and its relationship with demographic factors, disease severity, and exercise frequency in patients with rheumatoid arthritis. *Phys Ther.* 1994;74:32–39.

Vandervoort AA, Chesworth BM, Cunningham DA, et al. An outcome measure to quantify passive stiffness of the ankle. *Can J Public Health.* 1992;83(suppl 2): S19–S23.

Treatment

Abu-Samrah S, Bayham AG, Cluck RN, et al. Practice patterns for treating rheumatoid arthritis. *Am J Managed Care.* 1999;5:S870–879.

Ayling J, Marks R. Efficacy of paraffin wax baths for rheumatoid arthritic hands. *Physiotherapy.* 2000;86:190–201.

Bell MJ, Lineker SC, Wilkins AL, et al. A randomized controlled trial to evaluate the efficacy of community-based physical therapy in the treatment of people with rheumatoid arthritis. *J Rheumatol.* 1998;25:231–237.

Biundo JJ, Hughes GM. Rheumatoid arthritis: Part 1. Practical guidelines on rest, ambulatory aids, and exercise programs. *Consultant.* 1997;37:2958–2968.

Brozik M, Rosztoczy I, Meretey K, et al. Interleukin 6 levels in synovial fluids of patients with different arthritises: correlation with local IgM rheumatoid factor and systemic acute phase protein production. *J Rheumatol.* 1992;19:63–68.

Brus H, van de Laar M, Taal E, et al. Compliance in rheumatoid arthritis and the role of formal patient education. *Semin Arthritis Rheum.* 1997;26:702–710.

Buljina AI, Taljanovic MS, Hunter TB. Physical and exercise therapy for treatment of the rheumatoid hand. *Arthritis Rheum.* 2001;45:392–397.

Chang RW, ed. *Rehabilitation of Persons with Rheumatoid Arthritis.* Gaithersburg, Md. Aspen Publishers; 1996.

David C, Lloyd J. *Rheumatological Physiotherapy.* London, England: CV Mosby Co; 1999.

Dhondt W, Willaeys T, Verbruggen LA, et al. Pain threshold in patients with rheumatoid arthritis and effect of manual oscillations. *Scand J Rheumatol.* 1999;28:88–93.

Engh CA, Culpepper WJ. Long-term results of the use of the anatomic medullary locking prostesis in total hip arthroplasty. *J Bone Joint Surg.* 1997;79:177–184.

Falus A, Lakatos T, Smolen J. Dissimilar biosynthesis of interleukin-6 by different areas of synovial membrane of patients with rheumatoid arthritis and osteoarthritis. *Scand J Rheumatol.* 1992;21:116–119.

Ganz SB, Harris LL. General overview of rehabilitation in the rheumatoid patients. *Rheumatol Dis Clin North Am.* 1998;24:181–201.

Grabois M, Garrison SJ, Hart KA, Lehmkuhl LD. *Physical Medicine and Rehabilitation: The Complete Approach.* Malden, Mass: Blackwell Science; 2000.

Hayes KW. Heat and cold in the management of rheumatoid arthritis. *Arthritis Care Res.* 1993;6:3:156–166.

Helewa A, Smythe HA. Physical therapy in rheumatoid arthritis. In: Wolfe F, Pincus T, eds. *Rheum Arthritis.* New York, NY: Marcel Dekker, Inc; 1994:415–433.

Hirohata S, Inoue T, Ito K. Development of rheumatoid arthritis after chronic hepatitis caused by hepatitis C virus infection. *Intern Med.* 1992;31:493–495.

Hirohata S, Lipsky PE. Regulation of B cell function by bucillamine, a novel disease-modifying antirheumatic drug. *Clin Immunol Immunopathol.* 1993;66:1:43–51.

Iversen MD, Fossel AH, Daltroy LH. Rheumatologist–patient communication about exercise and physical therapy in the management of rheumatoid arthritis. *Arthritis Care Res.* 1999;12:180–192.

Lechner DE. Rehabilitation of the knee with arthritis. In: Greenfield BH, ed. *Rehabilitation of the Knee: A Problem-Solving Approach.* Philadelphia, Pa: FA Davis Co;1993:206–241.

Leiby KW, Neece PJ, Phipps SH, et al. A comparison of two methods of resistance training on ipsilateral/contralateral hip abduction strength. *J Sports Phys Ther.* 1995;21:52.

Lewis CB, Knortz KA, eds. *Orthopedic Assessment and Treatment of the Geriatric Patient.* St. Louis, Mo: CV Mosby Co;1993.

Li Y, McClure PW, Pratt N. The effect of hamstring muscle stretching on standing posture and on lumbar and hip motions during forward bending. *Phys Ther.* 1996;76:836–849.

Lineker SC, Bell MJ, Wilkins AL, et al. Improvements following short term home based physical therapy are maintained at one year in people with moderate to severe rheumatoid arthritis. *J Rheumatol.* 2001;28:165–168.

Long WT, Borr LD, Healy B, Perry J. Functional recovery of noncemented total hip arthroplasty. *Clin Orthop Related Res.* 1993;288:73–77.

MacSween A, Brydson G, Creed G, et al. A preliminary validation of the 10-metre incremental shuttle walk test as a measure of aerobic capacity in women with rheumatoid arthritis. *Physiotherapy.* 2001;87:38–44.

Maravic M, Bozonnat MC, Sevezan A. Preliminary evaluation of medical outcomes (including quality of life) and costs in incident RA cases receiving hospital-based multidisciplinary management. *Joint Bone Spine.* 2000;67:425–433.

Marion JL, Alexander JE, Butcher JE, MacDonald PB. Effect of a water exercise program on walking gait, flexibility, strength, self-reported disability and other psycho-social measures of older individuals with arthritis. *Physiotherapy Can.* 2001;53:203–211.

Marks R, Ghanagaraja S, Ghassemi M. Ultrasound for osteo-arthritis of the knee: a systematic review. *Physiotherapy.* 2000;86:452–463.

Marks RM, Merson MS. Foot and ankle issues in rheumatoid arthritis. *Bull Rheumatol Dis.* 1997;46:1–3.

Neumann DA, Cook TM, Sholty RL, et al. An electromyographic analysis of hip abductor muscle activity when subjects are carrying loads in one or both hands. *Phys Ther.* 1992;72:207–217.

Rijken PM, Dekker J. Clinical experience of rehabilitation therapists with chronic diseases: a quantitative approach. *Clin Rehabil.* 1998;12:143–150.

Roos EM, Roos HP, Lohmander LS, et al. *J Orthop Sports Phys Ther.* 1998;28:88–96.

Shinohara S, Hirohata S, Inoue T, et al. Phenotypic analysis of peripheral blood monocytes isolated from patients with rheumatoid arthritis. *J Rheumatol.* 1992;19:211–215.

Shrader JA, Siegel KL. Postsurgical hindfoot deformity of a patient with rheumatoid arthritis treated with custom-made foot orthoses and shoe modifications. *Phys Ther.* March 1997;77(3):296–305.

Shumway-Cook A, Gruber W, Baldwin M, Liao S. The effect of multidimensional exercise on balance, mobility, and fall risk in community-dwelling older adults. *Phys Ther.* 1997;77:46–57.

Stenstrom CH. Radiologically observed progression of joint destruction and its relationship with demographic factors, disease severity, and exercise frequency in patients with rheumatoid arthritis. *Phys Ther.* 1994;74:32–39.

Stenstrom CH, Arge B, Sundbom A. Home exercise and compliance in inflammatory rheumatic diseases—a prospective clinical trial. *J Rheumatol.* 1997;24:470–476.

Stewart M. Researches into the effectiveness of physiotherapy in rheumatoid arthritis of the hand. 1996;82:666–672.

Stokes BA, Helewa A, Linekar SC. Total assessment of rheumatoid polyarthritis—a postgraduate training program for physical and occupational therapists: a 20-year success story. *J Rheumatology.* 1997;24:1634–1638.

Swezey RL. Rehabilitation of the rheumatoid arthritic patient. *Ryumachi.* 1997;37:144–145.

Tomkins GS, Jacobs JJ, Kull LR, et al. Primary total hip arthroplasty with a porous-coated acetabular component: seven to ten year results. *J Bone Joint Surg.* 1997;79:169–176.

Tsuchiya N, Endo T, Matsuta K, et al. Detection of glycosylation abnormality in rheumatoid IgG using N-acetylglucosamine-specific Psathyrella velutina lectin. *J Immunol.* 1993; 151:1137–1146.

Tsuchiya N, Endo T, Shiota M, et al. Distribution of glycosylation abnormality among serum IgG subclasses from patients with rheumatoid arthritis. *Clin Immunol Immunopathol.* 1994;70:1:47–50.

Tsuchiya N, Murayama T, Yoshinoya S, et al. Antibodies to human cytomegalovirus 65-kilodalton Fc-binding protein in rheumatoid arthritis: idiotypic mimicry hypothesis of rheumatoid factor production. *Autoimmunity.* 1993;15:1:39–48.

Vliet Vlieland TPM, Zwinderman AH, Vandenbrouke JP, et al. A randomized clinical trial of in-patient multidisciplinary treatment versus routine out-patient care in active rheumatoid arthritis. *Br J Rheumatol.* 1996;35:475–482.

Wadsworth CT. Elbow, forearm, wrist and hand. In: Myers RS, ed. *Saunders Manual of Physical Therapy Practice.* Philadelphia, Pa: WB Saunders Co;1995:888–891.

Westby MD, Wade JP, Rangno KK, et al. A randomized controlled trial to evaluate the effectiveness of an exercise program in women with rheumatoid arthritis taking low dose prednisone. *J Rheumatol.* 2000;27:1674–1680.

Wright FV, Helewa A, Goldsmith CH, Doshi N. Observation variation in an audit of charts of patients with Rheumatoid Arthritis. *Physiotherapy Can.* 1992;44:26–33.

Yamamoto K, Sakoda H, Nakajima T, et al. Accumulation of multiple T cell clonotypes in the synovial lesions of patients with rheumatoid arthritis revealed by a novel clonality analysis. *Int Immunol.* 1992;4:1219–1223.

Chapter 4
Endocrine Disorders

Diabetes Mellitus

DESCRIPTION

Diabetes mellitus (DM) is a disorder resulting in hyperglycemia due to a diminished effectiveness or secretion of insulin. Severe complications from DM include atherosclerotic coronary disease, nephropathy, peripheral arterial disease, peripheral neuropathy, and retinopathy. Clients with DM are at risk for diabetic ketoacidosis and nonketotic hyperglycemic-hyperosmolar coma. Over half of lower extremity amputations are a result of complications from diabetes.

DM is classified as insulin-dependent DM (IDDM, Type I DM) or non-insulin-dependent DM (NIDDM, Type II DM) on the basis of the tendency toward diabetic ketoacidosis, as well as other diagnostic criteria.

CAUSE

DM has varied etiology relating to genetic factors or environmental influences. DM can also occur secondary to the following disorders: endocrine disease, pancreatic disease, presence of beta-cell toxin, acanthosis nigricans, lipotrophic diabetes, and genetic disorders specific to insulin function.

ASSESSMENT

Note: See APTA's Guide to Physical Therapist Practice. 2nd ed. *Physical Therapy.* 2001;81.

Cardiopulmonary Preferred Practice Patterns: A, B

Integumentary Preferred Practice Patterns: A, B

Musculoskeletal Preferred Practice Patterns: C, J

Neuromuscular Preferred Practice Pattern: G

AREAS
- History
- Cardiovascular, including pulse and blood pressure
- Pulmonary
- Neurological, including sensation, especially peripheral, and any retinopathy
- Vascular: any claudication
- Strength, including active motion
- Mobility, including active range of motion
- Skin: color changes, especially in lower legs and feet
- Functional level

INSTRUMENTS/PROCEDURES
- efficacy measure for diabetic program
- Sickness Impact Profile (SIP)
- Physical Performance Test (PPT)
- Functional Reach Test (FR)

Special Tests to Which the Physical Therapist May or May Not Have Access
- glucose fasting levels
- ketone levels

Mobility
- subtalar joint motion testing
- ankle dorsiflexion testing

Neurological
- sensation with Semmes-Weinstein monofilaments

PROBLEMS
- Classic signs of DM: polyuria, polydipsia, quick weight loss, ketouria, and extreme elevation of fasting and plasma glucose levels.
- Client may develop severe complications from DM, including atherosclerotic coronary disease, nephropathy, peripheral arterial disease, peripheral neuropathy, and retinopathy.

TREATMENT/MANAGEMENT
- Establish general program of exercise for fitness.
- Educate client about skin care—especially of the feet—and prevention of open wounds. Emphasize the need to keep skin clean and dry, and inspect frequently for signs of breakdown.
- Assess need for orthotics—especially for feet—and recommend proper footwear.
- Consider prescribing an accommodative shoe that has a rocker sole and a shock-absorbing insert.
- Early wound care may include warm soaks or whirlpool and relief of pressure. Consider use of modalities such as ultrasound, transcutaneous electrical nerve stimulation (TENS; high-voltage), pulsating diathermy, and low-voltage microcurrent stimulation, with negative treatment electrode followed by positive treatment electrode.

Notes: Proper self-care of skin includes removal of excess callus with gentle sanding technique instead of using a sharp instrument. Skin should be hydrated daily with a quick soaking or bathing process followed by use of lotion. Nails should be trimmed straight across on a monthly basis using professional help.

PRECAUTIONS/CONTRAINDICATIONS
- If a client has coronary disease in addition to diabetes, the clinician should be aware that beta blockers can mask the typical signs of impending insulin shock. If blood glucose level is lower than 70 mg/dl or higher than 240 mg/dl, the client should not exercise.
- When a client with diabetes is exercising, the increased glucose induced by exercise needs to be offset by the amount of insulin being administered. Administration directly into a muscle that will be exercised can increase absorption and effect of insulin. An insulin reaction can be caused by exercising at the peak action time of insulin (3 hours after regular insulin injection or 6 hours after Neutral Protamine Hagedorn (NPH) insulin injection).
- Excessive exercise may lead to dehydration and increase the risk of ketosis in a client with diabetes. If ketones are present in the urine, the client should not exercise.
- If the client has an eye condition, such as retinopathy, exercise can worsen the condition.

DESIRED OUTCOME/PROGNOSIS
- The client will alter glucose intolerance with exercise.
- The client will prevent ulcerations from diabetic peripheral vascular disease.
- The client will prevent end-stage kidney disease.

Note: Success depends on medical strategy for modification with diet control and medication.

REFERENCES

Assessment

American Physical Therapy Association. Guide to physical therapist practice. 2nd ed. *Phys Ther*. 2001;81.

Byl N, Pfalzer LA. Integumentary system screening, examination, and assessment. In: Myers RS, ed. *Saunders Manual of Physical Therapy Practice*. Philadelphia, Pa: WB Saunders Co; 1995:582.

Certo C. Cardiovascular. In: Myers RS, ed. *Saunders Manual of Physical Therapy Practice*. Philadelphia, Pa: WB Saunders Co; 1995:243.

Treatment

Adelowo OO, Odusan O. Soft tissue rheumatism among Nigerians. *Afr J Med Sci*. 1997;26:183–184.

Amato AA, Aarohn RJ. *Diabetic Lumbosacral Polyradiculoneuropathies*. 2001;3:139–146.

Bruen KJ, Blair KC, Haynie SD. Addressing risk factors and functional mobility in diabetic wound care. *Phys Ther Case Rep*. 1998;1:227–241.

Diamond JE, Mueller MJ, Delitto A. Effect of total contact cast immobilization on subtalar and talocrural joint motion in patients with diabetes mellitus. *Phys Ther*. 1993;73:310–315.

Grabois M, Garrison SJ, Hart KA, Lehmkuhl LD. *Physical Medicine and Rehabilitation: The Complete Approach*. Malden, Mass: Blackwell Science; 2000.

Hean LB, Tan KEK. Physical activity level among patients with diabetes mellitus. *Physiotherapy Singapore*. 2000;3:61–63.

Horlocker TT, O'Driscoll SW, Dinapoli RP. Recurring brachial plexus neuropathy in a diabetic patient after shoulder surgery and continuous interscalene block. *Anesth Analg*. 2000;91:688–690.

Kwon OY, Mueller MJ. Walking patterns used to reduce forefoot plantar pressures in people with diabetic neuropathies. *Phys Ther*. 2001;81:828–835.

Lundeberg TC, Erikssan SV, Malm M. Electrical nerve stimulation improves healing of diabetic ulcers. *Ann Plast Surg*. 1992;29:328–331.

McCulloch JM. The role of physiotherapy in managing patients with wounds. *J Wound Care*. 1998;7:241–244.

McPoil TG, Yamada W, Smith W, et al. The distribution of plantar pressures in American Indians with diabetes mellitus. *J Am Podiatr Med Assoc*. 2001;91:280–287.

Morcuende JA, Dobbs MB, Crawford H, et al. Diabetic muscle infarction is a rare complication of diabetes mellitus. *Iowa Orthop*. 2000;20:65–74.

Mueller MJ. Identifying patients with diabetes mellitus who are at risk for lower-extremity complications: use of Semmes-Weinstein monofilaments. *Phys Ther*. 1996;76:68–71.

Myers, RS, ed. *Saunders Manual of Physical Therapy Practice*. Philadelphia, Pa: WB Saunders Co; 1995:220, 243, 236, 414, 581–582, 629, 1190.

Naftulin S, Fast A, Thomas M. Diabetic lumbar radiculopathy: sciatica without disc herniation. *Spine*. 1993;18:2419.

Ogilvie-Harris DJ, Myerthall S. The diabetic frozen shoulder. *Arthroscopy*. 1997;13:1–8.

Reddy GK, Stehno-Bittel L, Hanade S, et al. The biomechanical integrity of bone in experimental diabetes. *Diabetes Res Clin Pract*. 2001;54:1–8.

Rijken PM, Degger J. Clinical experience of rehabilitation therapists with chronic diseases; a quantitative approach. *Clin Rehabil.* 1998;12:143–150.

Salsich GB, Mueller MJ. Relationships between measures of function, strength and walking speed in patients with diabetes and transmetatarsal amputation. *Clin Rehabil.* 1997; 11:60–67.

Sinacore DR. Healing times of pedal ulcers in diabetic immunosuppressed patients after transplantation. *Arch Phys Med Rehabil.* 1999;80:935–940.

Sinacore DR. Severe sensory neuropathy need not precede Charcot arthropathies of the foot or ankle: implications for the rehabilitation specialist. *Physiotherapy Theor Prac.* 2001;17:39–50.

Sinacore DR, Mueller MJ. Neuropathic plantar ulcers in patients with diabetes mellitus. *PT Magazine Phys Ther.* 1998;6:58–60.

Van Rooijen AJ, Rheeder P, Eales CJ. Black female patients with Type 2 Diabetes Mellitus: knowledge, attitudes and physical activity. *S Afr J Physiotherapy.* 2001;57:20–27.

Chapter 5

Hand Injuries

Colles Fracture

DESCRIPTION

Colles fracture is the most common fracture of the forearm/wrist/hand area. Colles fracture occurs at the distal 2 inches of the radius, leaving a dorsally angulated fracture, and may include ulnar fracture as well. It occurs most frequently in the elderly. A Smith fracture, or "reverse Colles," leaves a volarly angulated fracture of the radius. Other fractures in this area include scaphoid, metacarpal, and phalangeal fractures.

CAUSE

A Colles fracture results from falling onto an outstretched hand when the wrist is extended. A Smith fracture results from falling onto an outstretched hand when the wrist is flexed.

ASSESSMENT

> **Note:** See APTA's Guide to Physical Therapist Practice. 2nd ed. *Physical Therapy.* 2001;81.
>
> Musculoskeletal Preferred Practice Patterns: G, I

AREAS
- History, including occupation, hand dominance, details of injury, and psycho-social factors
- Pain
- Mobility, including active and passive range of motion (ROM), accessory motion, composite range of motion, and any fixed deformities
- Strength: compare with uninvolved hand, if applicable; power and precision
- Sensitivity
- Skin and soft tissue: trophic changes, edema, temperature, condition of nails
- Joint integrity and structural deviations
- Neurological, including deep tendon reflexes and sensation
- Functional level
- Vascular

INSTRUMENTS/PROCEDURES

See References for sources.

Functional Level
- Demerit Point System: Colles fractures
- Jebsen Test of Hand Function
- Physical Capacity Evaluation

Joint Integrity and Structural Deviations
1. orthopedic tests of the hand
    - Bunnell-Littler test
    - circle formation with tip opposition between thumb and index finger test
    - digit collateral ligamentous stress test
    - elbow collateral ligament test
    - Finklestein test
    - Froment's sign
    - lateral and medial epicondylitis test
    - lunate displacement test
    - oblique retinacular ligament test
    - trigger finger test
    - triquestrolunate test

- ulnar snuff box test
- Watson's test
2. photography of joint deformity

MOBILITY
- goniometry
- Guidelines for Measurement from the American Society for Surgery of the Hand (all motions measured from neutral starting position)

Neurological/Sensitivity
- carpal and cubital tunnels
- Dellon modification of Moberg test
- distal ulnar tunnel
- Minnesota manual dexterity test
- Minnesota rate of manipulation test
- Moberg pick-up test
- nerve conduction velocity test
- O'Connor finger dexterity test
- Phalen's test
- pinch test
- point localization
- Purdue pegboard test
- ridge sensiometer
- Seddon coin test
- sensitivity to deep pressure
- sensitivity to light touch (Semmes-Weinstein monofilaments)
- sensitivity to pain
- sensitivity to temperature
- sudomotor test
- Tinel's sign
- two-pound discrimination test
- vibratory test
- wrinkle test

Skin and Soft Tissue
1. edema
    - tape measure
    - volumetric measurements
2. temperature
    - palpation

Strength
- grasp
- grip: sphygmomanometer and Jamar grip dynamometer
- pinch

Vascular
- Allen's test
- modified Allen's test
- capillary refill
- volumetric measures

PROBLEMS
- The client often has pain.
- The client may have edema.
- The fracture may be unstable.
- The client may have complications with wound healing.

TREATMENT/MANAGEMENT
- Active ROM follows the period of immobilization, which is usually 4 to 6 weeks. Emphasize forearm, wrist, and thumb movements. Begin with gentle wrist flexion/extension and supination/pronation activities.
- Consider passive stretch to intrinsic musculature (ie, metacarpophalangeal extension with interphalangeal flexion).
- Stretch extrinsic flexor tendons (ie, combination extension of fingers and wrist).
- Use joint mobilization as indicated.
- Instruct in elevation and use of wrapping materials for edema of fingers and hand. Also consider retrograde massage for edema.

- Consider use of transcutaneous electrical nerve stimulation (TENS) or functional electrical stimulation for pain.
- Consider use of mild heat if stiffness is a problem.

PRECAUTIONS/CONTRAINDICATIONS
- Fingers must be observed for swelling after cast is applied.
- Uninjured parts should remain free and activity encouraged to prevent contracture. Metacarpal joints, in particular, should remain unrestricted for finger flexion and thumb opposition to little finger.

DESIRED OUTCOME/PROGNOSIS
- The client will have an increase in motion.
- The client will have increase in strength.
- The client will have a reduction of pain.
- The client will return to full function.

REFERENCES

Assessment

American Physical Therapy Association. Guide to physical therapist practice. 2nd ed. *Phys Ther.* 2001;81

Anthony MS. Sensory evaluation. In: Clark GL, Wilgis EF, Aiello B, et al, eds. *Hand Rehabilitation: A Practical Guide.* New York, NY: Churchill Livingstone; 1993:55–72.

Hackel ME, Wolfe GA, Bang SM, et al. Changes in hand function in the aging adult as determined by the Jebsen Test of Hand Function. *Phys Ther.* 1992;72:373–377.

Hamilton GF, McDonald C, Chenier TC. Measurement of grip strength: validity and reliability of the sphygmomanometer and Jamar grip dynamometer. *J Orthop Sports Phys Ther.* 1992;16:215–219.

LaStayo PC, Wheeler DL. Reliability of passive wrist flexion and extension goniometric measurements: a multicenter study. *Phys Ther.* 1994;74:162–174.

Rothstein JM, Roy SH, Wolf SL. *The Rehabilitation Specialist's Handbook.* Philadelphia, Pa: FA Davis Co; 1991:126–127.

Saidoff DC, McDonough AL. *Critical Pathways in Therapeutic Intervention.* Philadelphia, Pa: CV Mosby Co; 2002.

Tomberlin JP, Saunders HD. *Evaluation, Treatment and Prevention of Musculoskeletal Disorders. Vol 2: Extremities.* Chaska, Minn: The Saunders Group; 1994:164.

Tubiana R, Thomine JM, Mackin E. *Examination of the Hand and Wrist.* New York, NY: CV Mosby Co; 1996.

Wadsworth CT. Elbow, forearm, wrist, and hand. In: Myers RS, ed. *Saunders Manual of Physical Therapy Practice.* Philadelphia, Pa: WB Saunders Co; 1995:841–917.

Treatment

Bialocerkowski A. A home program is as effective as in-rooms in the management of distal radius fracture. *Australian Journal of Physiotherapy.* 2001;47:68.

Bianchi S. Partial transient osteoporosis of the hand. *Skeletal Radiol.* 1999;28:324–329.

Bryan BK, Kohnke EN. Therapy after skeletal fixation in the hand and wrist. *Hand Clin.* 1997;13:761–776.

Colbert B, Fye L, Bielefeld T, et al. Hand therapy: roles for PT's and OT's. *PT-Magazine Phys Ther.* 1997;5:10.

Crosby CA, Wehbe MA. Early motion protocols in hand and wrist rehabilitation. *Hand Clin.* 1996;12:31–41.

Cyr LM, Ross RG. How controlled stress affects healing tissues. *J Hand Ther.* 1998;11:125–130.

Flowers KR. Digital diagnoses in a digital world. *J Hand Ther.* 1999;12:185–186.

Margles SW. Early motion in the treatment of fractures and dislocation in the hand and wrist. *Hand Clin.* 1996;12:65–72.

Michlovitz S. Physical therapy after hand injuries. *Hand Clin.* 1999;15:261–273.

Miller DS. Medical management of pain for early motion in hand and wrist surgery. *Hand Clin.* 1996;12:139–147.

Miller RE. Hand care in the new millennium: therapist's commentary. *J Hand Ther.* 1999; 12:182–183.

Popescu V, Burdea G, Bouzit M, et al. PC-based telerehabilitation system with force feedback. *Stud Health Technol Information.* 1999;62:261–267.

Randall T, Portney L, Harris BA. Effects of joint mobilization on joint stiffness and active motion of the metacarpal-phalangeal joint. *J Orthop Sports Phys Ther.* 1992;16:30–36.

Russell CR. Bone and joint injury in the hand: therapist's commentary. *Journal of Hand Therapy.* 1999;12:121–122.

Wadsworth CT. Elbow, forearm, wrist, and hand. In: Myers RS, ed. *Saunders Manual of Physical Therapy Practice.* Philadelphia, Pa: WB Saunders Co; 1995:841–917.

Weinstock TB. Management of fractures of the distal radius: Therapist's commentary. *J Hand Ther.* 1999;12:99–102.

Wynn KE. The challenges and complexities of hand rehabilitation. *PT-Magazine Phys Ther.* 1997;5:58–67.

de Quervain's Disease

Also known as *repetitive trauma of the hand.*

DESCRIPTION

de Quervain's disease is a type of tenosynovitis or inflammation of the abductor pollicis longus and extensor pollicus brevis tendons' sheath. Other hand conditions that can be caused by repetitive trauma include trigger finger and ganglia.

CAUSE

Etiology is unknown. de Quervain's disease may be caused by repetitive microtrauma or extreme trauma, strain, unaccustomed exercise, or the effects of aging. Specifically, overuse of activities combining thumb and wrist movements may be implicated.

ASSESSMENT

Note: See APTA's Guide to Physical Therapist Practice. 2nd ed. *Physical Therapy.* 2001;81.

Musculoskeletal Preferred Practice Patterns: D, E, F, I

AREAS

- History, including occupation, hand dominance, details of injury, and psycho-social factors
- Pain
- Mobility, including active and passive range of motion (ROM), accessory motion, composite range of motion, and any fixed deformities
- Strength: compare with uninvolved hand, if applicable; power and precision
- Sensibility
- Skin and soft tissue: trophic changes, edema, temperature, condition of nails
- Joint integrity and structural deviations
- Neurological, including deep tendon reflexes, sensation
- Functional level
- Vascular

INSTRUMENTS/PROCEDURES

See References for sources.

Functional Level
- impairment ratings
- Jebsen Test of Hand Function
- physical capacity evaluation

Joint Integrity and Structural Deviations
1. orthopedic tests of the hand
    - Bunnell-Littler test
    - circle formation with tip opposition between thumb and index finger test
    - digit collateral ligamentous stress test
    - elbow collateral ligament test
    - Finklestein test
    - Froment's sign
    - lateral and medial epicondylitis test
    - lunate displacement test
    - oblique retinacular ligament test
    - retinacular test
    - trigger finger test
    - triquestrolunate test
    - ulnar snuff box test
    - Watson's test
2. photography of joint deformity

Mobility
- goniometry
- Guidelines for Measurement from the American Society of Surgery of the Hand (all motions measured from neutral starting position)

Neurological/Sensibility
- carpal and cubital tunnels
- Dellon modification of Moberg test
- distal ulnar tunnel
- Minnesota manual dexterity test
- Minnesota rate of manipulation test
- Moberg pick-up test
- nerve conduction velocity test
- O'Connor finger dexterity test
- Phalen's test
- pinch test
- point localization
- Purdue pegboard test
- ridge sensiometer
- Seddon coin test
- sensitivity to deep pressure
- sensitivity to light touch (Semmes-Weinstein monofilaments)
- sensitivity to pain

- sensitivity to temperature
- sudomotor test
- Tinel's sign
- two-point discrimination test
- vibratory test
- wrinkle test

Skin and Soft Tissue
1. edema
   - tape measure
   - volumetric measures
2. temperature
   - palpation

Strength
- grasp
- grip: sphygmomanometer and Jamar grip dynamometer
- pinch

Vascular
- Allen's test
- modified Allen's test
- capillary refill
- volumetric measures

PROBLEMS
- The client often has pain in wrist with activity.
- The client may have decreased use of hand due to pain.
- The client often has swelling and tenderness around the wrist, first extensor compartment, or radial styloid process.
- The client often has decreased ROM in direction of ulnar deviation.
- The client may have accompanying nerve irritation.

TREATMENT/MANAGEMENT

ACUTE PHASE
- Instruct client in use of ice.
- Fit client with resting forearm splint.
- After 1 to 2 weeks, consider use of physical agents and modalities such as heat, phonophoresis, ultrasound, and friction massage.
- Begin mild stretching for wrist motion and active exercise.
- Consider soft tissue mobilization for neural problems.
- Educate client on benefits of activity modification of aggravating activities to prevent reinjury.

POSTSURGICAL REHABILITATION

Active exercise usually begins 2 to 3 days post surgery after dressings are removed.

PRECAUTIONS/CONTRAINDICATIONS

de Quervain's disease must be differentiated from osteoarthrosis of the trapezium.

DESIRED OUTCOME/PROGNOSIS
- The client will experience a decrease in symptoms.
- The client will progress to an increased functional level.
- The client will be instructed in avoiding aggravation of the condition and reinjury.

REFERENCES

Assessment

American Physical Therapy Association. Guide to physical therapist practice. 2nd ed. *Phys Ther.* 2001;81

Anthony MS. Sensory evaluation. In: Clark GL, Wilgis EF, Aiello B, et al, eds. *Hand Rehabilitation: A Practical Guide.* New York, NY: Churchill Livingstone; 1993:55–72.

Hackel ME, Wolfe GA, Bang SM, et al. Changes in hand function in the aging adult as determined by the Jebsen Test of Hand Function. *Phys Ther.* 1992;72:373–377.

Hamilton GF, McDonald C, Chenier TC. Measurement of grip strength: validity and reliability of the sphygmomanometer and Jamar grip dynamometer. *J Orthop Sports Phys Ther.* 1992;16:215–219.

LaStayo PC, Wheeler DL. Reliability of passive wrist flexion and extension goniometric measurements: a multicenter study. *Phys Ther.* 1994;74:162–174.

Rothstein JM, Roy SH, Wolf SL. *The Rehabilitation Specialist's Handbook.* 2nd ed. Philadelphia, Pa: FA Davis Co; 1999.

Tomberlin JP, Saunders HD. *Evaluation, Treatment and Prevention of Musculoskeletal Disorders. Vol 2: Extremities.* Chaska, Minn: The Saunders Group; 1994:164.

Tubiana R, Thomine JM, Mackin E. *Examination of the Hand and Wrist.* New York, NY: CV Mosby Co; 1996.

Wadsworth CT. Elbow, forearm, wrist, and hand. In: Myers RS, ed. *Saunders Manual of Physical Therapy Practice.* Philadelphia, Pa: WB Saunders Co; 1995:841–917.

Ward RS. Impairment rating. *Clin Manage.* 1992;12:5:38–45.

Treatment

Anderson M, Tichenor CJ. A patient with de Quervain's tenosynovitis: a case report using an Australian approach to manual therapy. *Phys Ther.* 1994;74:314–326.

Randall T, Portney L, Harris BA. Effects of joint mobilization on joint stiffness and active motion of the metacarpal-phalangeal joint. *J Orthop Sports Phys Ther.* 1992;16:30–36.

Tomberlin JP, Saunders HD. *Evaluation, Treatment and Prevention of Musculoskeletal Disorders. Vol 2: Extremities.* Chaska, Minn: The Saunders Group; 1994:141–182.

Dupuytren's Contracture

Also known as *Flexion contracture.*

DESCRIPTION

Dupuytren's contracture is a spontaneous thickening of the palmar fascia that leads to flexion contracture, which is usually painless but prevents full use of fingers. It may also appear as a nodular lesion in the adipose tissue. There is an increased incidence in men over women, over the age of 40.

CAUSE

The fibrous thickening has an unknown etiology. Dupuytren's contracture may be affected by repeated microtrauma. This disorder can also accompany shoulder-hand syndrome, diabetes, epilepsy, and alcoholism. There appears to be an inherited tendency toward the disorder among those of European ancestry.

ASSESSMENT

Note: See APTA's Guide to Physical Therapist Practice. 2nd ed. *Physical Therapy.* 2001;81.

Musculoskeletal Preferred Practice Patterns: D, I

AREAS
- History, including occupation, hand dominance, details of injury, and psycho-social factors
- Pain
- Mobility, including active and passive range of motion (ROM), accessory motion, composite range of motion, and any fixed deformities
- Strength: compare with uninvolved hand, if applicable; power and precision
- Sensibility
- Skin and soft tissue: trophic changes, edema, temperature, and condition of nails
- Joint integrity and structural deviations
- Neurological, including deep tendon reflexes and sensation
- Functional level
- Vascular

INSTRUMENTS/PROCEDURES

See References for sources.

Functional Level
- Jebsen Test of Hand Function
- Physical Capacity Evaluation

Joint Integrity and Structural Deviations
1. orthopedic tests of the hand
    - Bunnell-Littler test
    - circle formation with tip opposition between thumb and index finger test
    - digit collateral ligamentous stress test
    - elbow collateral ligament test
    - Finklestein test
    - Froment's sign
    - lateral and medial epicondylitis test
    - lunate displacement test
    - oblique retinacular ligament test
    - retinacular test
    - trigger finger test
    - triquestrolunate test
    - ulnar snuff box test
    - Watson's test
2. photography of joint deformity

Mobility
- goniometry
- Guidelines for Measurement from the American Society for Surgery of the Hand (all motions measured from neutral starting position)

Neurological/Sensibility
- carpal and cubital tunnels
- Dellon modification of Moberg test
- distal ulnar tunnel
- Minnesota manual dexterity test

- Minnesota rate of manipulation test
- Moberg pick-up test
- nerve conduction velocity test
- O'Connor finger dexterity test
- Phalen's test
- pinch test
- point localization
- Purdue pegboard test
- ridge sensiometer
- Seddon coin test
- sensitivity to deep pressure
- sensitivity to light touch (Semmes-Weinstein monofilaments)
- sensitivity to pain
- sensitivity to temperature
- sudomotor test
- Tinel's sign
- two-point discimination test
- vibratory test
- wrinkle test

Skin and Soft Tissue
1. edema
   - tape measure
   - volumetric measures
2. temperature
   - palpation

Strength
- grasp
- grip: sphygmomanometer and Jamar grip dynamometer
- pinch

Vascular
- Allen's test
- modified Allen's test
- capillary refill
- volumetric measures

PROBLEMS
- There is flexion contracture of the palmar aponeurosis.
- Often, the contractures affect the metacarpal phalangeal and proximal interphalangeal joints of the ring or little finger.
- The client often is affected on both hands.
- The client may have loss of hand function because of stiffness.
- The client may have a lump in palmar aponeurosis.
- After surgery, the client may have complications such as edema, decreased ROM of the whole hand, and recurrence of flexion contracture.

TREATMENT/MANAGEMENT

REHABILITATION FOR CONTRACTURE OR STIFFNESS
1. Consider use of massage with soft tissue mobilization techniques and joint mobilization.
2. Encourage use of splints—dynamic or static—between therapy sessions.
3. Use passive ROM and stretching techniques combined with heat, followed by active exercise.
4. Encourage active mobilization.
5. Progress to resistive exercise. Begin with isometric exercises and progress to resistive isotonic exercises.
6. Graded resistive activity can progress using manual resistance PNF techniques or external resistance or weight and isoflex exercises.
7. Instruct in home program of self-stretching with automobilization techniques or reverse-stretching techniques.

REHABILITATION FOLLOWING SURGICAL RELEASE; FASCIECTOMY

1. Provide whirlpool for wound care combined with active flexion and extension exercises.
2. Post whirlpool, one suggested routine has client elevate hand while performing fist-making exercise for 1 minute, followed by interval rest of 3 to 5 minutes to prevent edema.
3. Client may consult with physician for home program of soaking hand in water and regarding which type of dressings to use.
4. Fit client with dorsal splint after dressings are removed, as indicated. Splints must be carefully fitted and readjusted as indicated. Instruct client in proper use and fit of splints. See Precautions.
5. Instruct client on proper positioning to prevent swelling, such as keeping hand elevated above level of heart after surgery. Avoid extreme elbow flexion for proper venous flow. Keep hand elevated during sleep if possible.
6. Severe pitting edema may indicate the need for intermittent compression treatment. Mechanical compression can be followed by manual retrograde massage.
7. Elastic wraps or elastic glove may also be used to assist with edema.
8. Additional antiedema exercises may be recommended, such as elevation of arms and making a fist, on a suggested schedule of 10 times every hour while awake.
9. Consider intermittent compression if edema is severe. Amount of pressure is adjusted as condition warrants. Mechanical massage may be followed by retrograde massage with lanolin.
10. Instruct client in passive and active exercise.
11. Active hand exercises may include:
    - thumb opposition, abduction, and extension
    - finger abduction, adduction, extension, and flexion to thenar eminence
    - fist making
    - wrist flexion and extension
    - intrinsic extension
    - finger blocking: isolation of distal flexion with proximal joints held firm

    Frequency of exercise: 10 repetitions, 3 to 4 times per day, is one recommended schedule, with increased precision as client increases in motion. Can add tendon gliding exercises at this time.
12. Client may begin putty-squeezing exercises at 4 to 6 weeks postoperatively, if indicated.
13. Provide modification of scar tissue with direct pressure, serial or dynamic splints, and ROM or stretching techniques. Scar management may be enhanced with massage with lotion and pressure forms for scars.
14. Instruct client in desensitization techniques if hypersensitive over healed area.

PRECAUTIONS/CONTRAINDICATIONS

GENERAL

- Suspect reflex sympathetic dystrophy if client reports edema and stiffness combined with extreme pain.
- Do not allow overexercise, which can lead to increased pain and edema.
- Avoid squeezing exercises.
- Avoid overstretching the capsules in the finger joints.
- Fingers should always be stretched individually. If stretching multijoint muscles, do not elongate all joints simultaneously.

- When using a splint, clients should be taught to look for signs of too much pressure, such as color changes in fingertips, feelings of tingling or numbness, or increased edema.
- When splinting, the traction must be perpendicular to the involved segment.

POSTOPERATIVELY

- Avoid having hand in a dependent position when in whirlpool.
- Exercise should not begin after surgery until from day 3 to day 21, as indicated.
- Avoid contaminating the wound area with lanolin or lotion during massage.
- Intermittent external compression can be used with open wounds if sterile dressings are in place.

DESIRED OUTCOME/PROGNOSIS

- The client will restore joint play and full range of motion of the involved hand.
- The client will have an increase in strength and endurance of the involved hand.
- The client will return to former activities/work.

Postoperatively:

- Through therapy, the client will reduce or prevent edema.
- There will be a modification of scar tissue.
- Recovery time is variable but function is usually limited for at least 6 weeks postoperatively.

Notes: To maintain gains from surgery and achieve optimal results, therapy is critical and is usually needed for 1 month or more. The use of nighttime splints may be indicated for approximately 6 months.

Any diminished sensation usually resolves itself spontaneously.

REFERENCES

Assessment

American Physical Therapy Association. Guide to physical therapist practice. 2nd ed. *Phys Ther.* 2001;81

Anthony MS. Sensory evaluation. In: Clark GL, Wilgis EF, Aiello B, et al, eds. *Hand Rehabilitation: A Practical Guide.* New York, NY: Churchill Livingstone; 1993:55-72.

Hackel ME, Wolfe GA, Bang SM, et al. Changes in hand function in the aging adult as determined by the Jebsen Test of Hand Function. *Phys Ther.* 1992;72:373-377.

Hamilton GF, McDonald C, Chenier TC. Measurement of grip strength: validity and reliability of the sphygmomanometer and Jamar grip dynamometer. *J Orthop Sports Phys Ther.* 1992;16:215-219.

LaStayo PC, Wheeler DL. Reliability of passive wrist flexion and extension goniometric measurements: a multicenter study. *Phys Ther.* 1994;74:162-174.

Rothstein JM, Roy SH, Wolf SL. *The Rehabilitation Specialist's Handbook.* 2nd ed. Philadelphia, Pa: FA Davis Co; 1999.

Saidoff DC, McDonough AL. *Critical Pathways in Therapeutic Intervention.* Philadelphia, Pa: CV Mosby Co; 2002.

Tomberlin JP, Saunders HD. *Evaluation, Treatment and Prevention of Musculoskeletal Disorders. Vol 2: Extremities.* Chaska, Minn: The Saunders Group; 1994:164.

Tubiana R, Thomine JM, Mackin E. *Examination of the Hand and Wrist.* New York, NY: CV Mosby Co; 1996.

Wadsworth CT. Elbow, forearm, wrist, and hand. In: Myers RS, ed. *Saunders Manual of Physical Therapy Practice*. Philadelphia, Pa: WB Saunders Co; 1995:841–917.

Treatment

Clark GL, Wilgis EF, Aiello B, et al, eds. *Hand Rehabilitation: A Practical Guide*. New York, NY: Churchill Livingstone; 1993.

Randall T, Portney L, Harris BA. Effects of joint mobilization on joint stiffness and active motion of the metacarpal-phalangeal joint. *J Orthop Sports Phys Ther*. 1992;16:30–36.

Stanley BG, Tribuzi SM. *Concepts in Hand Rehabilitation*. Philadelphia, Pa: FA Davis Co; 1992.

Wadsworth CT. Elbow, forearm, wrist, and hand. In: Myers RS, ed. *Saunders Manual of Physical Therapy Practice*. Philadelphia, Pa: WB Saunders Co; 1995:841–917.

Gamekeeper's Thumb (Sprains and Dislocations of the Hand)

DESCRIPTION

Gamekeeper's thumb is the forceful rupture of the ulnar collateral ligament or volar plate insertion at the first metacarpal (MP) joint. Other areas prone to sprains and dislocations are the lunate bone, the second to fifth MP joints, the proximal interphalangeal (PIP) joints, and distal interphalangeal (DIP) joints.

CAUSE

First-MP-joint dislocation or sprain often happens during a fall such as skiing. When the skiier lands on an abducted thumb, the joint is forced into hyperextension.

ASSESSMENT

Note: See APTA's Guide to Physical Therapist Practice. 2nd ed. *Physical Therapy.* 2001;81.

Musculoskeletal Preferred Practice Patterns: D, I

AREAS
- History, including occupation, hand dominance, details of injury, and psychosocial factors
- Pain
- Mobility, including active and passive range of motion (ROM), accessory motion, composite range of motion, and any fixed deformities
- Strength, compare with uninvolved hand, if applicable; power and precision
- Sensibility
- Skin and soft tissue: trophic changes, edema, temperature, condition of nails
- Joint integrity and structural deviations
- Neurological, including deep tendon reflexes and sensation
- Functional level
- Vascular

INSTRUMENTS/PROCEDURES

See References for sources.

Functional Level
- Jebsen Test of Hand Function
- Physical Capacity Evaluation

Joint Integrity and Structural Deviations
1. orthopedic tests of the hand
   - Bunnell-Littler test
   - circle formation with tip opposition between thumb and index finger test
   - digit collateral ligamentous stress test
   - elbow collateral ligament test
   - Finklestein test
   - Froment's sign
   - lateral and medial epicondylitis test
   - lunate displacement test
   - oblique retinacular ligament test
   - retinacular test
   - trigger finger test
   - triquestrolunate test
   - ulnar snuff box test
   - Watson's test
2. photography of joint deformity

MOBILITY
- goniometry
- Guidelines for Measurement from the American Society for Surgery of the Hand (all motions measured from neutral starting position)

NEUROLOGICAL/SENSIBILITY
- carpal and cubital tunnels
- Dellon modification of Moberg test
- distal ulnar tunnel
- Minnesota manual dexterity test
- Minnesota rate of manipulation test
- Moberg pick-up test
- nerve conduction velocity test
- O'Connor finger dexterity test
- Phalen's test
- pinch test
- point localization
- Purdue pegboard test
- ridge sensiometer
- Seddon coin test
- sensitivity to deep pressure
- sensitivity to light touch (Semmes-Weinstein monofilaments)
- sensitivity to pain
- sensitivity to temperature
- sudomotor test
- Tinel's sign
- two-point discrimination test
- vibratory test
- wrinkle test

Skin and Soft Tissue
1. edema
   - tape measure
   - volumetric measures
2. temperature
   - palpation

Strength
- grasp
- grip: sphygmomanometer and Jamar grip dynamometer
- pinch

Vascular
- Allen's test
- modified Allen's test

- capillary refill
- volumetric measures

PROBLEMS
- The client often has pain and inflammation.
- The client often has joint instability if there is complete rupture.
- The client may have loss of function.

TREATMENT/MANAGEMENT

PARTIAL RUPTURE
- Initiate gentle ROM.
- Gradually progress to strengthening thumb exercises.

COMPLETE RUPTURE
- A period of immobilization is usually 2 to 6 weeks, following manual or open reduction.
- After immobilization, begin treatment as for partial rupture.

PRECAUTIONS/CONTRAINDICATIONS
- If the adductor aponeurosis is caught between the ligament and the proximal phalanx, an open reduction is generally indicated.

DESIRED OUTCOME/PROGNOSIS
- The client will have a reduction in symptoms.
- The client will resume normal hand function.

REFERENCES

Assessment

American Physical Therapy Association. Guide to physical therapist practice. 2nd ed. *Phys Ther.* 2001;81.

Anthony MS. Sensory evaluation. In: Clark GL, Wilgis EF, Aiello B, et al, eds. *Hand Rehabilitation: A Practical Guide.* New York, NY: Churchill Livingstone; 1993:55–72.

Hackel ME, Wolfe GA, Bang SM, et al. Changes in hand function in the aging adult as determined by the Jebsen Test of Hand Function. *Phys Ther.* 1992;72:373–377.

Hamilton GF, McDonald C, Chenier TC. Measurement of grip strength: validity and reliability of the sphygmomanometer and Jamar grip dynamometer. *J Orthop Sports Phys Ther.* 1992;16:215–219.

LaStayo PC, Wheeler DL. Reliability of passive wrist flexion and extension goniometric measurements: a multicenter study. *Phys Ther.* 1994;74:162–174.

Rothstein JM, Roy SH, and Wolf SL. *The Rehabilitation Specialist's Handbook.* 2nd ed. Philadelphia, Pa: FA Davis Co; 1999.

Tomberlin JP, Saunders HD. *Evaluation, Treatment and Prevention of Musculoskeletal Disorders. Vol 2: Extremities.* Chaska, Minn: The Saunders Group; 1994:164.

Tubiana R, Thomine JM, Mackin E. *Examination of the Hand and Wrist.* New York, NY: CV Mosby Co; 1996.

Wadsworth CT. Elbow, forearm, wrist, and hand. In: Myers RS, ed. *Saunders Manual of Physical Therapy Practice.* Philadelphia, Pa: WB Saunders Co; 1995:841–917

Treatment

Burnett WR. Rehabilitation techniques for ligament injuries of the hand. *Hand Clin.* 1992;8: 803–815.

Randall T, Portney L, Harris BA. Effects of joint mobilization on joint stiffness and active motion of the metacarpal-phalangeal joint. *J Orthop Sports Phys Ther.* 1992;16:30–36.

Tendon Injuries

DESCRIPTION

Tendon injuries such as avulsion injuries, tendon lacerations, and crush injuries disrupt tendons as well as nearby soft tissues, nerve, or bone.

CAUSE

Hand injuries usually have a thermal, traction, crush, or chemical mode of injury. Burns, sudden muscular contraction against resistance, trauma, and sharp cuts may lead to tendon injury.

ASSESSMENT

Note: See APTA's Guide to Physical Therapist Practice. 2nd ed. *Physical Therapy.* 2001;81.

Musculoskeletal Preferred Practice Pattern: D

AREAS
- History, including occupation, hand dominance, details of injury, and psycho-social factors
- Pain
- Mobility, including active and passive range of motion (ROM), accessory motion, composite range of motion, and any fixed deformities
- Strength: compare with uninvolved hand, if applicable; power and precision
- Sensibility
- Skin and soft tissue: trophic changes, edema, temperature, condition of nails
- Joint integrity and structural deviations
- Neurological, including deep tendon reflexes and sensation
- Functional level
- Vascular

INSTRUMENTS/PROCEDURES

See References for sources.

Functional Level
- Jebsen Test of Hand Function
- Physical Capacity Evaluation

Joint Integrity and Structural Deviations
1. orthopedic tests of the hand
   - Bunnell-Littler test
   - circle formation with tip opposition between thumb and index finger test
   - digit collateral ligamentous stress test
   - elbow collateral ligament test
   - Finklestein test

- Froment's sign
- lateral and medial epicondylitis test
- lunate displacement test
- oblique retinacular ligament test
- retinacular test
- trigger finger test
- triquestrolunate test
- ulnar snuff box test
- Watson's test
2. photography of joint deformities

MOBILITY
- goniometry
- Guidelines for Measurement from the American Society for Surgery of the Hand (all motions measured from neutral starting position)

Neurological/Sensibility
- carpal and cubital tunnels
- Dellon modification of Moberg test
- distal ulnar tunnel
- Minnesota manual dexterity test
- Minnesota rate of manipulation test
- Moberg pick-up test
- nerve conduction velocity test
- O'Connor finger dexterity test
- Phalen's test
- pinch test
- point localization
- Purdue pegboard test
- ridge sensiometer
- Seddon coin test
- sensitivity to deep pressure
- sensitivity to light touch (Semmes-Weinstein monofilaments)
- sensitivity to pain
- sensitivity to temperature
- sudomotor test
- Tinel's sign
- two-point discrimination test
- vibratory test
- wrinkle test

Skin and Soft Tissue
1. edema
    - tape measure
    - volumetric measures
2. temperature
    - palpation

Strength
- grasp
- grip: sphygmomanometer and Jamar grip dynamometer
- pinch

Vascular
- Allen's test
- modified Allen's test
- capillary refill
- volumetric measures

PROBLEMS
- The pain is usually localized.
- There is usually immediate functional loss of hand usage.

TREATMENT/MANAGEMENT

Treatment depends on zone of injury. Zones of injury are divided into flexor zones, extensor zones, and the zones of the thumb. See Tables 5.1, 5.2, and 5.3.

TABLE 5.1
Flexor Zones of the Hand

Zone	Locator Descriptions
1	Includes the fingertips, distal interphalangeal (DIP) joint, and distal half between the DIP and proximal interphalangeal (PIP) joint
2	Includes the proximal half between the DIP and PIP joint, the PIP joint, and the metacarpal phalangeal (MCP) point to the palmar crease
3	Includes the space between the palmar crease to a line drawn across the palm at the distal point where the thumb joins the hand
4	Includes the space between the line drawn across the palm at the distal point where the thumb joins the hand to the crease at the wrist
5	Begins at the crease at the wrist up the forearm

Source: Reed K. *Quick Reference to Occupational Therapy.* Austin, Tex: PRO-ED Inc; 1991:266.

TABLE 5.2
Extensor Zones of the Hand

Zone	Locator Descriptions
1	Distal interphalangeal joints (DIP) of joints 2 to 5
2	Space between the DIP and proximal interphalangeal (PIP) joints of digits 2 to 5
3	PIP joints of digits 2 to 5
4	Space between the PIP joints and the metacarpal phalangeal (MCP) joints of digits 2 to 5
5	MCP joints
6	Space between the MCP joints and the carpal bones of the wrist
7	Carpal bones of the wrist

Source: Reed K. *Quick Reference to Occupational Therapy.* Austin, Tex: PRO-ED Inc; 1991:267.

TABLE 5.3
Zones of the Thumb

Zone	Locator Descriptions
T1	Interphalangeal (IP) joint
T2	Space between the IP joint and the metacarpal phalangeal (MCP) joint
T3	MCP joint
T4	Space between the MCP joint and the carpal bones of the wrist
T5	Area of the carpal bones on the thumb

Source: Reed K. *Quick Reference to Occupational Therapy.* Austin, Tex: PRO-ED Inc; 1991:267.

Rehabilitation of the flexor tendons after surgery is described in Table 5.4 following. Rehabilitation of the extensor tendons after surgery is described in Table 5.5 following.

PRECAUTIONS/CONTRAINDICATIONS
- Do not overstress healing tendon.

DESIRED OUTCOME/PROGNOSIS
- The client will return to normal function.

TABLE 5.4
Rehabilitation of Flexor Tendons after Surgical Repair

Time Post Surgery	Treatment
Day 0 to day 3	Elevation
Day 4 to week 3.5	Wear dorsal protective splint; passive flexion, active extension, composite and isolated joint movement 8 times every 2 hours; edema control
Week 3.5 through week 5	Switch to wrist cuff with dynamic traction or adapt splint; gentle active finger flexion, active wrist extension with finger flexion, active finger extension with wrist flexion, composite wrist and finger extension to neutral 10 times every hour
Week 6 through week 8	Discontinue splint or cuff active wrist flexion and extension; digital blocking exercise; differential tendon gliding 12 times per hour; begin scar management; use contracture control measures as needed; consider passive wrist and digit extension or extension splinting (week 7)
Week 9 through week 12	Progress to resistive exercise and work therapy

Source: Reprinted with permission from CT Wadsworth. Elbow, forearm, wrist, and hand. *Saunders Manual of Physical Therapy Practice.* Philadelphia, Pa: WB Saunders Co; 1995:841–917.

TABLE 5.5
Rehabilitation of Extensor Tendons after Surgical Repair

Zone	Time Post Surgery	Treatment
1, 2	Day 0 to day 3	Elevation
	Day 4 through week 7	Splint DIP joint in hyperextension (0 to 10 degrees)
	Week 8 through week 9	Decrease use of splint, gentle active DIP flexion (20 to 40 degrees)
	Week 10 through week 11	Full ROM and function
3, 4	Day 0 through day 3	Elevate hand
	Day 4 through week 6	Splint PIP joint (0 degrees); start DIP joint extension for central slip injury
	Week 7 through week 8	Decrease use of splint, begin gentle active PIP joint flexion and extension (MP joint in extension)
	Week 9 through week 10	Isolated PIP active extension with increasing resistance
5, 6	Day 0 through day 3	Elevate hand
	Day 4 through week 4	Volar forearm-hand splint (40 degrees wrist extension, 40 degrees wrist flexion, IP joint extension)
	Week 4	Active MP joint exercise, "clawing" exercise
	Week 5	Put splint in neutral position for 2 weeks; wrist ROM with finger extension, intrinsic muscle and "clawing" exercise
	Week 7 through week 9	Begin light resistive exercise
	Week 10 through week 11	Begin progressive resistive exercise
7	Day 0 through day 3	Elevate hand
	Day 4 through week 4	Volar forearm-hand splint (40 degrees wrist extension, 40 degrees MP flexion, IP joint extension if tendons injured)
	Week 4	Wrist flexion exercise (fingers extended) and finger flexion (wrist extended)
	Week 5 through week 6	Use splint with heavy activity; begin composite flexion and extension of wrist and fingers
	Week 7 through week 9	Begin light resistive exercise
	Week 10 through week 11	Begin progressive resistive exercise
Thumb 1, 2	Day 0 through day 3	Elevate hand
	Day 4 through week 6	Splint at IP joint (0 degrees)
	Week 7 through 8	Begin gentle active exercise
	Week 7 through week 9	Decrease use of splint
	Week 9 through week 11	Progress to full ROM and function
Thumb 3, 4	Day 0 through day 3	Elevate hand
	Day 4 through week 7	Splint MP joint (0 degrees) and wrist (30 degrees)
	Week 5 through week 6	Begin ROM
	Week 7 through week 8	Progress to full ROM and function
Thumb 5	Day 0 through day 3	Elevate hand
	Day 4 through week 4	Splint wrist in extension (40 degrees) and thumb extended
	Week 5 through week 6	Start active ROM
	Week 7 through week 8	Progress to full ROM and function

Source: Reprinted with permission from CT Wadsworth. Elbow, forearm, wrist, and hand. *Saunders Manual of Physical Therapy Practice.* Philadelphia, Pa: WB Saunders Co; 1995:841–917.

REFERENCES

Assessment

American Physical Therapy Association. Guide to physical therapist practice. 2nd ed. *Phys. Ther.* 2001;81.

Anthony MS. Sensory evaluation. In: Clark GL, Wilgis EF, Aiello B, et al, eds. *Hand Rehabilitation: A Practical Guide.* New York, NY: Churchill Livingstone; 1993:55–72.

Hackel ME, Wolfe GA, Bang SM, et al. Changes in hand function in the aging adult as determined by the Jebsen Test of Hand Function. *Phys Ther.* 1992;72:373–377.

Hamilton GF, McDonald C, Chenier TC. Measurement of grip strength: validity and reliability of the sphygmomanometer and Jamar grip dynamometer. *J Orthop Sports Phys Ther.* 1992;16:215–219.

LaStayo PC, Wheeler DL. Reliability of passive wrist flexion and extension goniometric measurements: a multicenter study. *Phys Ther.* 1994;74:162–174.

Rothstein JM, Roy SH, Wolf SL. *The Rehabilitation Specialist's Handbook.* 2nd ed. Philadelphia, Pa: FA Davis Co; 1998.

Tomberlin JP, Saunders HD. *Evaluation, Treatment and Prevention of Musculoskeletal Disorders. Vol 2: Extremities.* Chaska, Minn: The Saunders Group; 1994:164.

Tubiana R, Thomine JM, Mackin E. *Examination of the Hand and Wrist.* New York, NY: CV Mosby Co; 1996.

Wadsworth CT. Elbow, forearm, wrist, and hand. In: Myers RS, ed. *Saunders Manual of Physical Therapy Practice.* Philadelphia, Pa: WB Saunders Co; 1995:841–917.

Treatment

Brandsma JW, Brand PW. Claw finger correction: considerations in choice of technique. *J Hand Surg.* 1992;17B:615–621.

Cyr LM, Ross RG. How controlled stress affects healing tissues. *J Hand Ther.* 1998;11:125–130.

Margles SW. Early motion in the treatment of fractures and dislocation in the hand and wrist. *Hand Clin.* 1996;12:65–72.

Miller DS. Medical management of pain for early motion in hand and wrist surgery. *Hand Clin.* 1996;12:139–147.

Randall T, Portney L, Harris BA. Effects of joint mobilization on joint stiffness and active motion of the metacarpal-phalangeal joint. *J Orthop Sports Phys Ther.* 1992;16:30–36.

Russell CR. Bone and joint injury in the hand: therapist's commentary. *J Hand Ther.* 1999; 12:121–122.

Schreuders TA, Stam HJ, Hovius SE. Training of muscle excursion after tendon transfer. *J Hand Ther.* 1996;9:243–245.

Silverman PM, Gordon L. Early motion after replantation. *Hand Clin.* 1996;12:97–107.

Steelman P. Treatment of flexor tendon injuries: therapist's commentary. *J Hand Ther.* 1999;12:149–151.

Wadsworth CT. Elbow, forearm, wrist, and hand. In: Myers RS, ed. *Saunders Manual of Physical Therapy Practice.* Philadelphia, Pa: WB Saunders Co; 1995:841–917.

Wehbe MA. Early motion after hand and wrist reconstruction. *Hand Clin.* 1996;12:25–29.

Chapter 6

Infectious Disease Conditions

Human Immunodeficiency Virus (HIV) Infection

DESCRIPTION

HIV is an infection resulting from a retrovirus that may lead to a spectrum of clinical manifestations. The spectrum ranges from being an asymptomatic carrier to having a debilitating and ultimately fatal disorder. Acquired immunodeficiency syndrome (AIDS) is a secondary immunodeficiency syndrome at the extreme end of HIV infection clinical presentations. AIDS can lead to a variety of symptoms, including infections, malignancies, and neurological dysfunction. There have been clients who have recovered from AIDS.

CAUSE

A retrovirus named human immunodeficiency virus (HIV); previously named human T-cell lymphotropic virus type III [HTLV-III], lymphadenopathy-associated virus [LAV], and AIDS-associated retrovirus [ARV]. HIV-1 and HIV-2—two related viruses—have also been discovered to cause AIDS. Transmission of the virus requires contact with bodily fluids containing the infected cells or plasma. These bodily fluids, or exudates, include blood, breast milk, saliva, semen, and vaginal secretions. Documented transmission via saliva or droplets of nuclei that would be produced from coughing has not been established. In pregnant women, HIV can be transmitted through the placenta or perinatally.

ASSESSMENT

Note: See APTA's Guide to Physical Therapist Practice. 2nd ed. *Physical Therapy.* 2001;81.

Musculoskeletal Preferred Practice Pattern: C

Neuromuscular Preferred Practice Pattern: E

Cardiovascular/Pulmonary Preferred Practice Pattern: C

AREAS

- History, including history of opportunistic infections and nature of social support system
- Pain
- Mobility, including joint active range of motion (ROM)
- Posture
- Gait, including any deviations
- Neurological: reflexes, sensation (light touch, pain, and temperature), proprioception, position, balance, cognition, vision, plus bowel and bladder function
- Cardiovascular/pulmonary: resting heart rates, target heart rate, blood pressure, MET level, and overall level of fitness
- Functional level: activities of daily living (ADLs) and possibly ability to roll, transfer, use assistive devices

INSTRUMENTS/PROCEDURES

See References for sources.

Special Tests to Which the Physical Therapist May or May Not Have Access
- body composition: percent body fat measurement
- electrophysiologic testing
- Laboratory tests: enzyme-linked immunosorbent assay (ELISA) test, Western blot test, HIV culture, p24 antigen assay, polymerase chain reaction for HIV nucleic acid

Pain
- visual analog scale

PROBLEMS

- The client with neuromuscular manifestations of HIV may have peripheral neuropathy or myopathy.
- The client with AIDS dementia complex may show motor symptoms of loss of balance and lower extremity weakness and may report "clumsiness." This can lead to a decrease in joint mobility, difficulty ambulating, and deconditioning.
- The client may have incontinence, headaches, diminished cognition, aphasia, seizures, hemiparesis, hemisensory loss, difficulty breathing, visual disturbances, incoordination, cranial neuropathies, and pain.
- The client may have fibromyalgia, arthritis, and/or arthralgias.
- The client may have various skin problems. Some include Karposi's sarcoma lesions, herpes simplex, herpes zoster, and psoriasis.
- Many clients with AIDS have difficulty with at least 1 instrumental ADL and basic mobility.
- The client may be depressed or have other mood disorders.

TREATMENT/MANAGEMENT

Treatment involves:

- working with a team of specialists that may include physicians, pharmacists, psychologists, recreational therapists, social workers, speech-language pathologists, AIDS project volunteers, dieticians, family members/significant others, nurses, occupational therapists, and community pastoral care services
- educating both professionals and client about the disease and community resources, as needed

Note: Therapists should be aware of the variety of chemotherapeutic agents, which are rapidly expanding.

FITNESS

- Promote optimal fitness level with strength and conditioning activities.
- Maintain a flexible approach to treatment depending on client's stamina.
- Teach clients energy conservation measures, work-simplification techniques, and stress management.

EMOTIONS

- Give client "permission" to express feelings with statements such as, "It is common to be depressed about receiving a diagnosis of HIV."
- Express empathy through positive appropriate touch.

FUNCTION

- Assist client in gaining as much independence in function as possible. Provide ADL intervention and adaptive equipment as indicated. Assess and fit with splints, braces, or adaptive equipment.
- Provide mobility training.

GAIT

- Provide gait training with assistive devices as needed.

PAIN

- Assess for use of modalities to diminish pain. Consider use of transcutaneous electrical nerve stimulation (TENS), microcurrent electrical nerve stimulation (MENS), aquatics, relaxation exercises, and biofeedback for pain management.

Note: See Precautions.

JOINT MOBILITY
- Increase joint motion with stretching techniques, therapeutic exercise, postural training, functional movement patterns, and joint mobilization.

CENTRAL NERVOUS SYSTEM
- Provide perceptual-motor training.
- Consider use of facilitation and inhibition techniques for abnormal muscle tone.

RESPIRATORY
- Instruct in breathing exercises.
- Provide postural drainage and coughing techniques (except with Pneumocystis carinii pneumonia [PCP]).

SKIN
- Promote mobility.
- Prevention is a key component of treatment. Use pressure-relieving devices, proper skin care, good nutrition, and hydration.
- Instruct client and caregivers in proper positioning.
- Use whirlpool for wound care as indicated. Try to minimize use due to force. (See Precautions.)
- Consider use of occlusive dressings.

PRECAUTIONS/CONTRAINDICATIONS

GENERAL
- A client with hypersensitivity may not be able to tolerate electrotherapy, such as TENS. There is a report of reactivation of herpes simplex following TENS. Use modalities judiciously and monitor results.
- Therapists should practice universal precautions when in contact with mucous membranes or other surfaces in contact with bodily fluids. Precautions are indicated for any contact with blood and body fluids from *any* client.

Note: See Centers for Disease Control, Precautions (see References) for latest guidelines.

- Generally sharp or chemical debridement is contraindicated when T-cell count is under 50 mm3 or platelet count is under 50,000 mm3. Sharp debridement is contraindicated when neutrophil count is at 900 mm3 or higher.

Note: See Tucker in References for specific guidelines on wound care.

USE OF WHIRLPOOLS
- Follow guidelines from Centers for Disease Control (see References) for current standards.
- Wash hands and use gloves both before putting wound area in whirlpool and immediately after.
- Use other protective devices, such as mask, gown, and goggles, as directed by guidelines.
- When client is out of whirlpool wear sterile gloves for wound care.
- Discard disposable items in plastic bag and seal properly.

TO DISINFECT
- An agent such as sodium hypochlorite at 500 to 5000 ppm has been suggested to inactivate HIV rapidly. Consult manufacturer for recommendations. Sterilize as for any other infections.

Note: See References for additional guidelines.

DESIRED OUTCOME/PROGNOSIS

- The client will have a decrease in pain.
- The client will increase or maintain ROM.
- The client will increase or maintain normal muscle strength and movement patterns.
- The client will be functionally independent in ADLs.
- The client will ambulate independently with a normalized gait pattern.
- The client will breathe efficiently.
- The client will have intact skin with no breakdown.

REFERENCES

Assessment

American Physical Therapy Association. Guide to physical therapist practice. 2nd ed. *Phys Ther.* 2001;81

Galantino ML, Dellagatta R. HIV evaluation form. *Clin Manage Phys Ther.* 1990;10:6:30–36.

Galantino ML, McReynolds M. Managing pain in HIV. *Clin Manage Phys Ther.* 1992;12:6: 66–72.

Goodman C, Snyder TE. *Differential Diagnosis in Physical Therapy.* 2nd ed. Philadelphia, Pa: WB Saunders Co; 2000.

Treatment

Anonymous. Technical guidance on HIV counseling. Centers for Disease Control and Prevention. *MMWR* January 15, 1993:42:RR-2:11–17.

Balogun JA, Kaplan MT, Miller TM. The effect of professional education on the knowledge and attitudes of physical therapist and occupational therapist students about acquired immunodeficiency syndrome. *Phys Ther.* 1998;78:1073–1082.

Broner FA, Garland DE, Zigler JE. Spinal infections in the immunocompromised host. *Orthop Clin North Am.* 1996;27:37–46.

Butz L. Outpatient intervention in HIV. *Clin Manage Phys Ther.* 1992;12:6:51–53.

Coyne C. It need not be this way: AIDS and HIV. *Clin Manage Phys Ther.* 1992;12:6:51–53.

Dike L. Physiotherapists' perceptions of risk of HIV transmission in clinical practice. *Phys Ther.* 1993;79:3:178–185.

Galantino ML. *Clinical Assessment and Treatment of HIV: Rehabilitation of a Chronic Illness.* Thorofare, NJ: Slack; 1992.

Galantino ML, Jermyn RT, Tursi FJ, et al. Physical therapy management for the patient with HIV: lower extremity challenges. *Clin Podiatr Med Surg.* 1998;15:329–346.

Galantino ML, McReynolds M. The ever-changing challenge of HIV. *Clin Manage Phys Ther.* 1992;12:6:28–33.

Galantino ML, McReynolds M. Managing pain in HIV. *Clin Manage Phys Ther.* 1992;12:6: 66–72.

Grabois M, Garrison SJ, Hart KA, Lehmkuhl LD. *Physical Medicine and Rehabilitation: The Complete Approach.* Malden, Mass: Blackwell Science; 2000.

Hart M. More than just an infection: HIV. *Clin Manage Phys Ther.* 1992;12:6:42–50.

Hart M, Rogers EA. Acquired immunodeficiency syndrome. In: Fletcher GF, ed. *Rehabilitation Medicine: Contemporary Clinical Perspectives.* Philadelphia, Pa: Lea and Febiger; 1992:335–365.

Held SL. The effects of an AIDs education program on the knowledge and attitudes of a physical therapy class. *Phys Ther.* 1993;73:156–164.

Huba GJ, Brief DE, Cherin DA, et al. A typology of service patterns in end-stage AIDS care: relationships to the transprofessional model. *Home Health Care Serv Q.* 1998;17: 73–92.

Lang C. Community physiotherapy for people with HIV/AIDS. *Physiotherapy.* 1993;79:163–167.

Lang C. Experience of community physiotherapy for people with HIV infection. *Br J Occup Ther.* 1993;56:213–216.

Lang C. Using relaxation and exercise as part of the care of people living with HIV/AIDS. *Physiotherapy.* 1993;79:379–384.

Law V, Baldwin C. Nutritional support in HIV disease. *Physiotherapy.* 1993;79:394–399.

McClure J. The role of physiotherapy in HIV and AIDS. *Physiotherapy.* 1993;79:388–393.

Nixon S, Cott CA. Shifting perspectives: reconceptualizing HIV disease in a rehabilitation framework. *Physiotherapy Canada.* 2000;52:189–207.

Okoli U, King JD. Attitude towards people with HIV and AIDs. *Physiotherapy.* 1993;79:168–173.

Pillai G. Exercise and the immune system in HIV-infected individuals. *Physiotherapy Singapore.* 1998;1:86–87.

Potterton JL, Eales CJ. Prevalence of developmental delay in infants who are HIV positive. *S Afr J Physiotherapy.* 2001;57:11–15.

Reynolds JP. The polio of the 21st century: HIV and AIDS. *Clin Manage Phys Ther.* 1992;12:6:10.

Rogers EA. The interdisciplinary HIV team. *Clin Manage Phys Ther.* 1992;12:6:38–41.

Romani-Ruby C. HIV: ethical considerations. *Clin Manage Phys Ther.* 1992;12:6:62–65.

Rosensweet E, Fink CJ. Physical therapy for the patient with acquired immunodeficiency syndrome. *Clin Podiatr Med Surg.* 1992;9:883–893.

Sim J. Confidentiality and HIV status. *Physiotherapy.* 1997;83:90–96.

Smith K. Clinical features of HIV disease. *Physiotherapy.* 1993;79:375–378.

Smith K. HIV and the AIDS epidemic. *Physiotherapy.* 1993;79:3:159–162.

Smith K. HIV and the individual. *Physiotherapy.* 1993;79:371–375.

Tucker RS. Wound care in patients with HIV. *Clin Manage Phys Ther.* 1992;12:6:73–77.

Wicklund MP, Kissel JT. *Paraproteinemic Neuropathy.* 2001;3:147–156.

Williams B, Waters D, Partker K. *Am Fam Physician.* 1999;60:843–854.

Chapter 7

Injuries

Dislocation

DESCRIPTION

When a joint is dislocated, the articular surfaces are totally displaced. The joint structures that can be affected include the capsule, ligaments, tendons, bursae, nonarticular cartilage, and synovial fluid. The inflammation resulting from injury is often acute, subacute, or chronic. The inflammatory process may also lead to fibrous adhesions. A client may also have a chronically dislocating joint in which there is no acute ligamentous injury. The shoulder is the most commonly dislocated joint in adults, followed by the elbow. In children, the elbow is the most commonly dislocated joint.

Joint displacement can also occur to a lesser degree. Subluxation is a partial joint separation possibly related to damage of the capsule and ligaments.

CAUSE

Dislocations are often a result of disruptive forces from a long-lever-arm mechanism of injury. With smaller joints, dislocation is often due to the approximation of surrounding tissues.

ASSESSMENT

Note: See APTA's Guide to Physical Therapist Practice. 2nd ed. *Physical Therapy.* 2001;81.

Musculoskeletal Preferred Practice Patterns: D, I

Neuromuscular Preferred Practice Pattern: H

AREAS
- History
- Pain
- Posture, including symmetry and effect of injury on posture
- Skin and soft tissue: edema, temperature, color changes
- Gait, if applicable
- Joint integrity and structural deviations: crepitus, deformity, laxity
- Strength, including voluntary movements
- Mobility: active range of motion (ROM) within tolerance
- Functional level, including independence in activities of daily living (ADLs)

INSTRUMENTS/PROCEDURES
- subluxation measuring device

Special Tests to Which the Physical Therapist May or May Not Have Access
- x-rays

PROBLEMS
- The joint may appear misshapen.
- There is often a limitation of movement.
- There may be muscle spasm.
- The client often reports a tearing sensation.
- The client often reports intense pain initially that later eases.
- There is often a loss of function, and there may be muscle atrophy.

TREATMENT/MANAGEMENT
- Instruct client in proper positioning to avoid edema due to a dependent position.

- Initial treatment often involves reduction of the dislocation, which may have already been performed before the client sees a therapist. This is typically followed by a period of immobilization. Provide sling, traction, or bed rest as needed.
- Consider use of early mobilization with passive ROM and active-assistive ROM as indicated within pain tolerance and follow any precautions due to the direction of dislocation. Instruct client in movements allowed to prevent adhesions and atrophy.
- Progress to neuromuscular facilitation techniques, active movement, and resistive exercise.
- Modalities may include cold therapy, ultrasound, shortwave diathermy, and infrared.

PRECAUTIONS/CONTRAINDICATIONS
- Be aware of complications that often accompany dislocation, including fractures and injury to nerves, blood vessels, and surrounding tissues.

DESIRED OUTCOME/PROGNOSIS
- There will be a reduction of the joint dislocation.
- The client will experience a decrease in symptoms.
- There will be a maintenance of allowable movement and prevention of atrophy.
- The client will return to normal function.

Note: Surgical repair may be indicated when there is a complete ligamentous tear.

REFERENCES

Assessment

American Physical Therapy Association. Guide to physical therapist practice. 2nd ed. *Phys Ther.* 2001;81.

Buschbacher RM, ed. *Musculoskeletal Disorders: A Practical Guide for Diagnosis and Rehabilitation.* Boston, Mass: Andover Medical Publishers; 1994.

Daniels L, Worthingham C. *Muscle Testing Techniques of Manual Examination.* 6th ed. Philadelphia, Pa: WB Saunders Co; 1995.

Delitto A, Synder-Mackler L. The diagnostic process: examples in orthopedic physical therapy. *Phys Ther.* 1995;75:203–210.

Donatelli RA. *The Biomechanics of the Foot and Ankle.* 2nd ed. Philadelphia, Pa; 1996.

Hall CM, Brody TB. *Therapeutic Exercise: Moving Toward Function.* Philadelphia, Pa: Lippincott Williams and Wilkins; 1999.

Hertling D, Kessler RM. *Management of Common Musculoskeletal Disorders.* 3rd ed. Philadelphia, Pa: JB Lippincott Co; 1996:78,534.

Kendall FP, McCreary EK, Provance PG. *Muscles: Testing and Function.* 4th ed. Baltimore, Md: Williams and Wilkins; 1993.

Kisner C, Colby LA. *Therapeutic Exercise: Foundations and Techniques.* 3rd ed. Philadelphia, Pa: FA Davis Co; 1996:241–270.

Lesh SG. *Clinical Orthopedics for the Physical Therapist Assistant.* Philadelphia, Pa: FA Davis Co; 2000.

Malone TR, McPoil T, Nitz AJ, eds. *Orthopaedic and Sports Physical Therapy.* 3rd ed. St. Louis, Mo: CV Mosby Co; 1997.

Myers RS, ed. *Saunders Manual of Physical Therapy Practice.* Philadelphia, Pa: WB Saunders Co; 1995.

Rothstein JM, Roy SH, Wolf SL. *The Rehabilitation Specialist's Handbook*. 2nd ed. Philadelphia, Pa: FA Davis Co; 1998.

Schunk C, Reed K. *Clinical Practice Guidelines*. Gaithersburg, Md: Aspen Publishers; 2000.

Tomberlin JP, Saunders HD. *Evaluation, Treatment and Prevention of Musculoskeletal Disorders. Vol 2: Extremities*. Chaska, Minn: The Saunders Group; 1994.

Treatment

Becker HP, Rosenbaum D, Kriese T, et al. Gait asymmetry following successful surgical treatment of ankle fractures in young adults. *Clin Orthop Rel Res*. 1995;2:262–269.

Brumback RJ, Toal TR, Murphy-Zane MS, et al. Immediate weight-bearing after treatment of a comminuted fracture of the femoral shaft with a statically locked intramedullary nail. *J Bone Joint Surg Am*. 1999;81:1538–1544.

Cole BJ, Harner CD. The multiple ligament injured knee. *Clin Sports Med*. 1999;18:241–262.

Contesti LA. The radioulnar joints and forearm axis: therapist's commentary. *J Hand Ther*. 1999;12:85–91.

Lynch SA, Renstrom PA. Groin injuries in sport: treatment strategies. *Sports Med*. 1999;28:137–144.

Magarey M, Jones M. Clinical diagnosis and management of minor shoulder instability. *Aust J Physiotherapy*. 1992;38:269–280.

Margles SW. Early motion in the treatment of fractures and dislocations in the hand and wrist. *Hand Clin*. 1996;12:65–72.

McAtee SJ. Low-energy scapular body fracture: a case report. *Am J Orthop*. 1999;28:468–472.

Myers RS, ed. *Saunders Manual of Physical Therapy Practice*. Philadelphia, Pa: WB Saunders Co; 1995:823, 824, 886, 897–900.

Ogawa K, Yoshida A, Inokuchi W. Posterior shoulder dislocation associated with fracture of the humeral anatomic neck: treatment guidelines and long-term outcome. *J Trauma*. 1999;46:318–323.

Shamus JL, Shamus EC. A taping technique for the treatment of acromioclaicular joint sprains: a case study. *J Orthop Sports Phys Ther*. 1997;256:390–394.

Terada N, Yamada H, Seki T, et al. The importance of reducing small fractures of the coronoid process in the treatment of unstable elbow dislocation. *J Shoulder Elbow Surg*. 2000;9:344–346.

Tinetti ME, Baker DI, Gottschalk M, et al. Home-based multicomponent rehabilitation program for older persons after hip fracture: a randomized trial. *Arch Phys Med Rehabil*. 1999;80:916–922.

Tung TC, Chen HC, Hsiao CW, et al. Chronic volar dislocation of the metacarpophalangeal joint of the thumb: a case report and review of the literature. *J Trauma*. 1996;41:561–564.

Turnbull JR. Acromioclavicular joint disorders. *Med Sci Sports Exerc*. 1998;30:S26–32.

Weinstock TB. Management of fractures of the distal radius; therapist's commentary. *J Hand Ther*. 1999;12:99–102.

Fractures

DESCRIPTION

A fracture is defined as discontinuity of bone structure. A fracture that occurs in an otherwise normal bone is classified—in terms of the relationship of the fracture fragments to the external environment—as closed when the skin is intact or open (compound) when the skin has been injured.

CAUSE

A fracture can be caused by pathology or trauma.

- Pathological causes include congenital defects, dysplasias, infectious disease, metabolic disease, and neoplasms.
- Traumatic causes include direct or indirect force. Muscular force can also lead to fracture due to avulsion of the muscular attachment to the bone.

Stress fractures are also common and associated with inadequate training and musculoskeletal malalignment.

ASSESSMENT

Note: See APTA's Guide to Physical Therapist Practice. 2nd ed. *Physical Therapy.* 2001;81.

Musculoskeletal Preferred Practice Patterns: G,H, I

AREAS
- History
- Pain
- Posture, including symmetry, effect of injury on posture
- Skin and soft tissue: edema, temperature, and color changes
- Gait, if applicable—eg, ambulation outcome after hip fracture
- Joint integrity and structural deviations: crepitus, deformity, and laxity
- Strength, including voluntary movements
- Mobility, including active range of motion (ROM) within tolerance and precautions
- Functional level, including independence in activities of daily living (ADLs)

INSTRUMENTS/PROCEDURES

Classifications
- Salters fracture classification

Functional Level
- functional outcomes after hip fracture
- Harris Hip Score

Gait
- ambulation outcomes after hip fracture

Mobility
- passive stiffness of the ankle

Special Tests to Which the Physical Therapist May or May Not Have Access
- acetabular contact pressure testing
- ultrasound

PROBLEMS

GENERAL

- The client often has pain and tenderness.
- There is often a loss of function or abnormal movement.
- There may be swelling or hemorrhage.
- There may be crepitus.
- There is often deformity.

STRESS FRACTURE

- The client often has extreme pain at site of injury.
- The client often has skin irritation at site of injury.
- The client often reports relief of pain with rest.

TREATMENT/MANAGEMENT

- After the fracture has been properly immobilized—which usually occurs before the client reaches therapy—treatment focuses on restoration and preservation of function.
- Provide modalities for pain reduction such as transcutaneous electrical nerve stimulation (TENS), ice, ultrasound, or moist heat.
- Instruct in gait training with assistive devices such as crutches, as indicated.
- Instruct in respiratory care for clients at risk for respiratory problems, such as clients with a thoracic area injury or spinal cord injury.

During the immobilization period, consider the following:

- Protect the fracture area from any contraindicated WB forces.
  1. Encourage movement of noninvolved joints.
  2. Use isometric exercises for joint where movement is contraindicated.
  3. Encourage independence in ADLs.
  4. Instruct client in signs of proper use of cast/splint.

When full mobilization is allowed, consider the following:

1. Provide strengthening exercises for muscles, using resistive exercises and proprioceptive neuromuscular facilitation (PNF) patterns with resistance.
2. Provide training in restoration of function.
3. Provide mobilization as indicated with exercise, passive mobilization, and aquatic therapy.
4. Instruct client in care of skin after cast/splint is removed.

Treatment for stress fractures involves rest from pain-inducing activity. As symptoms allow, the client may engage in cardiovascular activities such as swimming or cycling, which allow for fitness without excessive weight bearing. Consider use of orthotics. Training or resumption of previous activities should be gradual after x-ray confirms no defects on the bone.

PRECAUTIONS/CONTRAINDICATIONS

- Stress fracture injury may not appear on x-ray until 2 to 3 weeks after onset of symptoms.
- Remain alert for local and generalized complications affecting skin, viscera, bone, joints, muscles, tendons, nerves, and arteries.
- Local complications can include, but are not limited to: lacerations, spinal cord injury, delayed union, avascular necrosis, infection, Sudeks atrophy, myositis ossificans, neuropraxia, thrombosis, and impaired arterial perfusion.
- General complications can include, but are not limited to: fat or pulmonary embolism and venous thrombosis.

DESIRED OUTCOME/PROGNOSIS

- The client will preserve function in noninjured areas.
- The client will restore function to injured areas.
- The client will have normal movement.

Notes: A good index of rehabilitation outcome is the recovery of independent ambulation.

In general, stress fractures may take a period of healing equal to the period of symptoms.

REFERENCES

Assessment

American Physical Therapy Association. Guide to physical therapist practice. 2nd ed. *Phys Ther.* 2001;81.

Buschbacher RM, ed. *Musculoskeletal Disorders: A Practical Guide for Diagnosis and Rehabilitation.* Boston, Mass: Andover Medical Publishers; 1994.

Daniels L, Worthingham C. *Muscle Testing Techniques of Manual Examination.* 6th ed. Philadelphia, Pa: WB Saunders Co; 1995.

Delitto A, Synder-Mackler L. The diagnostic process: examples in orthopedic physical therapy. *Phys Ther.* 1995;75:203–210.

Donatelli RA. *The Biomechanics of the Foot and Ankle.* 2nd ed. Philadelphia, Pa; 1996.

Givens-Heiss DL, Krebs DE, Riley PO, et al. In vivo acetabular contact pressures during rehabilitation: postacute phase. *Phys Ther.* 1992;72:700–710.

Hall CM, Brody TB. *Therapeutic Exercise: Moving Toward Function.* Philadelphia, Pa: Lippincott Williams and Wilkins; 1999.

Hertling D, Kessler RM. *Management of Common Musculoskeletal Disorders.* 3rd ed. Philadelphia, Pa: JB Lippincott Co; 1996:78, 534.

Kendall FP, McCreary EK, Provance PG. *Muscles: Testing and Function.* 4th ed. Baltimore, Md: Williams and Wilkins, 1993.

Kisner C, Colby LA. *Therapeutic Exercise: Foundations and Techniques.* 3rd ed. Philadelphia, Pa: FA Davis Co; 1996:241–270.

Krebs DE, Elbaum L, Riley PO, Hodge WA, Mann RW. Exercise and gait effects on in vivo hip contact pressures. *Phys Ther.* 1991;71:301–309.

Lesh SG. *Clinical Orthopedics for the Physical Therapist Assistant.* Philadelphia, Pa: FA Davis Co; 2000.

Malone TR, McPoil T, Nitz AJ, eds. *Orthopaedic and Sports Physical Therapy.* 3rd ed. St. Louis, Mo: CV Mosby Co; 1997.

Moffa Trotter ME, Anemaet WK. Home care for hip fracture survivors and fallers: The "Be HIP!" Program. *Top Geriatr Rehabil.* 1996;12:1:55–58.

Myers RS, ed. *Saunders Manual of Physical Therapy Practice.* Philadelphia, Pa: WB Saunders Co; 1995.

Rothstein JM, Roy SH, Wolf SL. *The Rehabilitation Specialist's Handbook.* 2nd ed. Philadelphia, Pa: FA Davis Co; 1998.

Schunk C, Reed K. *Clinical Practice Guidelines.* Gaithersburg, Md; 2000.

Strickland EM, Fares M, Krebs DE, et al. In vivo acetabular contact pressures during rehabilitation: acute phase. *Phys Ther.* 1992;72:691–699.

Tomberlin JP, Saunders HD. *Evaluation, Treatment and Prevention of Musculoskeletal Disorders. Vol 2: Extremities.* Chaska, Minn: The Saunders Group; 1994.

Vandervoort AA, Chesworth BM, Cunningham DA, Rechnitzer PA, Paterson DH, Koval JJ. An outcome measure to quantify passive stiffness of the ankle. *Can J Pub Health.* 1992; 83(suppl 2):S19–S23.

Treatment

Baker AW, McMahon J, Moos KF. Current consensus on the management of fractures of the mandibular condyle. *Int J Oral Maxilofac Surg.* 1998;27:258–266.

Bartosh RA, Dugdale TW, Neilsen R. Isolated musculocutaneous nerve injury complicating closed fracture of the clavicle: a case report. *Am J Sports Med.* 1992;20:356–359.

Bialocerkowski A. A home program is as effective as in-rooms in the management of distal radius fracture. *Aust J Physiotherapy.* 2001;47:68.

Bohannon RW, Andrews AW, Thomas MW. Walking speed: Reference values and correlates for older adults. *J Orthop Sports Phys Ther.* 1996;24:2:86–90.

Braun W, Wiedemann M, Rutter A, Kundel K, et al. Indications and results of nonoperative treatment of patellar fractures. *Clin Orthop.* 1993;289:197–201.

Brindle TJ, Coen M. Scapular avulsion fracture of a high school wrestler. *J Orthop Sports Phys Ther.* 1998;27:444–447.

Brownstein B, Bronner S. Patella fractures associated with accelerated ACL rehabilitation in patients with autogenous patella tendon reconstructions. *J Orthop Sports Med.* 1997; 26:168–172.

Burns A, Park K. Proximal femoral fractures in the female patient, a controlled trial: the role of the occupational therapist and the physiotherapist. *Br J Occup Ther.* 1992;55:397–400.

Camden P, Nade S. Fracture bracing the humerus. *Inj.* 1992;23:245–248.

Carter PR, Frederick HA, Laseter GF. Open reduction and internal fixation of unstable distal radius fractures with a low-profile plate: a multicenter study of 73 fractures. *J Hand Surg.* 1998;23:300–307.

Dai YT, Huang GS, Yang RS, et al. Effectiveness of a multidisciplinary rehabilitation program in elderly patients with hip fractures. *J Formos Med Assoc.* 2001;100:120–126.

Davis DS, Post WR. Segond fracture: lateral capsular ligament avulsion. *J Orthop Sport Phys Ther.* 1997;25:103–106.

Edwards SG, Whittle AP. Nonoperative treatment of ipsilateral fractures of the scapula and clavicle. *J Bone Joint Surg.* 2000;82:774–780.

Feldman MD. Arthroscopic excision of type II capitellar fractures. *Arthroscopy.* 1997;13: 743–748.

Felsenthal F, Garrison SJ, Steinberg FU, eds. *Rehabilitation of the Aging and Elderly Patient.* Baltimore, Md: Williams and Wilkins; 1994.

Gaffney KM. Avulsion injury of the serratus anterior: a case history. *Clin J Sports Med.* 1997;7:134–136.

Guccione AA, Fagerson TL, Anderson JJ. Regaining functional independence in the acute care setting following hip fracture. *Phys Ther.* 1996;76:818–826.

Gutierres M, Cabral T, Miranda A. Fractures of the posteromedial process of the talus: a report of two cases. *Int Orthop.* 1998;22:394–396.

Hakim RM, Gruen GS, Delitto A. Outcomes of patients with pelvic-ring fractures managed by open reduction internal fixation. *Phys Ther.* 1996;76:286–295.

Harada ND, Chun A, Chiu V, et al. Patterns of rehabilitation utilization after hip fracture in acute hospitals and skilled nursing facilities. *Med Care.* 2000;38:1119–1130.

Henry P, Panwitz B, Wilson JK. Rehabilitation of a post-surgical patella fracture: case report. *Physiotherapy*. 2000;86:139–142.

Hoenig H, Sloane R, Horner R, et al. What is the role of timing in the surgical and rehabilitative care of community-dwelling older persons with acute hip fracture? *Arch Int Med*. 1997;157:485–486.

Imura K, Ishii Y, Yagisawa K, et al. *Arch Orthop Trauma Surg*. 2000;120:369–371.

Jarnlo GB, Thorngren KG. Background factors to hip fractures. *Clin Orthop Related Res*. 1993;287:41–49.

Jones DL, Erhard RE. Diagnosis of trochanteric bursitis versus femoral neck stress fracture. *Phys Ther*. 1997;77:58–67.

Kay S, Haensel N, Stiller K. The effect of passive mobilisation following fractures involving the distal radius: a randomized study. *Aust J Physiotherapy*. 2000;46:93–101.

Kennedy EM. Hip fracture outcomes in peoples 50 and over—background paper. *U.S. Government Printing Office*. Washington, DC: 1994.

Koval KJ, Gallagher MA, Marsicano JG, et al. Functional outcome after minimally displaced fractures of the proximal part of the humerus. *J Bone Joint Surg*. 1997;79:203–207.

Levi SJ. Posthospital setting, resource utilization, and self-care outcome in older women with hip fracture. *Arch Phys Med Rehabil*. 1997;78:973–979.

Lewis CD, Bottomly JM, eds. *Geriatric Physical Therapy: A Clinical Approach*. Norwalk, Conn: Appleton and Lange; 1994.

Luz JG, Chilvarquer I. Remodelling of bilateral fractures of the mandibular condyle. *Acta Orthopaedica Belgica*. 1996;93:167–170.

Margles SW. Early motion in the treatment of fractures and dislocations in the hand and wrist. *Hand Clin*. 1996;12:65–72.

McAndrew M. The treatment of geriatric hip fractures. *Top Geriatr Rehabil*. 1996;12:32–37.

McClure PW, Flowers KR. Treatment of limited shoulder motion: a case study based on biomechanical considerations. *Phys Ther*. 1992;72:929–936.

McGarvey CL. Effect of a thermoplastic orthosis in the rehabilitation of a patient with a scapular fracture. *Phys Ther*. 1983;63:1289–1291.

Melchiorre PJ. Acute hospitalization and discharge outcome of neurologically intact trauma patients sustaining thoracolumbar vertebral fractures managed conservatively with thoracolumbosacral orthoses and physical therapy. *Arch Phys Med Rehabil: N Engl J Med*. 1999;340:389–390.

Michlovitz S. Rehabilitation after displaced intra-articular fracture of the distal radius. *Phys Ther Case Rep*. 2000;3:226–232.

Myers AH, Palmer MH, Engel BT, et al. Mobility in older patients with hip fractures: examining pre-fracture status, complications, and outcomes at discharge from the acute-care hospital. *J Orthop Trauma*. 1996;10:1996.

Myers RS, ed. *Saunders Manual of Physical Therapy Practice*. Philadelphia, Pa: WB Saunders Co; 1995:80, 115, 175, 632–633, 885, 906–907, 1259, 1274, 1290.

Nashi M, Ashby V, Muddu BN, et al. Is there any place for the physiotherapist service in the fracture clinic? *J Clin Effectiveness*. 1998;3:134–136.

Olson K. Rehabilitation: nonacute physical therapy. In: Hansen ST, Swiontkowski MF, eds. *Orthop Trauma Protocols*. New York, NY: Raven Press; 1993:65–72.

Parker MJ, Handoll HHG, Dynan Y. Mobilisation strategies after hip fracture surgery in adults. *Cochrane Libr*. 2000;4:13.

Puckree T, Moonasur R, Govender K. Bedrest alters respiratory muscle strength inpatients immobilized due to fractured femurs. *S Afr J Physiotherapy*. 2001;54:27–30.

Rapado A. General management of vertebral fractures. *Bone*. 1996;18(suppl 3):191S–196S.

Reigger-Krugh C. In: Malone TR, McPoil T, Nitz AJ, eds. *Orthop Sports Phys Ther*. 3rd ed. St. Louis, Mo: CV Mosby Co; 1997.

Ringsberg K, Johnell O, Obrant K. Balance and speed of walking of women with Colles' fractures. *Physiotherapy*. 1993;79:689–692.

Rush S. Rehabilitation following ORIF of the hip. *Top Geriatr Rehabil*. 1996;12:38–45.

Sennwald G. The effects of wrist distraction on carpal kinematice. *J Hand Surg*. 1999;24: 1344–1345.

Shaffer MA, Okereke E, Esterhai JL, et al. Effects of immobilization on plantar-flexion torque, fatigue resistance, and functional ability following an ankle fracture. *Phys Ther*. 2000; 80:769–780.

Sherrington C, Lord SR. Home exercise to improve strength and walking velocity after hip fracture; a randomized controlled trial. *Arch Phys Med Rehab*. 1997;78:208–212.

Sine R, Liss SE, Rousch RE, et al. *Basic Rehabilitation Techniques: A Self-Instructional Guide*. 4th ed. Gaithersburg, Md: Aspen Publishers; 2000.

Stetson WB, Friedman MJ, Fulkerson JP, et al. Fracture of the proximal tibia with immediate weightbearing after a Fulkerson osteomoty. *Am J Sports Med*. 1997;25:570–574.

Thomas RL. Management of hip fracture in the geriatric patient: A team approach in the institutional setting. *Top Geriatr Rehabil*. 1996;12:59–69.

Tinetti ME, Baker DI, Gottschalk M. Systematic home-based physical and functional therapy for older persons after hip fracture. *Arch Phys Med Rehabil*. 1997;78:1237–1247.

Vandenborne K, Elliott MA, Watler GA, et al. Longitudinal study of skeletal muscle adaptations during immobilization and rehabilitation. *Muscle Nerve*. 1998;21:1006–1012.

Varga TL. Acute physical therapy. In: Hansen ST, Swiontkowski MF, eds. *Orthopaedic Trauma Protocols*. New York, NY: Raven Press; 1993:61–64.

Wajswlner H. Management of rowers with rib stress fractures. *Aust J Physiotherapy*. 1996; 42:157–161.

Wakefield AE, McQueen MM. The role of physiotherapy and clinical predictors of outcome after fracture of the distal radius. *J Bone J Surg Br*. 2000;82:972–976.

Warden SJ, Bennell KL, McMeeken JM, et al. Can conventional therapeutic ultrasound units be used to accelerate fracture repair? *Phys Ther Rev*. 1999;4:117–126.

Weinstock TB. Management of fractures of the distal radius: therapist's commentary. *J Hand Ther*. 1999;12:99–102.

Weiss JM. Treatment of leg edema and wounds in a patient with severe musculoskeletal injuries. *Phys Ther*. 1998;78:1338–1339.

Head Injury

Also known as *traumatic brain injury*.

DESCRIPTION

Problems caused from head injury may be due to primary damage and/or secondary effects. Primary damage refers to the specific brain trauma. Secondary effects refers to the damage caused by metabolic and physiologic events occuring after the initial trauma.

Men are more frequently injured than women. More than 500,000 new cases of traumatic brain injury each year are due to a head injury. Out of that number, 70,000 clients develop disabilities that hinder a normal independent life.

Traumatic head injury is the number one cause of mortality in American children and young adults, with the typical victim being 15 to 24 years old.

CAUSE

Approximately half of all traumatic head injuries are caused by motor vehicle accidents. The remainder are attributed to falls (~21%), assaults and violence (~12%), and sport or recreation (~10%).

ASSESSMENT

Note: See APTA's Guide to Physical Therapist Practice. 2nd ed. *Physical Therapy.* 2001;81.

Neuromuscular Preferred Practice Pattern: I

AREAS

- History
- Psychosocial
- Posture, including alignment in supine, side-lying, and sitting positions
- Cognition, including behavioral status
- Communication, including any aphasia, dysarthria, or hearing problems
- Cardiovascular, including heart rate and blood pressure changes with activity
- Pulmonary, including ventilator dependency, infection, and need for suctioning
- Neurological, including sensation, proprioception, and reflexes—facial avoidance, rooting, asymmetric tonic neck reflex (ATNR), Babinski, tonic labyrinthine reflex, and associated movements
- Mobility, including passive range of motion (ROM) and trunk mobility, especially lumbar/pelvic rotation

Note: See Precautions when testing cervical ROM.

- Motor function, including tone, resistance to passive movement, spontaneous movement, and volitional movement
- Balance: static and dynamic
- Skin and soft tissue: discoloration, edema, and pressure sores
- Gait, if indicated, including symmetry, coordination, and any extension in standing
- Functional level, including activities of daily living (ADLs), bed mobility, and transfers
- Equipment, including use of intracranial pressure (ICP) bolt and monitor, adaptive equipment, assistive devices, splints, orthotics, or wheelchair

INSTRUMENTS/PROCEDURES

Balance
- clinical balance testing and clinical vestibular testing (functional testing and provocation of specific deficits)

Cardiovascular
- exercise testing

Cognition
- Rancho Los Amigos Levels of Cognitive Functioning (LOCF)
- Galveston Orientation and Amnesia Test
- Westmead Posttraumatic Amnesia Scale

Communication
- speech and language assessment

Disability
- Rappaport's Disability Rating Scale

Functional Level

- Action Research Arm Test
- Glasgow Coma Scale
- Institute of Medicine index
- Level of Rehabilitation Scale (LORS–II)

- Rivermeade ADL Assessment
- World Health Organization International Classification of Impairments, Disabilities, and Handicaps

Mobility

- mobility scale
- precasting assessment

Motor Function

- dynamometer

Neurological

- brain potentials
- finger-to-nose test

Special Tests to Which the Physical Therapist May or May Not Have Access

- auditory testing
- cerebral blood flow (CBF) mapping
- computed tomography (CT) scan
- computed sinusoidal harmonic acceleration
- dynamic platform posturography

- electroencephalograms (EEGs)
- electronystagmogram
- magnetic resonance imaging (MRI)
- platform fistula testing
- sensory organization testing

PROBLEMS

- The client often has a decreased level of consciousness.
- The client often has learning, memory, and information-processing deficits.
- The client may have receptive and expressive communication disorders.
- The client often has behavioral disorders.
- The client is often deconditioned, with general weakness and loss of flexibility.
- The client may have hemiparesis or bilateral hemiparesis.
- The client often has a balance deficit.
- The client may have unilateral or bilateral ataxia.
- The client often has a coordination deficit.
- The client may have an intention tremor.
- The client may have associated injuries.
- If unconscious, the client may have impaired mucociliary clearance.

TREATMENT/MANAGEMENT

ACUTE CARE

- Schedule frequent position changes.
- Assist to sitting, standing, or supported standing position.
- For chest PT, consider postural drainage, percussion, vibration and shaking, rib springing, or suction, as indicated.
- Use manual techniques to facilitate respiration, assisted sitting, and standing.
- Begin passive ROM.
- Consider use of splints or prophylactic short leg casts and passive standing using a tilt table.
- Consider continuous passive motion (CPM) for minimum time per day to achieve a beneficial effect.
- Begin functional mobility training after the client reaches a stable medical status.
- Consider sensory stimulation for clients in an unresponsive state.

REHABILITATION

Rehabilitation is based on the level of cognitive function (LOCF) (see Table 7.1 following).

LOCFs 1 to 3
- Evaluate the effectiveness of positioning devices. Consider casting if client is unresponsive for more than 2 weeks.
- Continue passive ROM to prevent contractures. Place in side-lying position for shoulder ROM slow, controlled stretches.
- Consider use of sensory stimulation or sensory regulation, usually in short sessions of 15 to 30 minutes via one or two modalities at a time. Stimulation may be auditory, visual, olfactory, gustatory, tactile, or vestibular.

LOCF 4
- Continue with LOCF 1 to 3, and add transfers, ambulation, and other functional activities.
- Encourage active mobility as soon as the client is able.

LOCFs 5 and 6
- Increase ROM.
- Increase physical conditioning.
- Treat hemiparesis, nerve injury, or ataxia as for a patient without brain injury (see Chapter 10: Neurological Disorders).

LOCFs 7 and 8
- Integrate cognitive, physical, and emotional skills.
- Continue problem-solving and planning activities for ADLs.
- Consider electrical stimulation.
- Address any need for strengthening with weights, proprioceptive neuromuscular facilitation (PNF), biofeedback, isokinetic exercisers, or sling suspension.
- To affect tone, consider inhibitory or facilitory techniques as indicated.
- Use coordination, balance, and sensation activities as indicated.

TABLE 7.1
Rancho Los Amigos Levels of Cognitive Functioning (LOCF) Following Head Injury

LOCF	Response
LOCF1–No response	Appears to be in a deep sleep/completely unresponsive to any stimuli
LOCF2–Generalized response	Reacts inconsistently and nonpurposefully to stimuli
LOCF3–Localized response	Reacts specifically but inconsistently to stimuli
LOCF4–Confused-agitated	Heightened state of activity. Behavior is bizarre, and verbalizations are frequently incoherent
LOCF5–Confused-inappropriate	Responds to simple commands somewhat consistently
LOCF6–Confused-appropriate	Goal-directed behavior possible under direction
LOCF7–Automatic-appropriate	Behavior appropriate but somewhat robotic
LOCF8–Purposeful-appropriate	Can recall and integrate past and recent events and respond to environment

Source: Reprinted with permission from P. Leahy Traumatic head injury. *Physical Rehabilitation: Assessment and Treatment.* Schmitz TJ and O'Sullivan SB. FA Davis Co; 1994:49.

- For pain, consider use of ultrasound, ice, or transcutaneous electrical nerve stimulation (TENS).
- Encourage activities to build endurance.
- For edema, consider mild electrical stimulation for swelling.
- Facilitate increased mobility with wheelchair, transfers, and bed mobility activities.
- For ambulation training, use external support and assistance as needed.
- For respiratory problems, consider deep breathing and coughing exercises.
- If possible, consider the use of a therapeutic pool or hippotherapy.

PRECAUTIONS/CONTRAINDICATIONS

- Do not test cervical ROM if ventriculostomy or Richmond bolt is present. Consult with medical staff on other restrictions when these devices are in place.
- Avoid prolonged pressure over shunt if present.
- Generally, the client is kept in a position with head elevated while in the acute phase.
- Passive ROM should be used with caution due to client's low level of consciousness in LOCFs 1 to 3.
- Footboard may have the counterproductive effect of increasing tone into a position of plantar flexion instead of the desired response of decreasing it.
- Secondary brain damage caused by late-occurring intracranial hematomas can turn a relatively mild injury into a life-threatening condition.
- A client's status may change quickly and dramatically. Maintain frequent communication with nurse.
- Sitting is contraindicated if the autoregulation of intracranial pressure or blood pressure is lost.
- Standing is contraindicated if unfixated, displaced fractures of long bones are present.
- Avoid ROM in area with arterial lines, and exercise caution to avoid dislodging other tubing when moving client.

DESIRED OUTCOME/PROGNOSIS

General

- The client's level of consciousness will increase.
- The client's musculoskeletal system will improve in flexibility.
- Contractures, respiratory distress, and skin breakdown will be prevented (loss of ROM may be so severe that it interferes with functional tasks if not prevented).
- Functional mobility training will increase the client's tolerance of upright posture and increase active movement.
- Client will achieve optimal function and minimize disability.

LOCF AS AN OUTCOME PREDICTOR OF FUNCTIONING

- LOCFs 1 to 3 may be considered a low level.
- LOCFs 4 to 6 may be considered midlevel.
- LOCFs 7 and 8 may be considered high level.

PHYSICAL LEVELS DEFINED BY IMPAIRMENT

- Minimal impairment: independent but with balance and coordination deficits
- Moderate impairment: ambulatory with assistance
- Severe impairment: dependent for ADLs

PREDICTED OUTCOME BASED ON COMBINED LOCF AND PHYSICAL LEVELS

- Low-level cognitive skill and minimal impairment: acutely ill but fair prognosis
- High-level cognitive skill, but severe physical disability: high need for adaptive equipment

- Midlevel cognitive skill and minimal impairment: good prognosis, but need to educate family regarding residual deficits

Notes: Outcome is influenced by preinjury level of function, degree of immediate damage to the brain (primary damage), and effect of secondary brain damage.

One study found that unilateral compensatory treatments are not justified physiologically. They should be superseded by treatments that guide axonal and dendritic development and facilitate the opening of new pathways. Long-term physical therapy may continue to enhance recovery.

One study reported on head injury survivors at 3 months after the injury and found the following:

- 4% in a vegetative state
- 8% severely disabled
- 22% moderately disabled
- 66% showing good recovery

There are very few absolute predictors of success. Prevention is the only real "cure" for head injury.

REFERENCES

Assessment

American Physical Therapy Association. Guide to physical therapist practice. 2nd ed. *Phys Ther.* 2001;81

Bryan VL. Management of residual physical deficits. In: Ashley MJ, Krych DK, eds. *Traumatic Brain Injury Rehabilitation.* New York, NY: CRC Press; 1995:131–186.

Cammack S, Eisenberg MG, eds. *Key Words in Physical Rehabilitation: A Guide to Contemporary Usage.* New York, NY: Springer Publishing Co; 1995:45.

DeLisa D. *Rehabilitation Medicine: Principle and Practice.* Philadelphia, Pa: Lippincott; 1998.

Grabois M, Garrison SJ, Hart KA, Lehmkuhl LD. *Physical Medicine and Rehabilitation: The Complete Approach.* Malden, Mass: Blackwell Science; 2000.

Krych DK, eds. *Traumatic Brain Injury Rehabilitation.* New York, NY: CRC Press; 1995:131–186.

O'Sullivan SB, Schmitz TJ, eds. *Physical Rehabilitation: Assessment and Treatment.* 3rd ed. Philadelphia, Pa: FA Davis Co; 1994:494.

Patla AE, Clous SD. Visual assessment of human gait: reliability and validity. *Rehabil Res.* 1998;1:87–96.

Roland PS, Otto E. Vestibular dysfunction after traumatic brain injury: evaluation and management. In: Ashley MJ, Krych DK, eds. *Traumatic Brain Injury Rehabilitation.* New York, NY: CRC Press; 1995:131–186.

Sine R, Liss SE, Rousch RE, et al. *Basic Rehabilitation Techniques: A Self-Instructional Guide.* 4th ed. Gaithersburg, Md: Aspen Publishers; 2000.

Swain BR, Sullivan SJ. Reliability of the scores for the finger-to-nose test in adults with traumatic brain injury. *Phys Ther.* 1993;73:71–78.

Williams G, Goldie P. Validity of motor tasks for predicting running ability in acquired brain injury. *Brain Inj.* 2001;15:831–841.

Treatment

Alderman N, Shepherd J, Youngson H. Increasing standing tolerance and posture quality following severe brain injury using a behaviour modification approach. *Physiotherapy.* 1992;78:335–343.

Bezner JR, Hunter DL. Wellness perception in persons with traumatic brain injury and its relation to functional independence. *Arch Phys Med Rehabil.* 2001;82:787–792.

Bryan VL. Management of residual physical deficits. In: Ashley MJ, Krych DK, eds. *Trauma Brain Inj Rehabil.* New York, NY: CRC Press; 1995:131–186.

Chua KSG, Kong K. Rehabilitation outcome following traumatic brain injury—the Singapore experience. *Int J Rehabil Res.* 1999;22:189–197.

Cifu DX, Kreutzer JS, Marwitz JH, et al. Functional outcomes of older adults with traumatic brain injury: a prospective, multicenter analysis. *Arch Phys Med Rehabil.* 1996;77: 883–888.

Denys P, Azouvi P, Denormandie P, et al. Late cognitive and behavioral improvement following treatment of disabling orthopaedic complications of a severe closed head injury. *Brain Inj.* 1996;10:149–153.

DeToledo JC, Haddad H. Progressive scoliosis in early, non-progressive CNS injuries: role of axial muscles. *Brain Inj.* 1999;13:39–43.

Durham DP. Occupational and physical therapists' perspective of the perceived benefits of a therapeutic home visit program. *Phys Occup Ther Geriatr.* 1992;10:3:15–33.

Geurts AD, Ribbers GM, Knoop JA, et al. Identification of static and dynamic postural instability following traumatic brain injury. *Arch Phys Med Rehabil.* 1996;77:639–644.

Goldstein B, Hammond M. Physical medicine and rehabilitation. *JAMA.* 1997;277:1891–1892.

Grabois M, Garrison SJ, Hart KA, Lehmkuhl LD. *Physical Medicine and Rehabilitation: The Complete Approach.* Malden, Mass: Blackwell Science; 2000.

Hall M, Brandys C, Yetman L. Multidisciplinary approaches to management of acute head injury. *J Neurosci Nurs.* 1992;24:4:199–204.

Horn LJ, Zasler ND, eds. *Medical Rehabilitation of Traumatic Brain Injury.* St. Louis, Mo: Mosby Year Book; 1996.

Kay RM, Dennis S, Rethlefsen S, et al. Impact of postoperative gain analysis on orthopaedic care. *Clin Orthop.* 2000;23:259–264.

Keren O, Reznik J, Groswasser Z, et al. Combined motor disturbances following severe traumatic brain injury: an integrative long-term approach. *Brain Inj.* 2001;15:633–638.

Kerrigan DC, Bang MS, Burke DT. An algorithm to assess stiff-legged gait in traumatic brain injury. *J Head Trauma Rehabil.* 1999;14:136–145.

Leahy P. Head trauma in adults: problems, assessment, and treatment. In: Lister MJ, ed. *Contemporary Management of Motor Control Problems: Proceedings of the II STEP Conference.* Fredricksburg, Va; Foundation for Physical Therapy; 1991:247–251.

Leahy P. Traumatic head injury. In: O'Sullivan SB, Schmitz TJ, eds. *Physical Rehabilitation: Assessment and Treatment.* 3rd ed. Philadelphia, Pa: FA Davis Co; 1994:491–508.

Lehmkuhl D. *Brain Injury Glossary.* Houston, Tex: HDI Publishers; 1992.

Lehmkuhl LD, Krawczyk L. Physical therapy management of the minimally responsive patient following traumatic brain injury: coma stimulation. *Neurol Rep.* 1993;17:10–17.

Linan E, O'Dell MW, Pierce JM. Continuous passive motion in the management of heterotopic ossification in a brain injured patient. *Am J Phys Med and Rehabilitation.* 2001; 80:614–617.

McGhee-Pierce S, Mayer NH, Whyte J. Computer-assisted exercise systems in traumatic brain injury: cases and commentary. *J Head Trauma Rehabil.* 2001;16:406–413.

McIlvoy L, Spain DA, Raque G, et al. Successful incorporation of the Severe Head Injury Guidelines into a phased-outcome clinical pathway. *J Neurosci Nurs.* 2001;33:72–78.

Montgomery J. *Phys Ther Trauma Brain Inj.* New York, NY: Churchill Livingstone; 1995.

Moseley AM. The effect of casting combined with stretching on passive ankle dorsiflexion in adults with traumatic head injuries. *Phys Ther.* 1997;77:240–247.

Murdock KR, Klein P. Physical therapy intervention for acute head injury. *Phys Ther Pract.* 1994;3:19–36.

Newton RA. Evaluation and treatment of balance problems associated with traumatic brain injury. *Phys Ther Pract.* 1994;3:218–226.

Orest M. Casting protocol for patients with neurological dysfunction. *PT-Magazine Phys Ther.* 1993;1:51–55.

Orest M. Patients with a low level of responsiveness. In: Myers RS, ed. *Saunders Manual of Physical Therapy Practice.* Philadelphia, Pa: WB Saunders Co; 1995:405–410.

Passler MA, Riggs RV. Positive outcomes in traumatic brain injury – vegetative state: patients treated with bromocriptine. *Arch Phys Med Rehabil.* 2001;82:311–315.

Rice-Oxley M, Turner-Stokes L. Effectiveness of brain injury rehabilitation. *Clin Rehabil.* 1999;13 suppl: 7–24.

Roland PS, Otto E. Vestibular dysfunction after traumatic brain injury: evaluation and management. In: Ashley MJ, Krych DK, eds. *Trauma Brain Inj Rehabil.* New York, NY: CRC Press; 1995:131–186.

Rosenthal M, Griffith ER, Bond MR, Miller JD. *Rehabilitation of the Adult and Child with Traumatic Brain Injury.* 3rd ed. Philadelphia: Pa: FA Davis; 1999.

Sine R, Liss SE, Rousch RE, et al. *Basic Rehabilitation Techniques: A Self-Instructional Guide.* 4th ed. Gaithersburg, Md: Aspen Publishers: 2000.

Spence C. The development of physiotherapeutic intervention with the head injured patient. *Ulster Med J.* 1998;67 suppl 1:56–62.

Stephenson R. A review of neuroplasticity: some implications for physiotherapy in the treatment of lesions of the brain. *Physiotherapy.* 1993;79:699–704.

Swain BR, Sullivan SJ. Longitudinal profile of early motor recovery following severe traumatic brain injury. *Brain Inj.* 1996;10:347–366.

Trettin H. Craniocerebral trauma caused by sports: pathogenic mechanism, clinical aspects and physical therapy with special reference to manual lymph drainage. *J Lymphol.* 1993;17:2:36–40.

Wales LR, Bernhardt JA. Case report: A case for slow to recover rehabilitation services following severe acquired brain injury. *Aust J Physiotherapy.* 2000;46:143–146.

Weingarden HP, Zeiling G, Heruti R et al. Hybrid functional electrical stimulation orthosis system for the upper limb: effects spasticity in chronic stable hemiplegia. *Am J Phys Med Rehabil.* 1998;77:276–281.

Woltersdorf MA. Beyond the sensorimotor strip. *Clin Manage Phys Ther.* 1992;12:3:63–69.

Balance-Related References

Bohannon R. Standing balance and function over the course of acute rehabilitation. *Arch Phys Med Rehabil.* 1995;76:994–996.

Chen H, Ashton-Miller J, Alexander N, et al. Effects of age and available response time on ability to stop over an obstacle. *J Gerontol.* 1994;49:M227–233.

DiFabio R, Seay R. Use of the "fast evaluation of mobility, balance, and fear" in elderly community dwellers: validity and reliability. *Phys Ther.* 1997;77:904–917.

Feltner M, MacRae P, McNitt-Gray J. Quantitative gait assessment as a predictor of prospective and retrospective falls in community-dwelling women. *Arch Phys Med Rehabil.* 1994;75:447–453.

Graham D, Newton RA. *Physiotherapy Res Intern.* 1999;4:293–301.

Haarda N, Chiu V, Damron-Rodriques J, et al. Screening for balance and mobility impairment in elderly individuals living in residential care facilities. *Phys Ther.* 1995;75:462–469.

Jeka J. Light touch contact as a balance aid. *Phys Ther.* 1997;77:476–487.

Lord S, Castell S. Effect of exercise on balance, strength and reaction time in older people. *Aust J Physiotherapy.* 1994;40:83–88.

Lord SR, Ward JA, Williams P. Effect of water exercise on balance and related factors in older people. *Aust J Physiotherapy.* 1993;42:1110–1117.

Maki B, Holliday P, Topper A. A prospective study of postural balance and risk of falling in an ambulatory and independent elderly population. *J Geriatr.* 1994;49:M72–M84.

Maki B, McIlroy W. The role of limb movement in maintaining upright stance: the "change-in-support" strategy. *Phys Ther.* 1997;77:488–507.

Orest MR, Blaisdell KA. Reliability testing of a timed functional performance protocol for adults with mild traumatic brain injury. *Physiotherapy Can.* 2000;52:131–137.

Swaine BR, Sullivan SJ. Interpreting reliability of early motor function measurement following head injury. *Physiotherapy Theory Pract.* 1999;15:155–164.

Winter D. *ABCs of Balance during Standing and Walking.* Waterloos, Ontario: Waterloo Biomechanics; 1995.

Woollacott M, Tang P. Balance control during walking in the older adult: research and its implications. *Phys Ther.* 1997;646–660.

Lower Extremity Amputation

DESCRIPTION

Amputation is the removal of a limb or appendage from the body. Levels of amputation are usually listed by anatomical consideration.

Note: Levels of amputation are from the Task Force on Standardization of Prosthetic and Orthotic Terminology:

- A below-knee (transtibial) amputation leaves a limb of between 20% and 50% of the original tibial length.
- A short below-knee amputation leaves a limb of less than 20% of tibial length.
- An above-knee (transfemoral) amputation leaves a limb of between 35% and 60% of femoral length.
- A long above-knee amputation leaves a limb of more than 60% of femoral length.

Note: Table 7.2 outlines other levels of lower extremity amputation.

TABLE 7.2
Levels of Lower Extremity Amputation/Disarticulation Sites

Level	Description
Toe disarticulation	Disarticulation at the metatarsal phalangeal joint
Syme's	Ankle disarticulation with attachment of heel pad to distal end of tibia; may include removal of malleoli and distal tibial/fibular flares
Knee disarticulation	Amputation through the knee joint; femur intact
Hip disarticulation	Amputation through hip joint; pelvis intact

Source: Reprinted with permission from O'Sullivan SB, Schmitz TJ. *Physical Rehabilitation.* FA Davis Co; 1994:376.

CAUSE

The main cause of amputation in the lower extremity is peripheral vascular disease, especially associated with smoking and diabetes. The next leading cause is trauma (eg, gunshot wound or motor vehicle accident) followed by malignant tumor, infections, and limb discrepancies.

ASSESSMENT

Note: See APTA's Guide to Physical Therapist Practice. 2nd ed. *Physical Therapy.* 2001;81.

Integumentary Preferred Practice Patterns: A, E

Musculoskeletal Preferred Practice Pattern: K

AREAS

- History
- Psychosocial, including depression and discharge plans
- Residual limb girth, length, shape, and level of amputation
- Skin and soft tissue, including edema and scars
- Vascular
- Neurological, including sensation
- Pain, including phantom pain and phantom sensation
- Pulmonary
- Mobility, including range of motion (ROM)
- Strength
- Balance
- Gait
- Functional level, including ADLs, bed mobility, transfers, wheelchair mobility and management, and elevations
- Equipment: assess prosthesis if available

INSTRUMENTS/PROCEDURES

See References for sources.

Equipment
- prosthetic requirements examination

Functional Level
- Barthel ADL index
- Functional Independence Measure
- Katz Index of ADLs
- Level of Rehabilitation Scale (LORS–II)
- PULSES profile
- Sickness Impact Profile

Gait
- gait recovery pattern assessment
- measurement of energy cost of walking

Mobility
- goniometry
- Get Up and Go Test

Strength
- manual muscle testing

PROBLEMS

- The client often has pain of intrinsic origin (eg, bone or vascular pain), or extrinsic origin (eg, pressure from a cast or phantom limb pain).
- There will be grief, and the client may experience depression.
- There may be adherent scar tissue.
- There may be edema in the residual limb.
- The client may have loss of strength, balance, and coordination.

- There may be functional loss.
- There may be medical complications.
- With forefoot amputation, the client may have balance loss, weight-bearing loss, proprioceptive loss, and loss of leverage.

TREATMENT/MANAGEMENT

TREATMENT POST SURGERY

Immediate postoperative care can include the following: deep breathing exercises, coughing, stump dressing care, positioning, exercise program, transfer procedures, and early ambulation.

Treatments for specific levels of amputation:

- *Toe disarticulation:* Cautiously mobilize (manually) any adherent scar tissue.
- *Forefoot amputation:* Stretch medial border of residual foot. Consider scar mobilization.
- *Ankle disarticulation (Syme's):* Stump end must be protected postsurgically. Client should not be allowed to bear weight without a heel pad.
- *Below-knee amputation:* Enhance weight bearing with slight flexion on stance to place weight-bearing on patellar tendon.
- *Knee disarticulation:* Emphasize hip extension.
- *Above-knee (transfemoral) amputation:* Prevent contractures. Before gait training, check for stump socket wall contact on all four sides. Prepare for gait training with stump exercises, balance exercise, and step practice.
- *Hip disarticulation:* Reduce edema in tissues surrounding the disarticulation. Exercise program before initiation of gait training should include uninvolved leg exercise, trunk range of motion (ROM), pelvic tilt, bilateral arm exercise, and scar mobilization.

GENERAL

- Instruct client to use firm support when lying and sitting. Have client use a firm mattress and provide with a wheelchair board.
- To prepare for ambulation, emphasize the following muscles: trunk extensors, abdominals, hip and knee extensors, hip and knee flexors. Use isometric exercises progressing to isotonic action.
- Teach the following transfers: bed to chair, with prosthesis, and with an overhead device.
- Promote early ambulation activities, including weight-bearing tolerance activities. Prior to receiving a prosthesis, clients with a unilateral amputation may use a three-point gait pattern.
- Assess socket position, suspension system, and alignment of temporary prosthetic device.
- Preparation for prosthetic fitting involves:
  1. educating the client about the prosthetic process
  2. facilitating stump maturation or healing of any stump skin problems; consider use of whirlpool, ultraviolet, suture line taping, bandaging, splinting, and reapplication of the rigid dressing
- Provide gait training by beginning with parallel bars. Progress with weight-shifting activities, heel-strike to foot-flat position, foot-flat to midstance position, and step-through. Monitor skin tolerance carefully.
- For edema, consider the use of elastic bandaging, shrinker sock application, rigid dressings, air splint, intermittent pressure pumping, pneumatic walking aid, and weight-bearing without an ambulation device.
- For any decrease in strength, consider a graded exercise regimen.

- For any decrease in ROM, consider the cautious use of heat or cold, as indicated; manual stretching techniques such as passive, active, and contract-relax; splinting with serial casting; active exercises; and ambulation with prosthesis.
- For any sensory impairment, consider desensitization with vibration, stroking, percussion, and touching. Increase proprioceptive awareness with biofeedback and education to prevent skin trauma.
- For stump pain, consider the use of positioning, desensitization techniques, thermal modalities, transcutaneous electrical nerve stimulation (TENS), and weight-bearing activities.

PROSTHETIC MANAGEMENT

Management of the prosthesis includes the following:
- educating the client on maintenance and usage
- performing the prescription assessment
- adding to the prosthetic prescription as indicated
- assessing the prosthesis
- promoting physical and emotional acceptance
- training the client in donning, doffing, balance and coordination, gait and activities of daily living (ADLs), transfers, climbing, maintenance, and monitoring of skin response to use of prosthesis

PRECAUTIONS/CONTRAINDICATIONS

- Clients with bilateral amputations who are often in a sitting position are more likely to develop flexion contractures. Pillows under a stump should probably be discarded.
- A postoperative plaster cast can allow early weight bearing, but if it loosens, it should not be pushed back onto the stump. The upward pushing effort can cause the suture line to split. Adjustments to a prosthetic device must be performed by an experienced professional.
- The residual stump should be elevated only if there is excessive postoperative bleeding. Circulatory impairment restricts the use of thermal modalities.
- A client with claudication pain should be counseled to walk within comfort level. After pain begins, the client should rest the leg completely before resuming. Closely monitor skin response to prosthesis.
- Bandages should never be applied in a circular motion; restricted circulation may result.
- Caution should be used when prescribing exercise for clients with cardiac disease or hypertension.

DESIRED OUTCOME/PROGNOSIS

BEFORE PROSTHETIC FITTING
- The client will achieve the highest level of function possible.
- The client will be physically and psychologically ready for prosthetic rehabilitation.
- The client will prevent or reduce edema of residual limb.
- The client will prevent contracture.
- The client will maintain or increase strength in affected and remaining extremities.
- The client will be independent in mobility and ADLs.

AFTER PROSTHETIC TRAINING
- The client will maintain full ROM.
- The client will reach achievable muscular strength.

- The client will be able to care for the residual limb properly.
- The client will reach residual limb shrinkage.
- The client will reach potential for independence with bed mobility, transfers, and ambulation without the prosthesis.
- The client will reach independence with a wheelchair.
- The client will be independent in use of prosthesis for ADLs, dressing, transfers, wearing, and ambulation.
- The client will be informed about available support.

Note: Achievement may be limited by age, strength, endurance level of amputation, length of time after amputation, general medical status, pain, motivation, contractures, and any joint pathology.

REFERENCES

Assessment

American Physical Therapy Association. Guide to physical therapist practice. 2nd ed. *Phys Ther.* 2001;81.

Baker PA, Hewison SR. Gait recovery pattern of unilateral lower limb amputees during rehabilitation. *Prosthet Orthot Int.* 1990;14:2:80–84.

Bohannon RW. Manual muscle testing of the limbs: consideration, limitations, and alternative. *Phys Ther Pract.* 1992;2:11–21.

Bohannon RW. Nature, implications, and measurement of limb muscle strength in patients with orthopaedic or neurologic disorders. *Phys Ther Pract.* 1992;2:22–31.

Cammack S, Eisenberg MG, eds. *Key Words in Physical Rehabilitation: A Guide to Contemporary Usage.* New York, NY: Springer Publishing Co; 1995:92.

Daniels L, Worthingham C. *Muscle Testing Techniques of Manual Examination.* 6th ed. Philadelphia, Pa: WB Saunders Co; 1995.

Kendall FP, McCreary EK, Provance PG. *Muscles, Testing and Function.* 4th ed. Baltimore, Md: Williams and Wilkins; 1993.

Patrick DG. Prosthetics. In: Myers RS, ed. *Saunders Manual of Physical Therapy Practice.* Philadelphia, Pa: WB Saunders Co; 1995:1124–1130.

Weaver CJ. Terminology: assisted gaits. *Clin Manage Phys Ther.* 1992;12:1:32–37.

Treatment

Barr AE, Siegel KL, Danoff JV, et al. Biomechanical comparison of the energy-storing capabilities of SACH and Carbon Copy II prosthetic feet during the stance phase of gait in a person with below-knee amputation. *Phys Ther.* 1992;72:344–354.

Condie E, Scott H. Slow rehabilitation of a traumatic lower limb amputee. *Physiotherapy Res Int.* 1998;3:233–238.

Davidson J, Champion S, Cousins R, et al. Rehabilitation of a quadruple amputee subsequent to electrical burns sustained whilst hang gliding. *Disability Rehabil.* 2001; 23:90–95.

Edelstein JE. Prosthetic assessment and management. In: O'Sullivan SB, Schmitz TJ, eds. *Phys Rehabil.* 3rd ed. Philadelphia, Pa: FA Davis Co; 1994:397–419.

Engstrom B, Van de Ven C. *Physiotherapy for Amputees.* 2nd ed. New York, NY: Churchill Livingstone; 1993.

Esquenazi A, DiGiacomo R. Rehabilitation after amputation. *J Am Podiatr Med Assoc.* 2001;91:13–22.

Glassey N. Physiotherapy following replantation: case study. *Physiotherapy.* 1999;85:109–112.

Johnston C. Current concepts in lower limb amputee management: a multidisciplinary approach. *JARNA.* 2000;3:10–14.

Levin A. How are physiotherapists using the Vessa Pneumatic Post-Amputation Mobility Aid? *Physiotherapy.* 1992;78:318–322.

May BJ. Assessment and treatment of individuals following lower extremity amputation. In: O'Sullivan SB, Schmitz TJ, eds. *Phys Rehabil.* 3rd ed. Philadelphia, Pa: FA Davis Co; 1994:533–576.

May BJ. *Amputations and Prosthetics: A Case Study Approach.* Philadelphia, Pa: FA Davis Co; 1996.

Mueller MJ. Identifying patients with diabetes mellitus who are at risk for lower-extremity complications: use of Semmes-Weinstein monofilaments. *Phys Ther.* 1996;76:68–71.

Palma T, Hoyle D. Lower-extremity amputation. *Clin Manage Phys Ther.* 1992;12:3:96–99.

Patrick DG. Prosthetics. In: Myers RS, ed. *Saunders Manual of Physical Therapy Practice.* Philadelphia, Pa: WB Saunders Co; 1995:1121–1182.

Penington G, Warminton S, Hull S, Freijah N. Rehabilitation of lower limb amputees and some implications for surgical management. *Aust N Z J Surg.* 1992;62:774–779.

Pernot HF, Winnubst GM, Cluitmans JJ, et al. Amputees in Limburg: incidence, morbidity and mortality, prosthetic supply, care utilization and functional level after one year. *Prosthet Orthot Int.* 2000;24:90–96.

Porter-Romatowski TL, Deckert MMJ. Hemicorporectomy: a case study from a physical therapy perspective. *Arch Phys Med Rehabil.* 1998;79:464–468.

Singh S, Evans L, Datta D, et al. The costs of managing lower limb-threatening ischaemia. *Eur J Vasuclar Endovascular Surg.* 1996;12:359–362.

Welchon JG, Armstrong DG, Harkless LB. Pedal manifestations of meningococcal septicemia. *J Am Podiatr Med Assoc.* 1996; 1996;86:129–131.

Spinal Cord Injuries: Paraplegia

DESCRIPTION

Paraplegia is the partial or complete loss of neurologic function due to a spinal injury. Injury may result in a lesion at the level of the thoracic or lumbar spinal cord or at the sacral roots. With a complete lesion, no sensory or motor function remains below the level of the lesion. Typically the level of the lesion is defined as the most distal uninvolved nerve root segment with normal function at the corresponding skeletal level.

Incomplete lesions include the Brown-Sequard syndrome, anterior cord syndrome, central cord syndrome, and posterior cord syndrome. Approximately 54% of spinal cord injuries occurring in the United States are classified as incomplete. This classification is given if there is any motor or sensory function intact more than three levels below the level of neurologic injury.

CAUSE

Traumatic spinal cord injuries often result from a fall, sporting activity, diving accident, motor vehicle accident, or gunshot wound. Complete lesions are caused by transection with a severing action or by severe compression. Incomplete lesions usually result from contusions. Nontraumatic damage may also occur, such as vascular impairment to the cord, but it is not as common as damage due to trauma. Eighty percent of all spinal cord injuries occur in people under the age of 40.

ASSESSMENT

Note: See APTA's Guide to Physical Therapist Practice. 2nd ed. *Physical Therapy.* 2001;81.

Neuromuscular Preferred Practice Pattern: H

AREAS
- History
- Psychosocial
- Pain
- Pulmonary, including muscle strength and tone of respiratory muscles, chest expansion and mobility, breathing pattern and respiratory rate, cough effectiveness, vital capacity, tidal volume, and posture
- Cardiovascular, including endurance and heart rate
- Skin and soft tissue
- Neurological, including sensation and reflexes
- Motor control, including muscle tone
- Strength
- Mobility, including passive range of motion (ROM)
- Gait, as indicated, including ambulation potential
- Functional assessment, including activities of daily living (ADLs)
- Equipment, including home environment

INSTRUMENTS/PROCEDURES

Functional Level
- Barthel ADL index
- Functional Independence Measure
- Katz Index of ADLs
- Level of Rehabilitation Scale (LORS–II)

Gait
- based on motor scores of muscular strength

Motor Control
- modified Ashworth scale of muscle spasticity

Special Tests to Which the Physical Therapist May or May Not Have Access
- sacral sparing
- spinal canal assessment
- hydrostatic weight measurement

Strength
- manual muscle testing
- shoulder torque
- the Frankel scale

The six-point scale for grading muscles is illustrated in Table 7.3.

PROBLEMS

PRIMARY
- The client will often have motor deficits and sensory loss.
- The client will often have impaired temperature control.

TABLE 7.3
Six-Point Scale for Grading Muscles: Paralysis to Movement Scale

Scale	Description
0	Total paralysis
1	Palpable or visible contraction
2	Active movement, full ROM with gravity eliminated
3	Active movement, full ROM against gravity
4	Active movement, full ROM against moderate resistance
5	(Normal) active movement, full ROM against full resistance
NT	Not testable

Source: Reprinted courtesy of the American Spinal Injury Association. Chicago, Illinois.

- The client may have respiratory impairment.
- The client may have spasticity.
- The client will often have bladder and bowel dysfunction.
- The client will often have sexual dysfunction.

SECONDARY
- The client may develop autonomic dysreflexia.
- The client may develop contractures.
- The client may develop deep-vein thrombosis.
- The client may develop heterotopic bone formation.
- The client often experiences postural hypotension.
- The client may develop pressure sores.
- The client often has some complaints of pain; sources can be nerve root, physical trauma, spinal cord, or musculoskeletal.

TREATMENT/MANAGEMENT

ACUTE PHASE

Strengthening of Selected Musculature
- Strengthen upper extremity muscles, with emphasis on triceps, latissimus dorsi, and shoulder depressors, and functional activities.
- Exercise techniques in the early phase may include manual resistance in straight-plane motions or upper extremity proprioceptive neuromuscular facilitation (PNF) patterns, progressing to resistive exercise with cuffed weights.
- Pulley weight systems and sports may be used in the later phases of rehabilitation. Bilateral activities should be emphasized.
- Biofeedback may be used to augment the exercise program. It is typically used as an adjunct to motor retraining but may also be used for management of autonomic problems.

Consider use of neuromuscular stimulation (NMS) to counteract the impact of immobilization. Functional neuromuscular stimulation (FMS) may also be used to produce extremity motions for functional activities, including standing and amputation. Upper extremity FMS may be used to enhance reconstructive surgery. NMS can decrease the risk of deep vein thrombosis in paralyzed gastric musculature.

ROM
- Except for areas contraindicated (see Precautions following), full ROM exercises should be performed daily. It is preferable for ROM to be done in both prone and supine positions, if possible.
- Use selective stretching to allow development of selected tightness in enhancing function. For example, a tenodesis grasp in a patient with a C-6 and C-7 quadriplegia is formed by allowing mild tightness of long finger flexors to develop. This improves grasp by allowing fingers to close upon wrist extension and the fingers to open upon wrist flexion with assistance from gravity.

Positioning
- After the fracture site is stabilized, gradual acclimation to an upright posture is indicated. To facilitate acclimation, the patient may need an abdominal binder, elastic stockings, and/or elastic wraps.
- Consider splints for wrists, hands, and fingers, as well as ankle splints or boots. Gradually increase tolerance to prone position.

Respiratory Care
- Respiratory care may include the following activities: deep breathing exercises, glossopharyngeal breathing (for high-level cervical lesions), airshift chest expansion and chest mobility, diaphragm-strengthening exercises, assisted coughing, and stretching of pectoral and chest wall muscles.
- Consider the use of an abdominal support.
- Intervention strategies may include postural drainage and chest PT techniques such as vibration and percussion.

SUBACUTE PHASE
- Continue respiratory management, ROM, and positioning.
- Expand resistive exercises for innervated muscles.
- Include interval training—with upper extremity aerobic activity—for cardiovascular training.
- Teach independence in mobilization.
- Mat programs may be initiated after patient is cleared for activity. Mat programs are varied and can include facilitating mastery of the components of functional skills. Component skills may involve activities such as rolling; transition to sidelying; prone-on-elbows, prone-on-hands, or supine-on-elbows position; pull-ups (with quadriplegia); transition to sitting (long and short); transition to quadriped position (in paraplegia); and kneeling (in paraplegia). Consider using group mat activities.
- Independent transfer training may be initiated after adequate sitting balance is achieved. Transfer training can include two-person lift, stand-pivot transfer, airlift, sliding board transfer, and lateral and forward transfers. Basic functional transfer activities include:
  1. wheelchair to bed, car, toilet, or chair
  2. chair to bath or floor (an advanced-level skill)
- Prescribe wheelchair and teach management skills. Basic wheelchair skills include weight shifting; propelling the wheelchair; managing brakes, armrests, and legrest/footrests; and picking up objects off the floor. Advanced wheelchair skills include wheelies, ramps and curbs, stairs, getting wheelchair into the car, and controlled falling.

Ambulation
- Determine if patient is a candidate for ambulation.
- Prescribe orthotics; usually ankle and/or knee bracing is adequate, but low thoracic lesions, level T-9 to T-12, will need knee-ankle-foot orthoses (KAFOs).

- Consider use of functional electrical stimulation (FES). This modality can assist with ambulation and endurance activities but is still in the experimental stage and not widely available.
- Ambulation training includes donning and doffing orthoses, sit-to-stand activities, trunk balancing, push-ups, turning around, jackknifing, and parallel bars activities. Teach gait patterns such as four-point, two-point, swing-to and swing-through patterns, elevation activities, and controlled falling. Levels of ambulation usually include the following: standing only, therapeutic ambulation, indoor/functional ambulation and community ambulation. FES or FNS units may be used to facilitate ambulation. FES does not restore gait to pre-injury levels. Gait is slow with large energy consumption and there is risk of triggering autonomic dysreflexia with lesions above T6.

Treatment of Pressure Sores

- Use topical therapy debridement and dressing technique for pressure sores, grade 3 or grade 4, a minimum of twice daily. See Table 7.4 for grades for pressure sores.
- Consider use of whirlpool, hyperbaric oxygen, electrical stimulation, and laser therapy.

Psychosocial Issues

- Although physical therapy deals primarily with the physical and functional losses that a patient experiences, therapists need to be aware of the psychosocial issues facing a spinal-cord-injured patient.
- Physical therapists should work closely with other team members to address psychosocial issues such as home modifications, community re-entry, driving, communication skills, feeding, hygiene, bladder training, dressing, and other ADLs.
- Address psychosocial issues, including normalization, promoting independence, positive atmosphere, and interactions with the rehabilitation team, education, and social support.
- Formal strategies for discharge include counseling, education, social skills training, bladder and bowel retraining for postacute management, recreation training, pharmaceutical planning, and postdischarge planning.
- Psychosexual treatment involves physical evaluation, education, behavioral treatment, counseling, and prescription of physical aids for penile erectile dysfunction.

TABLE 7.4
Grades of Pressure Sores

Grade	Description
1	Limited to superficial epidermis and dermal layers
2	Involves the epidermal and dermal layers and extends into the adipose tissue
3	Extends through the superficial structures and adipose tissue down to and including muscle
4	Destroys all soft tissue structures down to bone, with communication with bone or joint structures or both

Source: Reprinted courtesy of the National Spinal Cord Injury Association. Thorofare, NJ.

PRECAUTIONS/CONTRAINDICATIONS

- Avoid allowing the patient to maintain a posture in bed of constant shoulder flexion, adduction, internal rotation, elbow flexion, and forearm pronation.
- Redness over bony prominences should be gone within 30 minutes of the position change.
- Surgical intervention may be needed for pressure sores if conservative measures are not successful.
- Unresolved pressure sores may lead to chronic localized infection, osteomyelitis, sepsis, or even death.
- During the acute period, caution should be used during muscle strengthening to avoid stress at the fracture site, especially at the hips and trunk in paraplegia.
- Avoid asymmetric rotational stresses on the spine.
- Extreme ROM should be avoided, especially at the hip or knee (only 45 degrees of abduction should be allowed at the hip).
- Support medial side of the knee to avoid excessive stress.
- Do not combine flexion of the wrist and fingers.
- With paraplegia, trunk motion and some hip motions are contraindicated. In general, straight leg raises (SLR) greater than 60 degrees and hip flexion beyond 90 degrees should be avoided during the acute phase. Avoid overstretching of the low back because mild tightness facilitates transfer activity.
- It is critical to prevent secondary shoulder pain due to the importance of the shoulder in functional activities.
- Testing or monitoring of patients who may have impaired cardiovascular adaptation during exercise is indicated because of the demands of wheelchair propulsion.
- Symptoms of autonomic dysreflexia should be considered a medical emergency. Immediate assessment of the bladder drainage system should be performed. Symptoms may include sudden episodes of sweating on the head, neck and shoulders, increased blood pressure, lowered heart rate, and headache. Remove the cause immediately and consult physician about the use of antihypertensive medications.
- Some experts state that ambulation is contraindicated for 6 months post fracture stabilization.
- Contraindications for FNS or FES application in spinal-cord-injured patients include:
  1. peripheral lesions
  2. osteoporosis
  3. heterotopic ossifications
  4. contractures
  5. severe atrophy of muscles and no response to restrengthening
  6. pressure sores
  7. obesity
  8. severe spasticity
  9. inadequate sitting balance
  10. lack of patient interest

Notes: Electrical stimulation can have a negative impact on lower motor neuron lesions. Avoid use in muscles near the level of injury.

DESIRED OUTCOME/PROGNOSIS

ACUTE

- The client will improve ventilation, increase effectiveness of cough, prevent chest tightness and substitute breathing patterns, maintain adequate bronchial hygiene, and develop coordination of breathing with activity.

- The client will maintain ROM, especially alignment of fingers, thumb, and wrist for functional activities or dynamic splints, and will maintain alignment and prevent heel cord tightness.
- The client will maintain skin integrity and prevent pressure sores.
- The client will have improved bladder drainage.
- The client will maintain the strength of remaining musculature.

SUBACUTE

- The client will have increased responsibility for skin inspection.
- The client will have relief of pressure and maintenance of proper hygiene.
- There will be an increase in wheelchair mobility.
- The client will develop motor control and muscle re-education techniques.
- The client will regain postural control and balance.
- The client will improve cardiovascular response to exercise.
- The client will have functional skills, achieve stability, and progress to controlled mobility that leads to mobility skill.

Outcomes for ambulation are as follows:

- The client will achieve functional ambulation and increase tolerance to standing.
- For KAFO users, the desired outcome is to master a swing-through gait pattern.

PROGNOSIS

GENERAL

Prognosis for recovery, in general, relates directly to the extent of the spinal cord damage and the prevention of additional compromise during the acute phase. With a complete lesion, there is no expectation of motor improvement except what may accompany motor root return. Most incomplete lesions begin to show improvement after spinal shock has subsided.

GAIT

Gait training can take 3 to 6 weeks or longer.
FES long-term follow-up data are not available at this time. It remains undetermined whether FES-facilitated ambulation is more practical than wheelchair mobility.

PSYCHOSOCIAL

After a period of adjustment to the profound loss, most people adapt to spinal cord injury and may have a positive self-concept and be generally satisfied with life. Research offers conflicting reports on whether depression is more common among cord-injured people than the general population.

FERTILITY

Fertility generally remains unchanged in women. Complications from a pregnancy for spinal-cord-injured women may include:

- autonomic dysreflexia during labor (with lesions above T-7)
- lack of awareness of labor contractions due to sensory loss (with lesions above T-6)
- increased risk of anemia
- urinary tract infection
- decubiti
- deep-vein thrombosis
- rapid labor
- high incidence of premature labor

There is, however, no major threat and no increased need for cesarean delivery. Most women can vaginally deliver healthy babies.

Note: Male fertility is lower following spinal cord injury, with incidence of paternity at 5% or lower.

REFERENCES

Assessment

American Physical Therapy Association. Guide to physical therapist practice. 2nd ed. *Phys Ther.* 2001;81.

DeLisa D. *Rehabilitation Medicine: Principle and Practice.* Philadelphia, Pa: Lippincott; 1998.

Grabois M, Garrison SJ, Hart KA, Lehmkuhl LD. *Physical Medicine and Rehabilitation: The Complete Approach.* Malden, Mass: Blackwell Science; 2000.

Hooker SP, Greenwood JD, Hatae DT, Husson RP, Matthiesen TL, Waters AR. Oxygen uptake and heart rate relationship in persons with spinal cord injury. *Med Sci Sports Exerc.* 1993;25:1115–1119.

Patla AE, Clous SD. Visual assessment of human gait: reliability and validity. *Rehabil Res.* 1998;1:87–96.

Powers CM, Newsam CJ, Gronley JK, et al. Isometric shoulder torque in subjects with spinal cord injury. *Arch Phys Med Rehabil.* 1994;75:761–765.

Schmitz TJ. Traumatic spinal cord injury. In: O'Sullivan SB, Schmitz TJ, eds. *Phys Rehabil.* 3rd ed. Philadelphia, Pa: FA Davis Co; 1994:537.

Sine R, Liss SE, Rousch RE, et al. *Basic Rehabilitation Techniques: A Self-Instructional Guide.* 4th ed. Gaithersburg, Md: Aspen Publishers; 2000.

Waters RL, Adkins R, Yakura J, et al. Prediction of ambulatory performance based on motor scores derived from standards of the American Spinal Injury Association. *Arch Phys Med Rehabil.* 1994;75:756–760.

Treatment

American Spinal Injury Association. International standards for neurological and functional classification of spinal cord injury. Atlanta, Ga: ASIA; 1994.

Basso DM. Neuroanatomical substrates of functional recovery after experimental spinal cord injury: implications of basic science research for human spinal cord injury. *Phys Ther.* 2000;80:808–817.

Behrman AL, Harrkman AL. Locomotor training after human spinal cord injury: a series of case studies. *Phys Ther.* 2000;80:688–700.

Bohannon RW. Tilt table standing for reducing spasticity after spinal cord injury. *Arch Phys Med Rehabil.* 1993;74:1121–1122.

Bonaroti D, Akers JM, Smith BT, et al. Comparison of functional electrical stimulation to long leg braces for upright mobility for children with complete thoracic level spinal injuries. *Arch Phys Med Rehabil.* 1999;80:1047–1053.

Bradley-Popovich GE, Frounfelter GG. Self-adapted resistance exercises for an individual with paraplegia. *Phys Ther Case Rep.* 2000;3:141–147.

Bromley I. *Tetraplegia and Paraplegia: A Guide for Physiotherapy.* 5th ed. New York, NY: Churchill Livingstone; 1998.

Brouwer B, Hopkins-Russel H. Motor cortical mapping of proximal upper extremity muscles following spinal cord injury. *Spinal Cord.* 1997;35:205–212.

Carr JH, Shepherd RB, Ada L. *Physiotherapy.* 1995;81:421–429.

Craik RL. Spinal cord injury: the bridge between basic science and clinical practice. *Phys Ther.* 2000;80:671–672.

Craik RL. Spinal Cord Injury. *Phys Ther.* 2000;80:671–672.

Curtis KA, Roach KE, Appelgate EB, et al. Development of the Wheelchair Users' Shoulder Pain Index (WUSPI). *Paraplegia.* 1995;33:290–293.

Daylan M, Cardenas DD, Gerard B. Upper extremity pain after spinal cord injury. *Spinal Cord.* 1999;37:191–195.

DeBruin ED, Frey-Rindova P, Herzop RE, et al. Changes of tibia bone properties after spinal cord injury: effects of early intervention. *Arch Phys Med Rehabil.* 1999;80:214–220.

DeLisa D. *Rehabilitation Medicine: Principle and Practice.* Philadelphia, Pa: Lippincott; 1998.

Edelstein JE. Orthoses. In: Myers RS, ed. *Saunders Manual of Physical Therapy Practice.* Philadelphia, Pa: WB Saunders Co; 1995:1198–1203.

El Masry WS, Tsubo M, Katoh M, et al. A 1996 validation of the American Spinal Injury Association (ASIA) Motor Score and the National Acute Spinal Cord Injury Study (NASCIS) Motor Score. *Spine.* 1996;21:614–619.

Ferguson ACB, Granat MH. Evaluation of functional electrical stimulation for an incomplete spinal cord injured patient. *Physiotherapy.* 1992;78:253–256.

Gerhart KA. Personal perspectives. In: Whiteneck GG, Charlifue SW, Gerhart KA, et al, eds. *Aging With Spinal Cord Injury.* New York, NY: Demos Publications; 1993:343–352.

Gordon T, Mao J. Muscle atrophy and procedures for training after spinal cord injury. *Phys Ther.* 1994;74:50–60.

Grabois M, Garrison SJ, Hart KA, Lehmkuhl LD. *Physical Medicine and Rehabilitation: The Complete Approach.* Malden, Mass: Blackwell Science; 2000.

Granat MH, Ferguson ACB, Andrews BJ, et al. The role of functional electrical stimulation in the rehabilitation of patients with incomplete spinal cord injury-observed benefits during gait studies. *Paraplegia.* 1993;31:207–215.

Gunduz S, Kalyon TA, Dursun H, Mohur H, Bilgic F. Peripheral nerve block with phenol to treat spasticity in spinal cord injured patients. *Paraplegia.* 1992;30:808–811.

Harvey LA, Batty J, Fahey A. Reliability of a tool for assessing mobility in wheelchair-dependent paraplegics. *Spinal Cord.* 1998;36:427–431.

Hughes CJ, Weimar WH, Sheth PN, Brubaker CE. Biomechanics of wheelchair propulsion as a function of seat position and user-to-chair interface. *Arch Phys Med Rehabil.* 1992; 73:263–269.

Imle PC. Physical therapy for acute spinal cord injury. *Phys Ther Pract.* 1994;3:11–18.

Krawetz P, Nance P. Gait analysis of spinal cord injured subjects: effects of injury level and spasticity. *Arch Phys Med Rehabil.* 1996;77:635–638.

Lanig I, ed. *A Practical Guide to Health Promotion After Spinal Cord Injury.* Gaithersburg, Md: Aspen Publishers; 1996.

Marsolais EB, Kobetic R, Polando G, et al. The Case Western Reserve University hybrid gait orthosis. *J Spinal Cord Med.* 2000;23:100–108.

Mayer F, Billow H, Horstmann T, et al. Muscular fatigue, maximum strength and stress reactions for the shoulder musculature in paraplegics. *Int J Sports Med.* 1999;20:487–493.

Melia JL. Development of orthoses for people with paraplegia. *Physiotherapy.* 1997;83:23–25.

Morrison SA. Clinical pathways for individuals with spinal cord injury. *Phys Ther Case Rep.* 1998;1:129–139.

Muir GD, Steeves JD. Sensorimotor stimulation to improve locomotor recovery after spinal cord injury. *TINS.* 1997;20:72–77.

Nash MS, Jacobs PL. Cardiac structure and function in exercise trained and sedentary persons with paraplegia. *Med Sci Sports Exerc.* 1998;30:609–613.

Pease WS. Therapeutic electrical stimulation for spasticity: quantitative gait analysis. *Am J Phys Med Rehabil.* 1998;77:351–355.

Porter-Romatowski TL, Deckert J. Hemicorporectomy: a case study from a physical therapy perspective. *Arch Phys Med Rehabil.* 1998;79:464–468.

Priebe MM, Sherwood AM, Thornby JI, et al. Clinical assessment of spasticity in spinal cord injury: a multidimensional problem. *Arch Phys Med Rehabil.* 1996;77:713–716.

Riva G. Virtual reality in paraplegia: a VR-enhanced orthopaedic appliance for walking and rehabilitation. *Stud Health Technol Inform.* 1998;58:209–218.

Sampson EE, Burnham RS, Andrews BJ. Functional electrical stimulation effect on orthostatic hypotension after spinal cord injury. *Arch Phys Med Rehabil.* 2000;81:139–143.

Schmitz TJ. Traumatic spinal cord injury. In: O'Sullivan SB, Schmitz TJ, eds. *Physical Rehabilitation.* 3rd ed. Philadelphia, Pa: FA Davis Co; 1994:533–576.

Shields RK, Cook TM. Lumbar support thickness: effect on seated buttock pressure of individuals with and without spinal cord injury. *Phys Ther.* 1992;72:218–226.

Sighinolfi L, Carrodori S, Ghinelli F. Avascular necrosis of the femoral head: a side effect of highly active antiretroviral therapy (HAART) in HIV patients? *Infect.* 2000;28:254–255.

Sine R, Liss SE, Rousch RE, et al. *Basic Rehabilitation Techniques: A Self-Instructional Guide.* 4th ed. Gaithersburg, Md: Aspen Publishers; 2000.

Sinnott A, Mercer S. The weightbearing shoulder and long term paraplegia: A management issue. *N Z J Physiotherapy.* 2000;28:36–41.

Skold C. Spasticity in spinal cord injury: self-and clinically rated intrinsic fluctuations and intervention-induced changes. *Arch Phys Med Rehabil.* 2000;81:144–149.

Skold C, Levi R, Seiger A. *Arch Phys Med Rehabil.* 1999;80:1548–1557.

Solomonow M, Aquilar E, Reisin E, et al. Reciprocating gait orthosis powered with electrical muscles stimulation (RGO II). Part I: Performance evaluation of 70 paraplegic patients. *Orthop.* 1997;20:314–324.

Somers MF. *Spinal Cord Injury: Functional Rehabilitation.* Norwalk, Conn: Appleton & Lange; 1992.

Sorg RJ. HDL-cholesterol: exercise formula: results of long-term (6 year) strenuous swimming exercise in a middle-aged male with paraplegia. *J Orthop Sports Phys Ther.* 1993;17:195–199.

Suyama T, Nihei R, Kimura T, et al. Rehabilitation of spinal cord injury in the national rehabilitation center for the disabled of Japan: profile of a spinal service. *Spinal Cord.* 1997;35:720–724.

Trimble MH, Kukula CG, Behrman AL. *Neurosci Lett.* 1998;246:186–188.

Tuel SM, Cross LL, Meythaler JM, et al. Interdisciplinary management of hemicorporectomy after spinal cord injury. *Arch Phys Med Rehabil.* 1992;73:669–673.

Walker JB, Harris M. GM-1 ganglioside administration combined with physical therapy restores ambulation in humans with chronic spinal cord injury. *Neurosci Lett.* 1993;161:174–178.

Walter JS, Sola PG, Sacks J, et al. Indications for a home standing program for individuals with spinal cord injury. *J Spinal Cord Med.* 1999;22:152–158.

Waters RL, Sie ID, Adkins RH. The musculoskeletal system. In: Whiteneck GG, et al, eds. *Aging With Spinal Cord Injury.* New York, NY: Demos Publications; 1993;53–71.

Wickelgran I. Teaching the spinal cord to walk. *Sci.* 1998;279:319–321.

Wilson MS, Qureshy H, Protas EJ, et al. Equipment specification for supported treadmill ambulation training. *J Rehabil Res Dev.* 2000;37:415–422.

Yarkony GM, ed. *Spinal Cord Injury: Medical Management and Rehabilitation.* Gaithersburg, Md: Aspen Publishers; 1994.

Young JH. Implications of elbow arthrodesis for individuals with paraplegia. *Phys Ther.* 1993;73:194–201.

Spinal Cord Injuries: Tetraplegia (Quadriplegia)

DESCRIPTION

Quadriplegia is damage to the cervical spinal cord resulting in partial or complete motor and/or sensory function of all extremities and the trunk, including respiratory muscles.

CAUSE

Traumatic spinal cord injuries can result from a fall, sporting activity, diving accident, motor vehicle accident, or gunshot wound. Complete lesions are caused by a transection with a severing action or by severe compression. Incomplete lesions usually result from contusions. Nontraumatic damage can also occur, such as vascular impairment to the cord, but it is not as common as damage due to trauma. Eighty percent of all spinal cord injuries occur to people under the age of 40.

ASSESSMENT

Note: See APTA's Guide to Physical Therapist Practice. 2nd ed. *Physical Therapy.* 2001;81.

Neuromuscular Preferred Practice Pattern: H

AREAS
- History, including medications, gastrointestinal complaints, and visual disturbances
- Psychosocial, including behavior
- Communication
- Balance
- Pain
- Posture (sitting)
- Respiratory status and function, including muscle strength and tone of respiratory muscles, chest expansion and mobility, breathing pattern and respiratory rate, cough effectiveness, vital capacity, and tidal volume
- Cardiovascular, including endurance and heart rate
- Skin and soft tissue, including any edema
- Neurological, including sensation and DTRs
- Motor control, including muscle tone
- Strength, especially of shoulder flexors, abductors, elbow flexors and extensors, and wrist extensors
- Genitourinary, including bowel and bladder continence schedule
- Mobility, including passive range of motion (ROM)
- Gait: ambulation potential
- Functional assessment, including mobility and activities of daily living (ADLs)
- Equipment, including assistive devices and assessment of home environment

INSTRUMENTS/PROCEDURES

See References for sources.

Cardiovascular
- arm ergometry

Functional Level
- Barthel ADL index
- Functional Independence Measure
- Katz Index of ADLs
- Level of Rehabilitation Scale (LORS–II)

Gait
- based on motor scores of muscular strength

Motor Control
- modified Ashworth scale of muscle spasticity
- PENN Spasm Frequency Scale

Respiratory Status and Function
- maximal inspiratory pressure
- spirometric measurements

Special Tests to Which the Physical Therapist May or May Not Have Access
- sacral sparing
- spinal canal assessment
- hydrostatic weight assessment

Strength
- manual muscle testing
- shoulder torque

See Table 7.3 for the six-point scale for grading muscles in preceding section, "Spinal Cord Injuries: Paraplegia."

PROBLEMS

PRIMARY
- The client will often have motor deficits and sensory loss.
- The client will often have impaired temperature control.
- The client may have respiratory impairment.
- The client may have spasticity.
- The client will often have bladder and bowel dysfunction.
- The client will often have sexual dysfunction.

SECONDARY
- The client may develop autonomic dysreflexia.
- The client may develop contractures.
- The client may develop deep-vein thrombosis.
- The client may develop heterotopic bone formation.
- The client often experiences postural hypotension.
- The client may develop pressure sores.
- The client often has some complaints of pain; sources can be nerve root, physical trauma, spinal cord, or musculoskeletal (especially shoulder pain).

TREATMENT/MANAGEMENT

ACUTE PHASE

Strengthening of Selected Musculature
- Strengthen upper extremity muscles, with emphasis on anterior deltoids, shoulder extensors, biceps, and lower trapezius muscles. Focus on functional activities.
- Exercise techniques in the early phase can include manual resistance in straight-plane motions or upper extremity proprioceptive neuromuscular facilitation (PNF) patterns, progressing to resistive exercise with cuffed weights.
- Pulley weight systems and sports can be used in the later phases of rehabilitation. Bilateral activities should be emphasized.

ROM
- Except for areas contraindicated (see Precautions following), full ROM exercises should be performed daily. It is preferable for ROM to be done in both prone and supine positions if possible.

- Use selective stretching to allow development of selected tightness to enhance function. A tenodesis grasp, for example—in a patient with a C-6 and C-7 quadriplegia—is formed by allowing a mild tightness of the long finger flexors to develop. This improves grasp by allowing fingers to close upon wrist extension and the fingers to open upon wrist flexion (with assistance from gravity).

Positioning
- After the fracture site is stabilized, gradual acclimation to an upright posture is indicated. To facilitate acclimation, the patient may need an abdominal binder, elastic stockings, and/or elastic wraps.
- Consider splints for wrists, hands, and fingers, as well as ankle splints or boots. Gradually increase tolerance to prone position.

Respiratory Care
- Respiratory care can include the following activities: deep breathing exercises, glossopharyngeal breathing (for high-level cervical lesions), airshift chest expansion and chest mobility, diaphragm-strengthening exercises, assisted coughing, and stretching of pectoral and chest wall muscles.
- Consider the use of an abdominal support.
- Intervention strategies can include postural drainage and chest PT techniques such as vibration and percussion.

SUBACUTE PHASE
- Continue respiratory management, ROM, and positioning. Shoulder ROM (both glenohumeral and scapular thoracic) initiated within the first 2 weeks of injury may prevent shoulder pain.
- Expand resistive exercises for innervated muscles.
- Include interval training, with upper extremity aerobic activity, for cardiovascular training.
- Teach independence in mobilization.
- Mat programs can be initiated after patient is cleared for activity. Mat programs are varied and can include facilitating mastery of the components of functional skills. Component skills may involve activities such as rolling; transition to side-lying; prone-on-elbows, prone-on-hands, or supine-on-elbows position; pull-ups, and transition to sitting (long and short). Consider using group mat activities.
- Independent transfer training can be initiated after adequate sitting balance is achieved. Transfer training can include two-person lift, stand-pivot transfer, airlift, sliding board transfer, and lateral and forward transfers. Basic functional transfer activities include the following:
  1. wheelchair to mat
  2. removal of footplates
  3. chair to bed or car; chair to toilet or bath if patient has use of triceps
- Prescribe wheelchair and teach management skills. Basic wheelchair skills include weight shifting; propelling the wheelchair; managing brakes, armrests, and legrest/footrests; and picking up objects off the floor. Advanced wheelchair skills include wheelies, ramps and curbs, stairs, getting wheelchair into the car, and controlled falling.

Treatment of Pressure Sores
- Use topical therapy debridement and dressing technique for pressure sores, grade 3 or grade 4, a minimum of twice daily. See Table 7.4 for the grades of pressure sores in previous section, "Spinal Cord Injuries: Paraplegia."
- Consider use of whirlpool, hyperbaric oxygen, electrical stimulation, and laser therapy.

Psychosocial Issues
- Although physical therapy deals primarily with the physical and functional losses that a patient experiences, therapists need to be aware of the psychosocial issues facing a spinal-cord-injured patient.
- Physical therapists should work closely with other team members to address psychosocial issues such as home modifications, community re-entry, driving, communication skills, feeding, hygiene, bladder training, dressing, and other ADLs.
- Address psychosocial issues, including normalization, promoting independence, positive atmosphere and interactions with the rehabilitation team, education, and social support.
- Formal discharge strategies include counseling, education, social skills training, bladder and bowel retraining for postacute management, recreation training, pharmaceutical planning, and postdischarge planning.
- Psychosexual treatment involves physical evaluation, education, behavioral treatment, counseling, and prescription of physical aids for penile erectile dysfunction.

PRECAUTIONS/CONTRAINDICATIONS
- Avoid allowing the patient to maintain a posture in bed of constant shoulder flexion, adduction, internal rotation, elbow flexion, and forearm pronation.
- Redness over bony prominences should be gone within 30 minutes of the position change. Surgical intervention for pressure sores may be needed if conservative measures are not successful.
- Unresolved pressure sores may lead to chronic localized infection, osteomyelitis, sepsis, or even death.
- During the acute period, caution should be used during muscle strengthening to avoid stress at the fracture site, especially at the scapula and shoulder with quadriplegia.
- Avoid asymmetric rotational stresses on the spine.
- Extreme ROM should be avoided, especially at the hip or knee (ie, only 45 degrees of abduction should be allowed at hip). Overstretched trunk extensors, for instance, can lead to kyphosis and/or scoliosis
- Support medial side of the knee to avoid excessive stress.
- Do not combine flexion of the wrist and fingers.
- Testing or monitoring of patient who may have impaired cardiovascular adaptation during exercise is indicated during wheelchair propulsion.
- Symptoms of autonomic dysreflexia should be considered a medical emergency. Immediate assessment of the bladder drainage system should be performed.
- Dependence on upper extremities for mobility may lead to acceleration of degenerative changes in joints and upper extremity pain.

DESIRED OUTCOME/PROGNOSIS

ACUTE
- The client will improve ventilation, increase effectiveness of cough, prevent chest tightness and substitute breathing patterns, maintain adequate bronchial hygiene, and develop coordination of breathing with activity.
- The client will maintain ROM, especially alignment of fingers, thumb, and wrist for functional activities or dynamic splints, and will maintain alignment and prevent heel cord tightness.
- The client will maintain skin integrity and prevent pressure sores.
- The client will have improved bladder drainage.
- The client will maintain strength of remaining musculature.

SUBACUTE

- The client will have increased responsibility for skin inspection.
- The client will have relief of pressure and maintenance of proper hygiene.
- There will be an increase in wheelchair mobility.
- The client will develop motor control and muscle re-education techniques.
- The client will regain postural control and balance.
- The client will improve cardiovascular response to exercise.
- The client will have functional skills, achieve stability, and progress to controlled mobility leading to skill.

PROGNOSIS

GENERAL

In the past, the chances of reversing spinal cord injury were negligible. Recently, however, new medications such as methylprednisolone and 4-aminopyridine, have improved the outcomes for SCI. The use of transplantation and peripheral nerve grafts are under investigation.

Prognosis for recovery, in general, relates directly to the extent of the spinal cord damage and the prevention of additional compromise during the acute phase. With a complete lesion, there is no expectation of motor improvement except what may accompany motor root return. Most incomplete lesions begin to show improvement after spinal shock has subsided. The highest level to achieve independence in transfers are quadriplegics at the C-6 level. Muscle strength scores higher than 3 out of 5 in upper extremities may indicate a good prognosis for functional independence.

PSYCHOSOCIAL

After a period of adjustment to the profound loss, most people adapt to spinal cord injury and may have a positive self-concept and be generally satisfied with life. Research offers conflicting reports on whether depression is more common among cord-injured people than the general population.

AGING

Changes in the musculoskeletal system due to age may lead to changes in functional status.

REFERENCES

Assessment

American Physical Therapy Association. Guide to physical therapist practice. 2nd ed. *Phys Ther*. 2001;81.

Cromwell S. Patients with quadriplegia. In: Myers RS, ed. *Saunders Manual of Physical Therapy Practice*. Philadelphia, Pa: WB Saunders Co; 1995:396.

DeLisa D. *Rehabilitation Medicine: Principle and Practice*. Philadelphia, Pa: Lippincott; 1998.

Derrickson J, Ciesla N, Simpson N, Imle PC. A comparison of two breathing exercise programs for patients with quadriplegia. *Phys Ther*. 1992;72:763–769.

Grabois M, Garrison SJ, Hart KA, Lehmkuhl LD. *Physical Medicine and Rehabilitation: The Complete Approach*. Malden, Mass: Blackwell Science; 2000.

Hooker SP, Greenwood JD, Hatae DT, et al. Oxygen uptake and heart rate relationship in persons with spinal cord injury. *Med Sci Sports Exerc*. 1993;25:1115–1119.

Powers CM, Newsam CJ, Gronley JK, et al. Isometric shoulder torque in subjects with spinal cord injury. *Arch Phys Med Rehabil*. 1994;75:761–765.

Schmitz TJ. Traumatic spinal cord injury. In: O'Sullivan SB, Schmitz TJ, eds. *Phys Rehabil*. 3rd ed. Philadelphia, Pa: FA Davis Co; 1994:537.

Sine R, Liss SE, Rousch RE, et al. *Basic Rehabilitation Techniques: A Self-Instructional Guide*. 4th ed. Gaithersburg, Md: Aspen Publishers; 2000.

Stiller K, Simionato R, Rice K, Hall B. The effect of intermittent positive pressure breathing on lung volumes in acute quadriparesis. *Paraplegia*. 1992;30:2:121–126.

Waters RL, Adkins R, Yakura J, et al. Prediction of ambulatory performance based on motor scores derived from standards of the the American Spinal Injury Association. *Arch Phys Med Rehabil*. 1994;75:756–760.

Treatment

Allison GT, Singer KP. Assisted reach and transfers in individuals with tetraplegia: towards a solution. *Spinal Cord*. 1997;35:217–222.

American Physical Therapy Association. Guide to physical therapist practice. 2nd ed. *Phys Ther*. 2001;81.

Batavia M, Batavia AI. Pressure ulcer in a man with tetraplegia and a poorly fitting wheelchair: a case report with clinical and policy implications. *Spinal Cord*. 1999;37:140–141.

Blackmer J, Marshall S. Obesity and spinal cord injury: an observational study. *Spinal Cord*. 1997;35:245–247.

Bohannon RW. Tilt table standing for reducing spasticity after spinal cord injury. *Arch Phys Med Rehabil*. 1993;74:1121–1122.

Bromley I. *Tetraplegia and Paraplegia: A Guide for Physiotherapy*. 5th ed. New York, NY: Churchill Livingstone; 1998.

Carroll SG, Bird SF, Brown DJ. Electrical stimulation of the lumbrical muscles in an incomplete quadriplegic patient: case report. *Paraplegia*. 1992;30:223–226.

Carroll SG, Meeny CF. Electrical stimulation for restoring independent feeding in a man with quadriplegia. *Am J Occup Ther*. 1993;47:739–742.

Craik RL. Spinal cord injury: the bridge between basic science and clinical practice. *Phys Ther*. 2000;80:671–672.

Craik RL. Spinal Cord Injury. *Phys Ther*. 2000;80:671–672.

Cromwell S. Patients with quadriplegia. In: Myers RS, ed. *Saunders Manual of Physical Therapy Practice*. Philadelphia, Pa: WB Saunders Co; 1995:393–403.

Crowe J, MacKay-Lyons M, Morris H. A multi-centre, randomized controlled trial of the effectiveness of positioning on quadriplegic shoulder pain. *Physiotherapy Can*. 2000; 52:266–273.

Dallmeijer AJ, Hopman MT, Angenot EL, et al. *Scan J Rehabil Med*. 1997;29:181–186.

Daylan M, Cardenas DD, Gerard B. Upper extremity pain after spinal cord injury. *Spinal Cord*. 1999;37:191–195.

DeLisa D. *Rehabilitation Medicine: Principle and Practice*. Philadelphia, Pa: Lippincott; 1998.

Derrickson J, Ciesla N, Simpson N, Imle PC. A comparison of two breathing exercise programs for patients with quadriplegia. *Phys Ther*. 1992;72:763–769.

Drolet M, Noreau L, Vachon J, et al. Spasticity change during and following functional rehabilitation in individuals with spinal cord injury. *J Rehabil Outcomes Meas*. 2000;4: 1–14.

Edwards S. *Neurological Physiotherapy: a Problem-Solving Approach*. New York, NY: Churchill Livingstone; 1996.

Ferguson ACB, Granat MH. Evaluation of functional electrical stimulation for an incomplete spinal cord injured patient. *Physiotherapy*. 1992;78:253–256.

Gerhart KA. Changing the adaptive environment. Whiteneck GG, Charlifue SW, Gerhart KA, et al, eds. *Aging With Spinal Cord Injury*. New York, NY: Demos Publications; 1993: 343–351.

Goldstein B, Hammond M. Physical medicine and rehabilitation. *JAMA*. 1997;277:1891–1892.

Gordon T, Mao J. Muscle atrophy and procedures for training after spinal cord injury. *Phys Ther*. 1994;74:50–60.

Gouda JJ, Brown JA, Brinker RA. Delayed cervical epidural hemorrhage associated with silastic dural implant: case report. *Neurosurg*. 1997;41:943–945.

Grabois M, Garrison SJ, Hart KA, Lehmkuhl LD. *Physical Medicine and Rehabilitation: The Complete Approach*. Malden, Mass: Blackwell Science; 2000.

Gulati MS, Agin MA. *Journal of Spinal Cord Medicine*. 1996;19:12–16.

Hart C. Spinal cord injury statistics at the Natalspruit Hospital unit over an 11 year period. *S Afr J Physiotherapy*. 2000;56:13–15.

Harvey L. Principles of conservative management for a non-orthotic tenodesis grip in tetraplegics. *J Hand Ther*. 1996;9:238–242.

Harvey LA, Batty J, Fahey A. Reliability of a tool for assessing mobility in wheelchair-dependent. *Spinal Cord*. 1998;36:427–431.

Harvey L, Crosbie J. Effect of elbow flexion contractures on the ability of people with C5 and C6 tetraplegia to lift. *Physiotherapy Res Int*. 2001;6:106–117.

Hughes CJ, Weimar WH, Sheth PN, Brubaker CE. Biomechanics of wheelchair propulsion as a function of seat position and user-to-chair interface. *Arch Phys Med Rehabil*. 1992;73:263–269.

Hummelsheim H, Eickhof C. Repetitive sensorimotor training for arm and hand in a patient with locked-in syndrome. *Scand J Rehabil Med*. 1999;31:250–256.

Lanig I, ed. *A Practical Guide to Health Promotion After Spinal Cord Injury*. Gaithersburg, Md: Aspen Publishers; 1996.

Marson R, Edwards S. An unlikely case for successful rehabilitation. *Physiotherapy Res Int*. 1998;3:148–150.

Morrison SA. Clinical pathways for individuals with spinal cord injury. *Phys Ther Case Rep*. 1998;1:129–139.

Petrofsky JS. Microprocessor-based gait analysis system to retrain Trendelenburg gait. *Med Biol Eng Comput*. 2001;39:140–143.

Priebe MM, Sherwood Am, Thornby JI, et al. Clinical assessment of spasticity in spinal cord injury: a multidimensional problem. *Arch Phys Med Rehabil*. 1996;77:713–716.

Schmitz TJ. Traumatic spinal cord injury. In: O'Sullivan SB, Schmitz TJ, eds. *Phys Rehabil*. 3rd ed. Philadelphia, Pa: FA Davis Co; 1994:533–576.

Shields RK, Cook TM. Lumbar support thickness: effect on seated buttock pressure of individuals with and without spinal cord injury. *Phys Ther*. 1992;72:218–226.

Skold C. Spasticity in spinal cord injury: self- and clinically rated intrinsic fluctuations and intervention-induced changes. *Arch Phys Med Rehabil*. 2000.81:144–149.

Somers MF. *Spinal Cord Inj*. Norwalk, Conn: Appleton & Lange; 1992.

Tomaras CR, Grundmeyer RW, Chow TS, et al. Unusual foreign body causing quadriparesis: case report. *Neurosurgery*. 1997;40:1291–1293.

Walker JB, Harris M. GM-1 ganglioside administration combined with physical therapy restores ambulation in humans with chronic spinal cord injury. *Neurosci Lett.* 1993;161:2:174–178.

Waters RL, Sie IH, Adkins RH. The musculoskeletal system. In: Whiteneck GG, Chalifue SW, Gerhart KA, et al., eds. *Aging With Spinal Cord Injury.* New York, NY: Demos Publications; 1993:53–70.

Woods EN. An interview with Christopher Reeve. *PT-Magazine Phys Ther.* 1997;5:38–44.

Chapter 8

Musculoskeletal Disorders

Note: See also Chapter 9, Conditions in Back Pain, and Chapter 1, Conditions in Athletic Injuries.

Achilles Tendinitis

DESCRIPTION

Inflammation of the Achilles tendon.

CAUSE

Unknown etiology. Achilles tendinitis may be caused by the effects of aging, repetitive microtrauma, extreme trauma, strain, an inflexible gastrocsoleus complex, unaccustomed exercise, or malalignment of the foot structure. The tendon or the paratendon (a sleeve-like structure surrounding the Achilles tendon) becomes inflamed and painful. Tissue thickening also occurs in the area of the tendon. Abnormal alignment may predispose the tendon to injury. In the athlete, achilles tendinitis is associated with repetitive, high-impact sports such as basketball or running.

ASSESSMENT

Note: See APTA's Guide to Physical Therapist Practice. 2nd ed. *Physical Therapy.* 2001;81.

Musculoskeletal Preferred Practice Patterns: D, E, F, J

AREAS

- History
- Pain
- Posture, including anterial, lateral, and posterior view. May use biomechanical screen and static stance. Check lower extremity alignment, especially of the foot.
- Gait
- Strength
- Neurological, including sensation
- Joint integrity and structural deviations, including Q angle, patellar apprehension test, and tibial torsion
- Mobility, including active and passive range of motion (ROM); accessory motion, including FABER test, hip capsule tightness, sacroiliac compression, Ober's test, and modified Thomas' test.
- Skin and soft tissue: temperature, edema
- Equipment, including footwear

INSTRUMENTS/PROCEDURES

See References for sources.

Gait
- dynamic assessment of foot mechanics
  1. dynamic plantar pressure distribution
  2. foot pressure EMED system
  3. F-Scan system
  3. pedabarograph
  4. three-dimensional kinematic analysis
- footprint analysis
- gait velocity measurement
- stance phase analysis

Joint Integrity and Structural Deviations
- tibial varum assessment

Mobility
- goniometry
- open and closed kinetic chain subtalar joint neutral positions

- subtalar and ankle joint measurements
- visual estimates of ankle joint active ROM

Strength
- instrumentation
- manual muscle testing

PROBLEMS
- The client often has pain proximal to the heel.
- Pain may be experienced at rest but is routinely associated with activity, especially weight bearing.
- The client may have tenderness.
- The ankle may be edematous; there is often localized swelling.
- The client may feel crepitus with active motion.

TREATMENT/MANAGEMENT

For the treatment of foot and ankle problems in general:

- Exercises progress from passive ROM to active assisted and active ROM to resisted ROM.
- Begin non-weight-bearing strengthening activities after pain-free ROM is achieved.
- Isometric, isotonic, and isokinetic exercise may be used.
- Consider eccentric loading.
- Progress to jogging, running, and athletic maneuvers as indicated.
- Address preventive measures, such as stretching, choice of shoes, inserts or pads, and use of adhesive strapping during athletic activities.

For Achilles tendinitis specifically, the foundation of treatment is indicated by the acronym PRICEMM (see Figure 8.1).

Protection

Rest: Eliminate aggravating activities

Ice

Compression

Elevation

Medication as prescribed

Modalities: high-voltage electrical stimulation, ultra-sound, ice, heat

FIGURE 8.1. PRICEMM acronym outlining general approach for pain and inflammation.

In addition:

- Use physical agents as indicated. Consider iotophoresis with 10% hydrocortisone for inflammation.
- Whirlpools should be cold.
- Soft tissue mobilization may be indicated. Consider use of friction massage as tolerated.
- Consider heel lift or orthotics. Consider an ankle-foot arthosis (AFO) with limited-motion ankle joints placed in a shoe that also has a heel lift. A heel lift of between 12 and 15 mm thickness has been recommended.
- Modify daily activities as needed.
- Progress to active stretching that begins gently using a low-load, 10-second hold. Start with 10–20 repetitions BID.
- Use gastrocsoleus strengthening exercises, including eccentric exercises. May use Theraband for resistance with open kinetic chain exercise. Also consider use of isokinetic exercises and closed kinetic chain exercises in the final phase.
- Consider the use of a balance board, treadmill, stationary bike, and stairmaster.
- If available, use aquatic exercise progressing to weight-bearing activities.
- Ice may be indicated after activity. Suggested regimen of 20 minutes q2-3 hours.
- Assess footwear; consider counterforce straps and a flexible sole. Shoe heel should be well padded.
- Implement a home program of strength maintenance and flexibility. Home program may also include aerobics for fitness, such as walking.
- Consider protective taping for athletic activities.

Note: Specific protocol of strengthening regimens may be found in Alfredson, et al. (See References.)

PRECAUTIONS/CONTRAINDICATIONS

Achilles tendinits may lead to complete rupture of the tendon if the degenerative process is ignored or left untreated.

DESIRED OUTCOME/PROGNOSIS

- Symptoms, such as edema and inflammation, will be controlled and healing.
- The client will gain adequate flexibility and strength and reduce tension on the sural nerve and Achilles tendon.
- The client will return to normal function and activity, and recurrence will be prevented.

Notes: Most patients with acute Achilles tendinitis respond well to conservative therapy. Symptoms lasting longer than 6 to 8 weeks may mean that adhesions have formed in the tendoachilles region. Chronic Achilles tendinitis may need immobilization.

REFERENCES

Assessment

American Physical Therapy Association. Guide to physical therapist practice. 2nd ed. *Phys Ther.* 2001;81.

Buschbacher RM, ed. *Musculoskeletal Disorders: A Practical Guide for Diagnosis and Rehabilitation.* Boston, Mass: Andover Medical Publishers; 1994.

Daniels L, Worthingham C. *Muscle Testing Techniques of Manual Examination.* 6th ed. Philadelphia, Pa: WB Saunders Co; 1995.

Delitto A, Synder-Mackler L. The diagnostic process: examples in orthopedic physical therapy. *Phys Ther.* 1995;75:203–210.

Donatelli RA. *The Biomechanics of the Foot and Ankle.* 2nd ed. Philadelphia, Pa: FA Davis; 1996.

Hall CM, Brody TB. *Therapeutic Exercise: Moving Toward Function.* Philadelphia, Pa: Lippincott Williams and Wilkins; 1999.

Hertling D, Kessler RM. *Management of Common Musculoskeletal Disorders.* 3rd ed. Philadelphia, Pa: JB Lippincott Co; 1996:78, 534.

Jacobs K. *Ergonomics for Therapists.* 2nd ed. Boston, Mass: Butterworth Heinemann; 2000.

Kasman GS, Ram JR, Wolf Sl. *Clinical Applications in Surface Electromyography: Chronic Musculoskeletal Pain.* Bethesda, Md: Aspen Publishers; 1998.

Kendall FP, McCreary EK, Provance PG. *Muscles: Testing and Function.* 4th ed. Baltimore, Md: Williams and Wilkins; 1993.

Kisner C, Colby LA. *Therapeutic Exercise: Foundations and Techniques.* 3rd ed. Philadelphia, Pa: FA Davis Co; 1996:241–270.

Lesh SG. *Clinical Orthopedics for the Physical Therapist Assistant.* Philadelphia, Pa: FA Davis Co; 2000.

Malone TR, McPoil T, Nitz AJ, eds. *Orthopaedic and Sports Physical Therapy.* 3rd ed. St. Louis, Mo: CV Mosby Co; 1997.

Myers RS, ed. *Saunders Manual of Physical Therapy Practice.* Philadelphia, Pa: WB Saunders Co; 1995.

Picciano AM, Rowlands MS, Worrell T. Reliability of open and closed kinetic chain subtalar joint neutral positions and navicular drop test. *J Orthop Sports Phys Ther.* 1993;18: 553–558.

Rothstein JM, Roy SH, Wolf SL. *The Rehabilitation Specialist's Handbook.* 2nd ed. Philadelphia, Pa: FA Davis Co; 1998.

Saidoff DC, McDonough AL. *Critical Pathways in Therapeutic Intervention.* Philadelphia, Pa: CV Mosby Co; 2002.

Sammarco GJ. *Rehabilitation of the Foot and Ankle.* St. Louis, Mo: Mosby Year Book; 1995.

Schunk C, Reed K. *Clinical Practice Guidelines.* Gaithersburg, Md: Aspen Publishers; 2000.

Tomberlin JP, Saunders HD. *Evaluation, Treatment and Prevention of Musculoskeletal Disorders. Vol 2: Extremities.* Chaska, Minn: The Saunders Group; 1994.

Treatment

Alfredson H, Pietila T, Honsson P, et al. Heavy-load eccentric calf muscle training for the treatment of chronic Achilles tendinosis. *Am J Sports Med.* 1998;26:360–366.

Ballantyne BT, Kukulka CG, Soderberg GL. Motor unit recruitment in human medial gastrocnemius muscle during combined knee flexion and plantar flexion isometric contractions. *Exp Brain Res.* 1993;93:492–498.

Bruckner P. Sports medicine. Pain in the achilles region. *Aust Fam Phys.* 1997;26:463–465.

Draper DO, Sunderland S, Kirkendall DT, Richard M. A comparison of temperature rise in human calf muscles following applications of underwater and topical gel ultrasound. *J Orthop Sports Phys Ther.* 1993;17:247.

Enwemeka CS. The biomechanical effects of GA-As laser photostimulation on tendon health. *Phys Ther.* 1992;72:S67.

Fahlstrom M, Bjornstig U, Lorentzon R. Acute Achilles tendon rupture in badminton players. *Am J Sports Med.* 1998;26:467–470.

Grabois M, Garrison SJ, Hart KA, Lehmkuhl LD. *Physical Medicine and Rehabilitation: The Complete Approach*. Malden, Mass: Blackwell Science; 2000.

Hoffman M, Payne VG. The effects of proprioceptive ankle disk training on healthy subjects. *J Orthop Sports Phys Ther*. 1995;21:90–99.

Hunter G. The conservative management of Achilles tendinopathy. *Phys Ther Sport*. 2000; 1:6–14.

Jette AM. Using health-related quality of life measures in physical therapy outcomes research. *Phys Ther*. 1993;73:528–537.

Kasman GS, Ram JR, Wolf SI. *Clinical Applications in Surface Electromyography: Chronic Musculoskeletal Pain*. Bethesda, Md: Aspen Publishers; 1998.

Leard J, Massie DL, Brautigam J, Buschbacher R. Lower leg, ankle, and foot. In: Buschbacher RM, ed. *Musculoskeletal Disorders: A Practical Guide for Diagnosis and Rehabilitation*. Boston, Mass: Andover Medical Publishers; 1994:216–235.

McCrory JL, Martin DF, Lowery RP, et al. Etiologic factors associated with Achilles tendinitis in runners. *Medicine and Science in Sports and Exercise*. 1999;31:1374–1381.

McCulloch MU, Brunt D, Vander-Linden D. The effect of foot orthotics and gait velocity on lower limb kinematics and temporal events of stance. *J Orthop Sports Phys Ther*. 1993;17:1:2–10.

McPoil TC, Hunt GC. Evaluation and management of foot and ankle disorders: Present problems and future directions. *J Orthop Sports Phys Ther*. 1995;21:381–388.

Roebroeck ME, Dekker J, Oostendorp RA. The use of therapeutic ultrasound by physical therapists in Dutch primary health care. *Phys Ther*. 1998;78:470–478.

Rogers MM. Dynamic foot biomechanics. *J Orthop Sports Phys Ther*. 1995;21:306–316.

Sahrmann SA. *Diagnosis and Exercise Management of Musculoskeletal Pain Syndromes*. St. Louis, Mo: CV Mosby Co.

Sammarco GJ. *Rehabilitation of the Foot and Ankle*. St. Louis, Mo: CV Mosby Year Book; 1995.

Sioli MW. Achilles tendinitis. *Orthopedic Clinics of North America*. 1994;25:177–182.

Swenson C, Sward L, Karlsson J. Cryotherapy in sports medicine. *Scand J Med Sci Sports*. 1996;6:193–200.

ter Haar G. Therapeutic ultrasound. *Europ J Ultrasound*. 1999;9:3–9.

Tomaro JE, Butterfield SI. Biomechanical treatment of traumatic foot and ankle injuries with the use of foot orthotics. *J Orthop Sports Phys Ther*. 1995;21:373–380.

Tomberlin JP, Saunders HD. *Evaluation, Treatment and Prevention of Musculoskeletal Disorders. Vol 2: Extremities*. Chaska, Minn: The Saunders Group; 1994:265–306.

Vandervoort AA, Chesworth BM, Cunningham DA, et al. An outcome measure to quantify passive stiffness of the ankle. *Can J Public Health*. 1992;83(suppl 2):S19–S23.

Adhesive Capsulitis

Also known as *frozen shoulder* or *periarthritis*.

DESCRIPTION

Adhesive capsulitis is the inflammation of the shoulder capsule. Adhesive capsulitis leads to inflammation between the joint capsule and the shoulder's articular cartilage. Shoulder pain from adhesive capsulitis may be due to one pathologic process or a combination of disorders of adhesive capsulitis, tendinitis, and bursitis.

CAUSE

No specific cause of adhesive capsulitis may be determined. Possible causes are immobilization, reflex sympathetic dystrophy, trauma, alteration in scapulohumeral alignment, rheumatoid arthritis, and rarely, degenerative joint disease. It occurs in middle-aged and older persons more frequently than in the young. Women are more often affected than men.

ASSESSMENT

Note: See APTA's Guide to Physical Therapist Practice. 2nd ed. *Physical Therapy*. 2001;81.

Integumentary Preferred Practice Pattern: A

Musculoskeletal Preferred Practice Patterns: D, E, F, G, J

AREAS

- History
- Pain
- Posture
- Joint integrity and structural deviations
- Skin and soft tissue
- Movements, including active and passive range of motion
- (ROM) and accessory motion
- Strength
- Neurological
- Circulation
- Functional level: use of arm

INSTRUMENTS/PROCEDURES

See References for sources.

Functional Level
- Functional Index Questionaire
- Shoulder Pain and Disability Index (SPADI)
- Disabilities of the Arm, Shoulder, and Hand (DASH)
- Short Form-36 (SF-36) Health Survey

Joint Integrity/Structural Deviations and Neurological Involvement
- acromioclavicular instability test
- anterior apprehension test
- anterior drawer sign
- anterior stability test
- active impingement test
- Adson's test
- Allen's test
- clunk test
- costoclavicular syndrome test
- drop arm test
- Feagin test
- fulcrum test
- Gilchrist sign
- glenohumeral stability tests and glenoid labrum integrity tests*
- Halstead maneuver
- Hawkins–Kennedy impingement tests*
- hyperabduction syndrome test
- jerk test
- lateral scapular glide
- Lippmans test
- locking test impingement*
- Ludington's test bicipital* tendinitis*
- Neer's test impingement*
- Norwood stress test
- posterior apprehension test
- posterior drawer sign
- push-pull test
- quadrant test
- relocation test
- Roo's test (EAST test)
- Rockwood test
- Rowe test
- Speed's test (bicep's test)
- sulcus sign
- suprascapular nerve entrapment test
- supraspinatus test*

- transverse humeral ligament rupture test
- upper limb tension test

- upper quarter screen
- Yergason's test bicipital tendinitis*

Pain
- body chart
- visual analog scale

Special Tests to Which the Physical Therapist May or May Not Have Access
- electromyography (EMG)

Strength
- isokinetic evaluation
- manual muscle testing

Temperature
- thermography

PROBLEMS
- The client often reports gradual increase in pain and stiffness.
- The client often has decreased active and passive motion in shoulder in a capsular pattern, especially in external rotation and abduction. The restriction leads to an inability to reach behind the back with hand.
- The client may have some decreased ROM in flexion and internal rotation.
- There is often painless resisted motion.
- The client may have difficulty with activities of daily living due to decreased functional usage.
- The client often has disturbed sleep secondary to pressure on involved side in acute phase.
- The client often has pain at extremes of shoulder ROM or with lifting, especially overhead.
- There may be decreased shoulder strength.

TREATMENT/MANAGEMENT

ACUTE
- Use ice or superficial heat as indicated.
- Consider gentle joint mobilization.
- Maintain and try to increase ROM.
- Begin strength training with isometric exercises, progressing to isotonic and then resistive exercises.
- Instruct client in posture training. Emphasize avoidance of kyphotic and protracted shoulder postures.

CHRONIC
- Consider use of ultrasound if indicated.
- Consider joint mobilization and automobilization techniques.

PRECAUTIONS/CONTRAINDICATIONS
- Brachial plexus peripheral entrapment at the thoracic outlet or the shoulder can be mistakenly identified as musculoskeletal pain of the shoulder.
- Avoid self-stretching into abduction until sufficient gains in external rotation are reached to prevent traumatization of subacromial tissues.

Note: Ill-timed or overly aggressive therapy can extend the symptoms.

DESIRED OUTCOME/PROGNOSIS

- The client will experience a decrease in symptoms.
- Painless functional ROM will be restored (regaining full movement may not be possible).
- The client will increase shoulder movement and be independent in self-mobilization techniques.
- The client will be independent in a home ROM plan to maintain progress.

Notes: Therapy for 3 to 4 months should bring satisfactory results. Improvement, however, usually follows a nonlinear pattern of recovery. Some report spontaneous recovery on an average of 12 months to 2 years after onset. When frozen shoulder is caused by sympathetic dystrophy, it can be very resistant to conservative management.

REFERENCES

Assessment

American Physical Therapy Association. Guide to physical therapist practice. 2nd ed. *Phys Ther.* 2001;81.

Boublik M, Hawkins RJ. Clinical examination of the shoulder complex. *J Orthop Sports Phys Ther.* 1993;18:379–385.

Buschbacher RM, ed. *Musculoskeletal Disorders: A Practical Guide for Diagnosis and Rehabilitation.* Boston, Mass: Andover Medical Publishers; 1994.

Daniels L, Worthingham C. *Muscle Testing Techniques of Manual Examination.* 6th ed. Philadelphia, Pa: WB Saunders Co; 1995.

Delitto A, Synder-Mackler L. The diagnostic process: examples in orthopedic physical therapy. *Phys Ther.* 1995;75:203–210.

Hall CM, Brody TB. *Therapeutic Exercise: Moving Toward Function.* Philadelphia, Pa: Lippincott Williams and Wilkins; 1999.

Hertling D, Kessler RM. *Management of Common Musculoskeletal Disorders.* 3rd ed. Philadelphia, Pa: JB Lippincott Co; 1996:78, 534.

Jacobs K. *Ergonomics for Therapists.* 2nd ed. Boston, Mass: Butterworth Heinemann; 2000.

Kasman GS, Ram JR, Wolf Sl. *Clinical Applications in Surface Electromyography: Chronic Musculoskeletal Pain.* Bethesda, Md: Aspen Publishers; 1998.

Kendall FP, McCreary EK, Provance PG. *Muscles: Testing and Function.* 4th ed. Baltimore, Md: Williams and Wilkins, 1993.

Kisner C, Colby LA. *Therapeutic Exercise: Foundations and Techniques.* 3rd ed. Philadelphia, Pa: FA Davis Co; 1996:241–270.

Lesh SG. *Clinical Orthopedics for the Physical Therapist Assistant.* Philadelphia, Pa: FA Davis Co; 2000.

Malone TR, McPoil T, Nitz AJ, eds. *Orthopaedic and Sports Physical Therapy.* 3rd ed. St. Louis, Mo: CV Mosby Co; 1997.

Myers RS, ed. *Saunders Manual of Physical Therapy Practice.* Philadelphia, Pa: WB Saunders Co; 1995.

Rothstein JM, Roy SH, Wolf SL. *The Rehabilitation Specialist's Handbook.* 2nd ed. Philadelphia, Pa: FA Davis Co; 1998.

Saidoff DC, McDonough AL. *Critical Pathways in Therapeutic Intervention.* Philadelphia, Pa: CV Mosby Co; 2002.

Schunk C, Reed K. *Clinical Practice Guidelines.* Gaithersburg, Md: Aspen Publishers; 2000.

Tomberlin JP, Saunders HD. *Evaluation, Treatment and Prevention of Musculoskeletal Disorders. Vol 2: Extremities.* Chaska, Minn: The Saunders Group; 1994.

Wilk KE, Arrigo CA, Andrews JR. Isokinetic testing of the shoulder abductors and adductors: windowed vs non-windowed data collection. *J Orthop Sports Phys Ther.* 1992;15:107–112.

Winkel D. *Diagnosis and Treatment of the Upper Extremities.* Gaithersburg, Md: Aspen Publishers; 1997.

Treatment

Ballantyne BT, O'Hare SJ, Paschall JL, et al. Electromyographic activity of selected shoulder muscles in commonly used therapeutic exercises. *Phys Ther.* 1993;73:668–682.

Culham E, Peat M. Functional anatomy of the shoulder complex. *J Orthop Sports Phys Ther.* 1993;18:342–350.

Davies G, Dickoff-Hoffman S. Neuromuscular testing and rehabilitation of the shoulder complex. *J Orthop Sports Phys Ther.* 1993;18:449–458.

Ekelund AL, Rydell N. Combination treatment for adhesive capsulitis of the shoulder. *Clin Orthop.* 1992;282:105–109.

Grabois M, Garrison SJ, Hart KA, Lehmkuhl LD. *Physical Medicine and Rehabilitation: The Complete Approach.* Malden, Mass: Blackwell Science; 2000.

Griggs SM, Ahn A, Green A. Idiopathic adhesive capsulitis. A prospective functional outcome study of nonoperative treatment. *J Bone J Surg Am.* 2000;82-A:1398–1407.

Grubbs N. Frozen shoulder syndrome: a review of literature. *J Orthop Sports Phys Ther.* 1993;18:479–487.

Keyser KA. Clinical profiles. Differential diagnosis of shoulder pain: Parsonage Turner syndrome. *Phys Ther Case Rep.* 2000;3:120–124.

Liaw SC. The effect and timing of physiotherapy on change in range of motion and function in frozen shoulder. *Physiotherapy Singapore.* 2000;3:82–86.

Mao CY, Jaw WC, Cheng HC. Frozen shoulder: correlation between the response to physical therapy and follow-up shoulder arthrography. *Arch Phys Med Rehabil.* 1997;78:857–859.

Rizk ET, Gavant ML, Pinals RS. Treatment of adhesive capsulits (frozen shoulder) with arthrographic capsular distension and rupture. *Arch Phys Med Rehabil.* 1994;75:803–807.

Schenkman M, Rugo de Cartaya V. Kinesiology of the shoulder complex. *J Orthop Sports Phys Ther.* 1993;18:442–448.

Schneider G. Restricted shoulder movement: capsular contracture or cervical referral—a clinical study. *Aust J Physiotherapy.* 1989;35:2:97–100.

Simmons TC, Skyhair MJ. Rehabilitation of the shoulder. In: Nickel VL, Botte MJ, eds. *Orthop Rehabil.* New York, NY: Churchill Livingstone; 1992:747.

Tomberlin JP, Saunders HD. *Evaluation, Treatment and Prevention of Musculoskeletal Disorders. Vol 2: Extremities.* Chaska, Minn: The Saunders Group; 1994:91.

Wilk KE, Arrigo CA. An integrated approach to upper extremity exercises. In Timm K, ed. Exercise Principles. *Orthop Phys Ther Clin North Am.* 1992;2:337–360.

Wilk KE, Arrigo CA, Andrew JR. Current concepts: The stabilising structures of the glenohumeral joint. *J Orthop Sports Phys Ther.* 1997;25:364–379.

Lateral Epicondylitis and Medial Epicondylitis

DESCRIPTION

Lateral epicondylitis is also known as *tennis elbow* or *backhand tennis elbow*. In lateral humeral epicondylitis, the lateral forearm muscles (or their tendinous attachments) are strained close to their origin on the lateral epicondyle of the humerus. Tennis elbow occurs more frequently in men than women.

Medial epicondylitis is also known as *golfer's elbow, forehand tennis elbow, baseball elbow,* and *suitcase elbow.* In medial epicondylitis, the ventral forearm muscles and their attachments are strained.

CAUSE

Etiology is uncertain. The tissues may undergo degenerative changes called angiofibroblastic tendonosis.

Lateral epicondylitis may be caused by repetitive wrist action against resistance during extension and supination. *Medial epicondylitis* may be caused by repetitive stress during forceful wrist flexion and pronation.

Note: Table 8.1 lists examples of overuse injury risk factors.

ASSESSMENT

Note: See APTA's Guide to Physical Therapist Practice. 2nd ed. *Physical Therapy.* 2001;81.

Musculoskeletal Preferred Practice Patterns: D, E, F, J

AREAS
- History
- Pain
- Joint integrity and structural deviations
- Mobility: active and passive range of motion (ROM) and accessory motion
- Strength: any muscle weakness and biomechanical abnormality in rest of upper extremity that may be contributing to condition
- Neurological, including sensation and upper limb tension tests
- Skin and soft tissue, including edema
- Functional level, including activities of daily living (ADLs)

TABLE 8.1
Overuse Injury Risk Factors

Musculoskeletal Factors	Intrinsic Factors	Extrinsic Factors
	Malalignment	Training errors
	Muscular Imbalance	Equipment
	Inflexibility	Environment
	Muscular Weakness	Technique
	Instability	Sports-imposed Deficiencies

Source: Adapted with permission from Buschbacher RM. *Musculoskeletal Disorders: A Practical Guide for Diagnosis and Rehabilitation.* Boston, Mass: Andover Medical Publishers; 1994:163.

INSTRUMENTS/PROCEDURES

See References for sources.

Joint Integrity and Structural Deviations/Neurological Involvement

The following neurological and orthopedic tests for the elbow may be performed:

- elbow flexion test
- golfer's elbow test
- ligamentous instability tests
- modification of passive extension-adduction tests
- neural tissue tension test
- pinch test
- pronator teres syndrome
- Tinel's sign
- tennis elbow tests
- varus stress test
- valgus stress test

Pain

- Nirschl Pain Phase Scale

Special Tests to Which the Physical Therapist May or May Not Have Access

- integrated electromyography (IEMG)

Strength

- grip test dynamometer
- isokinetic testing
- manual muscle testing

PROBLEMS

LATERAL EPICONDYLITIS

- The client often has localized tenderness medial and distal to the lateral epicondyle or at the lateral epicondyle.
- The client may have pain that extends along the extensor muscle distally.
- Often, pain is associated with gripping or repetitive motion.
- The client may also have neck pain or symptoms involving the radial nerve.
- The client may have decreased wrist extension with wrist flexed and ulnarly deviated and with fingers flexed.

MEDIAL EPICONDYLITIS

- The client often has tenderness at the medial epicondyle.
- The client often has pain and loss of strength with gripping or repetitive motion.
- The client may complain of neck pain or symptoms involving the median or ulnar nerve.

TREATMENT/MANAGEMENT

GENERAL TREATMENT APPROACH

Note: Figure 8.2 following displays useful treatments.

- Implement rehabilitative exercises, aerobic exercise, and general conditioning.
- Initially use isometric strengthening of elbow flexors and wrist extensors.
- Emphasize the pronators and supinators for lateral injury and the wrist flexors for medial injury.
- Progress to isotonic exercise and then to resistive exercise.
- Isoflex resistance tubing may begin after patient can perform exercise tolerating a 3# weight. Flexibility exercises can be started after 80% of normal strength is achieved.

LATERAL EPICONDYLITIS

- Consider use of modalities—such as cryotherapy or high-voltage galvanic stimulation—for inflammation and electrical stimulation for mobilization. Ultrasound or phonophoresis may also promote healing.

Protection

Rest: Eliminate aggravating activities

Ice

Compression

Elevation

Medication as prescribed

Modalities: high-voltage electrical stimulation, ultra-sound, ice, heat

---

FIGURE 8.2. PRICEMM acronym outlining general approach for pain and inflammation.

- Provide friction massage to site of lesion.
- Use soft tissue mobilization to lateral forearm.
- Eliminate aggravating condition and avoid strong gripping activities in acute stage.
- Consider bracing to modify these conditions and combine with gentle ROM exercise when the brace is off.
- Include flexibility stretching exercises and strengthening as tolerated, including both eccentric and concentric exercises.
- Emphasize high-repetition, low-resistance exercises. May use freeweight elastic tubing if desired.
- Perform grip-strengthening exercises in functional power grip position.
- Consider appropriate neck, shoulder, and posture exercises.
- Consider ergonomic changes necessary to prevent injury recurrence.
- Ultrasound and friction massage may be useful in chronic conditions.
- Treatment following surgery usually includes gentle active ROM for approximately 3 weeks. Gradually progress to increase in ROM and resistance for strengthening exercises.

MEDIAL EPICONDYLITIS
- Generally, use the same treatments as with lateral tennis elbow, but direct them to the appropriate location.
- Avoid extreme repetitive flexion (if nerve is subluxating).
- Emphasize forearm flexor strength and endurance.
- Consider protection with elbow pad.

PRECAUTIONS/CONTRAINDICATIONS
- Progress cautiously with exercises to avoid aggravation of condition.
- Some other conditions that can cause similar pain and may be labeled as tennis elbow include pulled or pushed elbow, pinched synovial fringe, meniscal lock, periosteal bruise, and rotated elbow.

- Pain over the posterior aspect of the elbow may signal posterior tennis elbow; a rare condition.

DESIRED OUTCOME/PROGNOSIS
- The client will experience control of pain, edema, or spasm.
- The client will maintain soft tissue and joint mobility.
- The client will restore strength and extensibility to the muscle tendon complex.
- Therapy will promote maturation of the healed area of the tendon.
- The client will progress to functional recovery.
- The client will have restoration of normal, painless use of the involved arm.
- The client will prevent recurrence.

Notes: In lateral epicondylitis, rehabilitation usually lasts a minimum of 3 months. A patient who ranks phase 5 or less on the Nirschl Pain Phase Scale may respond better to the rehabilitation program. Exercise appears to be the critical factor in recovery.

In medial epicondylitis, if the client does not respond to the conservative management after 3 to 4 months, surgery may need to be considered.

REFERENCES

Assessment

American Physical Therapy Association. Guide to physical therapist practice. 2nd ed. *Phys Ther.* 2001;81.

Buschbacher RM, ed. *Musculoskeletal Disorders: A Practical Guide for Diagnosis and Rehabilitation.* Boston, Mass: Andover Medical Publishers; 1994.

Daniels L, Worthingham C. *Muscle Testing Techniques of Manual Examination.* 6th ed. Philadelphia, Pa: WB Saunders Co; 1995.

Delitto A, Synder-Mackler L. The diagnostic process: examples in orthopedic physical therapy. *Phys Ther.* 1995;75:203–210.

Hall CM, Brody TB. *Therapeutic Exercise: Moving Toward Function.* Philadelphia, Pa: Lippincott Williams and Wilkins; 1999.

Hertling D, Kessler RM. *Management of Common Musculoskeletal Disorders.* 3rd ed. Philadelphia, Pa: JB Lippincott Co; 1996;78, 534.

Jacobs K. *Ergonomics for Therapists.* 2nd ed. Boston, Mass: Butterworth Heinemann; 2000.

Kasman GS, Ram JR, Wolf SI. *Clinical Applications in Surface Electromyography: Chronic Musculoskeletal Pain.* Bethesda, Md: Aspen; 1998.

Kendall FP, McCreary EK, Provance PG. *Muscles: Testing and Function.* 4th ed. Baltimore, Md: Williams and Wilkins, 1993.

Kisner C, Colby LA. *Therapeutic Exercise: Foundations and Techniques.* 3rd ed. Philadelphia, Pa: FA Davis Co; 1996:241–270.

Lesh SG. *Clinical Orthopedics for the Physical Therapist Assistant.* Philadelphia, Pa: FA Davis Co; 2000.

Malone TR, McPoil T, Nitz AJ, eds. *Orthopaedic and Sports Physical Therapy.* 3rd ed. St. Louis, Mo: CV Mosby Co; 1997.

Myers RS, ed. *Saunders Manual of Physical Therapy Practice.* Philadelphia, Pa: WB Saunders Co; 1995.

Rothstein JM, Roy SH, Wolf SL. *The Rehabilitation Specialist's Handbook.* 2nd ed. Philadelphia, Pa: FA Davis Co; 1998.

Saidoff DC, McDonough AL. *Critical Pathways in Therapeutic Intervention.* Philadelphia, Pa: CV Mosby Co; 2002.

Schunk C, Reed K. *Clinical Practice Guidelines*. Gaithersburg, Md: Aspen Publishers; 2000.

Stratford PW, Levy DR, Gowland C. Evaluative properties of measures used to assess patients with lateral epicondylitis at the elbow. *Physiotherapy Can.* 1993;45:160–164.

Tomberlin JP, Saunders HD. *Evaluation, Treatment and Prevention of Musculoskeletal Disorders. Vol 2: Extremities*. Chaska, Minn: The Saunders Group; 1994.

Winkel D. *Diagnosis and Treatment of the Upper Extremities*. Gaithersburg, Md: Aspen Publishers; 1997.

Treatment

Almekinders LC, Almekinders SV. Outcome in the treatment of chronic overuse sports injuries: a retrospective study. *J Orthop Sports Phys Ther.* 1994;19:157–161.

Grabois M, Garrison SJ, Hart KA, Lehmkuhl LD. *Physical Medicine and Rehabilitation: The Complete Approach*. Malden, Mass: Blackwell Science; 2000.

Hertling D, Kessler RM. *Management of Common Musculoskeletal Disorders*. 3rd ed. Philadelphia, Pa: JB Lippincott Co; 1996:216.

Kisner C, Colby LA. *Therapeutic Exercise: Foundations and Techniques*. 3rd ed. Philadelphia, Pa: FA Davis Co; 1996:280–283.

Klaiman MD, Shroader JA, Danoff JV, et al. Phonophoresis versus ultrasound in the treatment of common musculoskeletal conditions. *Med Sci Sports Exerc.* 1998;30:1349–1355.

Louden J. Lateral epicondylitis. *Phys Ther Case Rep.* 2000;3:163–170.

Stroyan M, Wilk K. The functional anatomy of the elbow complex. *J Orthop Sports Phys Ther.* 1993;17:279–288.

Tomberlin JP, Saunders HD. *Evaluation, Treatment and Prevention of Musculoskeletal Disorders. Vol 2: Extremities*. Chaska, Minn: The Saunders Group; 1994:113–138.

Vasseljen O. Low-level laser versus traditional physiotherapy in the treatment of tennis elbow. *Physiotherapy.* 1992;78:329–334.

Wadsworth CT. Elbow, forearm, wrist, and hand. In: Myers RS, ed. *Saunders Manual of Physical Therapy Practice*. Philadelphia, Pa: WB Saunders Co; 1995:841–917.

Wadsworth CT, Nelson DH, Burns LT, et al. Effect of the counterforce armband on wrist extension and grip strength and pain in subjects with tennis elbow. *J Orthop Sports Phys Ther.* 1989;11:192–197.

Wilder RP, Nirschl PR, Sobel J. Elbow and forearm. In: Buschbacher RM, ed. *Musculoskeletal Disorders: A Practical Guide for Diagnosis and Rehabilitation*. Boston, Mass: Andover Medical Publishers; 1994:153–169.

Yaxley GA, Jull GA. Adverse tension in the neural system: a preliminary study of tennis elbow. *Aust J Physiotherapy.* 1993;39:1:15–22.

Hammer Toes

DESCRIPTION

Hammer toes are a deformity of the metatarsophalangeal joint resulting in flexion of the proximal interphalangeal joint.

CAUSE

Hammer toes are often caused by wearing ill-fitting shoes. Malalignment of the joint surfaces leads to subluxations, capsular and synovial impingement, and destruction of joint cartilage.

ASSESSMENT

Note: See APTA's Guide to Physical Therapist Practice. 2nd ed. *Physical Therapy.* 2001;81.

Musculoskeletal Preferred Practice Pattern: I

AREAS
- History
- Posture
- Pain
- Gait
- Equipment, including footwear
- Strength
- Neurological

- Joint integrity and structural deviations
- Mobility, including active and passive range of motion (ROM) and accessory motion
- Skin and soft tissue, including edema

INSTRUMENTS/PROCEDURES

See References for sources.

Mobility
- goniometry

Skin: Edema
- palpation

PROBLEMS
- The client often finds the condition painful.

TREATMENT/MANAGEMENT

In treatment of foot and ankle problems in general:
- Exercises progress from passive ROM to active-assisted and active ROM to resisted ROM.
- Begin non-weight-bearing strengthening activities after pain-free ROM is achieved.
- Isometric, isotonic, and isokinetic exercise may be used.
- Consider eccentric loading.
- Progress to jogging, running, and athletic maneuvers as indicated.
- Address preventive measures, such as stretching, choice of shoes, and use of adhesive strapping during athletic activities.

Specifically for hammer toes:
- Fit with shoes with a deep toe box.
- Use muscle-strengthening exercises for foot intrinsic muscles.

PRECAUTIONS
- No precautions are identified.

DESIRED OUTCOME/PROGNOSIS
- The client will experience relief of pressure on the dorsum of the flexed joints.

Note: Surgery may be indicated in severe cases.

REFERENCES

Assessment

American Physical Therapy Association. Guide to physical therapist practice. 2nd ed. *Phys Ther*. 2001;81.

Buschbacher RM, ed. *Musculoskeletal Disorders: A Practical Guide for Diagnosis and Rehabilitation*. Boston, Mass: Andover Medical Publishers; 1994.

Daniels L, Worthingham C. *Muscle Testing Techniques of Manual Examination*. 6th ed. Philadelphia, Pa: WB Saunders Co; 1995.

Delitto A, Synder-Mackler L. The diagnostic process: examples in orthopedic physical therapy. *Phys Ther*. 1995;75:203–210.

Donatelli RA. *The Biomechanics of the Foot and Ankle*. 2nd ed. Philadelphia, Pa: FA Davis Co; 1996.

Hall CM, Brody TB. *Therapeutic Exercise: Moving Toward Function*. Philadelphia, Pa: Lippincott Williams and Wilkins; 1999.

Hertling D, Kessler RM. *Management of Common Musculoskeletal Disorders*. 3rd ed. Philadelphia, Pa: JB Lippincott Co; 1996:78, 534.

Jacobs K. *Ergonomics for Therapists*. 2nd ed. Boston, Mass: Butterworth Heinemann; 2000.

Kasman GS, Ram JR, Wolf SI. *Clinical Applications in Surface Electromyography: Chronic Musculoskeletal Pain*. Bethesda, Md: Aspen Publishers; 1998.

Kendall FP, McCreary EK, Provance PG. *Muscles: Testing and Function*. 4th ed. Baltimore, Md: Williams and Wilkins; 1993.

Kisner C, Colby LA. *Therapeutic Exercise: Foundations and Techniques*. 3rd ed. Philadelphia, Pa: FA Davis Co; 1996:241–270.

Lesh SG. *Clinical Orthopedics for the Physical Therapist Assistant*. Philadelphia, Pa: FA Davis Co; 2000.

Malone TR, McPoil T, Nitz AJ, eds. *Orthopaedic and Sports Physical Therapy*. 3rd ed. St. Louis, Mo: CV Mosby Co; 1997.

Myers RS, ed. *Saunders Manual of Physical Therapy Practice*. Philadelphia, Pa: WB Saunders Co; 1995.

Rothstein JM, Roy SH, Wolf SL. *The Rehabilitation Specialist's Handbook*. 2nd ed. Philadelphia, Pa: FA Davis Co; 1998.

Saidoff DC, McDonough AL. *Critical Pathways in Therapeutic Intervention*. Philadelphia, Pa: CV Mosby Co; 2002.

Sammarco GJ. *Rehabilitation of the Foot and Ankle*. St. Louis, Mo: Mosby Year Book; 1995.

Schunk C, Reed K. *Clinical Practice Guidelines*. Gaithersburg, Md: Aspen Publishers; 2000.

Tomberlin JP, Saunders HD. *Evaluation, Treatment and Prevention of Musculoskeletal Disorders. Vol 2: Extremities*. Chaska, Minn: The Saunders Group; 1994.

Treatment

Buschbacher RM, ed. *Musculoskeletal Disorders: A Practical Guide for Diagnosis and Rehabilitation*. Boston, Mass: Andover Medical Publishers; 1994:216–235.

Edelstein JE. Physical therapy for elderly patients with foot disorders. *Top Geriatr Rehabil*. 1992;7:24–35.

Grabois M, Garrison SJ, Hart KA, Lehmkuhl LD. *Physical Medicine and Rehabilitation: The Complete Approach*. Malden, Mass: Blackwell Science; 2000.

Hertling D, Kessler RM. *Management of Common Musculoskeletal Disorders*. 3rd ed. Philadelphia, Pa: JB Lippincott Co; 1996:359–410.

Kisner C, Colby LA. *Therapeutic Exercise: Foundations and Techniques*. 3rd ed. Philadelphia, Pa: FA Davis Co; 1996:385–407.

McPoil TG, Hunt GC. Evaluation and management of foot and ankle disorders: present problems and future directions. *J Orthop Sports Phys Ther*. 1995;21:381–388.

Saltzman Cl, Nawoczenski DA. Complexities of foot architecture as a base of support. *Phys Ther*. 1995;21:354–360.

Tomaro JE, Butterfiedl SL. Biomechanical treatment of traumatic foot and ankle injuries with the use of foot orthotics. *J Orthop Sports Phys Ther*. 1995;21:373–380.

Tomberlin JP, Saunders HD. *Evaluation, Treatment and Prevention of Musculoskeletal Disorders. Vol 2: Extremities*. Chaska, Minn: The Saunders Group; 1994:265–305.

Hip Capsular Sprain

DESCRIPTION

Wrenching of the hip joint with disruption of the joint capsule.

CAUSE

Hip capsular sprain may have an insidious onset or be caused by minor trauma, such as a twisting motion.

ASSESSMENT

Note: See APTA's Guide to Physical Therapist Practice. 2nd ed. *Physical Therapy*. 2001;81.

Musculoskeletal Preferred Practice Patterns: E, F, J

AREAS

- History
- Pain
- Posture
- Joint integrity and structural deviations
- Gait
- Balance: unilateral stance
- Mobility: active and passive range of motion (ROM) and accessory motion
- Strength
- Neurological
- Skin and soft tissue, including edema
- Functional level

INSTRUMENTS/PROCEDURES

See References for sources.

Balance
- Berg Balance scale
- Balance Self-Perceptions test score

Functional Movement Tests
- Harris Hip Function Scale
- lumbopelvic rhythm with forward bending
- sit to stand, stairs, and squatting

Gait
- Dynamic Gait Index score

Joint Integrity and Structural Deviations

The following orthopedic tests may be performed:

- Craig's test
- Ely test
- FABER test
- hamstring tightness
- leg-length measurements
- Noble's compression test
- Ober's test

- piriformis test
- quadrant test
- Thomas' test
- Trendelenburg's sign
- Scour test for hip (flexion and adduction test)

Mobility
- arthrokinematic tests and osteokinematic ROMs
- goniometry
- muscular extensibility of the following muscles: medial and lateral hamstrings, iliopsoas, rectus femoris, TFL/ITB, hip adductors, hip rotators.

Posture
- clinical measurement of postural control
- pelvic tilt measurement

Skin: Edema
- palpation

Strength
- maximal isometric hip abductor muscles torques
- manual muscle testing and positional strength testing
- selective tissue tension tests

PROBLEMS
- The client will often have pain with weight bearing.
- The client may have decreased range of motion at hip.
- The client may be unable to tolerate weight bearing or may have shorter stride length.
- The client may have a decreased capacity for activities of daily living.

TREATMENT/MANAGEMENT
- Use modalities for pain relief and tissue management. Physical agents may include thermal modalities, cryotherapy, ultrasound, and phonophoresis.
- Consider gentle mobilization; progress as tolerated. Manual therapy techniques as indicated which may include soft tissue techniques, joint mobilization, and traction.
- Initiate ROM exercises early.
- The therapist may use external support, such as hip spica wrap and cane, crutches, or walker for support with weight-bearing activities.
- Begin strengthening exercises as tolerated. These can include active and resistive exercise. Consider proprioceptive neuromuscular facilitation (PNF) or aquatic therapy. Cardiovascular conditioning may include bike, treadmill, or Nordic track.
- Home program may include closed-kinetic chain functional exercises and flexibility exercises.

DESIRED OUTCOME/PROGNOSIS
- The client will return to pain-free activities of daily living.
- The client will prevent any further capsular stiffness and degenerative changes.
- Acute symptoms may resolve spontaneously; any lingering capsular tightness may lead to further hip problems.
- Prognosis may be affected by the presence of severe degenerative changes or hip contracture.

REFERENCES

Assessment

American Physical Therapy Association. Guide to physical therapist practice. 2nd ed. *Phys Ther.* 2001;81.

Buschbacher RM, ed. *Musculoskeletal Disorders: A Practical Guide for Diagnosis and Rehabilitation.* Boston, Mass: Andover Medical Publishers; 1994.

Daniels L, Worthingham C. *Muscle Testing Techniques of Manual Examination.* 6th ed. Philadelphia, Pa: WB Saunders Co; 1995.

Delitto A, Synder-Mackler L. The diagnostic process: examples in orthopedic physical therapy. *Phys Ther.* 1995;75:203–210.

Hall CM, Brody TB. *Therapeutic Exercise: Moving Toward Function.* Philadelphia, Pa: Lippincott Williams and Wilkins; 1999.

Hertling D, Kessler RM. *Management of Common Musculoskeletal Disorders.* 3rd ed. Philadelphia, Pa: JB Lippincott Co; 1996:78, 534.

Jacobs K. *Ergonomics for Therapists.* 2nd ed. Boston, Mass: Butterworth Heinemann; 2000.

Kasman GS, Ram JR, Wolf SI. *Clinical Applications in Surface Electromyography: Chronic Musculoskeletal Pain.* Bethesda, Md: Aspen Publishers; 1998.

Kendall FP, McCreary EK, Provance PG. *Muscles: Testing and Function.* 4th ed. Baltimore, Md: Williams and Wilkins; 1993.

Kisner C, Colby LA. *Therapeutic Exercise: Foundations and Techniques.* 3rd ed. Philadelphia, Pa: FA Davis Co; 1996:241–270.

Lesh SG. *Clinical Orthopedics for the Physical Therapist Assistant.* Philadelphia, Pa: FA Davis Co; 2000.

Malone TR, McPoil T, Nitz AJ, eds. *Orthopaedic and Sports Physical Therapy.* 3rd ed. St. Louis, Mo: CV Mosby Co; 1997.

Myers RS, ed. *Saunders Manual of Physical Therapy Practice.* Philadelphia, Pa: WB Saunders Co; 1995.

Rothstein JM, Roy SH, Wolf SL. *The Rehabilitation Specialist's Handbook.* 2nd ed. Philadelphia, Pa: FA Davis Co; 1998.

Saidoff DC, McDonough AL. *Critical Pathways in Therapeutic Intervention.* Philadelphia, Pa: CV Mosby Co; 2002.

Schunk C, Reed K. *Clinical Practice Guidelines.* Gaithersburg, Md: Aspen Publishers; 2000.

Tomberlin JP, Saunders HD. *Evaluation, Treatment and Prevention of Musculoskeletal Disorders. Vol 2: Extremities.* Chaska, Minn: The Saunders Group; 1994.

Treatment

Boyd KT, Peirce NP, Batt ME. Common hip injuries in sport. *Sports Med.* 1997;25:273–288.

Butcher JD, Salzman KL, Lillegard WA. Lower extremity bursitis. *Am Fam Phys.* 1996; 54(2):468.

Grabois M, Garrison SJ, Hart KA, Lehmkuhl LD. *Physical medicine and Rehabilitation: The Complete Approach.* Malden, Mass: Blackwell Science; 2000.

Hertling D, Kessler RM. *Management of Common Musculoskeletal Disorders.* 3rd ed. Philadelphia, Pa: JB Lippincott Co; 1996:272–297.

Kendall FP, McCreary EK, Provance PG. *Muscles: Testing and Function.* 4th ed. Baltimore, Md: Williams and Wilkins; 1993.

Kisner C, Colby LA. *Therapeutic Exercise: Foundations and Techniques.* 3rd ed. Philadelphia, Pa: FA Davis Co; 1996:317–344.

Kornberg C, McCarthy T. The effect of neural stretching technique on sympathetic outflow to the lower limbs. *J Orthop Sports Phys Ther.* 1992;16:269–274.

Richarson JK, Iglarsch AZ. *Clinical Orthopedic Physical Therapy.* Philadelphia, Pa: WB Saunders Co; 1994.

Tomberlin JP, Saunders HD. *Evaluation, Treatment and Prevention of Musculoskeletal Disorders. Vol 2: Extremities.* Chaska, Minn: The Saunders Group; 1994:200.

Iliopectineal Bursitis

DESCRIPTION

Acute or chronic inflammation of the iliopectineal bursa. Iliopectineal bursitis is less common than trochanteric bursitis.

CAUSE

Onset is insidious but can be associated with osteoarthritis. Iliopectineal bursitis may be caused by tightness in the iliopsoas muscle.

ASSESSMENT

Note: See APTA's Guide to Physical Therapist Practice. 2nd ed. *Physical Therapy.* 2001;81.

Musculoskeletal Preferred Practice Pattern: E

AREAS

- History
- Pain
- Posture
- Joint integrity and structural deviations
- Gait
- Mobility: active and passive range of motion (ROM) and accessory motion
- Strength
- Neurological
- Skin and soft tissue: edema
- Functional level

INSTRUMENTS/PROCEDURES

See References for sources.

Joint Integrity and Structural Deviations
- Craig's test
- Ely test
- FABER test
- hamstring tightness
- leg-length measurements
- Noble's compression test
- Ober's test
- piriformis test
- quadrant test
- Thomas' test
- Trendelenburg's sign

Mobility
- goniometry

Posture
- clinical measurement of postural control
- pelvic tilt

Skin: Edema
- palpation

Strength
- maximal isometric hip abductor muscles torques
- manual muscle testing

PROBLEMS
- This condition closely resembles trochanteric bursitis, but pain is with hip flexion against resistance or passive hip extension.
- The client often has pain in the groin area.
- There may be pain that radiates to the L-2 or L-3 segment level.

TREATMENT/MANAGEMENT
- Use modalities, such as ice, ultrasound, and iontophoresis, as indicated.
- Avoid aggravating activities.
- Discuss sleep posture adaptations with pillows.
- Assess for muscular imbalance and stretch (iliotibial band tightness), and strengthen accordingly.

Note: Refer to section on osteoarthritis if this condition is an aggravating factor.

DESIRED PROGNOSIS/OUTCOME
- The client will return to pain-free activities of daily living.
- Inflammation and pain will decrease, and recurrence will be prevented.
- Ultrasound may offer effective relief in 3 to 6 sessions.

REFERENCES

Assessment

American Physical Therapy Association. Guide to physical therapist practice. 2nd ed. *Phys Ther.* 2001;81.

Buschbacher RM, ed. *Musculoskeletal Disorders: A Practical Guide for Diagnosis and Rehabilitation.* Boston, Mass: Andover Medical Publishers; 1994.

Daniels L, Worthingham C. *Muscle Testing Techniques of Manual Examination.* 6th ed. Philadelphia, Pa: WB Saunders Co; 1995.

Delitto A, Synder-Mackler L. The diagnostic process: examples in orthopedic physical therapy. *Phys Ther.* 1995;75:203–210.

Hall CM, Brody TB. *Therapeutic Exercise: Moving Toward Function.* Philadelphia, Pa: Lippincott Williams and Wilkins; 1999.

Hertling D, Kessler RM. *Management of Common Musculoskeletal Disorders.* 3rd ed. Philadelphia, Pa: JB Lippincott Co; 1996:78, 534.

Jacobs K. *Ergonomics for Therapists.* 2nd ed. Boston, Mass: Butterworth Heinemann; 2000.

Kasman GS, Ram JR, Wolf SI. *Clinical Applications in Surface Electromyography: Chronic Musculoskeletal Pain.* Bethesda, Md: Aspen Publishers; 1998.

Kendall FP, McCreary EK, Provance PG. *Muscles: Testing and Function.* 4th ed. Baltimore, Md: Williams and Wilkins; 1993.

Kisner C, Colby LA. *Therapeutic Exercise: Foundations and Techniques.* 3rd ed. Philadelphia, Pa: FA Davis Co; 1996:241–270.

Lesh SG. *Clinical Orthopedics for the Physical Therapist Assistant.* Philadelphia, Pa: FA Davis Co; 2000.

Malone TR, McPoil T, Nitz AJ, eds. *Orthopaedic and Sports Physical Therapy*. 3rd ed. St. Louis, Mo: CV Mosby Co; 1997.

Myers RS, ed. *Saunders Manual of Physical Therapy Practice*. Philadelphia, Pa: WB Saunders Co; 1995.

Rothstein JM, Roy SH, Wolf SL. *The Rehabilitation Specialist's Handbook*. 2nd ed. Philadelphia, Pa: FA Davis Co; 1998.

Saidoff DC, McDonough AL. *Critical Pathways in Therapeutic Intervention*. Philadelphia, Pa: CV Mosby Co; 2002.

Schunk C, Reed K. *Clinical Practice Guidelines*. Gaithersburg, Md: Aspen Publishers; 2000.

Tomberlin JP, Saunders HD. *Evaluation, Treatment and Prevention of Musculoskeletal Disorders. Vol 2: Extremities*. Chaska, Minn: The Saunders Group; 1994.

Treatment

Grabois M, Garrison SJ, Hart KA, Lehmkuhl LD. *Physical Medicine and Rehabilitation: The Complete Approach*. Malden, Mass: Blackwell Science; 2000.

Hicklin SP, DePretis MC. Lower extremity: hip. In: Myers RS, ed. *Saunders Manual of Physical Therapy Practice*. Philadelphia, Pa: WB Saunders Co; 1995:955–999.

Kornberg C, McCarthy T. The effect of neural stretching technique on sympathetic outflow to the lower limbs. *J Orthop Sports Phys Ther*. 1992;16:269–274.

Tomberlin JP, Saunders HD. *Evaluation, Treatment and Prevention of Musculoskeletal Disorders. Vol 2: Extremities*. Chaska, Minn: The Saunders Group; 1994:200.

Interdigital Neuroma

Also known as *Morton's neuroma* or *metatarsalgia*.

DESCRIPTION

Neuroma is a benign fibrous tissue formation. Interdigital neuroma usually occurs at the third plantar interdigital nerve, although other locations are possible. Interdigital neuroma is more likely to be unilateral than bilateral and is more common in women than men.

CAUSE

This condition may begin with a lack of neural mobility and progress to the formation of a neuroma. It may be caused by excessive compression and the shearing force accompanying weight bearing. Undue pronation during the stance phase of weight bearing has also been implicated.

ASSESSMENT

Note: See APTA's Guide to Physical Therapist Practice. 2nd ed. *Physical Therapy*. 2001;81.

Musculoskeletal Preferred Practice Pattern: E

AREAS
- History
- Posture
- Pain
- Gait
- Strength
- Neurological
- Joint integrity and structural deviations

- Mobility, including active and passive range of motion (ROM) and accessory motion
- Skin and soft tissue
- Equipment, including footwear

INSTRUMENTS/PROCEDURES

See References for sources.

Gait
- dynamic assessment of foot mechanics
  1. dynamic plantar pressure distribution
  2. foot pressure EMED system
  3. pedabarograph
  4. three-dimensional kinematic analysis
- footprint analysis in gait documentation

PROBLEMS
- The client often has pain at the metatarsal head, especially the third or fourth, with weight bearing.
- The client may demonstrate extreme pronation of the subtalar joint.
- The client may have tenderness to touch at the third or fourth metatarsal head or at any metatarsal head.
- The metatarsal bone may demonstrate either hypomobility or hypermobility.
- Often the pain worsens with activity.

TREATMENT/MANAGEMENT
- Use physical agents, such as local ice application, as indicated.
- Consider joint mobilization for intermetatarsal joint.
- Use neural mobilization if indicated.
- Assess footwear. Consider custom-made shoes with support for proximal to metatarsal heads.
- Assess need for orthotics such as metatarsal arch pads.
- Assess and possibly change fitness training techniques as indicated.
- Use strengthening and flexibility exercises.
- If the client is postoperative, consider mobility exercises.

DESIRED OUTCOME/PROGNOSIS
- The client will experience control of symptoms.
- There will be an improved joint glide.
- Therapy will control forefoot hypermobility and excessive pronation.

Note: Sometimes surgical removal of the neuroma is indicated. Postoperative care may prevent scar tissue formation.

REFERENCES

Assessment

American Physical Therapy Association. Guide to physical therapist practice. 2nd ed. *Phys Ther.* 2001;81.

Buschbacher RM, ed. *Musculoskeletal Disorders: A Practical Guide for Diagnosis and Rehabilitation.* Boston, Mass: Andover Medical Publishers; 1994.

Daniels L, Worthingham C. *Muscle Testing Techniques of Manual Examination.* 6th ed. Philadelphia, Pa: WB Saunders Co; 1995.

Delitto A, Synder-Mackler L. The diagnostic process: examples in orthopedic physical therapy. *Phys Ther.* 1995;75:203–210.

Donatelli RA. *The Biomechanics of the Foot and Ankle.* 2nd ed. Philadelphia, Pa: FA Davis Co; 1996.

Hall CM, Brody TB. *Therapeutic Exercise: Moving Toward Function.* Philadelphia, Pa: FA Davis Co; Lippincott Williams and Wilkins; 1999.

Hertling D, Kessler RM. *Management of Common Musculoskeletal Disorders.* 3rd ed. Philadelphia, Pa: JB Lippincott Co; 1996:78, 534.

Jacobs K. *Ergonomics for Therapists.* 2nd ed. Boston, Mass: Butterworth Heinemann; 2000.

Kasman GS, Ram JR, Wolf SI. *Clinical Applications in Surface Electromyography: Chronic Musculoskeletal Pain.* Bethesda, Md: Aspen Publishers; 1998.

Kendall FP, McCreary EK, Provance PG. *Muscles: Testing and Function.* 4th ed. Baltimore, Md: Williams and Wilkins; 1993.

Kisner C, Colby LA. *Therapeutic Exercise: Foundations and Techniques.* 3rd ed. Philadelphia, Pa: FA Davis Co; 1996:241–270.

Lesh SG. *Clinical Orthopedics for the Physical Therapist Assistant.* Philadelphia, Pa: FA Davis Co; 2000.

Malone TR, McPoil T, Nitz AJ, eds. *Orthopaedic and Sports Physical Therapy.* 3rd ed. St. Louis, Mo: CV Mosby Co; 1997.

Myers RS, ed. *Saunders Manual of Physical Therapy Practice.* Philadelphia, Pa: WB Saunders Co; 1995.

Rothstein JM, Roy SH, Wolf SL. *The Rehabilitation Specialist's Handbook.* 2nd ed. Philadelphia, Pa: FA Davis Co; 1998.

Saidoff DC, McDonough AL. *Critical Pathways in Therapeutic Intervention.* Philadelphia, Pa: CV Mosby Co; 2002.

Sammarco GJ. *Rehabilitation of the Foot and Ankle.* St. Louis, Mo: Mosby Year Book; 1995.

Schunk C, Reed K. *Clinical Practice Guidelines.* Gaithersburg, Md: Aspen Publishers; 2000.

Tomberlin JP, Saunders HD. *Evaluation, Treatment and Prevention of Musculoskeletal Disorders. Vol 2: Extremities.* Chaska, Minn: The Saunders Group; 1994.

Treatment

Buschbacher RM, ed. *Musculoskeletal Disorders: A Practical Guide for Diagnosis and Rehabilitation.* Boston, Mass: Andover Medical Publishers; 1994:216–235.

Grabois M, Garrison SJ, Hart KA, Lehmkuhl LD. *Physical Medicine and Rehabilitation: The Complete Approach.* Malden, Mass: Blackwell Science; 2000.

Hertling D, Kessler RM. *Management of Common Musculoskeletal Disorders.* 3rd ed. Philadelphia, Pa: JB Lippincott Co; 1996:359–410.

Kisner C, Colby LA. *Therapeutic Exercise: Foundations and Techniques.* 3rd ed. Philadelphia, Pa: FA Davis Co; 1996:385–407.

McPoil TG, Hunt GC. Evaluation and management of foot and ankle disorders: present problems and future directions. *J Orthop Sports Phys Ther.* 1995;21:381–388.

Tomberlin JP, Saunders HD. *Evaluation, Treatment and Prevention of Musculoskeletal Disorders. Vol 2: Extremities.* Chaska, Minn: The Saunders Group; 1994:265–305.

Medial Tibial Stress Syndrome

Also known as *anterolateral* or *posteromedial shin splints* or *posterior tibialis tendinitis*.

DESCRIPTION

An overuse syndrome leading to damage of the anterior compartment muscles or postero-medial compartment muscles. The tibialis posterior tendon is the most commonly affected structure.

CAUSE

This overuse syndrome may be caused by irritation of the tibial periosteum. Tendinitis may also cause this complaint. Extreme pronation of the subtalar joint may cause this condition in the posteromedial compartment. Factors also influencing medial tibial stress syndrome include repetitive microtrauma, footwear, flexibility, muscle imbalance, and structural malalignment.

ASSESSMENT

Note: See APTA's Guide to Physical Therapist Practice. 2nd ed. *Physical Therapy.* 2001;81.

Musculoskeletal Preferred Practice Patterns: D, E, F, J

AREAS
- History
- Pain
- Posture: biomechanical screen, static stance, lower extremity alignment
- Gait: weight-bearing tolerance and use of assistive devices
- Strength: especially tibialis posterior
- Neurological
- Joint integrity and structural deviations: arch height
- Mobility, including active and passive range of motion (ROM) and accessory motion
- Skin and soft tissues
- Equipment, including footwear

INSTRUMENTS/PROCEDURES

See References for sources.

Gait
- dynamic assessment of foot mechanics
  1. dynamic plantar pressure distribution
  2. foot pressure EMED system
  3. pedabarograph
  4. three-dimensional kinematic analysis
- stance phase analysis
- gait velocity
- footprint analysis in gait documentation

Joint Integrity and Structural Deviations
- tibial varum assessment
- tinnels

Mobility
- assessment of ankle dorsiflexion
- goniometry
- visual estimates of ankle joint active ROM

Pain
- palpation

Strength
- isokinetic testing
- manual muscle testing

PROBLEMS

ANTEROLATERAL
- The client often has pain and tenderness at the lateral border and distal half of the medial tibial crest of the tibia.
- Often, the pain increases with active dorsiflexion and passive stretch of ankle dorsiflexors.

POSTEROMEDIAL
- The client often has shin pain posteromedially, 4 to 6 inches proximal to the medial malleolus with activity, especially weight bearing.
- There may be tenderness along the posteromedial border of the tibia, especially distally.
- The client may have a tendency toward excessive subtalor pronation.
- The client often has a tight soleus muscle.

TREATMENT/MANAGEMENT

For treatment of foot and ankle problems in general:
- Exercises progress from passive ROM to active assisted and active ROM to resisted ROM.
- Begin non-weight-bearing strengthening activities after pain-free ROM is achieved.
- Isometric, isotonic, and isokinetic exercise can be used.
- Eccentric loading should not be overlooked.
- Progress to jogging, running, and athletic maneuvers as indicated.
- Address preventive measures, such as stretching, choice of shoes, and use of adhesive strapping during athletic activities.

For medial tibial stress syndrome specifically:
- Use physical agents, such as ice, as indicated. Consider use of TENS and iontophoresis with 10% hydrocortisone on affected area. Heat may be considered in the subacute or recurrent phases.
- Consider use of compression. Consider use of myofascial release techniques.
- Avoid weight bearing; the client may need gait-assistive devices.
- Instruct in flexibility, strengthening exercises, and proprioceptive reeducation.
- Assess for orthotics and proper footwear with flexible, supportive insole, and a firm wide heel counter. Consider use of taping.
- Teach activity modification with return to activity as pain allows. Begin with limits of 1 hour of aerobic activity per day to a maximum of 3 to 4 times per week until tissues have recovered fully.

PRECAUTIONS/CONTRAINDICATIONS

Note: This condition can mimic tibial or fibular stress fracture, tibial stress reaction, or anterior compartment syndrome.

DESIRED OUTCOME/PROGNOSIS

- The client will experience control of symptoms such as edema, pain, and inflammation.
- The client will decrease stress with activity modification.
- There will be a decrease in excessive pronation, and shock will be absorbed with orthotics.
- Therapy will improve flexibility of the heel cord and the first metatarsal phalangeal joint to reduce excessive pronatatory forces.
- Therapy will strengthen the plantarflexors and inverters of the foot.
- The client will prevent recurrence.

REFERENCES

Assessment

American Physical Therapy Association. Guide to physical therapist practice. 2nd ed. *Phys Ther.* 2001;81.

Buschbacher RM, ed. *Musculoskeletal Disorders: A Practical Guide for Diagnosis and Rehabilitation.* Boston, Mass: Andover Medical Publishers; 1994.

Daniels L, Worthingham C. *Muscle Testing Techniques of Manual Examination.* 6th ed. Philadelphia, Pa: WB Saunders Co; 1995.

Delitto A, Synder-Mackler L. The diagnostic process: examples in orthopedic physical therapy. *Phys Ther.* 1995;75:203–210.

Hall CM, Brody TB. *Therapeutic Exercise: Moving Toward Function.* Philadelphia, Pa: Lippincott Williams and Wilkins; 1999.

Hertling D, Kessler RM. *Management of Common Musculoskeletal Disorders.* 3rd ed. Philadelphia, Pa: JB Lippincott Co; 1996:78, 534.

Jacobs K. *Ergonomics for Therapists.* 2nd ed. Boston, Mass: Butterworth Heinemann; 2000.

Kasman GS, Ram JR, Wolf SI. *Clinical Applications in Surface Electromyography: Chronic Musculoskeletal Pain.* Bethesda, Md: Aspen Publishers; 1998.

Kendall FP, McCreary EK, Provance PG. *Muscles: Testing and Function.* 4th ed. Baltimore, Md: Williams and Wilkins; 1993.

Kisner C, Colby LA. *Therapeutic Exercise: Foundations and Techniques.* 3rd ed. Philadelphia, Pa: FA Davis Co; 1996:241–270.

Lesh SG. *Clinical Orthopedics for the Physical Therapist Assistant.* Philadelphia, Pa: FA Davis Co; 2000.

Malone TR, McPoil T, Nitz AJ, eds. *Orthopaedic and Sports Physical Therapy.* 3rd ed. St. Louis, Mo: CV Mosby Co; 1997.

Myers RS, ed. *Saunders Manual of Physical Therapy Practice.* Philadelphia, Pa: WB Saunders Co; 1995.

Rothstein JM, Roy SH, Wolf SL. *The Rehabilitation Specialist's Handbook.* 2nd ed. Philadelphia, Pa: FA Davis Co; 1998.

Saidoff DC, McDonough AL. *Critical Pathways in Therapeutic Intervention.* Philadelphia, Pa: CV Mosby Co; 2002.

Schunk C, Reed K. *Clinical Practice Guidelines.* Gaithersburg, Md: Aspen Publishers; 2000.

Tomberlin JP, Saunders HD. *Evaluation, Treatment and Prevention of Musculoskeletal Disorders. Vol 2: Extremities.* Chaska, Minn: The Saunders Group; 1994.

Treatment

Ballantyne BT, Kukulka CG, Soderberg GL. Motor unit recruitment in human medial gastroc-nemius muscle during combined knee flexion and plantar flexion isometric contractions. *Exp Brain Res.* 1993;93:492–498.

Bennett JE, Reinking MF, Pluemer B, et al. Factors contributing to the development of medical tibial stress syndrome in high school runners. *J Orthop Sports Phys Ther.* 2001; 31:504–510.

Blackman P. Exercise-related lower leg pain-compartment syndromes. *Med Sci Sports Exerc.* 2000;32(suppl 3):S4–10.

Bruckner P. Exercise-related lower leg pain—an overview. *Med Sci Sports Exerc.* 2000; 32(suppl):S1–3.

Buschbacher RM, ed. *Musculoskeletal Disorders: A Practical Guide for Diagnosis and Rehabilitation.* Boston, Mass: Andover Medical Publishers; 1994:216–235.

Grabois M, Garrison SJ, Hart KA, Lehmkuhl LD. *Physical Medicine and Rehabilitation: The Complete Approach.* Malden, Mass: Blackwell Science; 2000.

Gross MT. Lower quarter screening for skeletal malalignment: suggestions for orthotics and shoewear. *J Orthop Sports Phys Ther.* 1995;21:389–405.

Hertling D, Kessler RM. *Management of Common Musculoskeletal Disorders.* 3rd ed. Philadelphia, Pa: JB Lippincott Co; 1996:359–410.

Kisner C, Colby LA. *Therapeutic Exercise: Foundations and Techniques.* 3rd ed. Philadelphia, Pa: FA Davis Co; 1996:385–407.

McCrory P. Exercise-related lower leg pain-neural. *Med Sci Sports Exerc.* 2000;32(suppl 3): S11–14.

McCulloch MU, Brunt D, Vander-Linden D. The effect of foot orthotics and gait velocity on lower limb kinematics and temporal events of stance. *J Orthop Sports Phys Ther.* 1993;17:2–10.

McPoil TG. Footwear. *Phys Ther.* 1988;68:1857–1865.

Tomberlin JP, Saunders HD. *Evaluation, Treatment and Prevention of Musculoskeletal Disorders. Vol 2: Extremities.* Chaska, Minn: The Saunders Group; 1994:265–305.

Varelas FL, Wessel J, Clement DB, Doyle DL, Wilery JP. Muscle function in chronic compartment syndrome of the leg. *J Orthop Sports Phys Ther.* 1993;18:586–589.

Youdas JW, Bogard CL, Suman VJ. Reliability of goniometric measurements and visual estimates of ankle joint active range of motion obtained in a clinical setting. *Arch Phys Med Rehabil.* 1993;74:1113–1118.

Patellar Tendinitis

Also known as *jumper's knee, popliteal tendinitis,* and *semimembranosus tendinitis.*

DESCRIPTION

Inflammation of patellar, popliteal, or semimembranosus tendons. There is often a higher incidence in clients involved in athletic activities.

CAUSE

Patellar tendinitis, popliteal tendinitis, and semimembranosus tendinitis are of unknown etiology, but overuse is considered an irritating factor. These conditions may be caused by the effects of aging, repetitive microtrauma, extreme trauma, strain, or unaccustomed exercise.

PATELLAR TENDINITIS

Patellar tendinitis (jumper's knee) is an overuse syndrome often caused by repetitive jumping and is often associated with tracking problems.

POPLITEAL AND SEMIMEMBRANOSUS TENDINITIS

Popliteal tendinitis and semimembranosus tendinitis are often associated with running. Downhill running and hyperpronation of the foot may lead to popliteal or bicipital tendinitis at the knee.

ASSESSMENT

Note: See APTA's Guide to Physical Therapist Practice. 2nd ed. *Physical Therapy.* 2001;81.

Musculoskeletal Preferred Practice Patterns: D, E, F, J

AREAS
- History
- Pain
- Posture, including static stance, and any pronation of feet and internal rotation at hip
- Joint integrity and structural deviations
- Mobility, including active and passive range of motion (ROM), and accessory motion
- Strength, including quadriceps and gluteus medius muscles and functional tests such as jumping, squatting, and stair descent.
- Neurological
- Skin and soft tissue, including edema
- Gait
- Functional level

INSTRUMENTS/PROCEDURES

See References for sources.

Functional Level
- Blazina classification for Functional Limitations Associated with Patellar Tendinitis
- modified Lysholm knee score

Joint Integrity and Structural Deviations

The following orthopedic tests of the knee may be used. *Note:* Those most recommended are marked with an asterisk.

- A-angle
- ALRI test
- AMRI test
- Apley grinding test
- apprehension test
- bounce home test
- brush or stroke (wipe) test
- Clark sign
- crepitus*
- crossover test
- dynamic Q-angle*
- Ely test
- external rotation test
- flexion rotation drawer sign
- fluctuation test
- gravity drawer test (posterior sag sign)
- hamstring length
- Helfet test
- Hughston plica test
- Hughston posterolateral drawer test
- Hughston test (jerk sign)

- hyperflexion-hyperextension test
- Jakob test (reverse pivot)
- Lachman's test
- lateral pull test
- limb-length discrepancy
- MacIntosh test (lateral pivot shift)
- McConnell test
- McMurray-Anderson test
- Noble's compression test
- Ober's test
- O'Donoghue test
- patellar tap
- patellar tilt
- patellofemoral grind test*

- Perkins test
- plica test
- posterior drawer sign
- posterior sag test
- quadriceps active test
- reverse pivot shift test
- Slocum test
- Steinman's test
- squat test
- Thomas' test*
- valgus stress test
- varus stress test
- Waldron test
- Wilson test

Skin and Soft Tissue: Edema
- thigh measurement

Special Tests to Which the Physical Therapist May or May Not Have Access
- arthrography and arthroscopy
- computed tomography (CT)
- joint aspiration
- magnetic resonance imaging (MRI)
- x-ray studies
- ultrasonography

Strength
- cable tensiometers
- isokinetic dynamometers
- strain gauge devices
- manual muscle testing

PROBLEMS

PATELLAR TENDINITIS
- The client often reports pain and tenderness at the inferior end of the patella.
- The client may have swelling.
- There is often pain when using the stairs and with any forceful knee extension.
- The client may complain of the knee getting stiff and sore with prolonged sitting.

POPLITEAL AND SEMIMEMBRANOSUS TENDINITIS
- The client often reports pain on the lateral aspect of the knee.

TREATMENT/MANAGEMENT

PATELLAR TENDINITIS
- Encourage rest.
- Use ice massage if indicated.
- Begin progressive resistive exercise strengthening program with emphasis on vastus medialis obliquus (VMO) and on eccentric exercises and assess for weakness of dorsiflexors.
- Implement flexibility exercises, including hamstring and gastrocnemius stretching.
- Consider phonophoresis with 10% hydrocortisone ointment. Other modalities include ultrasound or high-voltage pulsed monophasic current to the patellar tendon.
- Consider an orthosis, patellar taping, or infrapatellar straps.
- Consider patellofemoral knee sleeve for edema control and mobility reduction of patella tendon during activity.

- Consider use of manual therapy techniques.
- Advise client on modification of recreational and occupational activities.

POPLITEAL AND SEMIMEMBRANOSUS TENDINITIS
- Encourage rest.
- Try intermittent use of ice for at least the first 72-hour period, if indicated.
- Consider use of ultrasound.
- Begin flexibility and strengthening exercises.
- Assess training techniques and footwear.

PRECAUTIONS/CONTRAINDICATIONS
- X-rays should be consulted to rule out potential fractures.
- Carefully consider the nature of the problem before examination to avoid aggravating the condition with the test procedures.
- Avoid aggressive kinetic open-chain quadriceps exercise, which may aggravate tendinitis.
- Popliteal and semimembranosus tendinitis can mimic a meniscal injury.

DESIRED OUTCOME/PROGNOSIS
- The client will have a reduction in symptoms.
- The client will have pain-free full function of the knee.

Note: If tendinitis continues without treatment, the tendon may rupture.

REFERENCES

Assessment

American Physical Therapy Association. Guide to physical therapist practice. 2nd ed. *Phys Ther.* 2001;81.

Bandy WD, Timm KE. Relationship between peak torque, work, and power for knee flexion and extension in clients with grade I medial compartment sprains of the knee. *J Orthop Sports Phys Ther.* 1992;16:288–292.

Buschbacher RM, ed. *Musculoskeletal Disorders: A Practical Guide for Diagnosis and Rehabilitation.* Boston, Mass: Andover Medical Publishers; 1994.

Daniels L, Worthingham C. *Muscle Testing Techniques of Manual Examination.* 6th ed. Philadelphia, Pa: WB Saunders Co; 1995.

Delitto A, Synder-Mackler L. The diagnostic process: examples in orthopedic physical therapy. *Phys Ther.* 1995;75:203–210.

Hall CM, Brody TB. *Therapeutic Exercise: Moving Toward Function.* Philadelphia, Pa: Lippincott Williams and Wilkins; 1999.

Hertling D, Kessler RM. *Management of Common Musculoskeletal Disorders.* 3rd ed. Philadelphia, Pa: JB Lippincott Co; 1996:78, 534.

Jacobs K. *Ergonomics for Therapists.* 2nd ed. Boston, Mass: Butterworth Heinemann; 2000.

Kasman GS, Ram JR, Wolf SI. *Clinical Applications in Surface Electromyography: Chronic Musculoskeletal Pain.* Bethesda, Md: Aspen Publishers; 1998.

Kendall FP, McCreary EK, Provance PG. *Muscles: Testing and Function.* 4th ed. Baltimore, Md: Williams and Wilkins, 1993.

Kisner C, Colby LA. *Therapeutic Exercise: Foundations and Techniques.* 3rd ed. Philadelphia, Pa: FA Davis Co; 1996:241–270.

Lesh SG. *Clinical Orthopedics for the Physical Therapist Assistant.* Philadelphia, Pa: FA Davis Co; 2000.

Malone TR, McPoil T, Nitz AJ, eds. *Orthopaedic and Sports Physical Therapy.* 3rd ed. St. Louis, Mo: CV Mosby Co; 1997.

Myers RS, ed. *Saunders Manual of Physical Therapy Practice.* Philadelphia, Pa: WB Saunders Co; 1995.

Rothstein JM, Roy SH, Wolf SL. *The Rehabilitation Specialist's Handbook.* 2nd ed. Philadelphia, Pa: FA Davis Co; 1998.

Saidoff DC, McDonough AL. *Critical Pathways in Therapeutic Intervention.* Philadelphia, Pa: CV Mosby Co; 2002.

Schunk C, Reed K. *Clinical Practice Guidelines.* Gaithersburg, Md: Aspen Publishers; 2000.

Steiner LA, Harris BA, Krebs DE. Reliability of eccentric isokinetic knee flexion and extension measurements. *Arch Phys Med Rehabil.* 1993;74:1327–1335.

Tomberlin JP, Saunders HD. *Evaluation, Treatment and Prevention of Musculoskeletal Disorders. Vol 2: Extremities.* Chaska, Minn: The Saunders Group; 1994.

Treatment

Afzali L, Kuwabara F, Zachazewski J, Browne P, Robinson B. A new method for the determination of the characteristic shape of an isokinetic quadriceps femoris muscle torque curve. *Phys Ther.* 1992;72:585–595.

Blazina ME, Kerlan RK, Jobe FW. Jumper's knee. *Orthop Clin North Am.* 1993;4:665–678.

Buschbacher RM, ed. *Musculoskeletal Disorders: A Practical Guide for Diagnosis and Rehabilitation.* Boston, Mass: Andover Medical Publishers; 1994:206–208.

Caylor D, Fites R, Worrell TW. The relationship between quadriceps angle and anterior knee pain syndrome. *J Orthop Sports Phys Ther.* 1993;17:11–16.

Charteris J. An isometric normative database to facilitate restoration of function in knee-injured active young adults. *S Afr J Physiotherapy.* 1993;49:2:28–34.

Cook JL, Khan KM, Purdam CR. Conservative treatment of patellar tendinopathy. *Phys Ther Sport.* 2001;2:54–65.

Delitto A. Lower extremity: knee. In: Myers RS, ed. *Saunders Manual of Physical Therapy Practice.* Philadelphia, Pa: WB Saunders Co; 1995:1001–1029.

DiVeta JA, Vogelbach WD. The clinical efficacy of the A-angle in measuring patellar alignment. *J Orthop Sports Phys Ther.* 1992;16:136–139.

Duri ZAA, Aichroth PM. Patella tendinitis: clinical and literature review. *Knee Surg Sports Traumatology Arthroscopy.* 1995;95–100.

Grelsamer RP, McConnell J. *The Patella: A Team Approach.* Gaithersburg, Md: Aspen Publishers; 1998.

Grabois M, Garrison SJ, Hart KA, Lehmkuhl LD. *Physical Medicine and Rehabilitation: The Complete Approach.* Malden, Mass: Blackwell Science; 2000.

Karst GM, Jewett PD. EMG analysis of exercise proposed for differential activation of medial and lateral quadricep femoris muscle components. *Phys Ther.* 1993;73: 286–299.

Kisner C, Colby LA. *Therapeutic Exercise: Foundations and Techniques.* 3rd ed. Philadelphia, Pa: FA Davis Co; 1996:345–384.

McConnell J. Fat pad irritation—a mistaken patellar tendinitis. *Sport Health.* 1991;9:7–9.

Myers RS, ed. *Saunders Manual of Physical Therapy Practice.* Philadelphia, Pa: WB Saunders Co; 1995:1352.

Powers CM, Maffucci R, Hampton S. Rearfoot posture in subjects with patellofemoral pain. *J Orthop Sports Med.* 1995:22:155–160.

Puniello MS. Iliotibial band tightness and medial patellar glide in patients with patello-femoral dysfunction. *J Orthop Sports Phys Ther.* 1993;17:144–148.

Richards DP, Ajemian SV, Wiley P, et al. Knee joint dynamics predict patellar tendinitis in elite volleyball players. *Am J Sports Med.* 1996;676–683.

Tomberlin JP, Saunders HD. *Evaluation, Treatment and Prevention of Musculoskeletal Disorders. Vol 2: Extremities.* Chaska, Minn: The Saunders Group; 1994:217–264.

Wilk KE, Andrew JR. The effects of pad placement and angular velocity on tibial displacement during isokinetic exercise. *J Orthop Sports Phys Ther.* 1993;17:24–30.

Patellofemoral Stress Syndrome

Also known as *patellofemoral instability, patellar tracking dysfunction,* or *patellofemoral pain syndrome.*

DESCRIPTION

Patellofemoral stress syndrome is a condition in which the patella does not follow the normal path of tracking between the femoral condyles but articulates against the femur instead. This syndrome occurs more frequently in adolescent girls and in clients with anterior cruciate ligament problems.

CAUSE

The most common cause of patellofemoral problems is repetitive trauma. Patellofemoral stress syndrome can also be caused by patella alta (high-riding patella), plicas, or tightness in any of the following structures: hamstrings, heel cords, vastus lateralis, iliotibial tract, or lateral retinaculum. Weakness of the vastus medialis and a Q angle (angle between the long axis of the thigh and patella tendon) greater than 15 degrees can also be the cause. Another common cause is a lateral pull of the patella combined with excessive pronation. While the lower leg turns medially during pronation, the three quadriceps muscles pull laterally on the patella. This pulling causes the patella to articulate against the femur.

ASSESSMENT

Note: See APTA's Guide to Physical Therapist Practice. 2nd ed. *Physical Therapy.* 2001;81.

Musculoskeletal Preferred Practice Patterns: A, D, E, F, G, H, I, J

AREAS
- History
- Pain
- Posture, including any pronation of feet or internal rotation at femurs
- Joint integrity and structural deviations
- Mobility, including active and passive ROM, and accessory motion
- Strength: note especially any vastus medialis obliquus (VMO) weakness
- Neurological
- Skin and soft tissue
- Gait

INSTRUMENTS/PROCEDURES

See References for sources.

Functional Level
- Lysholm knee rating scale
- Victorian Institute of Sport Assessment (VISA)

Joint Integrity and Structural Deviations

The following orthopedic tests of the knee may be performed:

- A-angle
- ALRI
- AMRI
- Apley grinding test
- apprehension test
- bounce home test
- brush or stroke (wipe) test
- Clark sign
- crepitus
- crossover test
- Ely test
- external rotation test
- flexion rotation drawer sign
- fluctuation test
- gravity drawer test (posterior sag sign)
- hamstring length
- Helfet test
- Hughston plica test
- Hughston posterolateral drawer test
- Hughston test (jerk sign)
- hyperflexion-hyperextension test
- Jakob test (reverse pivot)
- Lachman's test
- lateral pull test
- limb-length discrepancy
- MacIntosh test (lateral pivot shift)
- McConnell test
- McMurray-Anderson test
- Noble's compression test
- Ober's test
- O'Donoghue test
- patellar tap
- patellar tilt
- patellofemoral grind test
- Perkins test
- plica test
- posterior drawer sign
- posterior sag test
- quadriceps active test
- reverse pivot shift test
- Slocum test
- Steinman's test
- step-down test
- squat test
- valgus stress test
- varus stress test
- Waldron test
- Wilson test

Pain
- palpation

Skin and Soft Tissue: Edema
- thigh measurement

Special Tests to Which the Physical Therapist May or May Not Have Access
- arthrography and arthroscopy
- computed tomography (CT) scan
- magnetic resonance imaging (MRI)
- x-ray studies
- joint aspiration
- ultrasonography

Strength
- dynamometer
- eccentric isokinetic knee flexion and extension measurements
- manual muscle testing
- Nautilus
- Orthotron II
- simple strain-gauge measure of isometric torque
- work measurements

PROBLEMS
- The client often complains of anterior knee pain.
- The client often finds pain worsens with weight bearing or standing immediately after prolonged sitting.

- The client may report episodes of the kneecap "going out" and a feeling of weakness.
- The client may report hearing crepitus (ie, noise) in the joint.
- The client may complain of swelling around the patella on medial side.

TREATMENT/MANAGEMENT

- Most knee conditions can be treated conservatively with ice, stretch, massage, and exercise.
- Consider patellar taping or infrapatellar straps during acute stage.
- Consider immobilization from 3 to 7 days to several weeks if dislocated. Immobilization is followed by strengthening program.
- While immobilized, the client may be on crutches with partial weight bearing.
- The client may want to wear a brace in the early stage of rehabilitation.
- Begin with closed kinematic chain exercises done in pain-free ROM. Closed kinematic chain exercise can include biking, stairs, or balance exercises on a board. If using cycling, instruct in proper seat height with knee angle of about 24 degrees when foot is in the downstroke position.
- Treat any edema.
- Stretching exercise should be included if tightness is found in piriformis, hamstring, gastrocsoleus muscles, or iliotibial band (ITB).
- Implement VMO reeducation through electrical stimulation, biofeedback, and patellofemoral taping. Role of VMO is critical to proper tracking of patella.
- Assess foot and ankle mechanics for proper footwear and orthosis.
- Include balance and proprioceptive training in the treatment program.
- Home program may include an emphasis on VMO training, flexibility, and muscle performance.

PRECAUTIONS/CONTRAINDICATIONS

- X-rays should be consulted to rule out potential fractures.
- Consult orthopedic surgeon if major ligament damage or meniscal tear is suspected or if hemarthosis or sudden effusion of joint develops.
- Carefully consider the nature of the problem before examination to avoid aggravating the condition with the test procedures.
- Open-chain exercises may predispose patella to lateral subluxation.
- Popliteal and semimembranosis tendinitis and patellar tendinitis can mimic a meniscal injury.
- Inflamed plica can sometimes be mistaken for a meniscal tear or patellofemoral dysfunction.

Notes: If client has pain during everyday activities and becomes progressively worse, the rehabilitation process will be lengthy and there should be a prolonged period of rest. Surgery may be required.

DESIRED OUTCOME/PROGNOSIS

- Any acute dislocation of the patella will be reduced, and further dislocation will be prevented.
- Clients who cannot function without taping after 8 weeks of treatment should consider patellar bracing.
- The client will experience a reduction in symptoms and increased patellar stability. Patients usually respond well to a conservative program.

Note: For continued success, the therapist must treat the source of the pain and not just the symptoms.

REFERENCES

Assessment

American Physical Therapy Association. Guide to physical therapist practice. 2nd ed. *Phys Ther.* 2001;81.

Bandy WD, Timm KE. Relationship between peak torque, work, and power for knee flexion and extension in clients with grade I medial compartment sprains of the knee. *J Orthop Sports Phys Ther.* 1992;16:288–292.

Bennell K, Bartam S, Crossley K, et al. Outcome measures in patellofemoral pain syndrome: test retest reliability and inter-relationships. *Phys Ther Sport.* 2000;1:32–41.

Buschbacher RM, ed. *Musculoskeletal Disorders: A Practical Guide for Diagnosis and Rehabilitation.* Boston, Mass: Andover Medical Publishers; 1994.

Daniels L, Worthingham C. *Muscle Testing Techniques of Manual Examination.* 6th ed. Philadelphia, Pa: WB Saunders Co; 1995.

Delitto A, Synder-Mackler L. The diagnostic process: examples in orthopedic physical therapy. *Phys Ther.* 1995;75:203–210.

Hall CM, Brody TB. *Therapeutic Exercise: Moving Toward Function.* Philadelphia, Pa: Lippincott Williams and Wilkins; 1999.

Hertling D, Kessler RM. *Management of Common Musculoskeletal Disorders.* 3rd ed. Philadelphia, Pa: JB Lippincott Co; 1996:78,534.

Jacobs K. *Ergonomics for Therapists.* 2nd ed. Boston, Mass: Butterworth Heinemann; 2000.

Kendall FP, McCreary EK, Provance PG. *Muscles: Testing and Function.* 4th ed. Baltimore, Md: Williams and Wilkins, 1993.

Kisner C, Colby LA. *Therapeutic Exercise: Foundations and Techniques.* 3rd ed. Philadelphia, Pa: FA Davis Co; 1996:241–270.

Lesh SG. *Clinical Orthopedics for the Physical Therapist Assistant.* Philadelphia, Pa: FA Davis Co; 2000.

Malone TR, McPoil T, Nitz AJ, eds. *Orthopaedic and Sports Physical Therapy.* 3rd ed. St. Louis, Mo: CV Mosby Co; 1997.

Myers RS, ed. *Saunders Manual of Physical Therapy Practice.* Philadelphia, Pa: WB Saunders Co; 1995.

Rothstein JM, Roy SH, Wolf SL. *The Rehabilitation Specialist's Handbook.* 2nd ed. Philadelphia, Pa: FA Davis Co; 1998.

Saidoff DC, McDonough AL. *Critical Pathways in Therapeutic Intervention.* Philadelphia, Pa: CV Mosby Co; 2002.

Schunk C, Reed K. *Clinical Practice Guidelines.* Gaithersburg, Md: Aspen Publishers; 2000.

Steiner LA, Harris BA, Krebs DE. Reliability of eccentric isokinetic knee flexion and extension measurements. *Arch Phys Med Rehabil.* 1993;74:1327–1335.

Tomberlin JP, Saunders HD. *Evaluation, Treatment and Prevention of Musculoskeletal Disorders. Vol 2: Extremities.* Chaska, Minn: The Saunders Group; 1994.

Watson C, Propps M, Galt W, et al. Reliability of measurements obtained using McConnell's classification of patellar orientation in symptomatic and asymptomatic subjects. *J Orthop Sports Phys Ther.* 1999;29:378–385.

EMG

Cram JR, Kasman GS. *Introduction to Surface Electromyograph.* Gaithersburg, Md: Aspen Publishers; 1998.

Kasman GS, Ram JR, Wolf SI. *Clinical Applications in Surface Electromyography: Chronic Musculoskeletal Pain.* Bethesda, Md: Aspen Publishers; 1998.

Levitt R, Deisinger JA, Remondet Wall J, et al. EMG feedback-assisted postoperative rehabilitation of minor arthroscopic knee surgeries. *J Sports Med Phys Fitness.* 1995;35:218–223.

Soderberg GL, ed. *Selected Topics in Surface Electromyography for Use in the Occupational Setting: Expert Perspective.* Washington, DC: US Dept of Health and US Services; 1992. NIOSH publication 91–100.

Treatment

Afzali L, Kuwabara F, Zachazewski J, Browne P, Robinson B. A new method for the determination of the characteristic shape of an isokinetic quadriceps femoris muscle torque curve. *Phys Ther.* 1992;72:585–595.

Arnell TK, Stothart JP, Kumar S. The effectiveness of functional foot orthoses as a treatment for patellofemoral stress syndrome: the clients' perspective. *Physiotherapy Can.* 2000; 52:153–157.

Arrol B, Ellis-Pegler E, Edwards A, et al. Patellofemoral pain syndrome: a critical review of the clinical trials on nonoperative therapy. *Am J Sports Med.* 1997;25:207–212.

Blond L, Hansen L. Patellofemoral pain syndrome in athletes: a 5.7 year retrospective follow-up study of 250 athletes. *Med Sci Sports Exerc.* 1998;30:1572–1577.

Buschbacher RM, ed. *Musculoskeletal Disorders: A Practical Guide for Diagnosis and Rehabilitation.* Boston, Mass: Andover Medical Publishers; 1994:206–208.

Caylor D, Fites R, Worrell TW. The relationship between quadriceps angle and anterior knee pain syndrome. *J Orthop Sports Phys Ther.* 1993;17:11–16.

Charteris J. An isometric normative database to facilitate restoration of function in knee-injured active young adults. *S Afr J Physiotherapy.* 1993;49:2:28–34.

Crossley K, Bennell K, Green S, et al. A systematic review of physical interventions for patellofemoral pain syndrome. *Clin J Sports Med.* 2001;11:103–110.

Cuddeford T, Williams AK, Medeiros JM. Electromyographic activity of the vasus medialis oblique and vastus lateralis muscles during selected exercises. *J Orthop Sports Phys Ther.* 1996;4:10–15.

DiVeta JA, Vogelbach WD. The clinical efficacy of the A-angle in measuring patellar alignment. *J Orthop Sports Phys Ther.* 1992;16:136–139.

Eng JJ. Evaluation of soft foot orthotics in the treatment of patellofemoral pain syndrome. *Phys Ther.* 1993;73:62–68.

Gilleard W, McConnell J, Partson D. The effect of patellar taping on the onset of vastus medialis obliquus and vasatus lateralis muscle activity in persons with patellofemoral pain. *Phys Ther.* 1998;78:25–32.

Grabois M, Garrison SJ, Hart KA, Lehmkuhl LD. *Physical Medicine and Rehabilitation: The Complete Approach.* Malden, Mass: Blackwell Science; 2000.

Gryzlo SM, Patek RM, Pink M, et al. Electromyographic analysis of knee rehabilitation exercises. *J Orthop Sports Phys Ther.* 1994;20:36–43.

Handfield T, Kramer J. Effect of McConnell taping on perceived pain and knee extensor torques during isokinetic exercise performed by patients with patellofemoral pain syndrome. *Physiotherapy Can.* 2000;52:39–44.

Harrison E, Quinney H, Magee D, et al. Analysis of outcome measures used in the study of patellofemoral pain syndrome. *Physiotherapy Can.* 1995;47:264–272.

Hertling D, Kessler RM. *Management of Common Musculoskeletal Disorders.* 3rd ed. Philadelphia, Pa: JB Lippincott Co; 1996:298–358.

Isear JA, Erickson JC, Worrell TW. EMG analysis of lower extremity muscle recruitment patterns during an unloaded squat. *Med Sci Sports Exerc.* 1997;29:532–539.

Johanson MA, Donatelli R, Greenfield BH. Rehabilitation of microtrauma injuries. In: Greenfield BH, ed. *Rehabilitation of the Knee: A Problem-Solving Approach.* Philadelphia, Pa: FA Davis Co; 1993:139–176.

Karst G, Jewett P. Electromyographic analysis of exercises proposed for differential activation of medial and lateral quadriceps femoris components. *Phys Ther.* 1993;73:286–295.

Karst G, Willett G. Onset timing of electromyographic activity in the vastus medialis oblique and vastus lateralis muscles in subjects with and without patellofemoral pain syndrome. *Phys Ther.* 1995;75:813–822.

Kisner C, Colby LA. *Therapeutic Exercise: Foundations and Techniques.* 3rd ed. Philadelphia, Pa: FA Davis Co; 1996:345–384.

LaPrade J, Culham E, Brower B. Comparison of five isometric exercises in the recruitment of the vasatus medialis oblique in persons with and without patellofemoral pain syndrome. *J Orthop Sports Phys Ther.* 1998;27:197–204.

MacIntyre DL, Hopkins PM, Harris SR. Evaluation of pain and functional activity in patellofemoral pain syndrome: reliability and validity of two assessment tools. *Physiotherapy Can.* 1995;47:164–172.

Mangine RE, ed. 2nd ed. *Physical Therapy of the Knee.* New York, NY: Churchill Livingstone; 1995.

McConnell J. Promoting effective segmental alignment. In: Crosbie J, McConnell J, eds. *Key Issues in Musculoskeletal Physiotherapy.* Oxford, England: Butterworth Heinemann; 1993.

McConnell JS. Management of patellofemoral problems. *Man Ther.* 1996;1:60–66.

Miyagawa H, Furukawa R, Shimono T, et al. Electromyographic analysis of knee muscles during the lateral step-up exercise. *J Phys Ther Sci.* 1993;5:45–50.

Morrish GM, Woledge RC. A comparison of the activation of muscles moving the patella in normal subjects and in patients with chronic patellofemoral problems. *Scand J Rehabil Med.* 1997;29:43–48.

Myers RS, ed. *Saunders Manual of Physical Therapy Practice.* Philadelphia, Pa: WB Saunders Co; 1995:1351.

Panni AS, Tartarone M, Maffulli N. Patellar tendinopathy in athletes. Outcomes of nonoperative and operative management. *Am J Sports Med.* 2000;28:392–397.

Powers CM, Landel R, Perry J. Timing and intensity of vastus muscle activity during functional activities in subjects with and without patellofemoral pain. *Phys Ther.* 1996;76:946–955.

Powers C, Landel R, Sosnick T, et al. The effects of patellar taping on stride characteristics and joint motion in subjects with patellofemoral pain. *J Orthop Sports Phys Ther.* 1997;26:286–291.

Puniello MS. Iliotibial band tightness and medial patellar glide in patients with patellofemoral dysfunction. *J Orthop Sports Phys Ther.* 1993;17:144–148.

Stiene HA, Brosky T, Reinking MF, et al. A comparison of closed kinetic chain and isokinetic joint isolation exercise in patients with patellofemoral dysfunction. *J Orthop Sports Phys Ther.* 1996;24:136–141.

Tomberlin JP, Saunders HD. *Evaluation, Treatment and Prevention of Musculoskeletal Disorders. Vol 2: Extremities.* Chaska, Minn: The Saunders Group; 1994:233.

Werner S, Arvidsson H, Arvidsson I, et al. Electrical stimulation of vastus medialis and stretching of lateral thigh muscles in patients with patello-femoral symptoms. *Knee Surg Sports Traumatology Arthroscopy.* 1993;1:85–92.

Wilk KE, Andrew JR. The effects of pad placement and angular velocity on tibial displacement during isokinetic exercise. *J Orthop Sports Phys Ther.* 1993;17:24–30.

Wilk KE, Davies GJ, Mangine RE, et al. Patellofemoral disorders: a classification system and clinical guidelines for nonoperative rehabilitation. *J Orthop Sports Phys Ther.* 1998; 28:307–322.

Witvrouw E, Sneyers C, Lysens R, et al. Comparative reflex response times of vastus medialis oblique and vastus lateralis in normal subjects and in subjects with patellofemoral pain syndrome. *J Orthop Sports Phys Ther.* 1996;24:160–165.

Orthotics

Eng JJ, Pierrynowski MR. The effects of soft foot orthotics on three dimensional lower limb kinematics during walking and running. *J Phys Ther.* 1994;74:45–53.

McCulloch MV, Brunt D, Vander Linden D. The effects of foot orthoses and gait velocity on lower limb kinematics and temporal events of stance. *J Orthop Sports Phys Ther.* 1993;17:2–10.

Reiley MA. *Guidelines for Prescribing Foot Orthotics.* Thorofare, NJ: Slack Inc; 1995:3–5.

Pes Cavus

DESCRIPTION

Pes cavus is a condition in which the foot is highly arched or abnormally supinated. A highly arched foot structure (either flexible or rigid) predisposes the patient to problems caused by a lack of shock absorption.

CAUSE

Abnormal supination is caused by the inability of the foot to pronate. This leads to prolonged supination during the stance phase of gait.

ASSESSMENT

> **Note:** See APTA's Guide to Physical Therapist Practice. 2nd ed. *Physical Therapy.* 2001;81.
>
> Musculoskeletal Preferred Practice Patterns: B, E

AREAS
- History
- Posture
- Pain
- Gait
- Strength
- Neurological
- Joint integrity and structural deviations
- Mobility, including active and passive range of motion (ROM) and accessory motion
- Skin and soft tissue
- Equipment, including footwear

INSTRUMENTS/PROCEDURES
See References for sources.

Gait
- dynamic assessment of foot mechanics
- dynamic plantar pressure distribution

- foot pressure EMED system
- pedabarograph
- three-dimensional kinematic analysis
- footprint analysis in gait documentation

Joint Integrity and Structural Deviations

The following orthopedic tests may be performed:

- Achilles tendon test
- anterior drawer sign
- Homan's sign
- Kleiger test
- talar tilt test
- Thompson test

PROBLEMS
- The client often complains of foot pain.
- The client may have related stress fracture, metatarsalgia, plantar fasciitis, and Achilles tendinitis.

TREATMENT/MANAGEMENT

For treatment of foot and ankle problems in general:

- Exercises progress from passive ROM to active assisted and active ROM to resisted ROM.
- Begin non-weight-bearing strengthening activities after pain-free ROM is achieved.
- Isometric, isotonic, and isokinetic exercise may be used.
- Eccentric loading should not be overlooked.
- Progress to jogging, running, and athletic maneuvers as indicated.
- Address preventive measures, such as stretching, choice of shoes, and use of adhesive strapping during athletic activities.

For pes cavus specifically:

- Consider rigid orthotic device with forefoot valgus post.
- Begin a lower extremity flexibility program of stretching, mobilization, and exercises.

PRECAUTIONS/CONTRAINDICATIONS
- No precautions are identified.

DESIRED OUTCOME/PROGNOSIS
- The client will have pain-free function of the foot.
- The client will experience a relief of foot pressure and lessen strain on lower extremities.

Notes: Flexible cavus foot responds well to orthotic foot control. Rigid cavus foot may need a special shock-absorbing material.

REFERENCES

Assessment

American Physical Therapy Association. Guide to physical therapist practice. 2nd ed. *Phys Ther.* 2001;81.

Buschbacher RM, ed. *Musculoskeletal Disorders: A Practical Guide for Diagnosis and Rehabilitation.* Boston, Mass: Andover Medical Publishers; 1994.

Daniels L, Worthingham C. *Muscle Testing Techniques of Manual Examination.* 6th ed. Philadelphia, Pa: WB Saunders Co; 1995.

Delitto A, Synder-Mackler L. The diagnostic process: examples in orthopedic physical therapy. *Phys Ther.* 1995;75:203–210.

Donatelli RA. *The Biomechanics of the Foot and Ankle.* 2nd ed. Philadelphia, Pa: FA Davis Co; 1996.

Hall CM, Brody TB. *Therapeutic Exercise: Moving Toward Function.* Philadelphia, Pa: FA Davis Co; Lippincott Williams and Wilkins; 1999.

Hertling D, Kessler RM. *Management of Common Musculoskeletal Disorders.* 3rd ed. Philadelphia, Pa: JB Lippincott Co; 1996:78, 534.

Jacobs K. *Ergonomics for Therapists.* 2nd ed. Boston, Mass: Butterworth Heinemann; 2000.

Kasman GS, Ram JR, Wolf SI. *Clinical Applications in Surface Electromyography: Chronic Musculoskeletal Pain.* Bethesda, Md: Aspen Publishers; 1998.

Kendall FP, McCreary EK, Provance PG. *Muscles: Testing and Function.* 4th ed. Baltimore, Md: Williams and Wilkins; 1993.

Kisner C, Colby LA. *Therapeutic Exercise: Foundations and Techniques.* 3rd ed. Philadelphia, Pa: FA Davis Co; 1996:241–270.

Lesh SG. *Clinical Orthopedics for the Physical Therapist Assistant.* Philadelphia, Pa: FA Davis Co; 2000.

Malone TR, McPoil T, Nitz AJ, eds. *Orthopaedic and Sports Physical Therapy.* 3rd ed. St. Louis, Mo: CV Mosby Co; 1997.

Myers RS, ed. *Saunders Manual of Physical Therapy Practice.* Philadelphia, Pa: WB Saunders Co; 1995.

Rothstein JM, Roy SH, Wolf SL. *The Rehabilitation Specialist's Handbook.* 2nd ed. Philadelphia, Pa: FA Davis Co; 1998.

Saidoff DC, McDonough AL. *Critical Pathways in Therapeutic Intervention.* Philadelphia, Pa: CV Mosby Co; 2002.

Sammarco GJ. *Rehabilitation of the Foot and Ankle.* St. Louis, Mo: Mosby Year Book; 1995.

Schunk C, Reed K. *Clinical Practice Guidelines.* Gaithersburg, Md: Aspen Publishers; 2000.

Tomberlin JP, Saunders HD. *Evaluation, Treatment and Prevention of Musculoskeletal Disorders. Vol 2: Extremities.* Chaska, Minn: The Saunders Group; 1994.

Treatment

Buschbacher RM, ed. *Musculoskeletal Disorders: A Practical Guide for Diagnosis and Rehabilitation.* Boston, Mass: Andover Medical Publishers; 1994:216–235.

Grabois M, Garrison SJ, Hart KA, Lehmkuhl LD. *Physical Medicine and Rehabilitation: The Complete Approach.* Malden, Mass: Blackwell Science; 2000.

Hertling D, Kessler RM. *Management of Common Musculoskeletal Disorders.* 3rd ed. Philadelphia, Pa: JB Lippincott Co; 1996:359–410.

Hunt GC, ed. *Physical Therapy of the Foot and Ankle.* 2nd ed. New York, NY: Churchill Livingstone; 1995.

Kisner C, Colby LA. *Therapeutic Exercise: Foundations and Techniques.* 3rd ed. Philadelphia, Pa: FA Davis Co; 1996.

McPoil TG, Hunt GC. Evaluation and management of foot and ankle disorders: present problems and future directions. *J Orthop Sports Phys Ther.* 1995;21:381–388.

Tomberlin JP, Saunders HD. *Evaluation, Treatment and Prevention of Musculoskeletal Disorders. Vol 2: Extremities.* Chaska, Minn: The Saunders Group; 1994:265–306.

Pes Planus

Also known as *flat foot, pronated foot,* and *pes planovalgus.*

DESCRIPTION

Pes planus results in a flattened medial longitudinal arch.

CAUSE

This condition may be caused by muscle weakness, ligamentous laxity, trauma, paralysis, or postural deformity. Pes planus may be congenital. Local structural disorder or structural deviations elsewhere contribute to the problem.

ASSESSMENT

Note: See APTA's Guide to Physical Therapist Practice. 2nd ed. *Physical Therapy.* 2001;81.

Musculoskeletal Preferred Practice Patterns: B, E

AREAS

- History
- Pain
- Posture
- Gait
- Strength
- Neurological, including sensation
- Joint integrity and structural deviations
- Mobility, including active and passive range of motion (ROM) and accessory motion
- Skin and soft tissue
- Equipment, including footwear

INSTRUMENTS/PROCEDURES

See References for sources.

Gait
- dynamic assessment of foot mechanics
  1. dynamic plantar pressure distribution
  2. foot pressure EMED system
  3. pedabarograph
  4. three-dimensional kinematic analysis

Joint Integrity and Structural Deviations

The following orthopedic tests for the lower extremities may be used:

- Achilles tendon test
- anterior drawer sign
- Homan's sign
- Kleiger test
- talar tilt
- Thompson test

PROBLEMS

- The client often has pain over the plantar aspect of the foot.
- Fatigue stress is often felt over the sole of the foot, especially on the medial side.
- Related knee pain is common.
- Forefoot pain is common.

TREATMENT/MANAGEMENT

- Begin strengthening exercises of the intrinsic foot muscles.
- Add flexibility exercises for the gastrocsoleus complex.
- Consider an orthotic device. Options may include an insert, such as the University of California Biomechanical Laboratory insert, a semirigid scaphoid pad insert, or a medial heel wedge (possibly in combination with a medial forefoot wedge) insert.
- Provide advice on appropriate activity level.
- Include proprioceptive balance training.
- Consider the use of strapping, usually a valgus correction strap attached to an ankle-foot orthosis.
- Use ultrasound and friction massage, if indicated.

DESIRED OUTCOME/PROGNOSIS

- The client will have the foot restored to normal alignment.
- The client will have pain-free function of the foot.
- Provide arch support and calcaneal control.

Notes: A rigid pes planus usually cannot be changed with an orthosis, although use of a heel wedge has been suggested. Selective reduction of abnormal stress reduces the frequency and/or magnitude of stress on the foot.

REFERENCES

Assessment

American Physical Therapy Association. Guide to physical therapist practice. 2nd ed. *Phys Ther.* 2001;81.

Bandy WD, Timm KE. Relationship between peak torque, work, and power for knee flexion and extension in clients with grade I medial compartment sprains of the knee. *J Orthop Sports Phys Ther.* 1992;16:288–292.

Buschbacher RM, ed. *Musculoskeletal Disorders: A Practical Guide for Diagnosis and Rehabilitation.* Boston, Mass: Andover Medical Publishers; 1994.

Daniels L, Worthingham C. *Muscle Testing Techniques of Manual Examination.* 6th ed. Philadelphia, Pa: WB Saunders Co; 1995.

Delitto A, Synder-Mackler L. The diagnostic process: examples in orthopedic physical therapy. *Phys Ther.* 1995;75:203–210.

Donatelli RA. *The Biomechanics of the Foot and Ankle.* 2nd ed. Philadelphia, Pa: FA Davis Co; 1996.

Hall CM, Brody TB. *Therapeutic Exercise: Moving Toward Function.* Philadelphia, Pa: Lippincott Williams and Wilkins; 1999.

Hertling D, Kessler RM. *Management of Common Musculoskeletal Disorders.* 3rd ed. Philadelphia, Pa: JB Lippincott Co; 1996:78, 534.

Jacobs K. *Ergonomics for Therapists.* 2nd ed. Boston, Mass: Butterworth Heinemann; 2000.

Kasman GS, Ram JR, Wolf Sl. *Clinical Applications in Surface Electromyography: Chronic Musculoskeletal Pain.* Bethesda, Md: Aspen Publishers; 1998.

Kendall FP, McCreary EK, Provance PG. *Muscles: Testing and Function.* 4th ed. Baltimore, Md: Williams and Wilkins; 1993.

Kisner C, Colby LA. *Therapeutic Exercise: Foundations and Techniques.* 3rd ed. Philadelphia, Pa: FA Davis Co; 1996:241–270.

Lesh SG. *Clinical Orthopedics for the Physical Therapist Assistant*. Philadelphia, Pa: FA Davis Co; 2000.

Malone TR, McPoil T, Nitz AJ, eds. *Orthopaedic and Sports Physical Therapy*. 3rd ed. St. Louis, Mo: CV Mosby Co; 1997.

Myers RS, ed. *Saunders Manual of Physical Therapy Practice*. Philadelphia, Pa: WB Saunders Co; 1995.

Rothstein JM, Roy SH, Wolf SL. *The Rehabilitation Specialist's Handbook*. 2nd ed. Philadelphia, Pa: FA Davis Co; 1998.

Saidoff DC, McDonough AL. *Critical Pathways in Therapeutic Intervention*. Philadelphia, Pa: CV Mosby Co; 2002.

Sammarco GJ. *Rehabilitation of the Foot and Ankle*. St. Louis, Mo: Mosby Year Book; 1995.

Schunk C, Reed K. *Clinical Practice Guidelines*. Gaithersburg, Md: Aspen Publishers; 2000.

Tomberlin JP, Saunders HD. *Evaluation, Treatment and Prevention of Musculoskeletal Disorders. Vol 2: Extremities*. Chaska, Minn: The Saunders Group; 1994.

Treatment

Buschbacher RM, ed. *Musculoskeletal Disorders: A Practical Guide for Diagnosis and Rehabilitation*. Boston, Mass: Andover Medical Publishers; 1994:216–235.

Edelstein JE. Orthoses. In: Myers RS, ed. *Saunders Manual of Physical Therapy Practice*. Philadelphia, Pa: WB Saunders Co; 1995:1189.

Hertling D, Kessler RM. *Management of Common Musculoskeletal Disorders*. 3rd ed. Philadelphia, Pa: JB Lippincott Co; 1996:359–410.

Hunt GC, ed. *Physical Therapy of the Foot and Ankle*. 2nd ed. New York, NY: Churchill Livingstone; 1995.

Kisner C, Colby LA. *Therapeutic Exercise: Foundations and Techniques*. 3rd ed. Philadelphia, Pa: FA Davis Co; 1996:385–407.

McPoil TG, Hunt GC. Evaluation and management of foot and ankle disorders: present problems and future directions. *J Orthop Sports Phys Ther*. 1995;21:381–388.

Tomberlin JP, Saunders HD. *Evaluation, Treatment and Prevention of Musculoskeletal Disorders. Vol 2: Extremities*. Chaska, Minn: The Saunders Group; 1994:265–305.

Piriformis Syndrome

DESCRIPTION

With the piriformis syndrome, the sciatic nerve is irritated by the overlying piriformis muscle. In 15% to 20% of the population, the nerve pierces the muscle. Piriformis syndrome is more common in women than men.

CAUSE

The sciatic nerve can be mechanically irritated when it is trapped between the muscle and the ischium or when it lies within the belly of the muscle.

ASSESSMENT

Note: See APTA's Guide to Physical Therapist Practice. 2nd ed. *Physical Therapy*. 2001;81.

Musculoskeletal Preferred Practice Patterns: I, F

AREAS

- History
- Pain
- Posture
- Joint integrity and structural deviations
- Gait
- Mobility, including active and passive range of motion
- (ROM), and accessory motion
- Strength
- Neurological
- Skin and soft tissue
- Functional level

INSTRUMENTS/PROCEDURES

See References for sources.

Joint Integrity and Structural Deviations

The following orthopedic tests for the lower quadrant may be performed:

- Craig's test
- Ely test
- FABER test
- hamstring tightness
- leg-length measurements
- Ober's test
- Noble's compression test
- piriformis test
- Thomas' test
- torque test
- Trendelenburg's sign
- quadrant test

Mobility
- goniometry
- hip flexibility

Posture
- clinical measurement of postural control
- pelvic tilt and the standing position

Special Tests to Which the Physical Therapist May or May Not Have Access
- electromyographic analysis of hip abductor musculature

Strength
- maximal isometric hip abductor muscles torques
- manual muscle test

PROBLEMS

- The client may complain of pain in posterior hip area.
- Often, resisted hip rotation (external) produces pain.
- The client may complain of pain in leg, lumbar spine, or pelvis.
- The client often has diminished tolerance to sitting and weight bearing.
- The client may have a decreased ROM in internal rotation with adduction.
- Normally, passive internal rotation produces pain.

TREATMENT/MANAGEMENT

- Use modalities, such as ice or ultrasound, as indicated.
- Encourage rest during acute stage.
- Consider soft tissue mobilization or neural mobilization techniques.
- Assess activities of daily living (ADLs) and posture, especially of the hip.
- Introduce gradual, gentle stretching of piriformis muscle in side-lying or sitting position.
- Maintain piriformis mobility with stretching to prevent recurrence.

DESIRED OUTCOME/PROGNOSIS

- The client will experience relief of symptoms.
- The client will experience decreased stress on muscle.

Notes: Addressing contributing factors and maintaining piriformis muscle mobility are critical to the prevention of recurrence.

In a report on 12 selected cases of chronic piriformis syndrome, 10 reported improvement post surgery.

REFERENCES

Assessment

American Physical Therapy Association. Guide to physical therapist practice. 2nd ed. *Phys Ther.* 2001;81.

Bandy WD, Timm KE. Relationship between peak torque, work, and power for knee flexion and extension in clients with grade I medial compartment sprains of the knee. *J Orthop Sports Phys Ther.* 1992;16:288–292.

Buschbacher RM, ed. *Musculoskeletal Disorders: A Practical Guide for Diagnosis and Rehabilitation.* Boston, Mass: Andover Medical Publishers; 1994.

Daniels L, Worthingham C. *Muscle Testing Techniques of Manual Examination.* 6th ed. Philadelphia, Pa: WB Saunders Co; 1995.

Delitto A, Synder-Mackler L. The diagnostic process: examples in orthopedic physical therapy. *Phys Ther.* 1995;75:203–210.

Hall CM, Brody TB. *Therapeutic Exercise: Moving Toward Function.* Philadelphia, Pa: Lippincott Williams and Wilkins; 1999.

Hertling D, Kessler RM. *Management of Common Musculoskeletal Disorders.* 3rd ed. Philadelphia, Pa: JB Lippincott Co; 1996:78, 534.

Jacobs K. *Ergonomics for Therapists.* 2nd ed. Boston, Mass: Butterworth Heinemann; 2000.

Kasman GS, Ram JR, Wolf SI. *Clinical Applications in Surface Electromyography: Chronic Musculoskeletal Pain.* Bethesda, Md: Aspen Publishers; 1998.

Kendall FP, McCreary EK, Provance PG. *Muscles: Testing and Function.* 4th ed. Baltimore, Md: Williams and Wilkins, 1993.

Kisner C, Colby LA. *Therapeutic Exercise: Foundations and Techniques.* 3rd ed. Philadelphia, Pa: FA Davis Co; 1996:241–270.

Lesh SG. *Clinical Orthopedics for the Physical Therapist Assistant.* Philadelphia, Pa: FA Davis Co; 2000.

Malone TR, McPoil T, Nitz AJ, eds. *Orthopaedic and Sports Physical Therapy.* 3rd ed. St. Louis, Mo: CV Mosby Co; 1997.

Myers RS, ed. *Saunders Manual of Physical Therapy Practice.* Philadelphia, Pa: WB Saunders Co; 1995.

Rothstein JM, Roy SH, Wolf SL. *The Rehabilitation Specialist's Handbook.* 2nd ed. Philadelphia, Pa: FA Davis Co; 1998.

Saidoff DC, McDonough AL. *Critical Pathways in Therapeutic Intervention.* Philadelphia, Pa: CV Mosby Co; 2002.

Schunk C, Reed K. *Clinical Practice Guidelines.* Gaithersburg, Md: Aspen Publishers; 2000.

Tomberlin JP, Saunders HD. *Evaluation, Treatment and Prevention of Musculoskeletal Disorders. Vol 2: Extremities.* Chaska, Minn: The Saunders Group; 1994.

Treatment

Coon B, Hart A, Nitz AJ. Piriformis Syndrome. *Phys Ther Case Rep.* 2000;3:220–225.

Grabois M, Garrison SJ, Hart KA, Lehmkuhl LD. *Physical Medicine and Rehabilitation: The Complete Approach.* Malden, Mass: Blackwell Science; 2000.

Hertling D, Kessler RM. *Management of Common Musculoskeletal Disorders.* 3rd ed. Philadelphia, Pa: JB Lippincott Co; 1996:272–297.

Hicklin SP, DePretis MC. Lower extremity: hip. In: Myers RS, ed. *Saunders Manual of Physical Therapy Practice.* Philadelphia, Pa: WB Saunders Co; 1995:976.

Kendall FP, McCreary EK, Provance PG. *Muscles: Testing and Function.* 4th ed. Baltimore, Md: Williams and Wilkins; 1993.

Kisner C, Colby LA. *Therapeutic Exercise: Foundations and Techniques.* 3rd ed. Philadelphia, Pa: FA Davis Co; 1996:317–344.

Kornberg C, McCarthy T. The effect of neural stretching technique on sympathetic outflow to the lower limbs. *J Orthop Sports Phys Ther.* 1992;16:269–274.

Tomberlin JP, Saunders HD. *Evaluation, Treatment and Prevention of Musculoskeletal Disorders. Vol 2: Extremities;* vol 2. Chaska, Minn: The Saunders Group; 1994:187–212.

Plantar Fasciitis

DESCRIPTION

Inflammation at the inner border of the plantar fascia that leads to pain.

CAUSE

The most irritating causative factor is overuse. Plantar fasciitis can also be triggered by excessive stretching. Flat feet and contracted heel cords are associated with this disorder. In runners, this condition can also be associated with limited range of motion (ROM) of the first metatarsal phalangeal (MTP) joint. Training errors, repetitive trauma, and hyperpronation (of the subtalar joint) have been implicated as well.

ASSESSMENT

Note: See APTA's Guide to Physical Therapist Practice. 2nd ed. *Physical Therapy.* 2001;81.

Musculoskeletal Preferred Practice Patterns: D, E, F, J

AREAS

- History
- Pain
- Posture
- Gait
- Strength
- Neurological, including sensation
- Joint integrity and structural deviations
- Mobility, including active and passive ROM and accessory motion
- Skin and soft tissue
- Equipment, including footwear

INSTRUMENTS/PROCEDURES

See References for sources.

Gait
- dynamic assessment of foot mechanics
  1. dynamic plantar pressure distribution
  2. foot pressure EMED system
  3. pedabarograph
  4. three-dimensional kinematic analysis
- footprint analysis in gait documentation

Joint Integrity and Structural Deviations
- tibial varum evaluation

Mobility
- goniometric subtalar and ankle joint measurements
- open and closed kinetic chain subtalar joint neutral positions and navicular drop test

Strength
- instrumentation
- manual muscle testing

PROBLEMS
- The client often has pain in heel with weight-bearing activities.
- Often, the pain increases with the first steps taken upon rising but is better after a few hours and then worse again.
- The client often has pain with passive dorsiflexion and great toe extension.
- There is often tenderness on the medial side of the heel and pain along the anteromedial aspect of the plantar surface of the calcaneus.
- The client may report that the foot is extremely stiff or hypermobile.

TREATMENT/MANAGEMENT

For general treatment of foot and ankle problems:
- Exercises progress from passive ROM to active assisted and active ROM to resisted ROM.
- Begin non-weight-bearing strengthening activities after pain-free ROM is achieved.
- Isometric, isotonic, and isokinetic exercise can be used.
- Consider eccentric loading.
- Progress to jogging, running, and athletic maneuvers as indicated.
- Address preventive measures, such as stretching, choice of shoes, and use of adhesive strapping during athletic activities.

For plantar fasciitis specifically:
- Use physical agents (eg, ice massage or immersion 3-4 times per day), as indicated. Iotophoresis with 10% hydrocortisone for 30 minutes to affected area may be considered. Phonophoresis and pulsed ultrasound may also be considered.
- Consider taping.
- Use foot orthotics during the healing phase.
- Consider long-term use of orthotics and inserts. One option is an insert that has a heel elevation, scaphoid pad, and a flexible top cover. May need medial forefoot and rearfoot posts.
- Mobilize immobile first MTP, if needed.
- Stretch gastrocsoleus complex in pain-free range flexibility program for lower extremities.

- Use strengthening exercise for gastrocnemius and arch musculature. Consider use of manual resistive exercises, closed chain exercises and elastic band exercises.
- Include gait training for stance stability and control of any excess pronation.
- Utilize neuromuscular and proprioceptive reeducation.
- Evaluate need for cardiovascular conditioning.
- Treat any neural tension.
- Try cross-friction massage with slow passive stretching. Consider myofascial release to gastrocnemius and soleus muscles.

PRECAUTIONS/CONTRAINDICATIONS
- Plantar fasciitis can mimic tibial nerve entrapment and/or medial plantar nerve entrapment, and these conditions should be ruled out. Pain under the plantar surface probably signals heel contusion, not plantar fasciitis.

DESIRED OUTCOME/PROGNOSIS
- The client will experience a reduction in symptoms and decreased stress on the plantar fascia.
- The client will prevent reinjury.

Notes: It is not unusual for plantar fasciitis to resist conservative therapy. All related elements must be addressed to promote successful treatment.

REFERENCES

Assessment

American Physical Therapy Association. Guide to physical therapist practice. 2nd ed. *Phys Ther.* 2001;81.

Bandy WD, Timm KE. Relationship between peak torque, work, and power for knee flexion and extension in clients with grade I medial compartment sprains of the knee. *J Orthop Sports Phys Ther.* 1992;16:288–292.

Buschbacher RM, ed. *Musculoskeletal Disorders: A Practical Guide for Diagnosis and Rehabilitation.* Boston, Mass: Andover Medical Publishers; 1994.

Daniels L, Worthingham C. *Muscle Testing Techniques of Manual Examination.* 6th ed. Philadelphia, Pa: WB Saunders Co; 1995.

Delitto A, Synder-Mackler L. The diagnostic process: examples in orthopedic physical therapy. *Phys Ther.* 1995;75:203–210.

Donatelli RA. *The Biomechanics of the Foot and Ankle.* 2nd ed. Philadelphia, Pa: FA Davis Co; 1996.

Hall CM, Brody TB. *Therapeutic Exercise: Moving Toward Function.* Philadelphia, Pa: Lippincott Williams and Wilkins; 1999.

Hertling D, Kessler RM. *Management of Common Musculoskeletal Disorders.* 3rd ed. Philadelphia, Pa: JB Lippincott Co; 1996:78, 534.

Jacobs K. *Ergonomics for Therapists.* 2nd ed. Boston, Mass: Butterworth Heinemann; 2000.

Kasman GS, Ram JR, Wolf SI. *Clinical Applications in Surface Electromyography: Chronic Musculoskeletal Pain.* Bethesda, Md: Aspen Publishers; 1998.

Kendall FP, McCreary EK, Provance PG. *Muscles: Testing and Function.* 4th ed. Baltimore, Md: Williams and Wilkins; 1993.

Kisner C, Colby LA. *Therapeutic Exercise: Foundations and Techniques*. 3rd ed. Philadelphia, Pa: FA Davis Co; 1996:241–270.

Lesh SG. *Clinical Orthopedics for the Physical Therapist Assistant*. Philadelphia, Pa: FA Davis Co; 2000.

Malone TR, McPoil T, Nitz AJ, eds. *Orthopaedic and Sports Physical Therapy*. 3rd ed. St. Louis, Mo: CV Mosby Co; 1997.

Myers RS, ed. *Saunders Manual of Physical Therapy Practice*. Philadelphia, Pa: WB Saunders Co; 1995.

Rothstein JM, Roy SH, Wolf SL. *The Rehabilitation Specialist's Handbook*. 2nd ed. Philadelphia, Pa: FA Davis Co; 1998.

Saidoff DC, McDonough AL. *Critical Pathways in Therapeutic Intervention*. Philadelphia, Pa: CV Mosby Co; 2002.

Sammarco GJ. *Rehabilitation of the Foot and Ankle*. St. Louis, Mo: Mosby Year Book; 1995.

Schunk C, Reed K. *Clinical Practice Guidelines*. Gaithersburg, Md: Aspen Publishers; 2000.

Tomberlin JP, Saunders HD. *Evaluation, Treatment and Prevention of Musculoskeletal Disorders. Extremities;* vol 2. Chaska, Minn: The Saunders Group; 1994.

Treatment

Ballantyne BT, Kukulka CG, Soderberg GL. Motor unit recruitment in human medial gastrocnemius muscle during combined knee flexion and plantar flexion isometric contractions. *Exp Brain Res*. 1993;93:492–498.

Buschbacher RM, ed. *Musculoskeletal Disorders: A Practical Guide for Diagnosis and Rehabilitation*. Boston, Mass: Andover Medical Publishers; 1994:216–235.

Cornwell M, McPoil T. Plantar fasciitis: etiology and treatment. *J Orthop Sports Phys Ther*. 1999;29:756–760.

Hertling D, Kessler RM. *Management of Common Musculoskeletal Disorders*. 3rd ed. Philadelphia, Pa: JB Lippincott Co; 1996:359–410.

Kisner C, Colby LA. *Therapeutic Exercise: Foundations and Techniques*. 3rd ed. Philadelphia, Pa: FA Davis Co; 1996:385–407.

McCulloch MU, Brunt D, Vander-Linden D. The effect of foot orthotics and gait velocity on lower limb kinematics and temporal events of stance. *J Orthop Sports Phys Ther*. 1993;17:2–10.

McPoil TG, Cornwall MW. The relationship between subtalor joint neutral position and rearfoot motion during walking. *Foot Ankle*. 1994;15:141–145.

McPoil TG, Cornwall MW. The relationship between static measurements of the lower extremity and the pattern of rearfoot motion during walking [abstract]. *Phys Ther*. 1994; 74:S:141.

McPoil TG, Hunt GC. Evaluation and management of foot and ankle disorders: Present problems and future directions. *J Orthop Sports Phys Ther*. 1995;21:381–388.

Monney M, Maffey-Ward L. All heel pain is not plantar fasciitis. *Physiotherapy Can*. 1995; 47:185–189.

Picciano AM, Rowlands MS, Worrell T. Reliability of open and closed kinetic chain subtalar joint neutral positions and navicular drop test. *J Orthop Sports Phys Ther*. 1993;18: 553–558.

Probe RA, Baca M, Adams R, et al. Night splint treatment for plantar fasciitis. A prospective randomized study. *Clin Orthop*. 1999;368:190–195.

Tomberlin JP, Saunders HD. *Evaluation, Treatment and Prevention of Musculoskeletal Disorders. Vol 2: Extremities*. Chaska, Minn: The Saunders Group; 1994:265–306.

Vandervoort AA, Chesworth BM, Cunningham DA, Rechnitzer PA, Paterson DH, Koval JJ. An outcome measure to quantify passive stiffness of the ankle. *Can J Public Health.* 1992;83(suppl 2):S19–S23.

Youdas JW, Bogard CL, Suman VJ. Reliability of goniometric measurements and visual estimates of ankle joint active range of motion obtained in a clinical setting. *Arch Phys Med Rehabil.* 1993;74:1113–1118.

Plica Syndrome

DESCRIPTION

The plica syndrome is a thickening of the medial synovial plica.
Note: Medial synovial plica is found in 60% of normal knees.

CAUSE

The thickening of the medial synovial plica combined with fibrotic changes causes anteromedial knee pain and noise.

ASSESSMENT

Note: See APTA's Guide to Physical Therapist Practice. 2nd ed. *Physical Therapy.* 2001;81.

Musculoskeletal Preferred Practice Pattern: I

AREAS

- History
- Posture
- Pain
- Joint integrity and structural deviations
- Mobility, including active and passive range of motion
- (ROM) and accessory motion
- Strength
- Neurological
- Skin and soft tissue
- Gait
- Functional level

INSTRUMENTS/PROCEDURES

See References for sources.

Functional Level
- modified Lysholm knee score

Joint Integrity and Structural Deviations

The following orthopedic tests for the knee may be performed:

- A-angle
- ALRI test
- AMRI test
- Apley grinding test
- apprehension test
- bounce home test
- brush or stroke (wipe) test
- Clark sign
- crossover test
- Ely test
- external rotation test
- flexion rotation drawer sign
- fluctuation test
- gravity drawer test (posterior sag sign)
- hamstring length
- Helfet test
- Hughston plica test
- Hughston posterolateral drawer test
- Hughston test (jerk sign)
- hyperflexion-hyperextension test
- Jakob test (reverse pivot)

- Lachman's test
- lateral pull test
- limb-length discrepancy
- MacIntosh test (lateral pivot shift)
- McConnell test
- McMurray-Anderson test
- Noble's compression test
- Ober's test
- O'Donoghue test
- patellar tap
- patellar tilt
- Perkins test
- plica test
- posterior drawer sign
- posterior sag
- quadriceps active test
- reverse pivot shift
- Slocum test
- Steinman's test
- squat test
- valgus stress test
- varus stress test
- Waldron test
- Wilson test

Mobility
- goniometric knee measurements

Special Tests to Which the Physical Therapist May or May Not Have Access
- arthrography and arthroscopy
- computed tomography (CT) scan
- magnetic resonance imaging (MRI)
- x-ray studies
- joint aspiration
- ultrasonography

Strength
- instrumentation
- manual muscle testing

PROBLEMS
- The client often complains of anteromedial knee pain.
- The client may report that pain worsens with running. Pain may also worsen with prolonged sitting but resolve after a few steps.
- In acute cases, the client may report clicking, swelling, catching, and a feeling of weakness.

TREATMENT/MANAGEMENT

ACUTE
- Encourage rest.
- Strengthen the quadriceps muscle, especially the articularis genu to assist with pulling synovial membrane away from the joint during knee extension.

PRECAUTIONS/CONTRAINDICATIONS
- X-rays should be consulted to rule out potential fractures.
- Consult orthopedic surgeon if major ligament damage or meniscal tear is suspected or if there is hemarthosis or sudden effusion of the joint.
- Carefully consider the nature of the problem before examination so the condition is not aggravated with the test procedures.

Note: Inflamed plica can sometimes be mistaken for meniscal tear or patellofemoral dysfunction.

DESIRED OUTCOME/PROGNOSIS
- The client will have a reduction in symptoms.
- The client will have full knee function.

Note: Conservative care reportedly offers good results but arthroscopic resection may be needed for unresponsive cases.

REFERENCES

Assessment

American Physical Therapy Association. Guide to physical therapist practice. 2nd ed. *Phys Ther*. 2001;81.

Bandy WD, Timm KE. Relationship between peak torque, work, and power for knee flexion and extension in clients with grade I medial compartment sprains of the knee. *J Orthop Sports Phys Ther*. 1992;16:288–292.

Buschbacher RM, ed. *Musculoskeletal Disorders: A Practical Guide for Diagnosis and Rehabilitation*. Boston, Mass: Andover Medical Publishers; 1994.

Daniels L, Worthingham C. *Muscle Testing Techniques of Manual Examination*. 6th ed. Philadelphia, Pa: WB Saunders Co; 1995.

Delitto A, Synder-Mackler L. The diagnostic process: examples in orthopedic physical therapy. *Phys Ther*. 1995;75:203–210.

Hall CM, Brody TB. *Therapeutic Exercise: Moving Toward Function*. Philadelphia, Pa: Lippincott Williams and Wilkins; 1999.

Hertling D, Kessler RM. *Management of Common Musculoskeletal Disorders*. 3rd ed. Philadelphia, Pa: JB Lippincott Co; 1996:78, 534.

Jacobs K. *Ergonomics for Therapists*. 2nd ed. Boston, Mass: Butterworth Heinemann; 2000.

Kasman GS, Ram JR, Wolf SL. *Clinical Applications in Surface Electromyography: Chronic Musculoskeletal Pain*. Bethesda, Md: Aspen Publishers; 1998.

Kendall FP, McCreary EK, Provance PG. *Muscles: Testing and Function*. 4th ed. Baltimore, Md: Williams and Wilkins; 1993.

Kisner C, Colby LA. *Therapeutic Exercise: Foundations and Techniques*. 3rd ed. Philadelphia, Pa: FA Davis Co; 1996:241–270.

Lesh SG. *Clinical Orthopedics for the Physical Therapist Assistant*. Philadelphia, Pa: FA Davis Co; 2000.

Malone TR, McPoil T, Nitz AJ, eds. *Orthopaedic and Sports Physical Therapy*. 3rd ed. St. Louis, Mo: CV Mosby Co; 1997.

Myers RS, ed. *Saunders Manual of Physical Therapy Practice*. Philadelphia, Pa: WB Saunders Co; 1995.

Rothstein JM, Roy SH, Wolf SL. *The Rehabilitation Specialist's Handbook*. 2nd ed. Philadelphia, Pa: FA Davis Co; 1998.

Saidoff DC, McDonough AL. *Critical Pathways in Therapeutic Intervention*. Philadelphia, Pa: CV Mosby Co; 2002.

Schunk C, Reed K. *Clinical Practice Guidelines*. Gaithersburg, Md: Aspen Publishers; 2000.

Steiner LA, Harris BA, Krebs DE. Reliability of eccentric isokinetic knee flexion and extension measurements. *Arch Phys Med Rehabil*. 1993;74:1327–1335.

Tomberlin JP, Saunders HD. *Evaluation, Treatment and Prevention of Musculoskeletal Disorders. Vol 2: Extremities*. Chaska, Minn: The Saunders Group; 1994.

Treatment

Afzali L, Kuwabara F, Zachazewski J, Browne P, Robinson B. A new method for the determination of the characteristic shape of an isokinetic quadriceps femoris muscle torque curve. *Phys Ther*. 1992;72:585–595.

Buschbacher RM, ed. *Musculoskeletal Disorders: A Practical Guide for Diagnosis and Rehabilitation*. Boston, Mass: Andover Medical Publishers; 1994:206–208.

Caylor D, Fites R, Worrell TW. The relationship between quadriceps angle and anterior knee pain syndrome. *J Orthop Sports Phys Ther.* 1993;17:11–16.

Charteris J. An isometric normative database to facilitate restoration of function in knee-injured active young adults. *S Afr J Physiotherapy.* 1993;49:2:28–34.

Delitto A. Lower extremity: knee. In: Myers RS, ed. *Saunders Manual of Physical Therapy Practice.* Philadelphia, Pa: WB Saunders Co; 1995:1001–1029.

DiVeta JA, Vogelbach WD. The clinical efficacy of the A-angle in measuring patellar alignment. *J Orthop Sports Phys Ther.* 1992;16:136–139.

Kisner C, Colby LA. *Therapeutic Exercise: Foundations and Techniques.* 3rd ed. Philadelphia, Pa: FA Davis Co; 1996:345–384.

Puniello MS. Iliotibial band tightness and medial patellar glide in patients with patellofemoral dysfunction. *J Orthop Sports Phys Ther.* 1993;17:144–148.

Tomberlin JP, Saunders HD. *Evaluation, Treatment and Prevention of Musculoskeletal Disorders. Vol 2: Extremities.* Chaska, Minn: The Saunders Group; 1994:233.

Wilk KE, Andrew JR. The effects of pad placement and angular velocity on tibial displacement during isokinetic exercise. *J Orthop Sports Phys Ther.* 1993;17:24–30.

Prepatellar Bursitis

Also known as *housemaid's knee.*

DESCRIPTION

Acute or chronic inflammation of the prepatellar bursa.

CAUSE

Unknown etiology. May be caused by trauma, such as a direct fall on the knee, or chronic overuse from persistent kneeling. Acute or chronic infection or arthritis can also be involved. This condition is the most common bursitis of the knee joint.

ASSESSMENT

Note: See APTA's Guide to Physical Therapist Practice. 2nd ed. *Physical Therapy.* 2001;81.

Musculoskeletal Preferred Practice Patterns: D, E, I, F

AREAS
- History
- Posture
- Pain
- Joint integrity and structural deviations
- Mobility, including active and passive range of motion
- (ROM) and accessory motion
- Strength
- Neurological
- Skin and soft tissue
- Gait
- Functional level

INSTRUMENTS/PROCEDURES

See References for sources.

Functional Level
- Lysholm knee score
- modified Lysholm knee score

Joint Integrity and Structural Deviations

The following orthopedic tests of the knee may be performed:

- A-angle
- ALRI test
- AMRI test
- Apley grinding test
- apprehension test
- bounce home test
- brush or stroke (wipe) test
- Clark sign
- crossover test
- Ely test
- external rotation test
- flexion rotation drawer sign
- fluctuation test
- gravity drawer test (posterior sag sign)
- hamstring length
- Helfet test
- Hughston plica test
- Hughston posterolateral drawer test
- Hughston test (jerk sign)
- hyperflexion-hyperextension test
- Jakob test (reverse pivot)
- Lachman's test
- lateral pull test
- limb-length discrepancy
- MacIntosh test (lateral pivot shift)
- McConnell test
- McMurray-Anderson test
- Noble's compression
- Ober's test
- O'Donoghue test
- patellar tap
- patellar tilt
- Perkins test
- plica test
- posterior drawer sign
- posterior sag test
- quadriceps active test
- Q-angle measurements
- reverse pivot shift
- Slocum test
- Steinman's test
- squat test
- valgus stress test
- varus stress test
- Waldron test
- Wilson test

Mobility
- goniometry

Special Tests to Which the Physical Therapist May or May Not Have Access
- x-ray studies
- joint aspiration
- magnetic resonance imagery (MRI)
- CT scan
- arthrography and arthroscopy

Strength
- instrumentation
- manual muscle testing

PROBLEMS
- The client often complains of anterior knee pain.
- The client may have an antalgic gait.
- The client may complain of weakness in quadriceps and tightness in hamstring and gastrocnemius/soleus muscles.

TREATMENT/MANAGEMENT
- Use physical modalities, such as ice, as indicated.
- Consider the use of compression.
- Avoid persistent kneeling or a direct fall on knee.

PRECAUTIONS/CONTRAINDICATIONS
- X-rays should be consulted to rule out any potential fractures.
- Carefully consider the nature of the problem before examination so the condition is not aggravated with the test procedures.

DESIRED OUTCOME/PROGNOSIS
- Relieve symptoms such as inflammatory response.
- The client will have pain-free knee function.

REFERENCES

Assessment

American Physical Therapy Association. Guide to physical therapist practice. 2nd ed. *Phys Ther.* 2001;81.

Bandy WD, Timm KE. Relationship between peak torque, work, and power for knee flexion and extension in clients with grade I medial compartment sprains of the knee. *J Orthop Sports Phys Ther.* 1992;16:288–292.

Buschbacher RM, ed. *Musculoskeletal Disorders: A Practical Guide for Diagnosis and Rehabilitation.* Boston, Mass: Andover Medical Publishers; 1994.

Daniels L, Worthingham C. *Muscle Testing Techniques of Manual Examination.* 6th ed. Philadelphia, Pa: WB Saunders Co; 1995.

Delitto A, Synder-Mackler L. The diagnostic process: examples in orthopedic physical therapy. *Phys Ther.* 1995;75:203–210.

Hall CM, Brody TB. *Therapeutic Exercise: Moving Toward Function.* Philadelphia, Pa: Lippincott Williams and Wilkins; 1999.

Hertling D, Kessler RM. *Management of Common Musculoskeletal Disorders.* 3rd ed. Philadelphia, Pa: JB Lippincott Co; 1996:78, 534.

Jacobs K. *Ergonomics for Therapists.* 2nd ed. Boston, Mass: Butterworth Heinemann; 2000.

Kasman GS, Ram JR, Wolf Sl. *Clinical Applications in Surface Electromyography: Chronic Musculoskeletal Pain.* Bethesda, Md: Aspen Publishers; 1998.

Kendall FP, McCreary EK, Provance PG. *Muscles: Testing and Function.* 4th ed. Baltimore, Md: Williams and Wilkins; 1993.

Kisner C, Colby LA. *Therapeutic Exercise: Foundations and Techniques.* 3rd ed. Philadelphia, Pa: FA Davis Co; 1996:241–270.

Lesh SG. *Clinical Orthopedics for the Physical Therapist Assistant.* Philadelphia, Pa: FA Davis Co; 2000.

Malone TR, McPoil T, Nitz AJ, eds. *Orthopaedic and Sports Physical Therapy.* 3rd ed. St. Louis, Mo: CV Mosby Co; 1997.

Myers RS, ed. *Saunders Manual of Physical Therapy Practice.* Philadelphia, Pa: WB Saunders Co; 1995.

Rothstein JM, Roy SH, Wolf SL. *The Rehabilitation Specialist's Handbook.* 2nd ed. Philadelphia, Pa: FA Davis Co; 1998.

Saidoff DC, McDonough AL. *Critical Pathways in Therapeutic Intervention.* Philadelphia, Pa: CV Mosby Co; 2002.

Schunk C, Reed K. *Clinical Practice Guidelines.* Gaithersburg, Md: Aspen Publishers; 2000.

Steiner LA, Harris BA, Krebs DE. Reliability of eccentric isokinetic knee flexion and extension measurements. *Arch Phys Med Rehabil.* 1993;74:1327–1335.

Tomberlin JP, Saunders HD. *Evaluation, Treatment and Prevention of Musculoskeletal Disorders. Vol 2: Extremities.* Chaska, Minn: The Saunders Group; 1994.

Treatment

Buschbacher RM, ed. *Musculoskeletal Disorders: A Practical Guide for Diagnosis and Rehabilitation.* Boston, Mass: Andover Medical Publishers; 1994:206–208.

Caylor D, Fites R, Worrell TW. The relationship between quadriceps angle and anterior knee pain syndrome. *J Orthop Sports Phys Ther.* 1993;17:11–16.

Charteris J. An isometric normative database to facilitate restoration of function in knee-injured active young adults. *S Afr J Physiotherapy.* 1993;49:2:28–34.

Delitto A. Lower extremity: knee. In: Myers RS, ed. *Saunders Manual of Physical Therapy Practice.* Philadelphia, Pa: WB Saunders Co; 1995:1001–1029.

DiVeta JA, Vogelbach WD. The clinical efficacy of the A-angle in measuring patellar alignment. *J Orthop Sports Phys Ther.* 1992;16:136–139.

Grabois M, Garrison SJ, Hart KA, Lehmkuhl LD. *Physical Medicine and Rehabilitation: The Complete Approach.* Malden, Mass: Blackwell Science; 2000.

Hertling D, Kessler RM. *Management of Common Musculoskeletal Disorders.* 3rd ed. Philadelphia, Pa: JB Lippincott Co; 1996.

Johanson MA, Donatelli R, Greenfield BH. Rehabilitation of microtrauma injuries. In: Greenfield BH, ed. *Rehabilitation of the Knee: A Problem-Solving Approach.* Philadelphia, Pa: FA Davis Co; 1993:139–176.

Kisner C, Colby LA. *Therapeutic Exercise: Foundations and Techniques.* 3rd ed. Philadelphia, Pa: FA Davis Co; 1996:345–384.

Tomberlin JP, Saunders HD. *Evaluation, Treatment and Prevention of Musculoskeletal Disorders. Vol 2: Extremities.* Chaska, Minn: The Saunders Group; 1994:233.

Retrocalcaneal Bursitis

DESCRIPTION

Acute or chronic inflammation of the retrocalcaneal bursa. This acute or chronic inflammation can appear in the superficial retrocalcaneal bursa between the skin and the Achilles tendons or in the deep bursae between the Achilles tendon and the calcaneus. It occurs more frequently in young women but may also be present in men. Retrocalcaneal bursitis can also occur in combination with Achiller tendinopathy.

CAUSE

Deep bursa irritation is caused by excessive compensatory subtalar joint pronation or direct trauma. Footwear can also cause irritation through compressive forces.

ASSESSMENT

Note: See APTA's Guide to Physical Therapist Practice. 2nd ed. *Physical Therapy.* 2001;81.

Musculoskeletal Preferred Practice Patterns: D, E, F, I

AREAS

- History
- Pain
- Posture
- Gait
- Strength
- Neurological
- Joint integrity and structural deviations
- Mobility: active and passive range of motion (ROM) and accessory motion
- Skin and soft tissue
- Equipment, including footwear

INSTRUMENTS/PROCEDURES

See References for sources.

Gait
- dynamic assessment of foot mechanics
  1. dynamic plantar pressure distribution
  2. foot pressure EMED system
  3. pedabarograph
  4. three-dimensional kinematic analysis
- gait velocity

Joint Integrity and Structural Deviations

The following orthopedic tests for the leg and foot may be performed:

- Achilles tendon test
- anterior drawer sign
- Homan's sign
- Kleiger test
- talar tilt
- Thompson test
- tibial varum evaluation

Mobility
- selected measures of ankle dorsiflexion
- goniometric measurements
- open and closed kinetic chain subtalar joint neutral positions and navicular drop test
- visual estimates of ankle joint active range of motion

Strength
- dynamometer
- manual muscle testing

PROBLEMS
- The client often complains of pain.
- The client often has swelling.
- The client may have inflammation over the posterior calcaneus.

TREATMENT/MANAGEMENT
- Use physical agents, such as ice, as indicated.
- Consider orthotics or supportive counters in the shoes.
- Implement heel cord stretching.
- Assess footwear.
- Encourage enforced rest if there is a partial tear.

PRECAUTIONS/CONTRAINDICATIONS
- Do not overstress the tendon for up to 6 weeks if it has been injected with a steroid anesthetic because it may be prone to rupture during this period.

DESIRED OUTCOME/PROGNOSIS
- The client will reduce superficial bursa irritation and decreased inflammation.
- The client will have normal function.

Note: Surgery may be indicated in severe cases.

REFERENCES

Assessment

American Physical Therapy Association. Guide to physical therapist practice. 2nd ed. *Phys Ther.* 2001;81.

Buschbacher RM, ed. *Musculoskeletal Disorders: A Practical Guide for Diagnosis and Rehabilitation.* Boston, Mass: Andover Medical Publishers; 1994.

Daniels L, Worthingham C. *Muscle Testing Techniques of Manual Examination.* 6th ed. Philadelphia, Pa: WB Saunders Co; 1995.

Delitto A, Synder-Mackler L. The diagnostic process: examples in orthopedic physical therapy. *Phys Ther.* 1995;75:203–210.

Donatelli RA. *The Biomechanics of the Foot and Ankle.* 2nd ed. Philadelphia, Pa: FA Davis Co; 1996.

Hall CM, Brody TB. *Therapeutic Exercise: Moving Toward Function.* Philadelphia, Pa: Lippincott Williams and Wilkins; 1999.

Hertling D, Kessler RM. *Management of Common Musculoskeletal Disorders.* 3rd ed. Philadelphia, Pa: JB Lippincott Co; 1996:78, 534.

Jacobs K. *Ergonomics for Therapists.* 2nd ed. Boston, Mass: Butterworth Heinemann; 2000.

Kasman GS, Ram JR, Wolf SI. *Clinical Applications in Surface Electromyography: Chronic Musculoskeletal Pain.* Bethesda, Md: Aspen Publishers; 1998.

Kendall FP, McCreary EK, Provance PG. *Muscles: Testing and Function.* 4th ed. Baltimore, Md: Williams and Wilkins; 1993.

Kisner C, Colby LA. *Therapeutic Exercise: Foundations and Techniques.* 3rd ed. Philadelphia, Pa: FA Davis Co; 1996:241–270.

Lesh SG. *Clinical Orthopedics for the Physical Therapist Assistant.* Philadelphia, Pa: FA Davis Co; 2000.

Malone TR, McPoil T, Nitz AJ, eds. *Orthopaedic and Sports Physical Therapy.* 3rd ed. St. Louis, Mo: CV Mosby Co; 1997.

Myers RS, ed. *Saunders Manual of Physical Therapy Practice.* Philadelphia, Pa: WB Saunders Co; 1995.

Rothstein JM, Roy SH, Wolf SL. *The Rehabilitation Specialist's Handbook.* 2nd ed. Philadelphia, Pa: FA Davis Co; 1998.

Saidoff DC, McDonough AL. *Critical Pathways in Therapeutic Intervention.* Philadelphia, Pa: CV Mosby Co; 2002.

Sammarco GJ. *Rehabilitation of the Foot and Ankle.* St. Louis, Mo: Mosby Year Book; 1995.

Schunk C, Reed K. *Clinical Practice Guidelines.* Gaithersburg, Md: Aspen Publishers; 2000.

Tomberlin JP, Saunders HD. *Evaluation, Treatment and Prevention of Musculoskeletal Disorders. Vol 2: Extremities.* Chaska, Minn: The Saunders Group; 1994.

Treatment

Buschbacher RM, ed. *Musculoskeletal Disorders: A Practical Guide for Diagnosis and Rehabilitation.* Boston, Mass: Andover Medical Publishers; 1994.

Hertling D, Kessler RM. *Management of Common Musculoskeletal Disorders.* 3rd ed. Philadelphia, Pa: JB Lippincott Co; 1996:359–410.

Hunt GC, ed. *Physical Therapy of the Foot and Ankle.* 2nd ed. New York, NY: Churchill Livingstone; 1995.

Kisner C, Colby LA. *Therapeutic Exercise: Foundations and Techniques.* 3rd ed. Philadelphia, Pa: FA Davis Co; 1996:385–407.

McCulloch MU, Brunt D, Vander-Linden D. The effect of foot orthotics and gait velocity on lower limb kinematics and temporal events of stance. *J Orthop Sports Phys Ther.* 1993;17:2–10.

McPoil TG, Hunt GC. Evaluation and management of foot and ankle disorders: present problems and future directions. *J Orthop Sports Phys Ther.* 1995;21:381–388.

Picciano AM, Rowlands MS, Worrell T. Reliability of open and closed kinetic chain subtalar joint neutral positions and navicular drop test. *J Orthop Sports Phys Ther.* 1993;18: 553–558.

Tomberlin JP, Saunders HD. *Evaluation, Treatment and Prevention of Musculoskeletal Disorders. Vol 2: Extremities.* Chaska, Minn: The Saunders Group; 1994:265–306.

Youdas JW, Bogard CL, Suman VJ. Reliability of goniometric measurements and visual estimates of ankle joint active range of motion obtained in a clinical setting. *Arch Phys Med Rehabil.* 1993;74:1113–1118.

Shoulder Bursitis

DESCRIPTION

Acute or chronic inflammation of the shoulder bursa. Bursitis of the shoulder may include the subacromial or subdeltoid bursas. Shoulder pain from bursitis may be due to one pathologic process or a combination of the following disorders: adhesive capsulitis, tendinitis, and bursitis.

CAUSE

Unknown etiology. Shoulder bursitis may be caused by trauma, chronic overuse, inflammatory arthritis, or acute or chronic infection.

ASSESSMENT

Note: See APTA's Guide to Physical Therapist Practice. 2nd ed. *Physical Therapy.* 2001;81.

Musculoskeletal Preferred Practice Patterns: D, E, F, G, J

AREAS

- History
- Pain
- Posture
- Joint integrity and structural deviations
- Skin and soft tissue
- Mobility: active and passive range of motion (ROM) and accessory motion
- Strength
- Neurological
- Vascular
- Functional level, including functional use of arm

INSTRUMENTS/PROCEDURES

See References for sources.

Joint Integrity and Structural Deviations/Neurological Involvement

The following neurological and orthopedic tests of the upper extremity may be performed:

- acromioclavicular instability test
- anterior apprehension sign
- anterior drawer sign
- anterior stability test

- active impingement test
- Adson's test
- Allen's test
- clunk test
- costoclavicular syndrome test
- drop arm test
- Feagin test
- fulcrum test
- Gilchrist sign
- Halstead maneuver
- Hawkins test
- hyperabduction syndrome test
- jerk test
- lateral scapular glide
- Lippmans test
- locking test
- Ludington's test
- Neer's test
- Norwood stress test
- posterior apprehension test
- posterior drawer sign
- push-pull test
- quadrant test
- relocation test
- Roo's test (EAST test)
- Rockwood test
- Rowe test
- Speed's test (bicep's test)
- sulcus sign
- suprascapular nerve entrapment test
- transverse humeral ligament rupture test
- upper limb tension test
- upper quarter screen
- Yergason's test

Pain
- body chart
- palpation
- visual analog scale

Special Tests to Which the Physical Therapist May or May Not Have Access
- electromyography (EMG)
- thermography

Strength
- isokinetic peak torque and work values
- isokinetic testing of the shoulder rotators
- manual muscle testing

PROBLEMS
- The client often has constant, intense pain, which may radiate down the arm.
- The client may have disturbed sleep because of pain.
- The client may be unable to use the arm secondary to pain.
- There is often a decreased ROM in active flexion and abduction.
- The client may have a decrease in internal and external rotation.

TREATMENT/MANAGEMENT

EXERCISE IN GENERAL
- Isokinetic rehabilitation can begin when the client's shoulder can tolerate resisted exercise through specific ROM.
- Progress exercise from submaximal isometrics to maximum-effort isometrics. Proceed from submaximal concentric isokinetics to isotonics. Proceed from maximal isokinetics through partial-range to full-ROM isokinetics at the submaximal level. Progress from isotonics at full ROM to maximal effort isokinetics at full ROM.

ACUTE
- Use ice or superficial heat as indicated.
- Consider external support for arm via sling.
- Begin gentle active assisted exercises and pendulum exercises.
- Use gentle joint mobilization techniques as indicated.

CHRONIC
- Use ultrasound as indicated.
- Consider joint mobilization.
- Begin a home program of strength training exercises and ROM exercises.
- Educate on proper usage to prevent recurrence.

PRECAUTIONS/CONTRAINDICATIONS
- Brachial plexus peripheral entrapment at the thoracic outlet or the shoulder can be mistakenly identified as shoulder tendinitis or musculoskeletal pain of the shoulder.
- Rule out pre-existing calcific rotator cuff tendinitis.
- Do not begin isokinetic exercise progression until after lesion is well healed and painless ROM is achieved.

DESIRED OUTCOME/PROGNOSIS
- The client will have an absence of pain at rest.
- The client will have active flexion to 90 degrees or more.
- Any chronic inflammatory process will be resolved, and full ROM, joint play, and strength will be restored.

Note: This condition is usually self-limiting after several weeks.

REFERENCES

Assessment

American Physical Therapy Association. Guide to physical therapist practice. 2nd ed. *Phys Ther.* 2001;81.

Ballantyne BT, O'Hare SJ, Paschall JL, et al. Electromyographic activity of selected shoulder muscles in commonly used therapeutic exercises. *Phys Ther.* 1993;73:668–682.

Buschbacher RM, ed. *Musculoskeletal Disorders: A Practical Guide for Diagnosis and Rehabilitation.* Boston, Mass: Andover Medical Publishers; 1994.

Corso G. Impingement relief test: an adjunctive procedure to traditional assessment of shoulder impingement syndrome. *J Orthop Sports Phys Ther.* 1995;22:183–192.

Daniels L, Worthingham C. *Muscle Testing Techniques of Manual Examination.* 6th ed. Philadelphia, Pa: WB Saunders Co; 1995.

Delitto A, Synder-Mackler L. The diagnostic process: examples in orthopedic physical therapy. *Phys Ther.* 1995;75:203–210.

Hall CM, Brody TB. *Therapeutic Exercise: Moving Toward Function.* Philadelphia, Pa: Lippincott Williams and Wilkins; 1999.

Hertling D, Kessler RM. *Management of Common Musculoskeletal Disorders.* 3rd ed. Philadelphia, Pa: JB Lippincott Co; 1996:78,534.

Jacobs K. *Ergonomics for Therapists.* 2nd ed. Boston, Mass: Butterworth Heinemann; 2000.

Kasman GS, Ram JR, Wolf SI. *Clinical Applications in Surface Electromyography: Chronic Musculoskeletal Pain.* Bethesda, Md: Aspen Publishers; 1998.

Kendall FP, McCreary EK, Provance PG. *Muscles: Testing and Function.* 4th ed. Baltimore, Md: Williams and Wilkins; 1993.

Kisner C, Colby LA. *Therapeutic Exercise: Foundations and Techniques.* 3rd ed. Philadelphia, Pa: FA Davis Co; 1996:241–270.

Lesh SG. *Clinical Orthopedics for the Physical Therapist Assistant.* Philadelphia, Pa: FA Davis Co; 2000.

Malone TR, McPoil T, Nitz AJ, eds. *Orthop Sports Phys Ther.* 3rd ed. St. Louis, Mo: CV Mosby Co; 1997.

Moseley JB, Jobe FW, Pink M, et al. EMG analysis of the scapular muscles during a shoulder rehabilitation program. *Am J Sports Med.* 1992;20:128–135.

Myers RS, ed. *Saunders Manual of Physical Therapy Practice.* Philadelphia, Pa: WB Saunders Co; 1995.

Rothstein JM, Roy SH, Wolf SL. *The Rehabilitation Specialist's Handbook.* 2nd ed. Philadelphia, Pa: FA Davis Co; 1998.

Saidoff DC, McDonough AL. *Critical Pathways in Therapeutic Intervention.* Philadelphia, Pa: CV Mosby Co; 2002.

Schunk C, Reed K. *Clinical Practice Guidelines.* Gaithersburg, Md: Aspen Publishers; 2000.

Tomberlin JP, Saunders HD. *Evaluation, Treatment and Prevention of Musculoskeletal Disorders. Vol 2: Extremities.* Chaska, Minn: The Saunders Group; 1994.

Wilk KE, Arrigo CA, Andrews JR. Isokinetic testing of the shoulder abductors and adductors: windowed vs non-windowed data collection. *J Orthop Sports Phys Ther.* 1992;15: 107–112.

Winkel D. *Diagnosis and Treatment of the Upper Extremities.* Gaithersburg, Md: Aspen Publishers; 1997.

Treatment

Boublik M, Hawkins RJ. Clinical examination of the shoulder complex. *J Orthop Sports Phys Ther.* 1993;18:379–385.

Culham E, Peat M. Functional anatomy of the shoulder complex. *J Orthop Sports Phys Ther.* 1993;18:342–350.

Davies G, Dickoff-Hoffman S. Neuromuscular testing and rehabilitation of the shoulder complex. *J Orthop Sports Phys Ther.* 1993;18:449–458.

Diamond W. Upper extremity: shoulder. In: Myers RS, ed. *Saunders Manual of Physical Therapy Practice.* Philadelphia, Pa: WB Saunders Co; 1995:802–822.

Frieman BG, Albert TJ, Fenlin JM. Rotator cuff disease: a review of diagnosis, pathophysiology, and current trends in treatment. *Arch Phys Med Rebabil.* 1994;75:604–609.

Grabois M, Garrison SJ, Hart KA, Lehmkuhl LD. *Physical Medicine and Rehabilitation: The Complete Approach.* Malden, Mass: Blackwell Science; 2000.

Greenfield B, Catlin PA, Coats PW, et al. Posture in patients with shoulder overuse injuries and healthy individuals. *J Orthop Sports Phys Ther.* 1995;21:287–295.

Grubbs N. Frozen shoulder syndrome: a review of literature. *J Orthop Sports Phys Ther.* 1993;18:479–487.

Haig SV. *Shoulder Pathophysiology: Rehabilitation and Treatment.* Gaithersburg, Md: Aspen Publishers; 1996.

Harrison AL, Barry-Greb T, Wojtowicz G. Clinical measurement of head and shoulder posture variables. *J Orthop Sports Phys Ther.* 1996;23:353–361.

Hertling D, Kessler RM. *Management of Common Musculoskeletal Disorders.* 3rd ed. Philadelphia, Pa: JB Lippincott Co; 1996:78,534.

Jobe FW, Pink M. Classification and treatment of shoulder dysfunction in the overhead athlete. *J Orthop Sports Phys Ther.* 1993;8:427–432.

Kamkar A, Irrgang JJ, Whitney SL. Non-operative management of secondary shoulder impingement syndrome. *J Orthop Sports Phys Ther.* 1993;17:212–224.

Kelly MJ, Clark WA, eds. *Orthopedic Therapy of the Shoulder*. Philadelphia, Pa: JB Lippincott Co; 1994.

Paine RM, Voight M. The role of the scapula. *J Orthop Sports Phys Ther*. 1993;18:386–391.

Schenkman M, Rugo de Cartaya V. Kinesiology of the shoulder complex. *J Orthop Sports Phys Ther*. 1993;18:442–448.

Simmons TC, Skyhair MJ. Rehabilitation of the shoulder. In: Nickel VL, Botte MJ, eds. *Orthop Rehabil*. New York, NY: Churchill Livingstone; 1992:747.

Tomberlin JP, Saunders HD. *Evaluation, Treatment and Prevention of Musculoskeletal Disorders. Vol 2: Extremities*. Chaska, Minn: The Saunders Group; 1994:73–111.

Wainner RS. Mangement of acute calcific tendonitis of the shoulder. *J Orthop Sports Phys Ther*. 1998;27:231–237.

Wilk KE, Arrigo CA. An integrated approach to upper extremity exercises. In Timm K, ed. Exercise Principles. *Orthop Phys Ther Clin North Am*. 1992;2:337–360.

Wilk KE, Arrigo Ca, Andrews JR. Current concepts: the stabilizing structures of the glenohumeral joint. *J Orthop Sports Phys Ther*. 1997;25:364–379.

Shoulder Tendinitis

DESCRIPTION

Shoulder tendinitis is the inflammation of a tendon. Shoulder pain from shoulder tendinitis may be due to one pathologic process or a combination of disorders: adhesive capsulitis, bursitis, and tendinitis.

CAUSE

Unknown etiology. Shoulder tendinitis may be caused by the effects of aging, repetitive microtrauma, extreme trauma, strain, or unaccustomed exercise. It occurs in young and old and almost equally in females and males.

ASSESSMENT

Note: See APTA's Guide to Physical Therapist Practice. 2nd ed. *Physical Therapy*. 2001;81.

Integumentary Preferred Practice Pattern: A

Musculoskeletal Preferred Practice Patterns: D, E, F, G, J

AREAS

- History
- Pain
- Posture
- Joint integrity and structural deviations
- Skin and soft tissue
- Mobility, including active and passive range of motion
- (ROM) and accessory motion
- Strength
- Neurological
- Vascular
- Functional level, including functional use of arm

INSTRUMENTS/PROCEDURES

See References for sources.

Joint Integrity and Structural Deviations/Neurological Involvement

The following neurological and orthopedic tests of the upper extremity may be performed:

- acromioclavicular instability test
- anterior apprehension test
- anterior drawer sign
- anterior stability test
- active impingement test
- Adson's test
- Allen's test
- clunk test
- costoclavicular syndrome test
- drop arm test
- Feagin test
- fulcrum test
- Gilchrist sign
- Halstead maneuver
- Hawkin's test
- hyperabduction syndrome test
- jerk test
- lateral scapular glide
- Lippmans test
- locking test
- Ludington's test
- Neer's test
- Norwood stress test
- posterior apprehension test
- posterior drawer sign
- push-pull test
- quadrant test
- relocation test
- Roo's test (EAST test)
- Rockwood test
- Rowe test
- Speed's test (bicep's test)
- sulcus sign
- suprascapular nerve entrapment test
- transverse humeral ligament rupture test
- upper limb tension test
- upper quarter screen
- Yergason's test

Pain
- body chart
- visual analog scale

Special Tests to Which the Physical Therapist May or May Not Have Access
- EMG
- thermography

Strength
- isokinetic peak torque and work values
- isokinetic testing of the shoulder rotators
- manual muscle testing

PROBLEMS
- The client often has intense lateral brachial pain, which may radiate into the arm.
- Often the pain is associated with increased arm usage and specific movements, especially reaching behind the back.
- The client often has pain with resisted motions, specifically shoulder abduction, internal and external rotation, elbow flexion, and forearm supination.

TREATMENT/MANAGEMENT
- Use physical modalities, such as ultrasound or friction massage, if indicated.
- Provide education in proper activity level.
- Begin strength training of rotator cuff muscles, progressing from isometric to isotonic to resistive exercise.
- Consider aquatic therapy.
- Teach automobilization techniques.
- Address total body fitness considerations.
- Prevent impingement via shoulder shrugs and push-ups with arm abducted to 90 degrees.

PRECAUTIONS/CONTRAINDICATIONS

- Brachial plexus peripheral entrapment at the thoracic outlet or the shoulder can be mistakenly identified as shoulder tendinitis or musculoskeletal pain of the shoulder.
- Avoid activities that require repeated arm elevation to 90 degrees or more.
- Rotator cuff muscles should be strong before initiating shoulder elevation above 90 degrees.
- It is preferable to perform exercises with arm close to side to avoid impingement in early phase of recovery.

DESIRED OUTCOME/PROGNOSIS

- The client will obtain pain relief.
- The client will be able to return to normal use of shoulder.
- There will be restoration of normal joint mechanics at shoulder.
- There will be restoration of normal strength and endurance.

Notes: If shoulder tendinitis is caused by a degenerative process, the pain will tend to be chronic. The condition may respond quite well to a treatment program but is unlikely to recover spontaneously. If the client has a surgical repair of the rotator cuff, the rehabilitation process is often slow. An athlete may average 12 to 14 months before obtaining prior activity status.

REFERENCES

Assessment

American Physical Therapy Association. Guide to physical therapist practice. 2nd ed. *Phys Ther.* 2001;81.

Buschbacher RM, ed. *Musculoskeletal Disorders: A Practical Guide for Diagnosis and Rehabilitation.* Boston, Mass: Andover Medical Publishers; 1994.

Daniels L, Worthingham C. *Muscle Testing Techniques of Manual Examination.* 6th ed. Philadelphia, Pa: WB Saunders Co; 1995.

Hall CM, Brody TB. *Therapeutic Exercise: Moving Toward Function.* Philadelphia, Pa: Lippincott Williams and Wilkins; 1999.

Hertling D, Kessler RM. *Management of Common Musculoskeletal Disorders.* 3rd ed. Philadelphia, Pa: JB Lippincott Co; 1996:78, 534.

Kasman GS, Ram JR, Wolf Sl. *Clinical Applications in Surface Electromyography: Chronic Musculoskeletal Pain.* Bethesda, Md: Aspen Publishers; 1998.

Kisner C, Colby LA. *Therapeutic Exercise: Foundations and Techniques.* 3rd ed. Philadelphia, Pa: FA Davis Co; 1996:241–270.

Lesh SG. *Clinical Orthopedics for the Physical Therapist Assistant.* Philadelphia, Pa: FA Davis Co; 2000.

Myers RS, ed. *Saunders Manual of Physical Therapy Practice.* Philadelphia, Pa: WB Saunders Co; 1995.

Rothstein JM, Roy SH, Wolf SL. *The Rehabilitation Specialist's Handbook.* 2nd ed. Philadelphia, Pa: FA Davis Co; 1998.

Saidoff DC, McDonough AL. *Critical Pathways in Therapeutic Intervention.* Philadelphia, Pa: CV Mosby Co; 2002.

Schunk C, Reed K. *Clinical Practice Guidelines.* Gaithersburg, Md: Aspen Publishers; 2000.

Tomberlin JP, Saunders HD. *Evaluation, Treatment and Prevention of Musculoskeletal Disorders. Vol 2: Extremities.* Chaska, Minn: The Saunders Group; 1994.

Wilk KE, Arrigo CA, Andrews JR. Isokinetic testing of the shoulder abductors and adductors: windowed vs non-windowed data collection. *J Orthop Sports Phys Ther.* 1992;15: 107–112.

Treatment

Almekinders LC, Almekinders SV. Outcome in the treatment of chronic overuse sports injuries: a retrospective study. *J Orthop Sports Phys Ther.* 1994;19:157–161.

Ballantyne BT, O'Hare SJ, Paschall JL, et al. Electromyographic activity of selected shoulder muscles in commonly used therapeutic exercises. *Phys Ther.* 1993;73:668–682.

Boublik M, Hawkins RJ. Clinical examination of the shoulder complex. *J Orthop Sports Phys Ther.* 1993;18:379–385.

Culham E, Peat M. Functional anatomy of the shoulder complex. *J Orthop Sports Phys Ther.* 1993;18:342–350.

Dacre JE, Beeney N, Scott DL. Injections and physiotherapy for the painful stiff shoulder. *Annals of the Rheumatic Diseases.* 1989;48:322–325.

Davies G, Dickoff-Hoffman S. Neuromuscular testing and rehabilitation of the shoulder complex. *J Orthop Sports Phys Ther.* 1993;18:449–458.

Diamond W. Upper extremity: shoulder. In: Myers RS, ed. *Saunders Manual of Physical Therapy Practice.* Philadelphia, Pa: WB Saunders Co; 1995:802–822.

Grabois M, Garrison SJ, Hart KA, Lehmkuhl LD. *Physical Medicine and Rehabilitation: The Complete Approach.* Malden, Mass: Blackwell Science; 2000.

Grubbs N. Frozen shoulder syndrome: a review of literature. *J Orthop Sports Phys Ther.* 1993;18:479–487.

Hertling D, Kessler RM. *Management of Common Musculoskeletal Disorders.* 3rd ed. Philadelphia, Pa: JB Lippincott Co; 1996;169–204, 532–541.

Jobe FW, Pink M. Classification and treatment of shoulder dysfunction in the overhead athlete. *J Orthop Sports Phys Ther.* 1993;8:427–432.

Kisner C, Colby LA. *Therapeutic Exercise: Foundations and Techniques.* 3rd ed. Philadelphia, Pa: FA Davis Co; 1996:241–270.

Moseley JB, Jobe FW, Pink M, et al. EMG analysis of the scapular muscles during a shoulder rehabilitation program. *Am J Sports Med.* 1992;20:128–135.

Schenkman M, Rugo de Cartaya V. Kinesiology of the shoulder complex. *J Orthop Sports Phys Ther.* 1993;18:442–448.

Simmons TC, Skyhair MJ. Rehabilitation of the shoulder. In: Nickel VL, Botte MJ, eds. *Orthop Rehabil.* New York, NY: Churchill Livingstone; 1992:747.

Smith ML. Differentiating angina and shoulder pathology pain. *Phys Ther Case Rep.* 1998;1: 210–212.

Tomberlin JP, Saunders HD. *Evaluation, Treatment and Prevention of Musculoskeletal Disorders. Vol 2: Extremities.* Chaska, Minn: The Saunders Group; 1994:73–111.

Wilk KE, Arrigo CA. An integrated approach to upper extremity exercises. In Timm K, ed. *Exercise Principles. Orthop Phys Ther Clin North Am.* 1992;9:337.

Wilk KE, Arrigo C. Current concepts in the rehabilitation of the athletic shoulder. *J Orthop Sports Phys Ther.* 1993;18:365–378.

Temporomandibular Joint (TMJ) Dysfunction

DESCRIPTION

The temporomandibular joint (TMJ) is subject to a variety of disorders, such as internal derangement and ankylosis as well as arthritis, dislocation, congenital anomalies, fractures, and neoplastic diseases. The more common lesions seen by physical therapists include TMJ internal derangement, dislocation, and arthritis.

CAUSE

Internal disk derangement can be caused by chronic muscle spasm, trauma, or changes in the articulating surfaces due to arthritis. Anklyosis is usually caused by trauma or infection but may be congenital or may occur with rheumatoid arthritis.

TMJ can also be affected by other craniomandibular disorders involving dentition. The masticatory system can be disrupted by malocclusion and stress.

ASSESSMENT

Note: See APTA's Guide to Physical Therapist Practice. 2nd ed. *Physical Therapy.* 2001;81.

Integumentary Preferred Practice Pattern: A

Musculoskeletal Preferred Practice Patterns: B, C, D, E, F, G, H, I

AREAS

- History, including screening history
- Pain
- Posture
- Cranial nerve exam
- Strength, including lips/cheek, tongue, and masticatory musculature
- Periarticular tissue and muscles, including:
  1. digastric
  2. masseter
  3. medial pterygoid
  4. mylohyoid
  5. lateral pterygoid
  6. levator scapula
  7. posterior cervical
  8. scaleni
  9. sternocleidomastoid
  10. temporalis
- Joint integrity and structural deviations of TMJ
- Mobility, including joint play and functional movement (opening, protrusion, and lateral deviation)
- Respiration, including normal diaphragmatic versus upper chest breathing
- Swallowing, including hyoid movement and tongue position
- Pain, including headaches

INSTRUMENTS/PROCEDURES

See References for sources.

Joint Integrity and Structural Deviations
- resting vertical dimension (anterior and posterior)
- condyle-meniscus relationship (opening click, closing click, force closing click, crepitus)
- TMJ loading
- upper quarter screen

Periarticular Tissue and Muscles
- palpation

Special Tests to Which the Physical Therapist May or May Not Have Access
- arthrography
- CT scan
- dental examination
- magnetic resonance imaging (MRI)
- occlusal examination
- x-rays

PROBLEMS

Problems that may be indicative of generalized TMJ dysfunction:
- cervical pain
- dizziness
- headache
- hyperalgesia
- symptoms in sinuses or eyes
- ringing in ears (tinnitus)

In TMJ derangement:

- The client may report a single click.
- The client may report an audible, reciprocal click when mandible opens.

In TMJ functional dislocation with reduction:

- The client has limited mouth opening.
- There is no report of audible noise with opening.
- The client may report joint catching or locking.
- The client often reports pain in jaw.

In TMJ functional dislocation with no reduction:

- The client reports limited jaw opening and restriction of movement to the unaffected side.
- The mandible is often pulled to the affected side.

In anklyosis:

- The client often reports painless restriction of movement.
- The condition is often chronic.

TREATMENT/MANAGEMENT

In general:

- Consider use of physical agents and modalities. Modalities may include moist heat, ultrasound, ice, vapocoolant sprays, electrical stimulation, electrogalvanic stimulation, transcutaneous electrical nerve stimulation (TENS), acupuncture point stimulation, soft tissue manipulation, massage, stretching, and joint mobilization through unloading in the closed pack position.
- Provide advice on TMJ joint protection:
  1. Open jaw within painless range.
  2. Avoid taking big bites of food and choose soft foods, when possible.
  3. Avoid clenching and grinding teeth.
- Prescribe exercise regimens, which may include:
  1. Passive range of motion (ROM) within client's pain-free range
  2. Active-assistive stretching exercises with gentle intermittent pressure
  3. Self-stretch home program
  4. Combined stretch and vapocoolant spray treatment
  5. Resistive exercises, usually for 10 repetitions, 5 times a day
  6. Isometric resisted jaw opening against fist

For displacements and dislocation with reduction:

- Consider fitting client with anterior repositioning appliance, which is worn continuously for several months as dictated by the extent of the damage.

For dislocation without reduction:

- Consider manipulation to reduce dislocation.
- Successful reduction is facilitated by relaxation of superior lateral pterygoid muscle, extreme forward condylar position, and increased disk space.
- Self-manipulation may be performed by moving the mandible in a side-to-side motion.
- Use modalities for pain as indicated such as ultrasound, phonophoresis, high-voltage pulsed current, and moist heat.

For arthritis:

- Consider use of appliance.
- Modalities for pain include moist heat and ultrasound.
- Use gentle active exercise for mandibular ROM.

PRECAUTIONS/CONTRAINDICATIONS

- Anterior displacement of disk that does not self-reduce is usually an indication for surgery.

DESIRED OUTCOME/PROGNOSIS

- The client will obtain optimal joint position to promote healing.
- The client will experience a reduction in symptoms.
- The client will have unrestricted mandibular function.

Note: The client may be a candidate for surgery if conservative treatment fails.

Post surgery:

- The client will experience a normalization of ROM.
- The client will experience the elimination of pain.
- The client will experience a reduction in inflammation.
- The client will have unrestricted mandibular function.

Notes: The majority of evidence is clinical without well-controlled studies. One study reports greater ROM with patients who receive physical therapy postoperatively.

REFERENCES

Assessment

American Physical Therapy Association. Guide to physical therapist practice. 2nd ed. *Phys Ther*. 2001;81.

Buschbacher RM, ed. *Musculoskeletal Disorders: A Practical Guide for Diagnosis and Rehabilitation*. Boston, Mass: Andover Medical Publishers; 1994.

Carmeli E, Sheklow SL, Bloomenfeld I. Comparative study of repositioning splint therapy and passive manual range of motion techniques for anterior displaced temporomandibular discs with unstable excursive reduction. *Physiotherapy*. 2001;87:26–36.

Conti PC, de Azevedo LR, de Souza NV. Pain measurement in TMD patients: evaluation of precision and sensitivity of different scales. *J Oral Rehabil*. 2001;28:534–539.

Daniels L, Worthingham C. *Muscle Testing Techniques of Manual Examination*. 6th ed. Philadelphia, Pa: WB Saunders Co; 1995.

Hall CM, Brody TB. *Therapeutic Exercise: Moving Toward Function*. Philadelphia, Pa: Lippincott Williams and Wilkins; 1999.

Hertling D, Kessler RM. *Management of Common Musculoskeletal Disorders*. 3rd ed. Philadelphia, Pa: JB Lippincott Co; 1996:78, 534.

Kasman GS, Ram JR, Wolf SI. *Clinical Applications in Surface Electromyography: Chronic Musculoskeletal Pain*. Bethesda, Md: Aspen Publishers; 1998.

Kisner C, Colby LA. *Therapeutic Exercise: Foundations and Techniques*. 3rd ed. Philadelphia, Pa: FA Davis Co; 1996:241–270.

Lesh SG. *Clinical Orthopedics for the Physical Therapist Assistant*. Philadelphia, Pa: FA Davis Co; 2000.

Myers RS, ed. *Saunders Manual of Physical Therapy Practice*. Philadelphia, Pa: WB Saunders Co; 1995.

Rothstein JM, Roy SH, Wolf SL. *The Rehabilitation Specialist's Handbook*. 2nd ed. Philadelphia, Pa: FA Davis Co; 1998.

Saidoff DC, McDonough AL. *Critical Pathways in Therapeutic Intervention*. Philadelphia, Pa: CV Mosby Co; 2002.

Schunk C, Reed K. *Clinical Practice Guidelines*. Gaithersburg, Md: Aspen Publishers; 2000.

Tomberlin JP, Saunders HD. *Evaluation, Treatment and Prevention of Musculoskeletal Disorders. Vol 2: Extremities*. Chaska, Minn: The Saunders Group; 1994.

Treatment

Au AR, Kineberg JJ. Isokinetic exercise management of temporomandibular joint clicking in young adults. *J Prosthet Dent*. 1993;70:33–38.

Austin BD, Shupe SM. The role of physical therapy in recovery after temporomandibular joint surgery. *J Oral Maxillofac Surg*. 1993;51:495–498.

Bertolucci LE. Physical therapy post-arthroscopic TMJ management [update]. *Cranio*. 1992; 10:130–137.

Bertolucci LE. Postoperative physical therapy in temporomandibular joint arthroplasty. *Cranio*. 1992;10:211–220.

Bourbon B. Craniomandibular examination and treatment. In: Myers RS, ed. *Saunders Manual of Physical Therapy Practice*. Philadelphia, Pa: WB Saunders Co; 1995:669–718.

Bradley JA. Acupuncture, acupressure, and trigger point therapy. In: Peat M, ed. *Current Physical Therapy*. Toronto: BC Decker; 1998:228–234.

Carmeli E, Shewlow SL, Bloomenfeld I. Comparative study of repositioning splint therapy and passive manual range of motion techniques for anterior displaced temporomandibular discs with unstable excursive reduction. *Physiotherapy*. 2001;87:26–36.

Casares G, Benito C, de la Hoz C. Treatment of TMJ static disk with arthroscopic lysis and lavage: a comparison between MRI arthroscopic findings and clinical results. *Cranio*. 1999;17:49–57.

Goodman C, Snyder TE. *Differential Diagnosis in Physical Therapy*. 2nd ed. Philadelphia, Pa: WB Saunders Co; 2000.

Grabois M, Garrison SJ, Hart KA, Lehmkuhl LD. *Physical Medicine and Rehabilitation: The Complete Approach*. Malden, Mass: Blackwell Science; 2000.

Gray RJ, Davies SJ. Occlusal splints and temporomandibular disorders: why, when, how? *Dent Update*. 2001;28:194–199.

Gray RJM, Quayle AA, Hall CA, et al. Physiotherapy in the treatment of temporomandibular joint disorders: a comparative study of four treatment methods. *Br Dent J*. 1994;176: 250–261.

Hansson T, Minor CAC, Taylor DLW. *Physical Therapy in Craniomandibular Disorders*. Chicago, Ill: Quintessence Publishing Co; 1992.

Hartley A. Temporomandibular assessment. In: Hartley A, ed. *Practical Joint Assessment: Upper Quadrant*. 2nd ed. St. Louis, Mo: CV Mosby Co;1995:1–41.

Hertling D. The temporomandibular joint. In: Herling D, Kessler RM, eds. *Management of Common Musculoskeletal Disorders*. 3rd ed. Philadelphia, Pa: JB Lippincott Co; 1996:411–447.

Kraus SL, ed. *TMJ Disorders: Management of Craniomandibular Complex*. 2nd ed. New York, NY: Churchill Livingstone; 1994.

Kronn E. The incidence of TMJ dysfunction in patients who have suffered a cervical whiplash injury following a traffic accident. *J Orofacial Pain*. 1993;7:209–213.

Kropmans TJ, Dijkstra PU, Stegenga B, et al. Therapeutic outcome assessment in permanent temporomandibular joint disc displacement. *J Oral Rehabil*. 1999;26:357–363.

Magee DJ. Temporomandibular joints. In: Magee DJ, et. *Orthop Phys Assess*. 2nd ed. Philadelphia, Pa: WB Saunders; 1992:71–89.

Mannheimer J. Physical therapy modalities and procedures. In: Pertes RA, Gross SG, eds. *Clin Manage Temporomandibular Disord Orofacial Pain*. Chicago, Ill: Quintessence Publishing; 1995:227–244.

Miller VJ, Zeltser R, Yoeli Z, et al. Ehlers-Danlos syndrome, fibromyalgia and temporomandibular disorder. *Cranio*. 1997;15:267–269.

Miyamoto H, Sakashita H, Miyata M, et al. *Aust Dent J*. 1998;43:301–304.

Myers S. (Appendix E). In: Myers RS, ed. *Saunders Manual of Physical Therapy Practice*. Philadelphia, Pa: WB Saunders Co; 1995:1331–1345.

Norkin CC, Lavangie PK. The temporomandibular joint. In: Norkin CC, Levangie PK, eds. *Joint Structure and Function: A Comprehensive Analysis*. 2nd ed. Philadelphia, Pa: FA Davis Co; 1992:193–206.

Palmieri C, Ellis E, Throckmorton G. *J Oral Maxillofac Surg*. 1999;57:764–775.

Suvinen TI, Hanes KR, Reade PC. Outcome of therapy in the conservative management of temporomandibular pain dysfunction disorder. *J Oral Rehabil*. 1997;24:718–724.

Waide FL, Bade DM, Lovasko J, Montana J. Clinical management of a patient following temporomandibular joint arthroscopy. *Phys Ther*. 1992;72:355–364.

Waide FL, Montana J, Bade DM, et al. Tolerance of ultrasound over the temporomandibular joint. *J Orthop Sports Phys Ther*. 1992;15:206–215.

Wang K. A report of 22 cases of temporomandibular joint dysfunction syndrome treated with acupuncture and laser radiation. *J Tradit Chin Med*. 1992;12:116–118.

Wilk BR, Stenback JT, McCain JP. Postarthroscopy physical therapy management of a patient with temporomandibular joint dysfunction. *J Orthop Sports Phys Ther*. 1993;18:473–478.

Yuasa H, Kurita K. Randomized clinical trial of primary treatment for temporomandibular joint disk displacement without reduction and without osseous changes: a combination of NSAIDs and mouth-opening exercise versus no treatment. *Oral Surg Oral Med Oral Pathol Oral Radiol and Endodontics*. 2001;91:671–675.

Trochanteric Bursitis

DESCRIPTION

Acute or chronic inflammation of the trochanteric bursa. Trochanteric bursitis is the most common bursitis in the hip area. This type of bursitis is seen often in dancers, gymnasts, and runners; those who use repetitive motion of hip flexion with external rotation. The condition is more common in women than men.

CAUSE

Unknown etiology. Trochanteric bursitis may be caused by trauma, chronic overuse, inflammatory arthritis, or acute or chronic infection. Onset is usually insidious but may be linked to a fall on the lateral hip or feeling a "snap" in the lateral hip. Factors influencing tendency toward condition include the following: iliotibial band tightness, muscular imbalance, postural imbalance, leg-length difference, and improper athletic footwear or running surface.

ASSESSMENT

Note: See APTA's Guide to Physical Therapist Practice. 2nd ed. *Physical Therapy.* 2001;81.

Musculoskeletal Preferred Practice Patterns: D, E, F, J

AREAS

- History
- Pain
- Posture
- Joint integrity and structural deviations
- Gait
- Mobility: active and passive range of motion
- (ROM) and accessory motion
- Strength
- Neurological
- Skin and soft tissue
- Functional level

INSTRUMENTS/PROCEDURES

See References for sources.

Joint Integrity and Structural Deviations

The following orthopedic tests for the lower extremity may be performed:

- Craig's test
- Ely test
- FABER test
- hamstring tightness
- leg-length measurements
- Ober's test
- Noble's compression test
- piriformis test
- Thomas' test
- torque test
- Trendelenburg's sign
- quadrant test

Mobility
- goniometry
- hip flexibility

Posture
- clinical measurement of postural control

Special Tests to Which the Physical Therapist May or May Not Have Access
- electromyographic (EMG) analysis of hip abductor musculature

Strength
- maximal isometric hip abductor muscles torques
- manual muscle testing

PROBLEMS

- The client often reports tenderness over area of lateral thigh and posterolateral trochanter. The area often has an increase in temperature.
- The client may have pain radiating to lumbosacral region on the same side.
- The client often has pain with sitting and weight-bearing activities, especially climbing the stairs.

- The client may be unable to tolerate side-lying position, so sleep is diminished.
- Often, pain is described as "deep" as opposed to "sharp."
- The client may have pain with adduction.
- Hip abduction with resistance is typically painful.

TREATMENT/MANAGEMENT

- Use modalities, such as ice, ultrasound, phonophoresis, and iontophoresis, if indicated.
- Avoid aggravating activities.
- Discuss sleep posture adaptations with pillows.
- Assess for muscular imbalance and stretch and strengthen accordingly (ie, iliotibial band tightness).

PRECAUTIONS/CONTRAINDICATIONS

- The pain pattern for trochanteric bursitis is very similar to that for an L-5 lesion.

DESIRED OUTCOME/PROGNOSIS

- The inflammation and pain will decrease, and recurrence will be prevented.
- Ultrasound may offer quite effective relief in 3 to 6 sessions. The key component of treatment is identifying the predisposing cause of injury.

Note: Chronic conditions may need surgical treatment.

REFERENCES

Assessment

American Physical Therapy Association. Guide to physical therapist practice. 2nd ed. *Phys Ther.* 2001;81.

Buschbacher RM, ed. *Musculoskeletal Disorders: A Practical Guide for Diagnosis and Rehabilitation.* Boston, Mass: Andover Medical Publishers; 1994.

Daniels L, Worthingham C. *Muscle Testing Techniques of Manual Examination.* 6th ed. Philadelphia, Pa: WB Saunders Co; 1995.

Hall CM, Brody TB. *Therapeutic Exercise: Moving Toward Function.* Philadelphia, Pa: Lippincott Williams and Wilkins; 1999.

Hertling D, Kessler RM. *Management of Common Musculoskeletal Disorders.* 3rd ed. Philadelphia, Pa: JB Lippincott Co; 1996:78, 534.

Kasman GS, Ram JR, Wolf Sl. *Clinical Applications in Surface Electromyography: Chronic Musculoskeletal Pain.* Bethesda, Md: Aspen Publishers; 1998.

Kisner C, Colby LA. *Therapeutic Exercise: Foundations and Techniques.* 3rd ed. Philadelphia, Pa: FA Davis Co; 1996:241–270.

Lesh SG. *Clinical Orthopedics for the Physical Therapist Assistant.* Philadelphia, Pa: FA Davis Co; 2000.

Myers RS, ed. *Saunders Manual of Physical Therapy Practice.* Philadelphia, Pa: WB Saunders Co; 1995.

Rothstein JM, Roy SH, Wolf SL. *The Rehabilitation Specialist's Handbook.* 2nd ed. Philadelphia, Pa: FA Davis Co; 1998.

Saidoff DC, McDonough AL. *Critical Pathways in Therapeutic Intervention.* Philadelphia, Pa: CV Mosby Co; 2002.

Schunk C, Reed K. *Clinical Practice Guidelines.* Gaithersburg, Md: Aspen Publishers; 2000.

Tomberlin JP, Saunders HD. *Evaluation, Treatment and Prevention of Musculoskeletal Disorders. Vol 2: Extremities.* Chaska, Minn: The Saunders Group; 1994.

Treatment

Hertling D, Kessler RM. *Management of Common Musculoskeletal Disorders.* 3rd ed. Philadelphia, Pa: JB Lippincott Co; 1996:272–297.

Hicklin SP, DePretis MC. Lower extremity: hip. In: Myers RS, ed. *Saunders Manual of Physical Therapy Practice.* Philadelphia, Pa: WB Saunders Co; 1995:975–976.

Jones DL, Erhard RE. Diagnosis of trochanteric bursitis versus femoral neck stress fracture. *Phys Ther.* 1997;77:58–67.

Kisner C, Colby LA. *Therapeutic Exercise: Foundations and Techniques.* 3rd ed. Philadelphia, Pa: FA Davis Co; 1996:317–344.

Kornberg C, McCarthy T. The effect of neural stretching technique on sympathetic outflow to the lower limbs. *J Orthop Sports Phys Ther.* 1992;16:269–274.

Tomberlin JP, Saunders HD. *Evaluation, Treatment and Prevention of Musculoskeletal Disorders. Vol 2: Extremities.* Chaska, Minn: The Saunders Group; 1994.

Chapter 9

Conditions in Back Pain

Note: See also Chapter 3, Connective Tissue Conditions, and Chapter 15, Women's Health Disorders.

Cervical Dysfunction/Thoracic Dysfunction

DESCRIPTION

Cervical dysfunction can lead to local, distant, or referred pain. It may include paresthesias, muscle weakness, and reflex or sensory loss.

Thoracic dysfunction is also known as *thoracic postural stabilizing syndrome*. Complaints vary by region but may include aching across the supraspinous fossa or along the spine of the scapula to the superior posterior border of the shoulder and posterolateral upper arm region. The client may feel anterior chest discomfort that may be confused with cardiac involvement and may have unilateral or bilateral low back pain with accompanying radiating pain. The T-7 level may refer pain into the mid- and upper abdominal area.

CAUSE

Cervical dysfunction may be caused by a pathologic process or a combination of abnormalities. Trauma, such as a motor vehicle accident, can also lead to cervical dysfunction. *Thoracic dysfunction* may be caused by hypomobility at the thoracic level or levels.

ASSESSMENT

CERVICAL DISC PATHOLOGY

Note: See APTA's Guide to Physical Therapist Practice. 2nd ed. *Physical Therapy.* 2001;81.

Musculoskeletal Preferred Practice Patterns: A, B, F, G, H, J

Neuromuscular Preferred Practice Pattern: F

CERVICAL STENOSIS

Note: See APTA's Guide to Physical Therapist Practice. 2nd ed. *Physical Therapy.* 2001;81.

Musculoskeletal Preferred Practice Pattern: G

CERVICAL/THORACIC GENERAL PAIN

Note: See APTA's Guide to Physical Therapist Practice. 2nd ed. *Physical Therapy.* 2001;81.

Cardiopulmonary Prefered Practice Pattern: B

Musculoskeletal Preferred Practice Patterns: B, C, D, E, F, G, H, I, J

Neuromuscular Preferred Practice Pattern: F

AREAS

- History, including nature of symptoms
- Posture, including resting posture
- Pain, including reproduction of symptoms
- Cervical spine: vertebral position
- Skin and soft tissues and associated structures such as peripheral joints, viscera, and paravertebral muscles
- Joint integrity and structural deviations
- Mobility: active cervical range of motion (ROM), combined movements, and repeated movements
- Strength

- Neurological: especially indicated if client has referred pain, weakness, paresthesia, signs of upper motor neuron lesion; include reflexes, sensation, Babinski's sign, and check for clonus
- Functional level

INSTRUMENTS/PROCEDURES

See References for sources.

Cervical Spine
- palpation examination of vertebral position
- mechanical diagnosis

Functional Level
- Neck Disability Index

Joint Integrity/Structural Deviations and Neurological Involvement

The following neurological and orthopedic tests of the cervical and thoracic region may be performed:

- adverse mechanical tension of the nervous system assessment
- brachial plexus tension test
- carpal tunnel test
- distraction test
- dizziness tests
- foraminal compression test
- ischemic vertigo
- Lhermitte's sign
- passive accessory intervertebral movement tests (PAIVMs)
- passive physiologic intervertebral movement tests (PPIVMs)
- scalenus anticus and thoracic outlet syndrome tests
- shoulder abduction test
- shoulder depression test
- slump test
- Spurling test
- upper limb tension test
- Valsalva test
- vertebral artery test

Mobility
1. craniovertebral hypermobility syndrome testing
2. ROM testing
   - tape measure
   - Myrin gravity reference goniometer

Pain
- visual analog scale

Posture
- cervical ROM device
- pendulum goniometer
- triaxial electrogoniometer

Skin and Soft Tissues
- palpation for temperature, tone, and tenderness

PROBLEMS

CERVICAL DYSFUNCTION

Acute Disk Bulge
- The client often has a sudden onset of severe pain in the neck. The problem may progress to muscle spasm.
- The client may be unable to rotate the neck unilaterally.
- The client often has limitation of rotation and flexion to one side but more movement to opposite side.

Cervical Degenerative Changes
- The client may have decreased motion in the neck.
- The client may have pain into the shoulders and arms.
- The client may have pain bilaterally; typically one side is more involved.
- The client may describe the pain as worse in the morning and again in the evening.
- There is often extreme restriction of motion into extension. The restriction is less with side bending, rotation, and flexion.
- The client may have pain at extremes of joint ROM.

Cervical Nerve Root Impingement
- The client often has unilateral pain in the neck, scapula, or arm.
- The client often has paresthesia into the fingers.
- The client may have sharp or aching arm pain.
- Often, the pain is intense and worse with weight bearing.

Localized Cervical Joint Restriction in Facet Joint (Zygapophyseal Joint)
- The client may have aching in the scapula, usually unilateral.
- The pain is typically worse at the end of the day.
- The pain is often worse with sustained muscular tension.
- The client often has pain with extremes of joint ROM in rotation and side bending.
- The client may have pain on extension.

THORACIC DYSFUNCTION
- The client often has a gradual onset of symptoms.
- The client may report symptoms after being in a prolonged stooped position with repetitive upper extremity work.
- The client may complain of central discomfort and tightness or a dull ache into the anterior lower thoracic rib cage.

T-4 Syndrome
- The client may have a feeling of tightness in the posterior mid-thoracic area.
- The client often has a dull pain with aching and discomfort and may have paresthesia in the arm.
- The client may also have posterior neck discomfort accompanied by a dull headache.

TREATMENT/MANAGEMENT

CERVICAL DYSFUNCTION

Disk Bulge

In acute cases:
- Often the position of comfort is a combined movement of extension and lateral flexion to the opposite side.
- Traction may make the condition more comfortable.
- To increase ROM and decrease pain, try a position of tolerable extension and manual traction. Begin ROM while applying traction to the symptom-free side.
- After achieving full ROM on the symptom-free side, begin on the painful side.
- Soft cervical support may be useful for a few days.
- After acute symptoms recede, more advanced therapy may be undertaken.

In subacute cases:
- Apply gentle manual traction, use a soft collar temporarily, and avoid flexion if painful.
- Use gentle mobilization techniques as tolerated.

- Moist warmth may be helpful.
- Correct muscle imbalance and any forward head posture.
- Teach self-treatment techniques.

Cervical Degenerative Changes
- Try positional traction.
- Provide activities of daily living (ADLs) instruction on how to avoid unwanted mechanical stress.
- Consider mobilization of adjacent segments.
- Relaxation exercises may reduce tension.
- Use external support collar if symptoms are acute.
- Strengthen muscle, beginning with isometric exercise in the pain-free range.

Cervical Nerve Root Impingement
- Traction may be used as tolerated.
- Consider passive mobilization.
- Consider McKenzie mechanical treatment and self-treatment if pain falls into one of the following categories: posture syndrome, dysfunction, or derangement.

Localized Cervical Joint Restriction in Facet Joint (Zygapophyseal Joint)
- Use manual traction with slow oscillation as a reciprocal relaxation technique.
- Mechanical traction may also be indicated.
- Spinal mobilization and manipulation are treatment options. Use gentle unilateral oscillatory pressure over appropriate zygapophyseal joints. Bilateral treatment may be necessary. Progress to firm pressure as tolerated.
- If no contraindications exist, use transverse thrust manipulation to open locked joint.
- Use unilateral oscillatory pressures for appropriate joint and consider use of ultrasound.
- Provide soft collar as needed.
- Instruct client in self-mobilization, strength, and coordination training if there is recurrent locking of the zygapophyseal joints.

THORACIC DYSFUNCTION
- Mobilize or manipulate appropriate hypomobile segments. Treat adjacent structures.

T-4 Syndrome
- Perform direct palpation of spinous processes at T-3 to T-6 level, using gentle oscillatory pressures and progressing to more forceful techniques as indicated.

PRECAUTIONS/CONTRAINDICATIONS

CERVICAL DYSFUNCTION
- Structural integrity must be known before treating the cervicothoracic spine.
- Any anatomical variation on normal can contraindicate therapy, especially passive movement.
- Prior to initiating mechanical treatment, upper cervical ligament integrity should be tested.
- Nerve root pain or musculoskeletal pain in the neck can actually be peripheral entrapment of the brachial plexus at the thoracic outlet.
- Vertebral arteries should be tested individually prior to using traction or mobilization techniques on the upper cervical spine. See the orthopedic tests listed in "Instruments" preceding.

- With existing degenerative joint disease, extension and extension with rotation can lead to further narrowing of the foramina and spinal canal and should be avoided.
- If neurological symptoms are present, the client should be reassessed frequently, perhaps at each treatment session.

THORACIC DYSFUNCTION

- Because these symptoms are often vague and nonspecific and because their on-set cannot be reproduced by movement, a potential visceral source of symptoms must be ruled out.

DESIRED OUTCOME/PROGNOSIS

CERVICAL DYSFUNCTION

- The client will have pain-free full cervical ROM.
- The client will have normal strength.
- The client will have normal cervical function.
- An acute disk bulge may sometimes resolve spontaneously in a few days.

THORACIC DYSFUNCTION

- The client will experience a reduction in symptoms.
- The client will have normal strength.
- The client will have normal thoracic function.

REFERENCES

Assessment

American Physical Therapy Association. Guide to physical therapist practice. 2nd ed. *Phys Ther.* 2001;81.

Buschbacher RM, ed. *Musculoskeletal Disorders: A Practical Guide for Diagnosis and Reha-bilitation.* Boston, Mass: Andover Medical Publishers; 1994.

Chok B, Gomez E. The reliability and application of the Neck Disability Index in physio-therapy. *Physiotherapy Singapore.* 2000;3:16–19.

Daniels L, Worthingham C. *Muscle Testing Techniques of Manual Examination.* 6th ed. Philadelphia, Pa: WB Saunders Co; 1995.

Delitto A, Synder-Mackler L. The diagnostic process: examples in orthopedic physical ther-apy. *Phys Ther.* 1995;75:203–210.

Edwards BC. *Manual of Combined Movements: Their Use in the Examination and Treatment of Mechanical Vertebral Column Disorders.* New York, NY: Churchill Livingstone; 1992.

Gogia P, Sabbahi M. Electromyographic analysis of neck muscle fatigue in patients with os-teoarthritis of the cervical spine. *Spine.* 1994;19:502–506.

Goodman C, Snyder TE. *Differential Diagnosis in Physical Therapy.* 2nd ed. Philadelphia, PA; WB Saunders Co; 2000.

Griegel-Morris P, Larson K, Mueller-Klaus K, Oatis CA. The incidence of common postural abnormalities in the cervical, shoulder, and thoracic regions and their association with pain in two age groups of healthy subjects. *Phys Ther.* 1992;72:425–431.

Hall CM, Brody TB. *Therapeutic Exercise: Moving Toward Function.* Philadelphia, Pa: Lippin-cott Williams and Wilkins; 1999.

Hertling D, Kessler RM. *Management of Common Musculoskeletal Disorders: Physical Therapy Principles and Methods.* 3rd ed. Philadelphia, Pa: JB Lippincott Co; 1996.

Highland T, et al. Changes in isometric strength and range of motion of the isolated cervical spine after eight weeks of clinical rehabilitation. *Spine.* 1992;17:S77–S82.

Jacobs K. *Ergonomics for Therapists.* 2nd ed. Boston, Mass: Butterworth Heinemann; 2000.

Kasman GS, Ram JR, Wolf SL. *Clinical Applications in Surface Electromyography: Chronic Musculoskeletal Pain.* Bethesda, Md: Aspen Publishers; 1998.

Kendall FP, McCreary EK, Provance PG. *Muscles: Testing and Function.* 4th ed. Baltimore, Md: Williams and Wilkins; 1993.

Kisner C, Colby LA. *Therapeutic Exercise: Foundations and Techniques.* 3rd ed. Philadelphia, Pa: FA Davis Co; 1996.

Lesh SG. *Clinical Orthopedics for the Physical Therapist Assistant.* Philadelphia, Pa: FA Davis Co; 2000.

Malone TR, McPoil T, Nitz AJ, eds. *Orthopaedic and Sports Physical Therapy.* 3rd ed. St. Louis, Mo: CV Mosby Co; 1997.

Myers RS, ed. *Saunders Manual of Physical Therapy Practice.* Philadelphia, Pa: WB Saunders Co; 1995.

Richardson J, Iglarsh ZA. *Clincial Orthopaedic Physical Therapy.* Philadelphia, Pa: WB Saunders Co; 1994.

Rheault W, Albright B, Byers C, et al. Intertester reliability of the cervical range of motion device. *J Orthop Sports Phys Ther.* 1992;15:147–150.

Riddle DL, Stratford PW. Use of generic versus region-specific functional status measures on patients with cervical spine disorders. *Phys Ther.* 1998;78:951–963.

Rothstein JM, Roy SH, Wolf SL. *The Rehabilitation Specialist's Handbook.* 2nd ed. Philadelphia, Pa: FA Davis Co; 1998.

Sandmark H, Nisell R. Validity of five common manual neck pain provoking tests. *Scand J Rehabil Med.* 1995;27:131–136.

Schunk C, Reed K. *Clinical Practice Guidelines.* Gaithersburg, Md: Aspen Publishers; 2000.

Tomberlin JP, Saunders HD. *Evaluation, Treatment and Prevention of Musculoskeletal Disorders. Vol 2: Extremities.* Chaska, Minn: The Saunders Group; 1994.

Westaway MD, Stratford PW, Binkley JM. The patient-specific functional scale: validation of its use in persons with neck dysfunction. *J Sports Phys Ther.* 1998;27:331–338.

Winkel D. *Diagnosis and Treatment of the Spine.* Gaithersburg, Md: Aspen Publishers; 1996.

Youdas JW, Garrett TR, Suman VJ, et al. Normal range of motion of the cervical spine: an initial goniometric study. *Phys Ther.* 1992;72:770–780.

Treatment

CERVICAL

Anderson M, Stevens B, Richards J, Jensen G. Cervical spine. In: Myers RS, ed. *Saunders Manual of Physical Therapy Practice.* Philadelphia, Pa: WB Saunders Co; 1995:727–787.

Axen K, Haas R, Schicchi J, Merrick J. Progressive resistance neck exercises using a compressible ball coupled with an air pressure gauge. *J Orthop Sports Phys Ther.* 1992; 16:275–280.

Curillo JA. Aquatic physical therapy approaches for the spine. *Orthop Phys Ther Clin North Am.* 1994;3:179–208.

Edgar D, et al. The relationship between upper trapezius muscle length and upper quadrant neural tissue extensibility. *Aust Physiotherapy J.* 1994;40:99–103.

Edwards BC. *Manual of Combined Movements: Their Use in the Examination and Treatment of Mechanical Vertebral Column Disorders.* New York, NY: Churchill Livingstone; 1992.

Goodman R, Frew L. Effectiveness of progressive strength resistance training for whiplash: a pilot study. *Physiotherapy Can.* 2000;52:211–214.

Grabois M, Garrison SJ, Hart KA, Lehmkuhl LD. *Physical Medicine and Rehabilitation: The Complete Approach.* Malden, Mass: Blackwell Science; 2000.

Grant R, ed. *Physical Therapy of the Cervical and Thoracic Spine.* 2nd ed. New York, NY: Churchill Livingstone; 1994.

Griegel-Morris P, Larson K, Mueller-Klaus K, Oatis CA. Incidence of common postural abnormalities in the cervical, shoulder, and thoracic regions and their association with pain in two age groups of healthy subjects. *Phys Ther.* 1992;72:425–431.

Gross AR, Aker PD, Quartly C. Manual therapy in the treatment of neck pain. *Rheumatol Dis Clin North Am.* 1996;22:579–598.

Hardin J Jr. Pain and the cervical spine. *Bull Rheum Dis.* 2001;50:1–4.

Hertling D, Kessler RM. *Management of Common Musculoskeletal Disorders: Physical Therapy Principles and Methods.* 3rd ed. Philadelphia, Pa: JB Lippincott Co; 1996.

Higbie EJ. Cervical pain and dysfunction. *Phys Ther Case Rep.* 2000;3:233–236.

Jordan A, Bendix T, Nielsen H, et al. Intensive training, physiotherapy, or manipulation for patients with chronic neck pain: a prospective, single-blinded, randomized clinical trial. *Spine.* 1998;23:311–318.

Koes BW, Bouter LM, van Mameren H, et al. A randomized clinical trial of manual therapy and physiotherapy for persistent back and neck complaints: subgroup analysis and relationship between outcome measures. *J Manipulative Physiol Ther.* 1993;16:211–219.

Levoska S, Keinanen-Kiukaaniemi S. Active or passive physiotherapy for occupational cervicobrachial disorders? A comparison of two treatment methods with a 1-year follow-up. *Arch Phys Med Rehabil.* 1993;74:425–430.

Magee DJ, Oborn-Barrett E, Turner S, et al. A systematic overview of the effectiveness of physical therapy intervention on soft tissue neck injury following trauma. *Physiotherapy Can.* 2000;52:111–130.

Mallone T, McPoil T, Nitz A. *Orthopedic and Sports Physical Therapy.* 3rd ed. St. Louis, Mo: Mosby Year Book; 1997.

Pearson N, Walmsley R. Trial into the effects of repeated neck retractions in normal subjects. *Spine.* 1995;20:1245–1251.

Pollack M, et al. Frequency and volume of resistance training: effect on cervical extension strength. *Arch Phys Med Rehabil.* 1993;74:1080–1086.

Richardson J, Iglarsh ZA. *Clincial Orthopaedic Physical Therapy.* Philadelphia, Pa: WB Saunders Co; 1994.

Ruth S, Kergerreis S. Facilitating cervical flexion using a Feldenkrais method: awareness through movement. *J Orthop Sports Phys Ther.* 1992;16:25–29.

Stump J, et al. A comparison of two modes of cervical exercise in adolescent male athletes. *J Manipulative Physiol Ther.* 1993;16:155–160.

Tan JC, Nordin M. Role of physical therapy in the treatment of cervical disk disease. *Orthop Clin North Am.* 1992;23:435–449.

Tasker T. Cervical headache. *Phys Ther Case Rep.* 2000;3:196–209.

Taylor J, Twomey L. Acute injuries to the cervical joints. *Spine.* 1993;18:1115–1122.

Treleavan J, et al. Cervical musculoskeletal dysfunction in post-concussional headache. *Cephalgia.* 1994;14:273–279.

Twomey LT, Taylor JR. The whiplash syndrome: pathology and physical treatment. *J Manual Manipulative Ther*. 1993;1:1:26–29.

Wallis BJ, Lord SM, Barnsley L, et al. Pain and psychological symptoms of Australian patients with whiplash. *Spine*. 1996;21:804.

THORACIC

Edmondston SJ, Singer KP. Thoracic spine: anatomical and biomechanicl considerations for manual therapy. *Manual Ther*. 1997;2:132–143.

Flynn TW. *The Thoracic Spine and Rib Cage: Musculoskeletal Evaluation and Treatment*. Boston, Mass: Butterworth Heinemann; 1996.

Grant R, ed. *Physical Therapy of the Cervical and Thoracic Spine*. 2nd ed. New York, NY: Churchill Livingstone; 1994.

Lee DG. Biomechanics of the thorax: a clinical model of in vivo function. *J Manual Manipulative Ther*. 1993;1:13.

Lee DG. *Manual Therapy for the Thorax—A Biomechanical Approach*. Delta, British Columbia, Canada: DOPC; 1994.

Lee DG. Biomechanics of the thorax. In: Grant R, ed. *Physical Therapy of the Cervical and Thoracic Spine*. New York, NY: Churchill Livingstone; 1994.

Low Back Pain

DESCRIPTION

Pain experienced in the lower lumbar, lumbosacral, or sacroiliac region of the back. Pain can also be accompanied by sciatica.

CAUSE

There are multiple causes of back pain. These can include (1) acute ligamentous sprain; (2) acute muscular strain or tear of paraspinous muscle; (3) chronic muscular strain secondary to faulty posture, poor conditioning, or mechanical factors such as pregnancy, obesity, or excessive use; (4) chronic fibromyalgia; (5) chronic osteoarthritis; (6) chronic ankylosing spondylosis; (7) congenital defects of the low lumbar and upper sacral spine; (8) ruptured or protruding intervertebral disk; (9) traumatic ligament rupture; (10) stress fracture of the pars interarticularis; (11) fracture, infection, or tumor involving the back, pelvis, or retroperitoneum; (12) spondylolisthesis with loss of substance in the pars interarticularis bilaterally and resultant forward slippage of one vertebra on another; (13) spinal stenosis with narrowing of spinal canal; (14) osteitis condensans ilii; and (15) visceral disease causing referred pain.

Risk factors that are strongly associated with low back pain include age, emotional distress, prior history of low back pain, job satisfaction, heavy or repetitive lifting, prolonged sitting or standing. Factors moderately associated include height, obesity, physical fitness, smoking, and vibration.

ASSESSMENT

GENERAL LOW BACK PAIN

Note: See APTA's Guide to Physical Therapist Practice. 2nd ed. *Physical Therapy*. 2001;81.

Cardiopulmonary Preferred Practice Pattern: B

Musculoskeletal Preferred Practice Patterns: D, C, D, E, F, G, H, I, J

Neuromuscular Preferred Practice Pattern: F

LUMBAR DISK PATHOLOGY

Note: See APTA's Guide to Physical Therapist Practice. 2nd ed. *Physical Therapy.* 2001;81.

Musculoskeletal Preferred Practice Patterns: A, B, E, F, G, J

POSTURAL DYSFUNCTION

Note: See APTA's Guide to Physical Therapist Practice. 2nd ed. *Physical Therapy.* 2001;81.

Musculoskeletal Preferred Practice Patterns: B, C, D, E, F, G, J

SI DYSFUNCTION

Note: See APTA's Guide to Physical Therapist Practice. 2nd ed. *Physical Therapy.* 2001;81.

Integumentary Preferred Practice Pattern: A

Musculoskeletal Preferred Practice Patterns: B, C, E, F, G, J

SPINAL STENOSIS

Note: See APTA's Guide to Physical Therapist Practice. 2nd ed. *Physical Therapy.* 2001;81.

Musculoskeletal Preferred Practice Patterns: F, G, J

SPONDYLOLISTHESIS

Note: See APTA's Guide to Physical Therapist Practice. 2nd ed. *Physical Therapy.* 2001;81.

Musculoskeletal Preferred Practice Patterns: B, G, J

AREAS

- History, including social/ psychological issues
- Pain
- Posture
- Gait
- Mobility, including active and passive range of motion (ROM)
- Joint integrity and structural deviations
- Neurological, including sensation and reflexes
- Strength
- Skin and soft tissue: palpation of trigger points
- Cardiovascular: endurance
- Functional level, including use of assistive devices and activities of daily living (ADLs)
- Health status

INSTRUMENTS/PROCEDURES

See References for sources.

Cardiovascular
- aerobic capacity testing

Evaluations
- algorithms and classification systems
- differential diagnosis

- McKenzie assessment algorithm
- National Institute for Occupational Safety and Health (NIOSH) Low Back Atlas of Standardized Tests and Measurements
- Toronto-Hamilton Lumbar Database (THLD)

Functional Level
- functional status exam

Gait
- visual gait assessment

Health Status
- Sickness Impact Profile
- Roland and Morris Disability Index
- Oswestry Low Back Pain questionnaire
- Waddell and Main Disability Index

Joint Integrity and Structural Deviations
1. low back orthopedic tests
    - bowstring test
    - Brudzinski's test
    - cram test
    - Ely test
    - femoral nerve traction test
    - Hoover sign
    - Kernig sign
    - Naffziger test
    - FABER test
    - popliteal pressure sign
    - prone knee flexion test (or reverse Lasegue test)
    - sitting root test
    - straight-leg-raising test
2. sacroiliac joint tests
    - Gillet test
    - palpation of anterior superior iliac spines (sitting, standing)
    - palpation of iliac crests (sitting, standing)
    - palpation of posterior superior iliac spines (sitting, standing)
    - prone knee flexion test
    - side-lying iliac compression test
    - sitting flexion test
    - standing flexion test
    - standing Gillet test
    - supine iliac gapping test
    - supine long sitting test

Mobility
- fingertip-to-floor measurements
- flexicurves
- goniometric measurement
- inclinometer
- double inclinometer
- Leighton flexometer
- modified fingertip-to-floor method
- optical methods
- PRIDE ROM
- radiologic ROM measures
- stiffness measures
- tape measure methods (Schober, modified Schober)
- three-dimensional digitizer

Neurological
- deep-tendon reflexes
- electromyography (EMG)

- motor tests
- sensory (dermatomal) tests

Outcome/Measures
- outcomes on ambulation, activity level, and pain
- outcome predictors

Pain
- Beck Depression Inventory
- Coping Strategy questionnaire
- Dallas Pain questionnaire
- McGill Pain questionnaire
- Modified Pain Rating chart
- pain drawings
- Pain Rating chart
- Oswestry Low Back Pain question-naire
- visual analog scale
- West Haven–Yale Multidimensional Pain Inventory
- Quebec Task Force (classification by pain patterns)

Posture
- photography

Special Tests to Which the Physical Therapist May or May Not Have Access
1. computed-tomography (CT) scan; CT-myelography, CT-discography, myelography, discography, facet arthrography, MRI, nuclear medicine, videofluoroscopy, ultrasound, angiography
2. electromyography (EMG)
3. ergonomics
   a. ergonomics or body mechanics examination
   b. mattress evaluation
   c. functional task performance
      - commercial lift testing units
      - commercial work evaluation systems
      - functional measurement laboratory
      - multiple-tasks obstacle course
      - progressive isoinertial lifeline evaluation (PILE)
      - physiological work performance testing

Strength
1. manual muscle testing
2. modified sphygmomanometer
3. partial sit-up/curl-up protocol
4. pressure biofeedback
5. Sorensen test
6. trunk strength testing
   - lifting dynamometers
   - isokinetic dynamometers
   - commercial trunk strength units

PROBLEMS

ANKYLOSING SPONDYLITIS
- The client often has decreased ROM of lumbar flexion and extension.
- The client often has decreased lumbar lordosis.
- The client may have restricted sacroiliac joint motion.
- The condition may involve stiffening of the entire spine and hips.

CHRONIC BACK PAIN
- The client may have altered muscle recruitment patterns.
- The client may have shortened muscle groups.

- The client may have reduced levels of endorphins.
- The client may have demineralization of spine.

DEGENERATIVE JOINT DISEASE (OSTEOARTHRITIS/SPONDYLOSIS)
- The client often has pain with movement.
- The client often has loss of active and passive mobility.
- The client may be hypermobile instead of hypomobile.

DISK HERNIATION
- The client may have neurological involvement (reflexes, myotome, and/or dermatome).
- The client may have pain and/or paresthesia distal to the knee.
- The client may find that mechanism of onset involves lumbar flexion.
- The client may have pain that is aggravated by sitting.

FACET-JOINT DERANGEMENT-ACUTE
- The client often has sudden onset of pain.
- The client typically has pain aggravated by movement.
- The client often has loss of active and passive motion in specific directions.

FRACTURE
- The client may have pain with active lumbar motion.
- The client may need radiographic confirmation.

HYPOMOBILITY DYSFUNCTION
- The client typically has less than normal accessory motion at one or more levels.
- The client often has less than normal flexion and/or extension ROM.
- The client often has pain and/or stiffness with no paresthesia.
- The client may have restricted passive intervertebral ROM.
- The client may have pain at end of ROM.
- The client often has limitation of movement in one or two directions only.
- The client typically has a reduction in lumbar spine lateral flexion associated with either extension or flexion.
- The client frequently has pain that is localized in the back but may be referred into the leg or abdominal areas.
- There may be no neurological signs.

INFECTION
- The client may have a fever.
- Confirmation with a bone scan is needed.

LIGAMENTOUS SPRAIN-ACUTE
- The client often has a loss of active and passive mobility.
- The client often has localized pain with movement.
- The client may experience distally radiating pain.

LOWER LUMBAR DISK HERNIATION (EXTRUSION)
WITH NERVE ROOT IMPINGEMENT
- The client may have unilateral leg pain, but bilateral pain is possible.
- The client often feels leg pain in the posterolateral thigh and the anterior lateral or posterior aspect of the lower leg.
- The client may have back pain alone; a combination of back and leg pain is less common.
- Frequently, lumbar extension will peripheralize pain. Extremity pain is often worse than back pain.

- The client often has mild segmental neurologic deficit, indicated by the presence of specific dermatome sensory loss or specific motor weakness.
- Rarely, rupture of the nerve root leads to decreased pain but increased neurological signs.

MUSCLE SPASM
- The client often has decreased ROM and pain and tenderness over the muscle.
- The client may have increased tone in muscles.
- The client may find that continued spasm becomes a source of additional pain due to a self-perpetuating cycle.

MUSCLE STRAIN–ACUTE
- The client may have localized swelling.
- The client typically has pain with movement.
- The client often has decreased and painful ROM.
- Frequently, passive movement is within normal limits.
- The client may show painful recovery from movement.
- The client may have unilateral pain.
- The client may have pain radiating distally.

NERVE ROOT ADHESION
- The client often has a minimum of one previous episode of back pain and/or current pain of at least 2 months' duration.
- The client typically finds that flexion and/or flexion with side flexion away from pain aggravates pain and/or paresthesia.
- The client may have reflex and/or motor deficit.

NERVE ROOT IRRITATION
- The client often has lower extremity pain aggravated by one or more lumbar movements.
- The client often has a subjective complaint of paresthesia.
- The client may have lower extremity pain distal to the knee.

POSTEROLATERAL DISK PROLAPSE–ACUTE
- The client may have sudden onset of unilateral lumbosacral pain.
- The client often reports that pain is severe, but pain may be dull and aching or knifelike.
- The client may have aching into the leg, usually unilateral.
- The pain is typically worse with sitting or sudden straining, and it may be hard to stand up.
- The client often has lumbar deformity with loss of lordosis.
- The client routinely has lumbar scoliosis (convexity on the involved side).
- There is often marked, painful restriction of spinal movement with decrease of extension mobility.
- Often the pain increases with repeated flexion and/or sustained flexion.
- Often the mechanism of onset involves flexion.

POSTURAL SYNDROME
- The client often finds that pain eases with activity.
- Typically, a standing or sitting posture is habitually beyond normal limits.
- The client may feel pain only during sustained positions of spine.

PREGNANCY/POSTPARTUM
- The client often has low back pain that worsens with fatigue, with static postures, and as the day progresses.
- The client may be more prone to injury.

- The client often has increased pelvic mobility.
- The client may have a combination of low back pain and dysfunction of the sacroiliac joint.
- The client may have gait dysfunction, pain, and tenderness of the sacroiliac joint.
- The client often has sacroiliac joint pain that is worse with prolonged posture or activity, unilateral weight bearing, or twisting activities.
- The pain may accompany pubic symphysial pain.

REFERRED VISCERAL
- Frequently, lumbar examination is negative and visceral findings are positive.

SACROILIAC JOINT DYSFUNCTION
- The client often complains of pain with sitting.
- The client often has pain when leaning forward.
- The client may have pain with increase in intra-abdominal pressure.
- The client often experiences a sudden onset of unilateral sacroiliac pain.
- The client may feel pain in the posterior thigh.
- The client may have anterior hip pain.
- The client may report paresthesia in the absence of neurological signs.
- There may be ipsilateral sacroiliac dysfunction present with L3–4 or L4–5 lesions.

SACROILIAC HYPOMOBILITY
- The client frequently has pelvic asymmetry.
- The client may have unilateral buttock and/or posterior thigh pain.
- The client may have restricted sacroiliac accessory motion.

SCHEURMANN'S DISEASE
- There may be thoracic kyphosis.
- Accessory motion may be restricted.

SCOLIOSIS
- There is often an observed spinal curve in the coronal plane.
- Scoliosis may be present in standing but alter its configuration on movement.
- There is often postural deviation that includes asymmetry in the shoulders, and the convex side of the curve shows a prominent scapula.
- There is unilateral hip protrusion and pelvic obliquity.
- Lumbar lordosis can be seen to increase with prominent erector spinae musculature on the side of the convexity.
- Diminished flexibility can be seen in spinal, abdominal, intercostal, and hip musculature and spinal ligaments.
- Weakness in musculature can be seen on the convex side of the curve. Abdominals, trunk extensors, and hip muscles may also weaken.

SEGMENTAL HYPERMOBILITY
- The client may report that sustained positions aggravate pain.
- Often accessory motion has a late onset of resistance and/or increased ROM.
- The client may have abnormal segmental spinal muscle activity patterns.
- The client may find that activity eases pain.
- The client may find that extension from a flexed position reproduces pain.
- Passive intervertebral ROM may indicate hypermobility.

SPINAL CONGENITAL ANOMALY

Sacralization of L-5 Transverse Processes, Abnormal Intervertebral Facets
- Radiographic confirmation is needed.

SPINAL STENOSIS

- The client often reports that extension reproduces and aggravates pain and/or paresthesia.
- Typically, flexion relieves pain.
- The client may have bilateral lower extremity pain.
- Often pain in one or both legs is brought on by walking.
- The client may find that pain is associated with weakness and/or paresthesias.
- Symptoms may be vague or diffuse.

SPONDYLOLISTHESIS

- The client may have pain coincidental with the level of radiographic results.
- The client may find that extension positions aggravate pain.
- The client may have a palpable step.

TUMOR

- The client may have constant pain.
- The client may find that low back pain is not relieved by rest.
- The pain may mimic musculoskeletal pain.
- The client may find that the pain increases at night.
- The pain may not be associated with activity.
- The pain may migrate or have insidious onset.

TREATMENT/MANAGEMENT

GENERAL TREATMENT CONSIDERATIONS

Therapists generally treat low back pain using exercise, education, and physical agents or modalities such as massage, heat, transcutaneous electrical nerve stimulation (TENS), interferential therapy, and shortwave diathermy. Additional approaches include manipulative and mechanical therapies: spinal manipulative therapy (SMT), mobilization, and traction (intermittent and autotraction). Active measures also include biofeedback, assessment of ADLs, and work hardening.

Exercise

Movement and exercise are critical to develop and maintain musculoskeletal strength. Types of exercise therapy include the following:

- Extension exercise can be useful to increase or maintain lordosis and to diminish and centralize pain.
- Flexion exercise can be useful in treating paravertebral musculature and the posterior facet syndrome.
- Proprioceptive neuromuscular facilitation (PNF) is used to produce increased muscular excitation or inhibition. In the lumbar spine, the psoas-iliacus muscle, hamstrings, quadratus lumborum, piriformis, lumbar spine extensors, and trunk extensors and flexors may be targeted.
- Muscle energy techniques are used to restore optimal static and dynamic posture.
- Stabilization exercise routines and posture education are used for instability.
- An aerobic fitness program may include brisk walking, cycling, aquatics, swimming, cross-country skiing, or low-impact aerobics.

Education

Education is important to facilitate recovery and prevent recurrence through information on back care strategies or through a back school. Goals of back schools, in general, include the following:

- Provision of information: anatomy, biomechanics, pain, drugs, sex, stress, physical fitness, holistic health, resources

- Rehabilitation/prevention: posture, awareness, movement, body/mind inter-relatedness, self-help techniques, physical interventions
- Teaching ergonomic principles: human considerations, environmental conditions, work dynamics, relevance of person to equipment

Manual Therapy

Manual therapy has several major physical therapist contributors, including Kaltenborn, Maitland, and McKenzie. All three advocate treatment strategies using mobilization and manipulation, exercise, and patient education. Differences include the following:

- Kaltenborn emphasizes testing intervertebral joint motion and treating through motion. He advocates traction, distraction, and soft tissue mobilization.
- Maitland emphasizes the pain-range-spasm relationship. Treatment also emphasizes continual assessment, adverse neural tissue mobilization, and traction.
- McKenzie's system classifies low back pain problems as postural, dysfunction, and derangement. Low back pain etiology may be caused by three predisposing factors: poor sitting posture, loss of extension, and frequency of flexion. Patient can self-treat using repeated movements.

Other therapists contributing to manual therapy approaches:

- Edwards: combined-movements techniques
- Grieve: major contributions as a clinician, teacher, and author
- Saunders: outlines a classification system based on anatomic structures
- Paris: developed structured training system

TREATMENT OF SPECIFIC CONDITIONS

Ankylosing Spondylitis
- Provide client education.
- Instruct client to avoid heavy lifting and occupations involving heavy lifting.
- Teach proper positioning.
- Educate client on exercises to avoid, such as flexion of spine and possibly hip flexion.
- Encourage client to sleep on firm mattress, avoiding sleeping in flexed, "fetal" position.
- Encourage client to use lumbar roll support when seated.
- Consider manual mobilization to promote extension.
- Provide physical agents and modalities, along with external support during acute flare-ups.

Chronic Back Pain
- Consider use of TENS.
- Promote overall fitness. A fitness program is critical for chronic low back pain.
- Encourage increased levels of activity as appropriate.

Degenerative Joint Disease
- Consider use of ultrasound, mobilization, traction, and exercise if client is hypomobile.
- Provide external support for hypermobility.
- Initiate muscle-strengthening exercises and postural training for either hypomobility or hypermobility.
- Provide physical agents and modalities for pain.
- Generally, exercise should proceed in a direction opposite the area of aggravation.
- Instruct in preventive measures and postures to relieve mechanical stress.

Disk Herniation

In the case of protrusion with neurological signs:
- Provide physical agents and modalities as indicated.
- Encourage rest.
- Avoid aggravation with postures causing increased intradiscal pressure—especially sitting and flexion.
- Consider use of heavy traction.
- Encourage client to maintain correct posture.
- Provide client education.
- Assess for external support.
- Consider trial of extension exercises.

In the case of extrusion:
- Consider use of TENS for pain.
- Consider trial of heavy traction if condition cannot be differentiated from nerve root syndrome.

Facet-Joint Derangement–Acute
- Use mobilization techniques as indicated.
- Consider manual or mechanical traction.

Fracture
- After healing, restore functional mobility and strength.

Hypomobility Dysfunction
- Use ultrasound as indicated.
- Use mobilization as indicated.
- Consider use of traction.

Muscle Spasm

In acute cases:
- Provide passive support, but avoid overdependence.
- Encourage elongation of muscle to tolerance via positioning. Use reverse muscle action techniques.
- Provide passive to active ROM in pain-free range.
- Consider use of ice or cold packs.

In subacute and chronic cases:
- Consider use of moist heat, diathermy, electrical stimulation, ice, cold packs, and/or massage.
- Progress exercise program as tolerated.
- Provide postural retraining with kinesthetic awareness.
- Teach client relaxation exercises.
- Provide education on condition.
- Search for underlying cause.

Muscle Strain

In acute cases:
- Encourage rest.
- Use ice and other physical agents and modalities, as well as muscle-setting techniques to elongate as tolerated.

In subacute cases:
- Begin gentle movement.
- Heat and massage may be added.
- Progress to full movement.

- Use gentle stretching techniques, graded isometric exercise, and resistive dynamic exercise.
- Correct posture abnormalities with kinesthetic training.
- Correct flexibility and strength imbalances.

Nerve Root Adhesion
- Use straight-leg stretch as tolerated.
- Use ultrasound as indicated.
- Consider unilateral traction.

Nerve Root Irritation
- Use physical agents and modalities as indicated.

Posterolateral Disk Derangement
- Reduce derangement with appropriate movement; client may find pain reduced with repeated extension.
- Maintain reduction with posture correction and restore function.
- Correct posture with education in prevention.
- Self-treatment with repeated movements may be tried first. Progress to mobilization and, if necessary, manipulation.
- Consider use of traction.
- Consider use of modalities for pain such as TENS, interferential, and diathermy.
- Client may find that a crook-lying position eases pain.

Postural Syndrome
- Teach postural exercises.
- Initiate general conditioning exercises.
- Offer physical agents and modalities as indicated.
- Use external support for severe cases.

Pregnancy/Postpartum

In cases of acute low back pain:

- Encourage decreased activity.
- Offer gentle heat and massage of muscle spasm while client is positioned side-lying.
- Provide obstetric back school.
- Initiate land-based or water-based exercise program.
- Use stabilization exercises as indicated.
- For diastasis recti, splint during stressful activity or abdominal exercise.

In cases of sacroiliac joint dysfunction:

- Provide education on vulnerability of the back.
- Offer posture and body mechanics education.
- Instruct client to avoid high heels and prolonged standing.
- Strengthen pelvic floor muscles and abdominal musculature.
- Teach proper relaxation positions.

Note: Avoid supine position for prolonged periods after 20 weeks gestation.

- Use gentle mobilization or muscle energy techniques.
- Provide external support to stabilize or relieve stress.
- Avoid unilateral weight bearing.
- Consider use of heel lift if needed for leg-length discrepancy.

In cases of pubic symphysis pain:

- Use moist heat or cold pack for pain.
- Avoid having legs spread in extremely wide position.
- Client may need crutches or walker for weight bearing.
- Provide binder around hips for support as tolerated.

- Consider gentle mobilization.
- Use muscle energy techniques as indicated.

Sacroiliac Hypermobility
- Provide external support.
- Encourage rest if condition is inflamed.

Sacroiliac Hypomobility
- Use ultrasound as indicated.
- Consider mobilization.
- Encourage rest and provide external support if condition is acute.

Scoliosis
- Exercise is used in conjunction with bracing, casting, or traction.
- Exercise alone for very mild idiopathic scoliosis may be useful.
- Consider lateral electrical surface stimulation or nighttime intermittent neuromuscular stimulation.

Note: See Chapter 12, Pediatric Disorders.

Segmental Hypermobility
- Initiate muscle-strengthening exercises and posture instruction.
- Provide external support.
- Use physical agents and modalities for pain relief as indicated.

Spinal Stenosis
- Provide patient education on avoiding irritation (client may rest or be in spinal flexion).
- Use lumbar bracing for support.
- Use modalities for pain.
- Flexibility exercises may be useful.

Spondylolisthesis
- Provide postural instruction.
- Begin abdominal exercises.
- Use physical agents and modalities for pain, as indicated.
- Provide external support if condition is severe.
- Assess for additional musculoskeletal conditions.

Tumor
- Consult with physician.

PRECAUTIONS/CONTRAINDICATIONS

CANCER

Cancer can mimic musculoskeletal complaints. Unexplained response to treatment or symptoms that cannot be categorized should lead you to suspect a more serious pathology.

Note: Modalities, manual therapy, and spinal traction may be contraindicated with tumor or neoplasm.

MANIPULATION
- The joint should not be forcibly thrust in a direction guarded by muscle spasm.
- Avoid manipulation with herniated nucleus pulposus protrusion with nerve root impingement.
- Use caution with degenerative joint disease. Due to the narrowed spinal canal, extension and extension with rotation could further narrow the canal and should be avoided.

MOBILIZATION

- Excessive force in young children may disrupt the epiphyseal plate, possibly leading to a secondary deformity. Pediatric therapists have been advised to be cautious in the use of joint mobilization.
- Avoid aggressive treatment of nerve root irritation if there is a history of severe trauma.

MODALITIES

- Modalities can be overused, particularly with musculoskeletal strain or sprain and inflammation. Pain relief through modalities should not cause you to ignore loss of motion and strength.

MOVEMENT

- Correction of lateral shift may cause increased back pain (a centralization effect) but should not cause increased leg pain. Discontinue extension exercise if this happens. Extension of spine is contraindicated if it does not decrease or centralize the pain, if bladder weakness is present or if there is paresthesia in the saddle region, or if the client is unable to assume position due to pain.
- Avoid flexion if it increases pain or peripheralizes the symptoms. Flexion positions and exercises may harm clients who have herniated nucleus pulposus with protrusion.
- If any increase in mobility increases pain or an inflammatory response, try another approach.
- Clients with pain and stiffness usually progress in improvement. If the client is not following patterns of improvement, this may be an alert to consider an organic disease or psychogenic disorder.

PREGNANCY–RELATED PRECAUTIONS

- Ultrasound or electrical stimulation over the sacral sulci is contraindicated during pregnancy.
- TENS for pain relief in pregnancy has not been approved by FDA and should be used only as a last resort. TENS has been used successfully, however, and the benefit may outweigh any potential risk.

Note: See Chapter 15, Women's Health Disorders.

- Special precautions should be taken when using mobilization during pregnancy. Adequate posturing of the client needs to be considered. Although some consider pregnancy a contraindication to mobilization, Maitland reports that clients can usually be treated with an appropriate mobilizing technique without any complication.

DESIRED OUTCOME/PROGNOSIS

- The client's pain and symptoms will decrease.
- The client will increase ROM, and function will be restored.
- Contracture and adhesion formation will be prevented or minimized.
- The client will avoid progression of disorder and recurrence.

Notes: Reportedly 70% to 80% of patients improve within 1 month of therapy. Recurrent back pain occurs in 30% of clients. Reports of recurrent pain vary from 11% to 30% after 1 month to 50% to 62% 1 year after an episode of acute back pain. The chance of successful rehabilitation decreases to 40% if the patient has had low back pain for more than 3 months. This is thought to be due to alteration of the client's affect. Often a specific cause for low back pain cannot be identified.

Activity-related pain is often nonspecific and is usually mechanical in origin. Ninety-two percent of clients are improved in 2 months.

In general, there is an absence of research to substantiate the use of one treatment over another. Physical agents and modalities do not alter the natural history of mechanical pain in the back.

REFERENCES

Assessment

American Physical Therapy Association. Guide to physical therapist practice. 2nd ed. *Phys Ther.* 2001;81.

Bigos S, Bowyer O, Braen G, et al. *Acute Low Back Problems in Adults: Clinical Practice Guideline.* Rockville, Md: US Dept of Health and Human Services, Public Health Service, Agency for Health Care Policy and Research; 1994. AHCPR Pub. No. 95–0643, Quick Reference Guide No. 14.

Binkley J, Finch E, Hall J, Black T, Gowland C. Diagnostic classification of patients with low back pain: report on a survey of physical therapy experts. *Phys Ther.* 1993;73:138–150.

Boland RA, Adams RD. Effects of ankle dorsiflexion on range and reliability of straight leg raising. *Aust J Physiotherapy.* 2000;46:191–200.

Buschbacher RM, ed. *Musculoskeletal Disorders: A Practical Guide for Diagnosis and Rehabilitation.* Boston, Mass: Andover Medical Publishers; 1994.

Daniels L, Worthingham C. *Muscle Testing Techniques of Manual Examination.* 6th ed. Philadelphia, Pa: WB Saunders Co; 1995.

Delitto A. Are measures of function and disability important in low back care? *Phys Ther.* 1994;74:452–462.

Delitto A, Cibulka MT, Erhard RE, Bowling RW, Tenhula JA. Evidence for use of an extension-mobilization category in acute low back syndrome: a prescriptive validation pilot study. *Phys Ther.* 1993;73:216–222.

Delitto A, Synder-Mackler L. The diagnostic process: examples in orthopedic physical therapy. *Phys Ther.* 1995;75:203–210.

D'Orarzio B. *Low Back Pain Handbook.* Boston, Mass: Butterworth Heinemann; 1999.

Dubb IBM, Driver HS. Ratings of sleep and pain in patients with low back pain after sleeping on mattresses of different firmness. *Physiotherapy Can.* 1993;45:26–28.

Edwards BC. *Manual of Combined Movements: Their Use in the Examination and Treatment of Mechanical Vertebral Column Disorders.* New York, NY: Churchill Livingstone; 1992.

Fenety A, Kumar S. Isokinetic trunk strength and lumbosacral range of motion in elite female field hockey players reporting low back pain. *J Orthop Sports Phys Ther.* 1992; 16:129–135.

Fischer K, Johnston M. Validation of the Oswestry Low Back Pain Disability questionnaire, its sensitivity as a measure of change following treatment and its relationship with other aspects of the chronic pain experience. *Physiotherapy Theory Pract.* 1997;13:67–80.

Fritz JM, Irrgang JJ. A comparison of a modified Oswestry Low Back Pain Disability questionnaire and the Quebec Back Pain Disability Scale. *Phys Ther.* 2001;81:776–788.

Gill C, Sandford J, Binkley J, Stratford P, Finch E. Low back pain: program description and outcome in a case series. *J Orthop Sports Phys Ther.* 1994;20:11–16.

Goodman C, Snyder TE. *Differential Diagnosis in Physical Therapy.* 2nd ed. Philadelphia, Pa: WB Saunders Co; 2000.

Graves JE, Fix CK, Pollock ML, Leggett SH, Foster DN, Carpenter DM. Comparison of two restraint systems for pelvic stabilization during isometric lumbar extension strength testing. *J Orthop Sports Phys Ther.* 1992;15:37–42.

Gronblad M, Hurri H, Kouri JP. Relationships between spinal mobility, physical performance tests, pain intensity and disability assessments in chronic low back pain patients. *Scand J Rehabil Med.* 1997;29;17–24.

Hall CM, Brody TB. *Therapeutic Exercise: Moving Toward Function.* Philadelphia, Pa: Lippincott Williams and Wilkins; 1999.

Hertling D, Kessler RM. *Management of Common Musculoskeletal Disorders.* 3rd ed. Philadelphia, Pa: JB Lippincott Co; 1996.

Iversen MD, Katz JN. Examination findings and self-reported walking capacity in patients with lumbar spinal stenosis. *Phys Ther.* 2001;81:1296–1306.

Jacobs K. *Ergonomics for Therapists.* 2nd ed. Boston, Mass: Butterworth Heinemann; 2000.

Kasman GS, Ram JR, Wolf SL. *Clinical Applications in Surface Electromyography: Chronic Musculoskeletal Pain.* Bethesda, Md: Aspen Publishers; 1998.

Kendall FP, McCreary EK, Provance PG. *Muscles: Testing and Function.* 4th ed. Baltimore, Md: Williams and Wilkins; 1993.

Kisner C, Colby LA. *Therapeutic Exercise: Foundations and Techniques.* 3rd ed. Philadelphia, Pa: FA Davis Co; 1996.

Kort HD, Hendriks ERH. A comparison of selected isokinetic trunk strength parameters of elite male judo competitors and cyclists. *J Orthop Sports Phys Ther.* 1992;16:92–96.

Lee CE, Simmonds MJ, Novy DM. Self-reports and clinician-measured physical function among patients with low back pain: a comparison. *Arch Phys Med Rehabil.* 2001; 82:227–231.

Lesh SG. *Clinical Orthopedics for the Physical Therapist Assistant.* Philadelphia, Pa: FA Davis Co; 2000.

Lindstrom I, Ohlund C, Eek C, Wallin L, Peterson L, Nachemson A. Mobility, strength, and fitness after a graded activity program for patients with subacute low back pain. *Spine.* 1992;17:641–652.

Maher C, Adams R. Reliability of pain and stiffness assessments in clinical manual lumbar spine examination. *Phys Ther.* 1994;801–811.

Malone TR, McPoil T, Nitz AJ, eds. *Orthopaedic and Sports Physical Therapy.* 3rd ed. St. Louis, Mo: CV Mosby Co; 1997.

Maricar NN. Treatment of discogenic back pain: a case study of physiotherapy intervention from subacute state to functional recovery. *Physiotherapy Singapore.* 2000;3:87–94.

Marras WS, Sommerich C. A three-dimensional motion model of loads on the lumbar spine. 1. Model structure. *Human Factors.* 1996;123–138.

Mayer TG, Mooney V, Gatchel RJ. *Contemporary Conservative Care for Painful Spinal Disorders.* Philadelphia, Pa: Lea and Febiger; 1993.

Miller SA, Mayer T, Cox R, Gatchel RJ. Reliability problems associated with the modified Schober technique for true lumbar flexion measurement. *Spine.* 1992;17:345–348.

Mitchell J. A new method of measuring the degree of lumbar spine curvature in pregnant women. *S Afr J Physiotherapy.* 1992;48:4:51–55.

Myers RS, ed. *Saunders Manual of Physical Therapy Practice.* Philadelphia, Pa: WB Saunders Co; 1995.

Nicholas MK, Wilson PH, Goyen J. Comparison of cognitive-behavioral group treatment and an alternative non-psychological treatment for chronic low back pain. *Pain.* 1992; 48:339–347.

Richardson J, Iglarsh ZA. *Clincial Orthopaedic Physical Therapy*. Philadelphia, Pa: WB Saunders Co; 1994.

Riddle DL, Lee KT, Stratford PW. Use of SF-36 and SF-12 health status measures: a quantitative comparison for groups versus individual patients. *Med Care*. 2001;39:867–878.

Riddle DL, Stratford PW, Binkley JM. Sensitivity to change of the Roland-Morris Back Pain questionnaire: part 2. *Phys Ther*. 1998;78:1197–1207.

Rothstein JM, Roy SH, Wolf SL. *The Rehabilitation Specialist's Handbook*. 2nd ed. Philadelphia, Pa: FA Davis Co; 1998.

Schunk C, Reed K. *Clinical Practice Guidelines*. Gaithersburg, Md: Aspen Publishers; 2000.

Simmonds MJ, Olson SL, Jones S, et al. Psychometric characteristics and clinical usefulness of physical performance tests in patients with low back pain. *Spine*. 1998;23:2412–2421.

Smith AL, Kolt GS, McConville JC. The effect of the Feldenkrais Method on pain and anxiety in people experiencing chronic low back pain. *NZ J Physiotherapy*. 2001;29:6–14.

Sparto PJ, Parnianpour M, Reinsel TE, et al. The effect of fatigue on multijoint kinematics, coordination, and postural stability during a repetitive lifting test. *J Orthop Sports Phys Ther*. 1997;25:3–12.

Squires MC, Latimer J, Adams RD, et al. Indenter head area and testing frequency effects on posteroanterior lumbar stiffness and subjects' rated comfort. *Man Ther*. 2001;6:40–47.

Sullivan MS, Shoaf LD, Riddle DL. The relationship of lumbar flexion to disability in patients with low back pain. *Phys Ther*. 2000;80:3:240–250.

Tomberlin JP, Saunders HD. *Evaluation, Treatment and Prevention of Musculoskeletal Disorders. Vol 2: Extremities*. Chaska, Minn: The Saunders Group; 1994.

Walker JM. The sacroiliac joint: a critical review. *Phys Ther*. 1992;72:903–916.

Williams R, Binkley J, Bloch R, Goldsmith CH, Minuk T. Reliability of the Modified-Modified Schober and double inclinometer methods for measuring lumbar flexion and extension. *Phys Ther*. 1993;73:33–44.

Winkel D. *Diagnosis and Treatment of the Spine*. Gaithersburg, Md: Aspen Publishers; 1996.

Treatment

Adams G, Sim J. A survey of UK manual therapists' practice of and attitudes towards manipulation and its complications. *Physiotherapy Res Int*. 1998;3:206.

Alaranta H. Intensive physical and psychosocial training program for patients with chronic low back pain—a controlled clinical trial. *Spine*. 1994;19:1339.

Alexander KM, LaPeir TL. Differences in static balance and weight distribution between normal subjects and subjects with chronic unilateral low back pain. *J Orthop Sports Phys Ther*. 1998;28:378–383.

Amundsen T, Weber H, Lilleas F, et al. Lumbar spinal stenosis: clinical and radiologic features. *Spine*. 1995;20:1178.

Aspden RM. Review of the functional anatomy of the spinal ligaments and the lumbar erector spinae muscles. *Clin Anatomy*. 1992;5:372–387.

Barker K, Atha J. Reducing the biomechanical stress of lifting by training. *Appl Ergonomics*. 1995;373–378.

Battie ME. Managing low back pain: attitudes and treatment preferences of physical therapists. *Phys Ther*. 1994;74:219.

Bendix AF, Bendix T, Labriola M, et al. Functional restoration for chronic low back pain. *Spine*. 1998;23:717.

Beurskens AJ, de Vet HC, Kike AJ, et al. Efficacy of traction for non-specific low back pain: a randomized clinical trial. *Lancet.* 1995;436:1596–1600.

Bigos S, Bowyer O, Braen G, et al. *Acute Low Back Problems in Adults: Assessment and Treatment.* US Department of Health and Human Services, Public Health Service, Agency of Health Care Policy and Research, Rockville, Maryland: AHCPR Pub. O. 95–0643.

Binkley J, Finch E, Hall J, Black T, Gowland C. Diagnostic classification of patients with low back pain: report on a survey of physical therapy experts. *Phys Ther.* 1993;73:138–150.

Blanda J, Bethem D, Moats W, et al. Defects of the pars interarticularis in athletes: A protocol for non-operative treatment. *J Spinal Disord.* 1993;6:406.

Boissonnault WG, ed. *Examination in Physical Therapy Practice: Screening for Medical Disease.* New York, NY: Churchill Livingstone; 1991.

Bullock-Saxton JE, Janda V, Bullock MI. Reflex activation of gluteal muscles in walking: an approach to restoration of muscle function for patients with low back pain. *Spine.* 1993;18:704–708.

Caling B, Lee M. Effect of direction of applied mobilization force on the posteroanterior response in the lumbar spine. *J Manipulative Physiol Ther.* 2001;24:71–78.

Cholewicke J, McGill S. Mechanical stability of the in vivo lumbar spine: implications for injury and chronic low back pain. *Clin Biomech.* 1996;11:1–15.

Cooper R, Stakes M, Sweet C, et al. Increased central drive during fatiguing contractions of the paraspinal muscles in patients with chronic LBP. *Spine.* 1993;18:610.

Cornefjord M, Katsuhiko S, Olmarker K, et al. A model for chronic nerve root compression studies. *Spine.* 1997;9:946–957.

Cresswell A, Oddsson L, Thorstenson A. The influence of sudden perturbations on trunk muscles activity and intra-abdominal pressure while standing. *Exp Brain Res.* 1994;98:336.

Curillo JA. Aquatic physical therapy approaches for the spine. *Orthop Phys Ther Clin North Am.* 1994;3:179–208.

D'Orazio BP. *Back Pain Rehabilitation.* Boston, Mass: Andover Medical Publishers; 1993.

D'Orazio BP. *Low Back Pain Handbook.* Boston, Mass: Butterworth Heinemann; 1999.

Danneels LA, Vanderstraeten GG, Cambier DC, et al. Effects of three different training modalities on the cross sectional area of the lumbar multifidus muscle in patients with chronic low back pain. *Br J Sports Med.* 2001;35:186–191.

Deen HG, Zimmerman RS, Lyons MK, et al. Use of the exercise treadmill to measure baseline functional status and surgical outcome in patients with severe lumbar spinal stenosis. *Spine.* 1998;23:244–248.

Delitto A, Cibulka MT, Erhard RE, Bowling RW, Tenhula J. Evidence for use of an extension-mobilization category in acute low back pain syndrome: a prescriptive validation pilot study. *Phys Ther.* 1993;73:216–228.

Delitto A, Erhard RE, Bowling RW. A treatment-based classification approach to low back syndrome: identifying and staging patients for conservative treatment. *Phys Ther.* 1995;75:470–498.

De Souza LH, Frank AO. Subjective pain experience of people with chronic back pain. *Physiotherapy Res Int.* 2000;5:207–219.

Dettori JR, Bullock SH, Sutlive TG, et al. The effects of spinal flexion and extension exercises and their associated postures in patients with acute low back pain. *Spine.* 1995;20:2303–2312.

DiFabio RP. Efficacy of Manual Therapy. *Phys Ther.* 1992;72:12:853–864.

DiFabio RP, Boissonnault W. Physical therapy and health-related outcomes for patients with common orthopedic disorders. *J Orthop Sports Phys Ther*. 1998;27:219–230.

Dodd T. The prevalence of low back pain in Great Britain in 1996. A report on research for the Department of Health using the ONS Omnibus Survey. London, England: The Stationary Office; 1997.

Donelson R, Aprill C, Medcalf R, Grant W. A prospective study of centralization of lumbar and referred pain. *Spine*. 1997;22:1115–1122.

DonTigny RL. Mechanics and treatment of the sacroiliac joint. *J Manipulative Physiol Ther*. 1993;3–12.

Edgerton V, Wolf S, Levendowski D, et al. Theoretical basis for patterning EMG amplitudes to assess muscle dysfuntion. *Med Sci Sports Exec*. 1996;28:744.

Edwards BC. *Manual of Combined Movements*. New York, NY: Churchill Livingstone; 1992.

Edwards BC, Zusman M, Hardcastle P et al. A physical approach to the rehabilitation of patients disabled by chronic LBP. *Med J Aust*. 1992;156:167.

Ehrmann-Feldman D, Rossignol M, Abenhaim L, et al. Physician referral to physical therapy in a cohort of workers compensated for low back pain. *Phys Ther*. 1996;76:150–157.

Ellis JJ, Spangnoli R. The hip and sacroiliac joint: prescriptive home exercise program for the dysfunction of the pelvic girdle and hip. In: Orthopedic Physical Therapy Home Study Course 971. LaCrosse, Wis: Orthopedic Section of the American Physical Therapy Association; 1997.

Erhard RE, Delitto A, Cibulka MT. Relative effectiveness of an extension program and a combined program of manipulation and flexion and extension exercises in patients with acute low back syndrome. *Phys Ther*. 1994;74:1093–1100.

Farrell JP, Jensen GM. Manual therapy: a critical assessment of role in the profession of physical therapy. *Phys Ther*. 1992;72:843–852.

Feurstein M, Beattie P. Biobehavioral factors affecting pain and disability and low back pain: mechanics and assessment. *Phys Ther*. 1995;267.

Fitzgerald GK, McClure PW, Beattie P, et al. Issues in determining effectiveness of manual therapy. *Phys Ther*. 1994;227–233.

Flores L, Gatchel RJ, Polatin PB. Objectification of functional improvement after nonoperative care. *Spine*. 1997;22:1622.

Fritz JM, Delitto A, Welch WC, et al. Lumbar spinal stenosis: a review of current concepts in evaluation, management, and outcome measurements. *Arch Phys Med Rehabil*. 1998;79:700–708.

Fritz JM, Erhard RE, Vignovic M. A nonsurgical treatment approach for patients with lumbar spinal stenosis. *Phys Ther*. 1997;77:962–973.

Frost H, Lamb SE, Shackleton CH. A functional restoration programme for chronic low back pain. *Physiotherapy*. 2000;86:285–293.

Gardener-Morse M, Stokes I, Laible J. Role of muscles in lumbar spine stability in maximum extension efforts. *J Orthop Res*. 1995;13:802–808.

Giles LG. Evidence-based clinical guidelines submitted to the Australian National Health and Medical Research Council for the management of acute low back pain: a critical review. *J Manipulative Physiol Ther*. 2001;24:131–139.

Giles LGF, Singer KP. *Clinical Anatomy and Management of Low Back Pain*. Oxford, England: Butterworth Heinemann; 1997.

Gill KP, Callaghan MJ. Measurement of lumbar proprioception in individuals with and without low back pain. *Spine*. 1998;23:371.

Goel V, Kong W, Han J, et al. A combined finite element and optimization investigation of lumbar spine mechanics with and without muscles. *Spine*. 1993;18:1531.

Grabiner M, Koh T, Ghazawi AE. Decoupling of bilateral paraspinal excitation in subjects with low back pain. *Spine.* 1992;17:1219.

Grabois M, Garrison SJ, Hart KA, Lehmkuhl LD. *Physical Medicine and Rehabilitation: The Complete Approach.* Malden, Mass: Blackwell Science; 2000.

Graver V. New dissertation: long-term results and predictors of outcome in lumbar disc surgery with special attention to the impact of hypofibrinolysis, psychological distress, and the extent of the surgical intervention. *Adv Physiotherapy.* 2000;2:93–95.

Hansen FR, Bendix T, Skov P, et al. Intensive, dynamic back-muscle exercises, conventional physiotherapy, or placebo-control treatment of low-back pain. *Spine.* 1993;18:98–108.

Hardcastle P. Repair of spondylolysis in young fast bowlers. *J Bone Joint Surg.* 1993;6:406.

Herzog W, Scheele D, Conway PJ. Electromyographic responses of back and limb muscles associated with spinal manipulative therapy. *Spine.* 1999;24:146.

Hides J, Stokes M, Saide M, et al. Evidence of lumbar multifidus muscles wasting ipsilateral to symptoms in patients with acute/subacute low back pain. *Spine* 1994;19:165.

Hides JA, Richardson CA, Jull GA. Multifidus muscle recovery is not automatic following resolution of acute first episode low back pain. *Spine.* 1996;21:2763–2769.

Hides JA, Richardson CA, Jull GA, Davies SE. Ultrasound imaging in rehabilitation. *Aust J Physiotherapy.* 1996;41:187–193.

Hilde G, Bo K. Effect of exercise in the treatment of chronic low back pain: a systematic review, emphasizing type and dose of exercise. *Phys Ther Rev.* 1998;3:107–117.

Hildebrandt J, Pfingsten M, Saur P, et al. Prediction of success from a multidisciplinary treatment program for chronic low back pain. *Spine.* 1997;22:990.

Hodges P, Richardson C. Feedforward contraction of transversus abdominus is not influenced by the direction of arm movement. *Exp Brain Res.* 1997;114:362–370.

Hodges PW, Richardson CA. Inefficient muscular stabilization of the lumbar spine associated with low back pain: a motor control evaluation of transversus abdominis. *Spine.* 1996;21:2640–2650.

Hodges PW, Richardson CA. Contraction of the abdominal muscles associated with movement of the lower limb. *Phys Ther.* 1997;77:132–144.

Hodges PW, Richardson CA. Delayed postural contraction of transversus abdominis in low back pain associated with movement of the lower limbs. *J Spinal Disord.* 1998;11:46–56.

Homer S, Mackintosh S. Injuries in young female elite athletes. *Physiotherapy.* 1992;78:804–808.

Hopper D, Elliott B. Lower limb and back injury patterns of elite netball players. *Sports Med.* 1993;16:148–162.

Indahl A, Velund L, Reikeraas O. Good prognosis for low back pain when left untampered: a randomized clinical trial. *Spine.* 1995;20:473–477.

Jackson DA. The history of and clinical findings in lumbar spinal stenosis: a brief review. *Phys Ther Rev.* 1998;3:163–167.

Janda V. Evaluation of muscular imbalance. In Liebenson C, ed. *Rehabilitation of the Spines: A Practitioner's Manual.* Philadelphia, Pa: Williams and Wilkins; 1996.

Jenner JR, Barry M. Low back pain. *BMJ.* 1995;929–932.

Jermyn RT. A nonsurgical approach to low back pain. *J Am Osteopath Assoc.* 2001;101:S6–11.

Jette AM, Smith K, Haley SM, Davis KD. Physical therapy episodes of care for patients with low back pain. *Phys Ther.* 1994;74:101–115.

Johannsen F, Remvig L, Kryger P, et al. Exercises for chronic low back pain: a clinical trial. *J Orthop Sports Phys Ther*. 1995;22:52–59.

Kaigle A, Holm S, Hansson T. Experimental instability in the lumbar spine. *Spine*. 1995;20:421.

Karas R, McIntosh G, Hall H, et al. The relationship between nonorganic signs and centralization of symptoms in the prediction of return to work for patients with low back pain. *Phys Ther*. 1997;74:1093–1100.

Kaser L, Mannion AF, Rhyner A, et al. Active therapy for chronic low back pain: part 2. Effects on paraspinal muscle cross-sectional area, fiber type size, and distribution. *Spine*. 2001;26:909–919.

Katilainen E, Valtonen S. Clinical instability after microdiscectomy. *Acta Neurosurg*. 1993;125:120.

Kellegren JH. The anatomical source of back pain. *Rheumatol Rehabil*. 1997;16:3–12.

Kerr DP, Walsh DM, Baxter GD. A study of the use of acupuncture in physiotherapy. *Complement Ther Med*. 2001;9:21–27.

Kessler RM, Hertling D. *Management of Common Musculoskeletal Disorders: Physical Therapy Principles and Methods*. 3rd ed. Philadelphia, Pa: Harper & Row; 1996.

Koes BW, Bouter LM, van Mameren H, et al. The effectiveness of manual therapy, physiotherapy, and treatment by the general practitioner for nonspecific back and neck complaints: a randomized clinical trial. *Spine*. 1992;17:1:28–35.

Koes BW, Bouter LM, van Mameren H, et al. Randomized clinical trial of manipulative therapy and physiotherapy for persistent back and neck complaints: results of one year follow up. *Br Med J*. 1992;304:601–605.

Kuukkanen T, Malkia E. Effects of a three-month therapeutic exercise programme on flexibility in subjects with low back pain. *Physiotherapy Res Int*. 2000;5:46–61.

Kuukkanen T, Malkia E. Muscular performance after a 3 month progressive physical exercise program and 9 month follow-up in subjects with low back pain: a controlled study. *Scand J Med Sci Sports*.

Lavender S, Marras W, Miller R. The development of response strategies in preparation for sudden loading to the torso. *Spine*. 1993;18:2097.

Lavendar S, Tsuang Y, Andersson G. Trunk muscle activation and co-contraction while resisting applied moments in a twisted posture. *Ergonomics*. 1993;36:1145.

Lee D. *The Pelvic Girdle*. New York, NY: Churchill Livingstone; 1999.

Lee RYW, Evans JH. Loads in the lumbar spine during traction therapy. *Aust J Physiotherapy*. 2001;47:102–108.

Li LC, Bombardier C. Physical therapy management of low back pain: an exploratory survey of therapist approaches. *Phys Ther*. 2001;81:1018–1028.

Lindgren K, Sihvonen T, Leino E, et al. Exercise therapy effects on functional radiographic findings and segmental electromyographic activity in lumbar spine instability. *Arch Phys Med Rehabil*. 1993;74:933.

Lindsay DM, Meeuwisse WH, Vyse A, et al. Lumbosacral dysfunctions in elite cross-country skiers. *J Orthop Sports Phys Ther*. 1993;18:580–585.

Lindstrom I. The effect of graded activity on patients with subacute low back pain: a randomized prospective clinical study with an operant-conditioning behavioural approach. *Phys Ther*. 1992;72:279–293.

Lindstrom I, Ohlund C, Eek C, Wallin L, Peterson L, Nachemson A. Mobility, strength, and fitness after a graded activity program for patients with subacute low back pain. *Spine*. 1992;17:641–652.

Lindstrom I, Ohlund C, Eek C, et al. The effect of graded activity on patients with subacute low back pain: a randomized prospective clinical study with an operant-conditioning behavioral approach. *Phys Ther.* 1992;72:279–293.

Lundon K, Boton K. Structure and function of the lumbar intervertebral disk in health, aging, and pathologic conditions. *J Orthop Sports Phys Ther.* 2001;31:291–303.

Magnusson ML, Bishop JB, Hasselquist L, et al. Range of motion and motion patterns in patients with low back pain before and after rehabilitation. *Spine.* 1998;23:2631–2639.

Malmivaara A. The treatment of acute low back pain—bed rest, exercises, or ordinary activity? *N Engl J Med.* 1995;332:351.

Manniche C. Clinical trial of postoperative dynamic back exercises after first lumbar discectomy. *Spine.* 1993:92.

Mannion AF, Junge A, Taimela S, et al. Active therapy for chronic low back pain: part 3. Factors influencing self-rated disability and its change following therapy. *Spine.* 2001;26: 920–929.

Mannion AF, Muntener M, Taimela S, et al. Comparison of three active therapies for chronic low back pain: results of a randomized clinical trial with one-year follow-up. *Rheumatol.* 2001;40:772–778.

Mannion AF, Taimela S, Muntener M, et al. Active therapy for chronic low back pain part 1. Effects on back muscle activation, fatigability, and strength. *Spine.* 2001;26:897–908.

May SJ. Patient satisfaction with management of back pain. Part 1: What is satisfaction? Review of satisfaction with medical management. Part 2: an explorative, qualitative study into patients' satisfaction with physiotherapy. *Physiotherapy.* 2001;87:4–20.

Mayer T, et al. Physical progress and residual impairment quantification after functional restoration, part I: lumbar mobility. *Spine.* 1994;19:389.

Mayer T, Polatin PB, Gatchel RJ. Functional restoration and other rehabilitation approaches to chronic musculoskeletal pain disability syndromes. *Crit Rev Phys Rehabil Med.* 1998;10:209.

Mayer TG, Mooney V, Gatchel RJ. *Contemporary Conservative Care for Painful Spinal Disorders.* Philadelphia, Pa: Lea and Febiger; 1993.

McGill S. A myoelectrically based dynamic three-dimensional model to predict loads on lumbar spine tissues during lateral bending. *J Biomech.* 1992;25:395.

McGill S. Low back exercises: evidence for improving exercise regimens. *Phys Ther.* 1998;78:754–765.

McGill SM. Low back stability: from formal description to issues for performance and rehabilitation. *Exerc Sport Sci Rev.* 2001;29:2–31.

Mimura M, Panjabi M, Oxland T, et al. Disc degeneration affects the multidirectional flexibility of the lumbar spine. *Spine.* 1994;19:1371.

Mohseni-Bandpei MA, Stephenson R, Richardson B. Spinal manipulation in the treatment of low back pain: a review of the literature with particular emphasis on randomized controlled clinical trials. *Phys Ther Rev.* 1998;3:185–194.

Mooney V, Andersson GBJ. Controversies—trunk strength testing in patient evaluation and treatment. *Spine.* 1994;19:2483–2485.

Nadler SF, Wu KD, Galski T, et al. Low back pain in college athletes: A prospective study correlating lower extremity overuse or acquired ligamentous laxity with low back pain. *Spine.* 1998;23:828.

Nagler W, Hausen HS. Conservative management of lumbar spinal stenosis: identifying patients likely to do well without surgery. *Postgrad Med.* 1998;103:69–83.

Noll E, Key A, Jensen G. Clinical reasoning of an experienced physiotherapist: insight into clinician decision-making regarding low back pain. *Physiotherapy Res Int.* 2001;6: 40–51.

Norris CM. Spinal stabilization. 1. Active lumbar stabilization—concepts. *Physiotherapy.* 1995:61–64.

Norris CM. Spinal stabilization. 5. An exercise program to enhance lumbar stabilization. *Physiotherapy.* 1995;138–146.

Nowasaki P, Delitto AA, Erhard RE. Lumbar spinal stenosis. *Phys Ther.* 1996;76:187–190.

O'Sullivan P, Twomey L, Allison G. Dynamic stabilization of the lumbar spine. *Crit Rev Phys Rehabil Med.* 1997;9:315.

O'Sullivan P, Twomey L, Allison G. Dysfunction of the neuro-muscular system in the presence of low back pain—implications for physical therapy management. *J Manual Manipulation Ther.* 1997;5:20.

O'Sullivan P, Twomey L, Allison G. Evaluation of specific stabilizing exercise in the treatment of chronic low back pain with radiological diagnosis of spondylolysis and spondylolisthesis. *Spine.* 1997;24:2959–2967.

O'Sullivan P, Twomey L, Allison G, et al. Altered patterns of abdominal muscle activation in patients with chronic back pain. *Aust J Physiotherapy.* 1997;43:91–98.

Oliver J. *Back Care: An Illustrated Guide.* Oxford, England: Butterworth Heinemann; 1994.

Parkhurst TM, Burnett CN. Injury and proprioception in the lower back. *J Orthop Sports Phys Ther.* 1994;19:282.

Peach JP, McGill SM. Kinematics and trunk muscle myoelectric activity in the chronic low back pain patient. *J of Phys Ther.* 1997.

Phuc V, Macmillan. The aging spine: clinical instability. *Miss South Med J.* 1994;87:S26–S35.

Pool-Goudzwaard AL, Vleeming A, Stoechart R, et al. Insufficient lumbopelvic stability: a clinical, anatomical and biomechanical approach to "a-specific" low back pain. *Man Ther.* 1998;3:12–20.

Porterfield JA, DeRosa C. *Mechanical Low Back Pain: Perspectives in Functional Anatomy.* 2nd ed. Philadelphia, Pa: WB Saunders Co; 1998.

Protas EJ. Aerobic exercise in the rehabilitation of individuals with chronic low back pain: A review. *Crit Rev Phys Rehabil Med.* 1996;8:283.

Pullen S. Myofascial pain: a review. *S Afr J Physiotherapy.* 1992;48:3:37–39.

Razmjou H, Cramer J, Yamada R. *Intertester Reliability of the McKenzie Evaluation of Mechanical Low Back Pain.* Chicago, Ill: North American Pain Society; 1999.

Richardson C, Jull G, Hodges P, et al. *Therapeutic Exercise for Spinal Segmental Stabilization in Low Back Pain: Scientific Basis and Clinical Approach.* Edinburgh, Scotland: Churchill Livingstone; 1999.

Richardson CA, Jull GA, Toppenberg RM, et al. Techniques for active lumbar stabilization for spinal protection: a pilot study. *Aust J Physiotherapy.* 1992;38:105.

Richardson CA, Jull GA. Muscle control–pain control: What exercises would you prescribe? *Man Ther.* 1995;1:2–10.

Richardson CA, Jull GA. An historical perspective on the development of clinical techniques to evaluate and treat the active stabilizing system of the lumbar spine. *Aust J Physiotherapy.* Monograph. 1995;1:5–13.

Riddle DL. Classification and low back pain: a review of the literature and critical analysis of selected systems. *Phys Ther.* 1998;78:708–737.

Rissanen A, Kalima H, Alaranta H. Effect of intensive training on the isokinetic strength and structure of lumbar muscles in patients with chronic low back strength and structure of lumbar muscles in patients with chronic low back pain. *Spine.* 1995;20:333–340.

Roberts L. *Physiotherapy.* Control issues and low back pain. 2001;87:149.

Robinson R. The new back school prescription: Stabilization training. Part 1. *Occup Med.* 1992;7:17–31.

Saal JA. The new back school prescription: Stabilization training II. *Occup Med.* 1992;7:33.

Sahrmann SA. *Diagnosis and Management of Musculoskletal Pain Syndromes.* St. Louis, Mo: CV Mosby Co; 1999.

Sato H, Kikuchi S. The natural history of radiographic instability of the lumbar spine. *Spine.* 1993;18:2075–2079.

Saur P, Ensink F, Frese K, et al. Lumbar range of motion: reliability and validity of the inclinometer techniques in the clinical measurement of trunk flexibility. *Spine.* 1996;21:1332.

Siddall PJ, Cousins MJ. Spine Update. Spinal pain mechanisms. *Spine.* 1997;22:98.

Skargren EI, Carlsson PG, Oberg BE. One year follow-up comparison of the cost effectiveness of chiropractic and physiotherapy as primary management for back pain. *Spine.* 1998;23:1875.

Soukup MG, Lonn J, Glomsrod B, et al. Exercises and education as secondary prevention for recurrent low back pain. *Physiotherapy Res Int.* 2001;6:27–39.

Stanley I, Miller J, Pinnington MA. Uptake of prompt access physiotherapy for new episodes of back pain presenting in primary care. *Physiotherapy.* 2001;87:60–67.

Steffen R, Nolte L, Pingel T. Importance of the back muscles in rehabilitation of postoperative segmental lumbar instability—a biomechanical analysis. *Rehabil.* 1994;33:164.

Steffen R, Nolte LP, Pingel TH. Rehabilitation of postoperative segmental lumbar instability. A biomechanical analysis of the rank of the back muscles. *Rehabil.* 1994;33:164–170.

Stokes M, Cooper R, Jayson M. Selective changes in multifidus dimensions in patients with chronic low back pain. *Eur Spine J.* 1992;1:38.

Storheim K. The effect of intensive group exercise in patients with chronic low back pain. *Adv Physiotherapy.* 2000;2:113–123.

Stratford PW, Binkley J, Soloman P, et al. Assessing change over time in patients with low back pain. *Phys Ther.* 1994;74:528.

Stuberg W. Manual therapy in pediatrics: some considerations. *PT Magazine of Phys Ther.* 1993;1:54–56.

Sufka A, Hauger B, Trenary M, et al. Centralization of low back pain and perceived functional outcome. *J Orthop Sports Phys Ther.* 1998;27:205–212.

Sullivan MS, Jues JM, Mayhew TP. Treatment categories for low back pain: a methodological approach. *J Orthop Sports Phys Ther.* 1996;24:359–364.

Taimela S, Osterman L, Alaranta H, Kijala AS. Long psychomotor reaction times in patients with chronic LBP. *Arch Phys Med Rehabil.* 1993;74:1161.

Taylor MM, Taylor JR, McCormick CC. Features associated with subluxation in lumbar facet joints: Anatomical and radiological comparisons. *Aust Soc Hum Biol.* 1992;5:359.

Taylor JR, Twomey LT. Structure and function of lumbar zygapophyseal joints. *J Orthop Med.* 1992;14:71.

Thelan D, Schultz A, Ashton-Miller J. Co-contraction of lumbar muscles during development of time-varying triaxial moments. *J Orthop Res.* 1995;13:390.

Timm K. A randomized-control study of active and passive treatments for chronic low back pain following L5 laminectomy. *J Orthop Sports Phys Ther.* 1994;20:276.

Trede FV. Physiotherapists' approaches to low back pain education. *Physiotherapy.* 2000;86:427–433.

Tokuhashi Y, Matsuzaki H, Sano S. Evaluation of clinical lumbar instability using the treadmill. *Spine*. 1993;18:2321.

Travell JG, Simons DG. *Myofascial Pain and Dysfunction: The Trigger Point Manual*. Baltimore, Md: Williams and Wilkins; 1992.

Tulder M, Assendelft W, Koes B, et al. Spinal radiological findings and non-specific low back pain. *Spine*. 1997;22:427.

Twomey L, Taylor J. Spine update: exercise and spinal manipulation in the treatment of low back pain. *Spine*. 1995;20:615–619.

Twomey LT. A rationale for the treatment of back pain and joint pain by manual therapy. *Phys Ther*. 1992;72:885–892.

Twomey LT, Taylor JR. *Physical Therapy of the Low Back*. 2nd ed. New York, NY: Churchill Livingstone; 1994.

Van Tulder MW, Koes BW, Bouter LM. Conservative treatment of acute and chronic nonspecific low back pain: A systematic review of randomized controlled trials of most common interventions. *Spine*. 1997;22:2128.

Verta L, Ronnemaa T. The association of mild-moderate isthmic lumbar spondylolisthesis and low back pain in middle-aged patients is weak and it only occurs in women. *Spine*. 1993;18:1496.

Vicenzian G, Twomey L. Side flexion induced lumbar spine conjuctrotation and its influencing factors. *Aust Physiotherapy*. 1993;39:4.

Vleeming A, Mooney V, Dorman T, et al. *Movement, Stability and Low Back Pain*. New York, NY: Churchill Livingstone; 1997.

Waddell G, Feder G, Lewis M. Systematic review of bed rest and advice to stay active for acute low back pain. *Br J Gen Pract*. 1997;47:647–652.

Walker JM. The sacroiliac joint: a critical review. *Phys Ther*. 1992;72:903–916.

Wallner-Schlotfeldt PJ. The predisposing factors to low back pain in workers. *S Afr J Physiotherapy*. 2000;56:33–38.

Walsh MJ. Evaluation of orthopedic testing of the low back for nonspecific lower back pain. *J Manipulative Physiol Ther*. 1998;21:232–236.

Watson TA, Walsh RM. Treatment of acute low back pain with an isometric multifidus contraction technique. *Phys Ther Case Rep*. 2000;3:267–273.

Werneke M, Hart D, Cook D. A descriptive study of the centralization phenomenon. *Spine*. 1999;24:676.

Werneke M, Hart D, Cook D. Centralization phenomenon as a prognostic factor for chronic low back pain and disability. *Spine Impress*. 1999;24:676–683.

Willen J, Danielsson B, Gaulitz A, et al. Dynamic effects on the lumbar spinal canal. *Spine*. 1997;24:2968–2976.

Wilke H, Wolf S, Claes L, et al. Stability increase of the lumbar spine with different muscle groups. *Spine*. 1995;20:192–198.

Wood K, Popp C, Transfeldt E, et al. Radiographic evaluation of instability in spondylolisthesis. *Spine*. 1994;19:1697.

Pregnancy-Related

Gleeson P, Pauls J. Obstetrical physical therapy: review of the literature. *Phys Ther*. 1988;68:1699–1702.

Pauls J. *Therapeutic Approaches to Women's Health: A Program of Exercise and Education*. Gaithersburg, Md: Aspen Publishers; 1995.

Paulsen TE. The conservative treatment of pain in the sacroiliac region during pregnancy: a case study. *S Afr J Physiotherapy*. 1993;49:1:14–17.

Polden M, Mantle J. *Physiotherapy in Obstetrics and Gynecology*. London, England: Butterworth Heinemann; 1990.

Samsford R, Bullock-Saxton J, Markwell S. *Women's Health: A Textbook for Physiotherapists*. Philadelphia, Pa: WB Saunders Co; 1999.

Stephenson RG, O'Connor L. *Obstetric and Gynecologic Care in Physical Therapy*. 2nd ed. Thorofare, NJ: Slack Inc; 2000.

Work Injury Management/Ergonomics

Apts DW. *Back Injury Prevention Handbook*. Chelsea, Mich: Lewis Publications; 1992.

Granata KP, Marras WS. The influence of trunk muscle coactivity on dynamic spinal loads. *Spine*. 1995;20:913.

Isernhagen S. Industrial physical therapy. *Orthop Phys Ther Clin North Am*. 1992;1:1.

Isernhagen S. Advancements in functional capacity evaluation. In: D'Orazio BP, ed. *Back Pain Rehabilitation*. Boston, Mass: Andover Medical Publishers; 1993.

King PM. Back injury prevention programs: a critical review of the literature. *J Occup Rehabil*. 1993;3:145–158.

Kjellman G, Oberg B, Hensing G, et al. A 12-year follow-up of subjects initially sicklisted with neck/shoulder or low back diagnoses. *Physiotherapy Res Int*. 2001;6:52–63.

Lahad A. The effectiveness of four interventions for the prevention of low back pain. *JAMA*. 1995;272:1286–1291.

Leamon TB. Research to reality: a consideration of validity of various criteria for the prevention of occupationally induced low back pain. *Ergonomics*. 1994;37:1959–1974.

Lechner DE. Work hardening and work conditioning interventions: do they affect disability? *Phys Ther*. 1994;74:472–493.

Lindstrom I, Ohlund C, Eek C, et al. The effect of graded activity on patients with subacute low back pain: a randomized prospective clinical study with an operant-conditioning behavioral approach. *Phys Ther*. 1992;72:279–293.

Magnussen M, Almqvist M, Roman, et al. Measurement of height loss during whole body vibrations. *J Spinal Dis*. 1992;5:198.

Maher CG. A systematic review of workplace interventions to prevent low back pain. *Aust J Physiotherapy*. 2000;46:259–269.

Marklin RW, Simoneau GC. Effect of setup configurations of split computer keyboards on wrist angle. *Phys Ther*. 2001;81:1038–1048.

Marras WS, Lavender SA, Leyrgans SE, et al. The role of dynamic three dimensional trunk motion in occupationally related low back pain disorders. *Spine*. 1993;18:617.

Resnick ML, Chaffin DB. Kinematics, Kinetics and psychophysical perceptions in symmetric and twisting, pushing and pulling tasks. *Hum Factors*. 1996;31:114.

Richardson B, Eastlake A. *Physiotherapy in Occupational Health: Management, Prevention, and Health Promotion in the Work Place*. Boston, Mass: Butterworth Heinemann; 1994.

Rothman J, Levine RE. *Prevention Practice: Strategies for Physical Therapy and Occupational Therapy*. Philadelphia, Pa: JB Saunders Co; 1992.

Saldana N. A computerized method for assessment of musculoskeletal discomfort in the workforce; a tool for surveillance. *Ergonomics*. 1994;37:1097–1112.

Waters TR, Putz-Anderson V. Ergonomic considerations for manual material handling and low back pain. In Erdil M Dickerson OB, eds. New York, NY: Reinhold; 1997.

Waters TR, Putz-Anderson V, Grag A, et al. Revised NIOSH equation of the design and evaluation of manual lifting tasks. *Ergonomics.* 1993;36:749.

Waters T, Putz-Anderson V, Garg A. *Application Manual for the Revised NIOSH lifting equation.* NIOSH Pub PB94, Rockville, Md: US Department of Health and Human Services, 1994.

Wilder DB, Mangusson ML, Fenwick J, Pope MH. The effect of posture and seat suspension design on disc comfort and back muscle fatigue during simulated truck driving. *Appl Ergonomic.* 1994;25:66.

Chapter 10

Neurological Disorders

Alzheimer's Disease

Also known as *Alzheimer-type dementia.*

DESCRIPTION

Alzheimer's disease is a gradual deterioration of the cerebral cortex, basal forebrain, and other areas of the brain. The most typical early symptom is memory loss. This disease is progressive, reaching an advanced state in 2 to 3 years.

CAUSE

Alzheimer's disease is caused by the degeneration of the brain cells, characterized by a smoothening and flattening of the sulci and gyri and by plaque formations.

ASSESSMENT

Note: See APTA's Guide to Physical Therapist Practice. 2nd ed. *Physical Therapy.* 2001;81.

Neuromuscular Preferred Practice Patterns: A, E

AREAS
- History
- Cognition, including orientation, level of recall, and cognitive and dementia screening, as indicated
- Posture
- Gait: including observational gait analysis (OGA)
- Mobility
- Neurological, including sensation
- Skin and soft tissues
- Functional level, including activities of daily living (ADLs)
- Environmental assessment

INSTRUMENTS/PROCEDURES
See References for sources.

Cognition
- Mini-Mental State exam
- Short Portable Mental Status Questionnaire (SPMSQ)

Functional Level
- Barthel ADL index
- Physical ADL (PADL)
- Structural Assessment of Independent Living Skills (SAILS)

Special Tests to Which the Physical Therapist May or May Not Have Access
- cerebral angiography
- computed tomography (CT)
- digital-subtraction angiography
- doppler flowmetry
- electroencephalography(EEG)
- electromyography (EMG)
- evoked potentials
- lumbar puncture (LP)
- magnetic resonance imaging and magnetic resonance angiography (MRI or MRA)
- positron emission tomography (PET)
- x-ray

PROBLEMS

- The client often has diminished motor planning skills. There may be cognitive inability to follow gait-training instructions.
- The client may have a decreased incentive to walk.
- There can be ataxia of gait.
- The client may have diminished coordination.
- The client may have diminished balance.
- The client may have a decreased ability to use assistive devices.
- The client often has a decreased awareness of safety issues.

TREATMENT/MANAGEMENT

- Treatment focuses on addressing symptoms and planning a realistic program.
- Work with a multidisciplinary team.
- Provide activities to stimulate coordination.
- Provide gait training as indicated.
- Assess safety factors related to client's living environment.

PRECAUTIONS/CONTRAINDICATIONS

- Stress safety issues with client and caregiver.

EXPECTED OUTCOME/PROGNOSIS

- The client will have an increased incentive to walk and improved motor planning skills.
- The client will maintain ability to use assistive devices as needed.
- The client will maintain coordination and balance.
- The client and any caregivers will have an increased awareness of safety issues.

REFERENCES

Assessment

American Physical Therapy Association. Guide to physical therapist practice. 2nd ed. *Phys Ther.* 2001;81.

DeLisa D. *Rehabilitation Medicine: Principle and Practice.* Philadelphia, Pa: Lippincott; 1998.

Grabois M, Garrison SJ, Hart KA, Lehmkuhl LD. *Physical Medicine and Rehabilitation: The Complete Approach.* Malden, Mass: Blackwell Science; 2000.

Patla AE, Clous SD. Visual assessment of human gait: reliability and validity. *Rehab Res.* 1998;1:87–96.

Sine R, Liss SE, Rousch RE, et al. *Basic Rehabilitation Techniques: A Self-Instructional Guide.* 4th ed. Gaithersburg, Md: Aspen Publishers; 2000.

Treatment

American Physical Therapy Association. Guide to physical therapist practice. 2nd ed. *Phys Ther.* 2001;81.

Chong RK, Horak FB. Sensory organization for balance: specific deficits in Alzheimer's but not in Parkinson's disease. *J Gerontol.* Series A, Biological Sciences and Medical Sciences. 1999;54:M129–135.

Chong RK, Jones CL, Horak FB. Postural set for balance control is normal in Alzheimer's but not in Parkinson's disease. *J Gerontol.* Series A, Biological Sciences and Medical Sciences. 1999;54:M129–135.

Everett T, Dennis M, Ricketts E. *Physiotherapy in Mental Health: A Practical Approach.* Boston, Mass: Butterworth Heinemann; 1995.

Forsyth E, Ritzline PD. An overview of the etiology, diagnosis, and treatment of Alzheimer's disease. *Phys Ther.* 1998;78:1325–1331.

Hamman RJ. Rehabilitation following hip fracture in patients with Alzheimer's disease and related disorders. *Am J Alzheimer's Dis.* 1997;12:209–211.

National Institute on Disability and Rehabilitation Research. *Digest of Data on Persons with Disabilities.* Washington, DC: US Dept of Education; 1992.

Pomeroy VM. The effect of physiotherapy input on mobility skills of elderly people with severe dementing illness. *Clin Rehabil.* 1993;7:163–170.

Amyotrophic Lateral Sclerosis

DESCRIPTION

Amyotrophic lateral sclerosis (ALS) is a progressive motor neuron disorder leading to eventual degeneration of corticospinal tracts and/or bulbar motor nuclei and/or anterior horn cells. ALS affects both upper and lower motor neurons, resulting in a combination of spasticity along with lowered tone, weakness, and atrophy. The initial signs are often muscle cramps and/or muscular fasciculations. The progression of muscular weakness and atrophy is asymmetric, but sensory systems, voluntary eye movements, and urinary sphincters remain unaffected. The disease is more common in men than women, generally beginning at age 55. The disease is fatal for 50% of clients within 3 to 4 years following onset.

CAUSE

The cause is unknown, but may be related to the destruction of motor neurons due to an increase in stimulation of glutamate, which produces nitric oxide and can lead to neuron toxicity.

ASSESSMENT

Note: See APTA's Guide to Physical Therapist Practice. 2nd ed. *Physical Therapy.* 2001;81.

Neuromuscular Preferred Practice Pattern: E

AREAS
- History, including medications and metabolic status
- Cardiovascular, including endurance to activities
- Cognition, including behavioral factors
- Posture
- Pain
- Mobility, including active and passive range of motion (ROM)
- Motor control, including strength
- Pulmonary status
- Skin and soft tissue, including edema and open wounds
- Neurological, including sensation
- Gait: including observational gait analysis (OGA)

- Functional level, including, but not limited to, activities of daily living (ADLs), bed mobility, sitting, transfers, and standing
- Equipment, including appliances and assistive devices, and environmental assessment of needs upon discharge

INSTRUMENTS/PROCEDURES

See References for sources.

Functional Level
- Barthel index
- Health-Related Quality of Life (HRQL) (Shields)
- Medical Outcome Study Short Form (SF-36)
- Tufts Quantitative Neuromuscular Exam (TQNE)
- PULSES profile

Motor Control
- maximum voluntary isometric contraction
- manual muscle testing
- motor unit estimating methodology

Pulmonary Status
- manual muscle testing
- palpation
- pulmonary tests

Special Tests to Which the Physical Therapist May or May Not Have Access
- electromyography (EMG)
- bioelectrical impedance analysis (BIA)
- dual x-ray absorptiometry (DEXA)

PROBLEMS
- The client typically complains first of painful muscle cramps after exercise or certain movements. These cramps may also occur at night.
- Fasciculations are also a common initial complaint of ALS.
- The client often complains of weakness and fatigue with accompanying muscle atrophy, initally in the small muscles of the hand and forearm. At onset, the weakness can be unilateral, but the other side will be affected soon after. Other muscles that can be involved in the early stages include the shoulder, serratus anterior, and pectoralis major muscles.
- Historically, the pelvic and lower extremity muscles weaken and atrophy at a later stage.
- If bulbar paralysis is present, there may be unilateral wasting of the tongue.
- In later stages, the client may have difficulty with dysphagia, dysarthria, and mastication.
- Pseudobulbar reflexes can be triggered, leading to complusive crying, compulsive laughing, and a brisk masseter reflex.
- Speech impairment may be present and may lead to total anarthria.
- In the final phase, the client may have paralysis and impaired breathing but is usually conscious.

TREATMENT/MANAGEMENT

When planning an exercise program, the therapist should regard the following:
- nature and rate of disease progression
- level of activity and physical condition of client
- level of client's fatigue
- psychological factors

The therapist should prescribe an exercise plan according to client's individual needs and modify accordingly. Exercise/treatment activities may include:

- General conditioning: mild to moderate exercise of multiple muscle groups via swimming, stationary bike, rowing, or walking
- Isometric exercise: for use when spasticity from upper motor neuron involvement is present and causes discomfort. Recommend that the client hold contraction for maximum of 5- to 10-second intervals unless the client fatigues earlier.
- Isotonic exercise
- Postural training
- Dynamic balance activities
- Active-assistive exercise
- Passive range of motion
- Instruct in breathing exercises for conditioning of primary muscles of inspiration such as diaphragm and external intercostals. Primary muscles of expiration include the abdominal and internal intercostal muscles. These may be strengthened through partial sit-ups, rolling from supine to side-lying, pelvic tilt, posterior neck flexion, huffing, slow controlled exhale, coughing, and general conditioning. Use manual assistive compression over lateral costal or epigastric regions if cough is weak. Consider postural drainage, especially for clients with bulbar dysfunction, if indicated. Vibration is usually tolerated better than percussion. Other respiratory techniques to consider include incentive spirometry to decrease atelectasis and manual techniques for chest wall mobility, such as stretching, squeezing, and posterior lifts.
- Provide gait training and assess need for ambulation aids and orthotics. Aids should ideally be lightweight yet stable.
- Provide functional training.

PRECAUTIONS/CONTRAINDICATIONS

- Endurance training is recommended when muscular weakness is minimal and should be performed at a submaximal level.
- Swimming is not recommended for clients with bulbar involvement due to risk of choking episodes.
- Isometric exercise may induce cramping in clients who do not have upper motor neuron symptoms.
- Isotonic and isokinetic exercise should be monitored closely to avoid overfatigue. Areas with extreme weakness are prone to cramping; resistive exercise should be avoided in these areas.

DESIRED OUTCOME/PROGNOSIS

- The client will function physically at the peak of his or her neuromuscular capacity.
- The client will ambulate independently with inhibition of unwanted tone.
- Contractures will be prevented.
- Breathing exercises will assist in conditioning of the primary muscles of inspiration and expiration to obtain maximal ventilatory muscle strength.
- Functional training will enable client to perform optimal ADLs.

Clinical studies addressing the effect of exercise on ALS are limited. Clients who demonstrate gains in strength through exercise are generally in the early or moderate stage of ALS, with the disease progressing slowly, and were inactive before the exercise program began.

REFERENCES

Assessment

American Physical Therapy Association. Guide to physical therapist practice. 2nd ed. *Phys Ther.* 2001;81.

DeLisa D. *Rehabilitation Medicine: Principle and Practice.* Philadelphia, Pa: Lippincott; 1998.

Grabois M, Garrison SJ, Hart KA, Lehmkuhl LD. *Physical Medicine and Rehabilitation: The Complete Approach.* Malden, Mass: Blackwell Science; 2000.

Patla AE, Clous SD. Visual assessment of human gait: reliability and validity. *Rehabil Res.* 1998;1:87–96.

Sine R, Liss SE, Rousch RE, et al. *Basic Rehabilitation Techniques: A Self-Instructional Guide.* 4th ed. Gaithersburg Md: Aspen Publishers; 2000.

Treatment

Dal Bello-Haas V, Kloos AD, Misumoto H. Physical therapy for a patients through six stages of amyotrophic lateral sclerosis. *Phys Ther.* 1998;78:1312–1324.

Grabois M, Garrison SJ, Hart KA, Lehmkuhl LD. *Physical Medicine and Rehabilitation: The Complete Approach.* Malden, Mass: Blackwell Science; 2000.

Jette DU, Slavin MD, Andres PL, et al. The relationship of lower-limb muscle force to walking ability in patients with amyotrophic lateral sclerosis. *Phys Ther.* 1999;79:672–681.

McComas AJ, Galea V, de-Bruin H. Motor unit populations in healthy and diseased muscles. *Phys Ther.* 1993;73:868–877.

Miller RG, Anderson FA, Bradley WG, et al. The ALS patient care database: goals, design, and early results. ALS C.A.R.E. Study Group. *Neurology.* 2000;54:53–57.

Munsat TL, Andres P, Skerry L. Therapeutic trials in amyotrophic lateral sclerosis. In: Rose FC, ed. *Amyotrophic Lateral Sclerosis.* New York, NY: Demos Publications; 1990:65–76.

Nau KL, Dick AR, Peters K, et al. Relative validity of clinical techniques for measuring the body composition of persons with amyotrophic lateral sclerosis. *J Neurol Sci.* 1997;152 suppl 1:S36–42.

Pandya S. Evaluation and management of patients with neuromuscular diseases. *Neurol Rep.* 1993;17:15–20.

Peruzzi AC, Potts AF. Physical therapy intervention for persons with amyotrophic lateral sclerosis. *Physiotherapy Can.* 1996;48:119–126.

Shields RK, Ruhland JL, Ross MA, et al. Analysis of health-related quality of life and muscle impairment in individuals with amyotrophic lateral sclerosis using the medical outcome survey and the Tufts Quantitative Neuromuscular Exam. *Arch Phys Med Rehabil.* 1998;79:855–862.

Slavin MD, Jette DU, Andres PL, et al. Lower extremity muscle force measures and functional ambulation in patients with amyotrophic lateral sclerosis. *Arch Phys Med Rehabil.* 1998;79:950–954.

Smith PS, Dal Bello-Haas V, Kloos AD, et al. Physical therapy for a patient through six stages of amyotrophic lateral sclerosis. *Phys Ther.* 1999;79:423–424.

Trail M, Nelson N, Van JN, et al. Wheelchair use by patients with amyotrophic lateral sclerosis: a survey of user characteristics and selection preferences. *Arch Phys Med Rehabil.* 2001;82:98–102.

Carpal Tunnel Syndrome

DESCRIPTION

Carpal tunnel syndrome (CTS) is a type of peripheral neuropathy leading to compression of the median nerve on the volar side of the wrist. This compression occurs between the forearm flexor muscle tendons and the transverse superficial carpal ligament and produces hand pain, tingling, and numbness. CTS is more common in women than men and more common after age 40.

CAUSE

The cause often remains undetermined, but the condition can stem from vascular insufficiency of the median nerve at the carpal tunnel or direct pressure on the nerve. Possible causes include structural changes, cumulative effect of overuse, trauma, and physiological disorders. Disorders such as arthritis, hypothyroidism, acromegaly, and myxedema have been associated with CTS. CTS is also associated with work that demands repeated forceful flexion of the wrist. The fluid changes that accompany pregnancy can also trigger CTS.

ASSESSMENT

Note: See APTA's Guide to Physical Therapist Practice. 2nd ed. *Physical Therapy.* 2001;81.

Musculoskeletal Preferred Practice Pattern: F

AREAS

See also: Chapter 5, Hand Injuries.

- History
- Posture
- Pain
- Joint integrity
- Soft tissue, including tenderness, mobility, circulation, and edema, especially volar swelling
- Skin, including condition of nails
- Mobility, including active and passive range of motion (ROM) and accessory motion
- Strength, including grip strength, and thenar atrophy
- Neurological, including sensation, dexterity, coordination, and median, radial, and ulnar nerve pressure reactions
- Functional level

INSTRUMENTS/PROCEDURES

See References for sources.

Functional
- Boston carpal tunnel questionnaire
- Nine-Hole Peg Test (NHPT)
- Jebsen-Taylor test (JTT)

Neurological
- Tinel's sign
- Phalen's sign

Special Tests to Which the Physical Therapist May or May Not Have Access
- nerve conduction studies
- cervical nerve root involvement testing

Strength
- manual muscle testing
- dynamometry

PROBLEMS
- The client typically has pain and paresthesias, or pins-and-needles sensation, into the first 3 or 4 fingers and on the radial aspect of the hand, along with the wrist and possibly the forearm and shoulder. This pain usually starts out gradually and may progress to a constant sensation.
- The client often has decreased sensation in the affected hand.
- The pain is often worse at night, waking the client during sleep.
- There may be weakness in hand muscles, especially the thenar muscles.
- The client may report "clumsiness" when using fingers.
- The client may complain of limitation in daily activities due to symptoms.
- The client may also have cervical symptoms.

TREATMENT/MANAGEMENT

The acronym **PRICEMM** outlines a general approach for pain and inflammation (see Figure 10.1).

Specifically:
- Recommend rest if disorder is linked to unaccustomed excessive use.
- Prescribe resting splint (neutral or up to 20 degrees of extension) for work and at night. A splint may only be needed at night, especially after the first few weeks of symptom relief (avoid pressure over median nerve at wrist).
- Consider use of physical agents and modalities, such as iontophoresis.
- Soft tissue mobilization, joint mobilization, and neural mobilization may be indicated.

Protection

Rest: Eliminate aggravating activities

Ice

Compression

Elevation

Medication as prescribed

Modalities: high-voltage electrical stimulation, ultra-sound, ice, heat

FIGURE 10.1. PRICEMM acronym outlining general approach for pain and inflammation.

- Education and activity modifications are very important. Adapt work positions and body mechanics to avoid aggravating symptoms. Consider work height, altered posture, frequent rest periods, early treatment, and ergonomic assessment as indicated.

For treatment post surgery, consider the following:

- elevation for 3 to 4 days
- early passive mobilization of hand and wrist—begin active finger exercises for the first few weeks; exercises may include making a full fist, making a flat fist, making a hook fist, and extending thumb
- mobilization of carpal bones
- neural tissue mobilization
- soft tissue mobilization of transverse carpal ligament and at incision site

PRECAUTIONS/CONTRAINDICATIONS

- Teach client how to don and doff splint without fastening straps too tightly, which can interfere with circulation.
- Consider referral to surgeon if there is rapid progression of symptoms that would necessitate the surgical release of the transverse carpal ligament.

DESIRED OUTCOME/PROGNOSIS

- The client will have pain-free full use of upper extremity.
- Postsurgically, therapy will prevent adhesions that would interfere with space needed for median nerve within the carpal tunnel.

Note: Early intervention assists in more effective management.

REFERENCES

Assessment

American Physical Therapy Association. Guide to physical therapist practice. 2nd ed. *Phys Ther.* 2001;81.

DeLisa D. *Rehabilitation Medicine: Principle and Practice.* Philadelphia, Pa: Lippincott; 1998.

Ghavanini MR. Carpal tunnel syndrome: reappraisal of five clinical tests. *Electromyography and Clinical Neurophysiology.* 1998;38:437–441.

Grabois M, Garrison SJ, Hart KA, Lehmkuhl LD. *Physical Medicine and Rehabilitation: The Complete Approach.* Malden, Mass: Blackwell Science; 2000.

Hertling D, Kessler RM. *Management of Common Musculoskeletal Disorders.* 3rd ed. Philadelphia, Pa: JB Lippincott Co; 1996.

Levine DW. A self-administered questionnaire for the assessment of severity of symptoms and functional status in carpal tunnel syndrome. *J Bone Joint Surg.* 1993;75A:1585–1592.

Patla AE, Clous SD. Visual assessment of human gait: reliability and validity. *Rehabil Res.* 1998;1:87–96.

Rothstein JM, Roy SH, Wolf SL. *The Rehabilitation Specialist's Handbook.* 2nd ed. Philadelphia, Pa: FA Davis Co; 1998.

Sine R, Liss SE, Rousch RE, et al. *Basic Rehabilitation Techniques: A Self-Instructional Guide.* 4th ed. Gaithersburg, Md: Aspen Publishers; 2000.

Tomberlin JP, Saunders HD. *Evaluation, Treatment and Prevention of Musculoskeletal Disorders. Vol 2: Extremities.* Chaska, Minn: The Saunders Group; 1994:233.

Weinstein S. Fifty years of somotosensory research: from the Semmes-Weinstein monofilaments to the Weinstein enhanced sensory test. *J Hand Ther.* 1993;6:11–22.

Treatment

Anonymous. Can laser therapy alleviate carpal tunnel syndrome? *Clin Laser Monthly.* 1994;12:59–60.

Armstrong TJ. A conceptual model for work-related neck and upper-limb musculoskletal disorders. *Scand J Work Environ Health.* 1993;19:73–84.

Baker D, Wilson JK. Bilateral carpal tunnel syndrome in a piano teacher. *Phys Ther Case Rep.* 1999;2:73–76.

Banta CA. A prospective, nonrandomized study of iotophoresis, wrist splinting, and anti-inflammatory medication in the treatment of early-mild carpal tunnel syndrome. *J Occup Med.* 1994;36:166–168.

Barthel HR, Miller LS, Deardorff WW, et al. Presentation and response of patients with upper extremity repetitive use syndrome to a multidisciplinary rehabilitation program: a retrospective review of 24 cases. *J Hand Ther.* 1998;11:191–199.

Bash DS, Farber RS. An examination of self-reported carpal tunnel syndrome symptoms in hand therapists, protective and corrective measures and job satisfaction. *Work: A Journal of Prevention, Assessment and Rehabilitation.* 1999;13:75–82.

Burke DT, Burke MM, Stewart GW, et al. Splinting for carpal tunnel syndrome: in search of the optimal angle. *Arch Phys Med Rehabil.* 1994;75:1241–1244.

Butterfield PG, Spencer PS, Redmond N, et al. Clinical and employment outcomes of carpal tunnel syndrome in Oregon workers; compensation recipients. *J Occup Rehabil.* 1997; 7:61–73.

Calandruccio JH, Jobe MT, Akin K. Rehabilitation of the hand and wrist. In: *Handbook of Orthopaedic Rehabilitation,* Brozman SB, ed. St. Louis, Mo: Mosby Year Book; 1996.

Deliss L. Ultrasound treatment for carpal tunnel syndrome. Emphasis must be on return of sensation and function. *BMJ.* 1998;317:601.

Engenbichler GR, Resch KL, Nicolakis P, et al. Ultrasound treatment for treating the carpal tunnel syndrome: randomized "sham" controlled trial. *Br Med J.* 1998;316:731–735.

Feuerstein M, Burrell LM, Miller VI, et al. Clinical management of carpal tunnel syndrome: a 12-year review of outcomes. *Am J Ind Med.* 1999;35:232–245.

Feuerstein M, Miller VL, Burrell LM, et al. Occupational upper extremity disorders in the federal workforce. Prevalence, health care expenditures, and patterns of work disability. *J Occup Environ Med.* 1998;40:546–555.

Fish DR, Morris-Allen DM. Musculoskeletal disorders in dentists. *NY State Dent J.* 1998;64: 44–48.

Franzblau A. Workplace surveillance for carpal tunnel syndrome: a comparison of methods. *J Occup Rehabil.* 1993;3:1–14.

Gleeson P, Pauls J. Carpal tunnel syndrome during pregnancy and lactation. *PT Magazine of Phys Ther.* 1993;9:52–54.

Grabois M, Garrison SJ, Hart KA, Lehmkuhl LD. *Physical Medicine and Rehabilitation: The Complete Approach.* Malden, Mass: Blackwell Science; 2000.

Headley BJ. Carpal tunnel syndrome. *Advance for Directors in Rehabilitation.* 1994;3:2:19–23.

Hertling D, Kessler RM. *Management of Common Musculoskeletal Disorders.* 3rd ed. Philadelphia, Pa: JB Lippincott Co; 1996.

Manente G, Torrieri F, Pineto F, et al. A relief maneuver in carpal tunnel syndrome. *Muscle Nerve.* 1999;22:1587–1589.

McAtamney L, Corlett EN. RULA: a survey method for the investigation of work-related upper limb disorders. *Appl Ergonomics*. 1993;24:91–99.

Nagai L, Eng J. Overuse injuries incurred by musicians. *Physiotherapy Can*. 1992;44:23–30.

Nathan PA, Meadows KD, Keniston RC. Rehabilitation of carpal tunnel surgery patients using a short surgical incision and an early program of physical therapy. *J Hand Surg*. 1993;18:1044–1050.

Nathan PA, Meadows KD, Keniston RC. Predictors of return to work after carpal tunnel release. *Am J Ind Med*. 1997;32:321–323.

Ozatas O, Turan B, Bora I, et al. Ultrasound therapy effect in carpal tunnel syndrome. *Arch Phys Med Rehabil*. 1998;79:1540–1544.

Parenmarck G, Alffram PE, Malmkvist AK. The significance of work tasks for rehabilitation outcome after carpal tunnel surgery. *J Occup Rehabil*. 1992;2:89–94.

Provinciali L, Giattini A, Splendiani G, et al. Usefulness of hand rehabilitation after carpal tunnel surgery. *Muscle and Nerve*. 2000;23:211–216.

Quarrier NF. Performing arts medicine: the musical athlete. *J Orthop Sports Phys Ther*. 1993;17:90–95.

Rozmaryn LM, Dovelle S, Rothman ER, et al. Nerve and tendon gliding exercises and the conservative management of carpal tunnel syndrome. *J Hand Ther*. 1998;11:171–179.

Saidoff DC, McDonough AL. *Critical Pathways in Therapeutic Intervention*. Philadelphia, Pa: CV Mosby Co; 2002.

Sailer SM, Lewis SB. Rehabilitation and splinting of common upper extremity injuries in athletes. *Clin Sports Med*. 1995;14:411–446.

Shirley KD, Lwenstein KL. The hand. *Orthop Phys Ther Clin North Am*. 1997;6:283–304.

Stolp-Smith KA, Pascoe MK, Ogburn PL Jr. Carpal tunnel syndrome in pregnancy: frequency, severity, and prognosis. *Arch Phys Med Rehabil*. 1998;79:1285–1287.

Sunders R, Anderson M. Early treatment intervention. *Orthop Phys Ther Clin North Am*. 1992;1:67–74.

Tittiranonda P, Rempel D, Armstrong T, et al. Effect of tour computer keyboards in computer users with upper extremity musculoskeletal disorders. *Am J Ind Med*. 1999;35:647–661.

Vanderpool HE, Friis EA, Smith BS, Harms KL. Prevalence of carpal tunnel syndrome and other work-related musculoskeletal problems in cardiac sonographers. *J Occup Med*. 1993;35:604–610.

Wadsworth C. Carpal tunnel syndrome: can you identify the contributing factors? *PT Magazine of Physical Therapy*. 1999;7:50–59.

Wadsworth CT. Elbow, forearm, wrist, and hand. In: Myers RS, ed. *Saunders Manual of Physical Therapy Practice*. Philadelphia, Pa: WB Saunders Co; 1995.

Chronic Pain

DESCRIPTION

Pain is typically classified as chronic when it continues for more than 3 to 6 months. The pain is no longer serving its role as a signal of biological injury or damage. Chronic pain is the pain that remains even after the initial damage has been physically healed. Even if little or no organic cause is identified, the pain is still quite "real." Clients with chronic pain may also display somatic symptoms such as weight change, sleep disturbance, and diminished libido. Depression is common. For many clients, the psychological state affects impairment more than any organic disease.

CAUSE

The cause of chronic pain is often unclear, but one system classifies the pathogenesis of pain as nociceptive, neuropathic, or psychogenic.

- *Nociceptive:* somatic or visceral pain caused by activation of pain-reactive nerve fibers
- *Neuropathic:* central, peripheral, or sympathetically mediated pain caused by damage to afferent nerve pathways
- *Psychogenic:* usually involves pain without an organic lesion and includes somatization disorder, psychogenic pain, and hypochondriasis; this category also includes syndromes in which there is an organic component. Musculoskeletal disorders in the spine leading to chronic pain include the following: postural pain, derangement, degenerative joint disease, facet joint pathology, compression fracture, spinal fusion, arachnoiditis, postoperative scarring, spondylolisthesis, piriformis syndrome, and cervical spine pain. Other pain syndromes include reflex sympathetic dystrophy, postherpetic neuralgia, amputation, and chronic abdominal pain.

ASSESSMENT

Note: See APTA's Guide to Physical Therapist Practice. 2nd ed. *Physical Therapy.* 2001;81.

Musculoskeletal Preferred Practice Patterns: B, D, E, F, I

Neuromuscular Preferred Practice Pattern: D

AREAS

- History, including mental status, daily schedule, work history, medical status, and surgical history
- Vital statistics: blood pressure, heart rate, pulse
- Pain, including aggravating factors, remitting factors, nature of pain over a 24-hour period, sleep, quality of pain
- Headache (if applicable)
- Posture
- Gait: including observational gait analysis (OGA)
- Mobility, including active and passive range of motion (ROM) and accessory movements
- Strength
- Coordination
- Neurological, including sensation, reflexes, dural tension signs, vertebral artery tests, and Babinski
- Skin and soft tissue
- Cardiovascular, including endurance and fitness level
- Functional level
- Health status

INSTRUMENTS/PROCEDURES

See References for sources.

Functional Level
- Functional Interference Estimate
- Functional Assessment Screening Questionnaire

- Personality-Physical-Cognitive (PPC) questionnaire
- visual analog scale

Headache
- Mood Adjective Checklist
- passive accessory intervertebral mobility (PAIVM) exam
- plumbline postural assessment

Health Status
- Sickness Impact Profile

Pain
- body pain diagrams
- box scale
- descriptor differential scale
- forceps algometer
- McGill Pain Questionnaire (MPQ)
- McGill Melzack Short Form
- Multidimensional Pain Inventory (MPI)
- Numeric Pain Rating Scale
- pain diary
- Pain Disability Index
- pain perception profile
- pain threshold measures
- Pain and Impairment Relationship Scale (PAIRS)
- palpation
- pressure dolorimeter
- Symptom Checklist 90 (SCL-90)
- verbal rating scale
- visual analog scale

Special Tests to Which the Physical Therapist May or May Not Have Access
- electromyography (EMG)

PROBLEMS
- The client has pain that may be accompanied by musculoskeletal and neuromuscular dysfunction.
- The client may have selected joint and soft tissue restriction.
- There may be areas of muscular weakness, instability, or imbalance.
- The client may have muscle spasm.
- The client may have related gait abnormalities.
- The client often has accompanying postural deviations.
- The client often has decreased independence in functional activities.
- The client often has decreased cardiovascular fitness.
- The client reports tension, and there is often difficulty with relaxation response.

TREATMENT/MANAGEMENT
Treatment should be designed with a client's individual needs in mind. Physical therapy is one component of a team approach that may also include behavior modification and family education.

Consider referral to vocational counseling, a support group, and counseling.

Recognize that pain-relieving techniques are often the secondary issue; the primary concern is the management of a client with chronic pain that also has a psychological or psychiatric component. Teach the client the concept that pain relief is not the primary goal, but part of working to criterion.

Consider the following strategy (and see Table 10.1):
- Provide information on origin of pain and exacerbating factors.
- Encourage the client to be an active participant in treatment.
- Consider behavioral factors when applying traditional physical therapy techniques, with emphasis on areas in which the client is motivated to attempt to improve function.
- Involve family and friends, as indicated.
- Provide a clear plan for cessation of treatment.

TABLE 10.1
Factors That Can Raise a Pain Threshold

Pain Factors	
Antidepressants	Mood Elevation
Analgesics	Relaxation
Anxiety Reduction	Rest/Sleep
Anxiolytics	Sympathy
Companionship	Symptom Relief
Diversional Activities	

Source: Reprinted with permission from Pflazer LA. Oncology: Examination, Diagnosis, and Treatment; Medical and Surgical Considerations. In: RS Myers, ed. *Saunders Manual of Physical Therapy and Practice.* Philadelphia, Pa: WB Saunders Co; 1995:839–852.

Individualize the client's treatment by choosing from the appropriate physical agents and modalities to modify pain, according to the following:

1. cold
   - ethyl chloride spray
   - ice massage
   - ice pack
   - chemical cold pack
2. combination cold/heat
   - contrast baths
3. electrical stimulation
   - alternating or direct current
   - high-voltage galvanic stimulation
   - iontophoresis
   - transcutaneous electrical nerve stimulation (TENS)
4. exercise
   - active
   - active-assistive
   - coordination
   - passive
   - proprioceptive neuromuscular facilitation
   - resistive
   - lifestyle modifications that include a general fitness exercise program
5. heat
   - hydrocollator packs, hydrotherapy, or paraffin bath for superficial heating
   - diathermy, microwave or shortwave, or ultrasound for deep heating
6. manual therapy
   - mobilization
   - muscle energy techniques
7. massage
   - effleurage
   - friction
   - petrissage
   - percussion
   - soft tissue mobilization
   - trigger point deactivation
   - vibration
   - accupressure
   - deep tissue massage
8. pacing
   - endurance activities
   - functional training

- work hardening (see also section "Low Back Pain," Chapter 9)
- proper body mechanics

9. relaxation
   - breathing techniques
   - EMG biofeedback
   - progressive relaxation
   - autogenic training
   - stress management
10. sensory training
    - desensitization
11. traction
    - intermittent
    - manual
    - positional
    - static

PRECAUTIONS/CONTRAINDICATIONS

- *Contrast baths:* contraindicated in clients with Berger's disease, Raynaud's disease, or sensory loss.
- *Cryotherapy:* contraindicated with Raynaud's disease.
- *Diathermy:* same as with other heat modalities.

Note: Diathermy should not be used over areas of poor circulation, malignancies, pregnant uterus, thrombophlebitis, or hemorrhagic diathesis. Use with special caution if sensation is diminished or if client is debilitated. Microwave diathermy is contraindicated in areas of eyes. Shortwave diathermy can be used, with caution, if contact lenses are taken off.

- *Electrical stimulation:* primarily contraindicated in a client with a cardiac disease that requires use of demand-type pacemakers or a client prone to arrhythmias due to electrical stimulation; contraindicated with phlebothrombosis and skin disorders.
- *Hydrocollator packs:* use cautiously. May be contraindicated over areas of inflammation, with areas with decreased sensation, or over open lesions.
- *Hydrotherapy:* use cautiously. May be contraindicated in clients with infections with swelling, peripheral vascular disease, or rash, or in clients who cannot withstand any increase in core temperature.
- *Massage:* use with caution. May be contraindicated with acute circulatory disorder, infection, malignancies, and select skin diseases.
- *Mobilization:* contraindicated with active disk prolapse with herniation with no neurologic signs, acute arthritis, hypermobility, malignancy, osteoporosis, fractures, osteomyelitis, ruptured ligaments, scoliosis, spondylosis, spondylolisthesis, and tuberculosis. Use with caution if client is debilitated, has ligamentous laxity, is pregnant, or has upper respiratory tract infection.
- *Paraffin baths:* use cautiously. May be contraindicated over areas of decreased circulation or sensation, infection, malignancies, or open lesions.
- *Traction:* contraindicated with acute trauma, acute inflammation, hemorrhage, malignancy, acute lumbago (as per source). Use cautiously with clients with neurological disorders.
- *Ultrasound:* contraindicated over areas of diminished circulation; over area of growth center of bone until growth is complete; over area of pacemaker implantation, healing fracture, pregnant uterus, or malignancy; over the eye; or over the spinal cord.

DESIRED OUTCOME/PROGNOSIS

- The client will be educated about pain reduction techniques.
- The client will eliminate or reduce pain. Caution client not to expect complete alleviation of the pain.
- Therapy will reduce stress on structures involved and promote healing.
- The client will control any edema formation and prevent secondary loss and disability.
- The client will restore function and increase stamina, endurance, and tolerance to functioning even when there is pain.
- The client will modify neuronal activity and stimulate release of endorphins.
- The client will promote autonomic homeostasis.
- The client will increase in movement awareness, muscle skill, strength, flexibility, and normalization strategies.
- The client will identify pain behaviors and work to eliminate them.
- Therapy will facilitate adaptation to any permanent disability.

Some clients do not seem to gain a favorable outcome from therapy. These clients may be affected by the following factors:

- incongruity between history and objective exam
- uncooperativeness with treatment
- unrealistic expectations
- litigation (this does not necessarily affect the outcome, but may be a factor)
- no interest in returning to work or ADLs

Notes: Functional improvement should be compared to client's baseline and not to the average person's schedule.

The most common types of pain treated at pain treatment centers are cervical pain, lower back pain, headache, nerve root injury, and myofascial syndromes.

REFERENCES

Assessment

American Physical Therapy Association. Guide to physical therapist practice. 2nd ed. *Phys Ther.* 2001;81.

DeLisa D. *Rehabilitation Medicine: Principle and Practice.* Philadelphia, Pa: JB Lippincott Co; 1998.

Delitto A, Strube MJ, Shulman AD, Minor SD. A study of discomfort with electrical stimulation. *Phys Ther.* 1992;72:410–424.

Echternack JL. Clinical evaluation of the patient in pain. *Phys Ther Pract.* 1993;2:3:14–16.

Differential Diagnosis

Goodman C, Snyder TE. *Differential Diagnosis in Physical Therapy.* 2nd ed. Philadelphia, Pa; WB Saunders Co; 2000.

Grabois M, Garrison SJ, Hart KA, Lehmkuhl LD. *Physical Medicine and Rehabilitation: The Complete Approach.* Malden, Mass: Blackwell Science; 2000.

Griegel-Morris P, Larson K, Mueller-Klaus K, Oatis CA. Incidence of common postural abnormalities in the cervical, shoulder, and thoracic regions and their association with pain in two age groups of healthy subjects. *Phys Ther.* 1992;72:425–431.

Headley BJ. Chronic pain management. In: O'Sullivan SB, Schmitz TJ, eds. *Physical Rehabilitation.* 3rd ed. Philadelphia, Pa: FA Davis Co; 1994.

Hogeweg JA, Langereis MJ, Bernards AT, et al. Algometry: measuring pain threshold, method and characteristics in healthy subjects. *Scand J Rehabil Med.* 1992;24:99–103.

Levoska S, Keinanen-Kiukaanniemi S, Bloigu R. Repeatability of measurement of tenderness in the neck-shoulder region by a dolorimeter and manual palpation. *Clin J Pain.* 1993;9:229–235.

Patla AE, Clous SD. Visual assessment of human gait: reliability and validity. *Rehabil Res.* 1998;1:87–96.

Rothstein JM, Roy SH, Wolf SL. *The Rehabilitation Specialist's Handbook.* 2nd ed. Philadelphia, Pa: FA Davis Co; 1998.

Simmonds M, Wessel J, Scudds R. The effect of pain quality on the efficacy of conventional TENS. *Physiotherapy Can.* 1992;44:35–40.

Sine R, Liss SE, Rousch RE, et al. *Basic Rehabilitation Techniques: A Self-Instructional Guide.* 4th ed. Gaithersburg, Md: Aspen Publishers; 2000.

Toomey TC, Mann JD, Hernandez JT, Abashian SW. Psychometric characteristics of a brief measure of pain-related functional impairment. *Arch Phys Med Rehabil.* 1993; 74:1305–1308.

Watson DH, Trott PH. Cervical headache: an investigation of natural head posture and upper cervical flexor muscle performance. *Cephalalgia.* 1993;13:272–284.

Treatment

Adams N, Ravey J, Taylor D. Psychological models of chronic pain and implication for practice. *Physiotherapy.* 1996;82:124–129.

Alexander KM, Kinney LaPier TL. Differences in static balance and weight distribution between normal subjects and subjects with chronic unilateral low back pain. *J Orthop Sports Phys Ther.* 1998;28:378–383.

American Physical Therapy Association. Guide to physical therapist practice. 2nd ed. *Phys Ther.* 2001;81.

Ashburn MA, Staats PS. Management of chronic pain. *Lancet.* 1999;353:1865–1869.

Askew R, Kibelstis C, Overbaugh S. Physical therapists' perception of patients' pain and its effect on management. *Physiotherapy Res Int.* 1998;3:37–57.

Barkin RL, Lubenow TR, Bruehl S, et al. Management of chronic pain. Part I. *Disease-A-Month.* 1996;42:389–454.

Barkin RL, Lubenow TR, Bruehl S, et al. Management of chronic pain. Part II. *Disease-A-Month.* 1996;42:457–507.

Bongers PM, deWinter CR, Kompier MA, et al. Psychosocial factors at work and musculoskeletal disease. *Scand J Work Environ Health.* 1993;297–312.

Chabal C, Fishbain DA, Weaver M, et al. Long-term transcutaneous electrical nerve stimulation (TENS) use: impact on medication utilization and physical therapy costs. *Clin J Pain.* 1998;14:66–73.

Clark WC. Pain and Suffering. In: Downey JA, Myers SJ, Gonzalez EG, et al, eds. *The Physiological Basis of Rehabilitation Medicine.* 2nd ed. Boston, Mass: Butterworth Heinemann; 1994:705.

Conaty J. Physiotherapy with alcohol and drug dependent patients: implications for general settings. *Physiotherapy Can.* 1992;44:31–34.

Cornwall J, Mercer S, Harris AJ. Pain of cortical origin-implications fot treatment. *NZ J Physiotherapy.* 2000;28:29–32.

Crook J, Tunks E. Pain clinics. *Rheum Dis Clin North Am.* 1996;22:599–611.

Ellis B. Short report: transcutaneous electrical nerve stimulation for pain relief: recent research finding sand implications for clinical use. *Phys Ther Rev.* 1998;3:3–8.

Feine JS, Widmer CG, Lund JP. Physical therapy: a critique. *Oral Surg.* 1997;83:123–127.

Ferrell BA, Josephson KR, Pollan AM, et al. A randomized trial of walking versus physical methods for chronic pain management. *Aging* (Milano). 1997;9:99–105.

Fishbain DA, Chabal C, Abbott A, et al. Transcutaneous electrical nerve stimulation (TENS) treatment outcome in long-term users. *Clin J Pain.* 1996;12:201–214.

Flicker PL, Flechenstein JL, Ferry K, et al. Lumbar muscle usage in chronic low back pain:magnetic resonance image evaluation. *Spine.* 1993:582.

French S, ed. *Physiotherapy: A Psychosocial Approach.* London, England: Butterworth Heinemann; 1992.

Gallager RM. Treatment planning in pain medicine. Integrating medical, physical, and behavioural therapies. *Med Clin North Am.* 1999;83:823–849.

Grabois M, Garrison SJ, Hart KA, Lehmkuhl LD. *Physical Medicine and Rehabilitation: The Complete Approach.* Malden, Mass: Blackwell Science; 2000.

Gridley L, vanden Dolder PA. The percentage improvement in pain scale as a measure of physiotherapy treatment effects. *Aust J Physiotherapy.* 2001;47:133–136.

Hadjistavropoulos HD, Clark J. Using outcome evaluations to assess interdisciplinary actue and chronic pain programs. *Joint Commision Journal on Quality Improvement.* 2001; 27:335–348.

Hadjistavropoulos HD, Hadjistravropoulos T, Quine A. Health anxiety moderates the effects of distraction versus attention to pain. *Behav Res Ther.* 2000;38:425–438.

Hanegan JL. Principles of nociception. In: Gersch MR, ed. *Electrotherapy in Rehabilitation.* Philadelphia, Pa: FA Davis Co; 1992.

Hankin HA, Spencer T, Kegerreis S, et al. Analysis of pain behavior profiles and functional disability in outpatient physical therapy clinics. *J Orthop Sports Phys Ther.* 2001; 31:90–95.

Harding V, Watson PJ. Increasing activity and improving function in chronic pain management. *Physiotherapy.* 2000;86:619–630.

Harding V, Williams ACD. Extending physiotherapy skills using a psychological approach: cognitive-behavioural management of chronic pain. *Physiotherapy.* 1995;81:681–688.

Harding VR, de C Williams A. Activities training: integrating behavioural and cognitive methods with physiotherapy in pain management. *J Occup Rehabil.* 1998:47–60.

Harman K. Neuroplasticity and the development of persistent pain. *Physiotherapy Can.* 2000;52:64–71.

Headley BJ. The use of biofeedback in pain management. *Phys Ther Pract.* 1993;2:2:49–56.

Herbert P, Rochman DL. Dealing with pain. *Rehab Management: the Interdisciplinary Journal of Rehabilitation.* 1998;11:56–59.

Hobden J. Easing away adolescent pain. *Physiotherpay Frontline.* 1999;5:17.

Jensen MP, Turner JA, Romano JM, et al. Comparative reliability and validity of chronic pain intensity measures. *Pain.* 1999;83:157–162.

King RB. Managing symptom magnification. In: D'Orazio BP, ed. *Back Pain Rehabilitation.* Boston, Mass: Andover Medical Publishers; 1993.

Kramis RC, Robers UJ, Gilletee RG. Non-nociceptive aspects of persistent musculoskeletal pain. *J Orthop Sports Phys Ther.* 1996;23:255–267.

Injury Specialists Physical Therapy Manual. Bridgeton, Mo: Physicians' Pain Management Center; 1994.

Lanes TC, Gauron EF, Spratt KF, et al. Long-term follow-up of patients with chronic back pain treated in a multidisciplianry rehabilitation program. *Spine*. 1995:801.

Leino P. Magni G. Depressive and distress symptoms as predictors of low back pain, neck-shoulder pain, and other musculoskeletal morbidity: a 10-year follow-up of metal industry employees. *Pain*. 1993:89–94.

Marcus DA. Treatment of nonmalignant chronic pain. *Am Fam Physician*. 2000;61:1331–1346.

Martensson L, Marklund B, Fridlund B. Evaluation of a biopsychosocial rehabilitation programme in primary healthcare for chronic pain patients. *Scand J Occup Ther*. 1999;6:157–165.

Martinez A, Simmonds MJ, Novey DM. Physiotherpay for patients with chronic pain: an operant-behavioural approach. *Physiotherapy Theory and Practice*. 1997;13:97–108.

McCombe WS, Mushi R. Physical therapy in the multidisciplinary pain treatment center. *Phys Ther Pract*. 1993;2:3:57–60.

McDonald AJR, Coates TW. The discovery of transcutaneous spinal electroanalgesia and its relief of chronic pain. *Physiotherapy*. 1995;81:653–661.

Meilman PW. Chronic pain: treatment considerations. In: D'Orazio BP, ed. *Back Pain Rehabilitation*. Boston, Mass: Andover Medical Publishers; 1993.

Nolan MF. Contemporary perspectives on pain and discomfort. *Phys Ther Pract*. 1993;2:3:1–6.

Nolan MF, Wilson MCB. Patient-controlled analgesia: a method for the controlled self-administration of opioid pain medications. *Phys Ther*. 1995;75:374–379.

Palmer GE. Application of a data base to a military pain clinic. Uniformed Services University of the Health Sciences: 1996:36.

Pflazer LA. Oncology: Examination, Diagnosis, and Treatment; Medical and Surgical Considerations. In: RS Myers, ed. *Saunders Manual of Physical Therapy and Practice*. Philadelphia, Pa: WB Saunders Co; 1995.

Prip K. *Physiotherapy to Torture Survivors*. Copenhagen, Denmark: International Rehabilitation Council for Torture Victims; 1994.

Rainville J, Sobel J, Hartigan C, et al. Decreasing disability in chronic back pain through aggressive spine rehabilitation. *J Rehabil Res Dev*. 1997;34:383–393.

Richardson CA, Jull GA. Muscle control, pain control. What exercies would you prescribe? *Man Ther*. 1995;1:1–2.

Rissanen A, Kalimo H, Alaranta H. Effect of intensive training on the isokinetic strength and structure of lumbar muscles in patients with chronic low back pain. *Spine*. 1995:333.

Robinson AJ. Transcutaneous electrical nerve stimulation for the control of pain in musculoskeletal disorders. *J Orthop Sports Phys Ther*. 1996;24:208–226.

Ryan WE, Krishna MK, Swanson CE. A prospective study evaluationg early rehabilitation in preventing back pain chronicity in mine worker. *Spine*. 1995:489.

Schramm DM. The management of chronic pain. *Rehab Management: the Interdisciplinary Journal of Rehabilitation*. 1995;8:45–53.

Simmonds M, Wessel J, Scudds R. The effect of pain quality of the efficacy of conventional TENS. *Physiotherapy Can*. 1992;44:35–40.

Sluka KA. Pain mechanisms involved in musculoskeletal disorders. *J Orthop Sports Phys Ther*. 1996;24;240–254.

Smith BH, Hopton JL, Chambers WA. Chronic pain in primary care. *Fam Pract*. 1999;16:475–482.

Smith LM. Physiotherapy. In: Tyrer SP, ed. *Psychology, Psychiatry, and Chronic Pain*. London, England: Butterworth Heinemann; 1992:179–187.

Smithers M. An assessment of the efficacy of physical thepray and physical modalities for the control of chronic musculoskeletal pain. *D.C. Tracts.* 1999;11:19–20.

Solomon PE. *Measurement of Pain Behaviour.* 1996;48:52–58.

Trumble EA, Krengel MP. Physical therapy. In: Raj PP, ed. *Pain Medicine: A Comprehensive Review.* New York, NY: CV Mosby Co; 1996:335–338.

VanDender J. Myofascial trigger points. *Physical Therapy.* 2001;81:1059–1060.

von Nieda K, Michlovitz S. The application of physical agents in the treatment of patients with pain. *Phys Ther Prac.* 1993;2:3:45–50.

Warren E. Addiction. In: French S, ed. *Physiotherapy: A Psychosocial Approach.* London, England: Butterworth Heinemann; 1992.

Wells PE, Frampton V, Bowsher D. *Pain Management by Physiotherapy.* 2nd ed. Boston, Mass: Butterworth Heinemann; 1994.

Zoidis JD. Managing chronic pain. *Rehab Management: the Interdisciplinary Journal of Rehabilitation.* 1996;9:30–33.

Headache

Arena JE, Bruno GM, Hannah SI, et al. A comparison of frontal electromyographic biofeedback training, trapezius electromyographic biofeedback training and progressive relaxation therapy in the treatment of tension headache. *Headache.* 1995;35:411–419.

Boline PD, Kassak K, Bronfort G, et al. Spinal manipulation vs. amitriptyline for the treatment of chronic tension-type headaches: a randomized clinical trial. *J Manipulative Physiol Ther.* 1995;18:148–154.

Diener I. The impact of cervicogenic headache on patients attending a private physiotherapy practice in Cape Town. *S Afr J Physiotherapy.* 2001;57:35–39.

Grant T, Niere K. Techniques used by manipulative physiotherapists in the management of headaches. *Aust J Physiotherapy.* 2000;46:215–222.

Griegel-Morris P, Larson K, Mueller-Klaus K, Oatis CA. Incidence of common postural abnormalitites in the cervical, shoulder, and thoracic regions and their association with pain in two age groups of healthy subjects. *Phys Ther.* 1992;72:425–431.

Hamill JM, Cook TM, Rosecrance JC. Effectiveness of a physical therapy regime in the treatment of tension-type headache. *Headache.* 1996;36:149–153.

Nicholson GG, Gaston J. Cervical headache. *J Orthop Sports Phys Ther.* 2001;31:184–193.

Schonensee SK, Jensen G, Nicholson G, et al. The effect of mobilization on cervical headaches. *J Orthop Sports Phys Ther.* 1995;21:184–196.

Stone RG, Wharton RG. Simultaneous multiple-modality therapy for tension headaches and neck pain. *Biomed Instrum Technol.* 1997;31:259–262.

Watson DH, Trott PH. Cervical headache: an investigation of natural head posture and upper cervical flexor muscle performance. *Cephalalgia.* 1993;13:272–284.

Facial Palsy

Also known as *Bell's palsy.*

DESCRIPTION

Facial palsy is a peripheral lesion of the seventh cranial nerve leading to unilateral facial weakness or paralysis. Sensory changes usually appear before motor changes. This type of peripheral nerve lesion is categorized as a neuropraxia, or localized blockage of the nerve conduction.

CAUSE

Facial palsy may be caused by pressure from inflammation of the seventh cranial nerve inside its canal. This inflammation can be caused by conditions affecting the middle ear, by herpes zoster of the geniculate ganglion, or by an immune disease. Facial palsy can also be idiopathic.

ASSESSMENT

Note: See APTA's Guide to Physical Therapist Practice. 2nd ed. *Physical Therapy.* 2001;81.

Neuromusculoskeletal Preferred Practice Pattern: D

Musculoskeletal Preferred Practice Pattern: F

AREAS
- History
- Communication, including speech
- Pain
- Strength, including active motion of facial muscles and facial expression—especially muscles used in raising eyebrows, smiling, and showing lower teeth
- Neurological, including facial nerve and sensation, especially ability to distinguish between sugar and salt
- Functional level

INSTRUMENTS/PROCEDURES

See References for sources.

Functional
- Facial Motion Assay
- House-Brackmann scale
- Facial Grading System (FGS)
- Facial Disability Index (FDI)
- Beck Anxiety Inventory
- Beck Depression Inventory

Neurological
- cranial nerve testing
- electromyography (EMG)

Special Tests to Which the Physical Therapist May or May Not Have Access
- nerve conduction velocity tests

Strength
- manual muscle testing

PROBLEMS
- The client may complain of pain behind the ear before rapidly developing unilateral facial weakness.
- The client will often have a unilateral loss of facial expression.
- The client will typically be unable to purse lips or smile.
- The client may complain of loss of taste.
- The client will often be unable to close eye.

TREATMENT/MANAGEMENT
- Instruct client in active and active assistive facial exercises.
- Consider use of neuromuscular facilitation techniques.
- Use surface EMG to facilitate relearning of facial motor control.

- Encourage use of mirror as feedback during facial motion exercises.
- Work with psychological or psychiatric services and support groups to address the disfigurement that accompanies facial palsy, if indicated.

PRECAUTIONS/CONTRAINDICATIONS
- Refer to occupational therapy and/or speech therapy if client has persistent difficulty with eating, drinking, or speech.

DESIRED OUTCOME/PROGNOSIS
- The client will restore form, movement, and function of face.

Note: The majority of clients with facial palsy recover in 4 weeks.

REFERENCES

Assessment

DeLisa D. *Rehabilitation Medicine: Principle and Practice*. Philadelphia, Pa: Lippincott; 1998.

Grabois M, Garrison SJ, Hart KA, Lehmkuhl LD. *Physical Medicine and Rehabilitation: The Complete Approach*. Malden, Mass: Blackwell Science; 2000.

Rothstein JM, Roy SH, Wolf SL. *The Rehabilitation Specialist's Handbook*. 2nd ed. Philadelphia, Pa: FA Davis Co; 1998.

Sine R, Liss SE, Rousch RE, et al. *Basic Rehabilitation Techniques: A Self-Instructional Guide*. 4th ed. Gaithersburg, Md: Aspen Publishers; 2000.

Treatment

American Physical Therapy Association. Guide to physical therapist practice. 2nd ed. *Phys Ther*. 2001;81.

Blatt PJ. Unilateral vestibular lesions secondary to acoustic neuroma: review and case studies. *Neurology Report*. 1996;20:30–40.

Bourbon B. Craniomandibular examination and treatment. In: Myers RS, ed. *Saunders Manual of Physical Therapy Practice*. Philadelphia, Pa: WB Saunders Co; 1995:698–699.

Brach JS, VanSwearingen JM. Not all facial paralysis is Bell's palsy: a case report. *Arch Phys Med Rehabil*. 1999;80:857–859.

Brach JS, VanSwearingen JM. Physical therapy for facial paralysis: a tailored treatment approach. *Phys Ther*. 1999;79:397–404.

Brach JS, VanSwearingen J, Delitto A, et al. Impairment and disability in patients with facial neuromuscular dysfunction. *Otolaryngology and Head and Neck Surgery*. 1997:11.

Brach JS, VanSwearingen JM, Lenert J, et al. Facial neuromuscular retraining for oral synkinesis. *Plast Reconstr Surg*. 1997;99:1922–1931.

Dyck PJ, Haase G, May M. When you suspect Bell's palsy. *Patient Care*. 1992;26;151–154.

Grabois M, Garrison SJ, Hart KA, Lehmkuhl LD. *Physical Medicine and Rehabilitation: The Complete Approach*. Malden, Mass: Blackwell Science; 2000.

Henkelmann T. Bell palsy. *Phys Ther*. 1999;79:705–706.

Isaacs ER, Bookout MR. Screening for pathologic origins of head and facial pain. In: Boissonnault WG, ed. *Examination in Physical Therapy Practice: Screening for Medical Disease*. New York, NY: Churchill Livingstone; 1991:185.

Kendall FP, McCreary EK, Provance PG. *Muscles: Testing and Function*. 4th ed. Baltimore, Md: Williams and Wilkins; 1993.

Labbe D, Huaualt M. Lengthening temporalis myoplasty and lop reanimation.

Novak CB, Ross B, Mackinnon SE, Nedzelski JM. Facial sensibility in patients with unilateral facial nerve paresis. *Otolaryngol Head Neck Surg.* 1993;109:506–513.

Pennock JD, Johnson PC, Manders EK, et al. Relationship between muscle activity of the frontalis and the associated brow displacement. *Plast Reconstr Surg.* 1999;104: 1789–1797.

Portney LG. Electromyography and nerve conduction velocity tests. In: O'Sullivan SB, Schmitz TJ, eds. *Physical Rehabilitation: Assessment and Treatment.* 3rd ed. Philadelphia, Pa: FA Davis Co; 1994:150.

Sakashita H, Miyata M, Miyamoto H, et al. Peripheral facial palsy after sagittal split ramus osteotomy for setback of the mandible. A case report. *Int J Oral Maxillofac Surg.* 1996;25:182–183.

Samii M, Matthies C. Management of 1000 vestibular schwannomas (acoustic neuromas): the facial nerve-preservation and restitution of function. *Neurosurgery.* 1997;40: 684–694.

VanSwearingen J. Tracing a clinical path for saving face. *Advance/Rehabilitation.* 1994;4: 10:45–47.

VanSwearingen JM, Brach JS. Validation of a treatment-based classification system for individuals with facial neuromotor disorders. *Phys Ther.* 1998;78:678–689.

VanSwearingen JM, Cohn JF, Bajaj-Luthro A. Specific impairment of smiling increases the severity of depressive symptoms in patients with facial neuromuscular disorders. *Aesthetic Plast Surg.* 1999;23:416–423.

VanSwearingen JM, Cohn JF, Turnbull J, et al. Psychological distress: linking impairment with disability in facial neuromotor disorders. *Otolaryngol Head Neck Surg.* 1998;118: 790–796.

Guillain-Barré Syndrome

Also known as *acute inflammatory demyelinating polyradiculoneuropathy.*

DESCRIPTION

Guillain-Barré syndrome (GBS) is an acute polyneuropathy leading to muscular weakness and mild sensory loss.

CAUSE

Cause is unknown, but the syndrome is thought to have an autoimmune basis. When GBS appears, it usually occurs within a few days or weeks following a respiratory tract infection, influenza, immunization, or surgery.

ASSESSMENT

Note: See APTA's Guide to Physical Therapist Practice. 2nd ed. *Physical Therapy.* 2001;81.

Cardiopulmonary Preferred Practice Patterns: B, F, G

Neuromuscular Preferred Practice Pattern: E

AREAS
- History, including medications and metabolic status
- Communication, including speech, reading, and writing

- Vision
- Cognition, including behavioral factors
- Pain
- Posture, including any asymmetry
- Pulmonary, including dyspnea and ventilator dependency
- Cardiovascular status, including endurance to activities
- Genitourinary status, including incontinence
- Mobility, including active and passive range of motion (ROM)
- Motor control, including tone (resting and dynamic), reflexes (tonic reflexes, righting reflexes, equilibrium responses), balance and postural reactions, and active movement control, including coordination, patterned movement, and isolated movement
- Strength, especially cranial nerve function; testing may be delayed until client is stable
- Neurological, including sensation and sensory component of cranial nerves I, V, and VII through X
- Skin and soft tissue, including atrophy, edema, pressure sores, or open wounds
- Functional level, including but not limited to activities of daily living (ADLs), bed mobility, sitting, transfers, standing, and gait, as indicated
- Equipment, including appliances and assistive devices, and environmental needs upon discharge

INSTRUMENTS/PROCEDURES

See References for sources.

Functional Level
- Barthel index
- PULSES profile

Strength
- manual muscle testing

PROBLEMS
- The client may have respiratory insufficiency if intercostal muscles are affected. In severe cases, the client can also have acute respiratory failure.
- The client often has bilateral muscular weakness, especially in the lower extremities, ranging from slight decline to total paralysis.
- Approximately 50% of clients have facial palsy, which can be bilateral.
- Approximately 50% of clients have paresthesia of feet that moves proximally, possibly felt in hands.
- The client typically has symptoms related to autonomic nervous system dysfunction, such as arrhythmia, tachycardia, orthostatic hypotension, hyperhydrosis, urine retention, and possibly diminished reflexes.

TREATMENT/MANAGEMENT
- Perform passive ROM and proper positioning.
- Instruct in exercises for strength and endurance.
- Provide gait training as indicated.
- Prescribe orthotics if needed.
- Perform respiratory therapy as indicated for enhanced elimination of secretions. Train respiration muscles for strength and endurance by breathing against mouthpiece that applies inspiratory resistance.
- Initiate exercises that progressively increase in difficulty from passive to active-assistive to active exercise as tolerated. Avoid fatigue. In the early stages, only 1

or 2 repetitions are indicated. Begin strengthening and aerobic exercises, but not to overexertion.
- Instruct client in modification of ADLs as needed. Include weight shifting, rolling, bed mobility skills, and transfer training. Teach client pressure relief techniques to avoid skin breakdown.
- Consider gait training with assistive devices as indicated.
- Assess needs for adaptive equipment for home environment.
- Instruct client in wheelchair independence if indicated.
- Reassess status frequently.

PRECAUTIONS/CONTRAINDICATIONS
- Limit physical activity in the acute phase to avoid exacerbating symptoms.
- Avoid overexertion during assessment.
- Be alert for signs of autonomic dysreflexia (sudden increase in blood pressure), orthostatic hypotension, or deep-vein thrombosis.

EXPECTED OUTCOME/PROGNOSIS
- The client will avoid secondary problems of contractures and decubitis ulcers.
- The client will return to normal activities of daily living.

Notes: Maximal paralysis typically peaks at 1 to 3 weeks after onset. Approximately 30% of clients experience residual weakness at 3 years post onset.

REFERENCES

Assessment

DeLisa D. *Rehabilitation Medicine: Principle and Practice.* Philadelphia, Pa: JB Lippincott Co; 1998.

Grabois M, Garrison SJ, Hart KA, Lehmkuhl LD. *Physical Medicine and Rehabilitation: The Complete Approach.* Malden, Mass: Blackwell Science; 2000.

Patla AE, Clous SD. Visual assessment of human gait: reliability and validity. *Rehabilitation Research.* 1998;1:87–96.

Rothstein JM, Roy SH, Wolf SL. *The Rehabilitation Specialist's Handbook.* 2nd ed. Philadelphia, Pa: FA Davis Co; 1998.

Sine R, Liss SE, Rousch RE, et al. *Basic Rehabilitation Techniques: A Self-Instructional Guide.* 4th ed. Gaithersburg, Md: Aspen Publishers; 2000.

Treatment

Grabois M, Garrison SJ, Hart KA, Lehmkuhl LD. *Physical Medicine and Rehabilitation: The Complete Approach.* Malden, Mass: Blackwell Science; 2000.

Kendall FP, McCreary EK, Provance PG. *Muscles: Testing and Function.* 4th ed. Baltimore, Md: Williams and Wilkins; 1993.

Meythaler JM. Rehabilitation of Guillain-Barré syndrome. *Arch Phys Med Rehabil.* 1997; 78: 872–879.

Meythaler JM, DeVivo MJ, Braswell WC. Rehabilitation outcomes of patients who have developed Guillain-Barré syndrome. *Am J Phys Med Rehabil.* 1997;76:411–419.

Pitetti KH, Barrett PH, Abbas D. Endurance exercise training in Guillain-Barré syndrome. *Arch Phys Med Rehabil.* 1993;74:761–765.

Umphred DA. *Neurological Rehabilitation.* 3rd ed. St. Louis, Mo: CV Mosby Co; 1995.

Huntington's Disease

Also known as *Huntington's chorea* or *Chronic Progressive chorea.*

DESCRIPTION

Huntington's disease (HD) is a neurodegenerative disease characterized by choreiform movements and progressive dementia. Usually beginning in a client's 40s, it affects men and women at similar rates of 6.5 per 100,000 people.

CAUSE

HD is an inherited autosomal-dominant neurodegenerative disease. The abnormal Huntington gene has been located on the short arm of chromosome 4.

ASSESSMENT

Note: See APTA's Guide to Physical Therapist Practice. 2nd ed. *Physical Therapy.* 2001;81.

Neurological Preferred Practice Pattern: E

Cardiovascular/Pulmonary Preferred Practice Patterns: B, E

AREAS

- History
- Communication
- Cognition, including orientation
- Posture
- Mobility
- Neurological, including sensation
- Skin and soft tissue
- Gait: including observational gait analysis (OGA)
- Functional level including activities of daily living (ADLs)
- Environmental needs

INSTRUMENTS/PROCEDURES

See References for sources.

Functional Level
- Barthel index
- PULSES profile

PROBLEMS

- The client may have memory loss, cognitive impairment, and personality changes.
- There may be dysarthria and dysphagia.
- The gait is typically ataxic, with choreiform or choreoathetoid movements.
- In later stages, the client often has rigidity and akinesia.

TREATMENT/MANAGEMENT

- Use range of motion (ROM) and strengthening exercises to promote joint stability.
- Offer facilitation and inhibition techniques.
- Biofeedback and relaxation techniques may be useful in the early stages of disease.
- At later stages of the disease, the choreiform movements of the mouth may be decreased with slow rocking and neutral warmth.
- Select adaptive equipment as needed for ADLs, or consult with an occupational therapist.
- Education and support are crucial, particularly for family members and caregivers.

DESIRED OUTCOME/PROGNOSIS
- The client will have stabilized proximal joint musculature.
- The client will function at the highest level possible.

REFERENCES

Assessment

DeLisa D. *Rehabilitation Medicine: Principle and Practice.* Philadelphia, Pa: JB Lippincott Co; 1998.

Grabois M, Garrison SJ, Hart KA, Lehmkuhl LD. *Physical Medicine and Rehabilitation: The Complete Approach.* Malden, Mass: Blackwell Science; 2000.

Patla AE, Clous SD. Visual assessment of human gait: reliability and validity. *Rehabil Res.* 1998;1:87–96.

Rothstein JM, Roy SH, Wolf SL. *The Rehabilitation Specialist's Handbook.* 2nd ed. Philadelphia, Pa: FA Davis Co; 1998.

Sine R, Liss SE, Rousch RE, et al. *Basic Rehabilitation Techniques: A Self-Instructional Guide.* 4th ed. Gaithersburg, Md: Aspen Publishers; 2000.

Treatment

Corcos DM. Strategies underlying the control of disordered movement. *Phys Ther.* 1991;71:25–38.

Ferraro-Herrera As, Kern HB, Nagler W. Autonomic dysfunction as the presenting feature of Guillain-Barre syndrome. *Arch Phys Med Rehabil.* 1997;78:777–779.

Grabois M, Garrison SJ, Hart KA, Lehmkuhl LD. *Physical Medicine and Rehabilitation: The Complete Approach.* Malden, Mass: Blackwell Science; 2000.

Imbriglio S, Peacock IW. Huntington's disease at mid-stage. *Clin Manage Phys Ther.* 1992; 12:5:62–72.

Meythaler JM. Rehabilitation of Guillain-Barré syndrome. *Arch Phys Med Rehabil.* 1997;78: 872–879.

Quinn L, Reilmann R, Marder K, et al. Altered movement trajectories and force control during object transport in Huntington's disease. *Movement Disorders.* 2001;16:469–480.

Viegas GV. Guillain-Barré syndrome. Review and presentation of a case with pedal manifestations. *J Am Podiatr Med Assoc.* 1997;87:209–218.

Late Effects of Poliomyelitis

Also known as *late motor neuron degeneration, postpolio progressive muscular atrophy, postpolio muscular atrophy, postpolio sequelae, postpolio syndrome, chronic anterior poliomyelitis,* and *forme fruste amyotrophic lateral sclerosis.*

DESCRIPTION

Late effects of poliomyelitis are symptoms that occur years after the onset of poliomyelitis, often 30 to 40 years after. Twenty-five percent or more of clients who contracted polio during the poliomyelitic epidemics of the 1940s and 1950s are reporting new symptoms. Symptoms may include choking and dysphagia (problems swallowing), cold sensitivity, difficulty breathing, diminished endurance, fatigue, pain, psychological problems, and weakness.

CAUSE

The cause of late effects of polio is not fully established, but effects are triggered when remaining motor units become gradually more dysfunctional.

ASSESSMENT

Note: See APTA's Guide to Physical Therapist Practice. 2nd ed. *Physical Therapy.* 2001;81.

Musculoskeletal Preferred Practice Pattern: A

Neuromuscular Preferred Practice Pattern: G

AREAS
- History, including medications and metabolic status
- Pain
- Posture
- Cardiovascular, including endurance to activities
- Pulmonary
- Mobility: active and passive range of motion (ROM)
- Motor function
- Strength
- Neurological, including sensation
- Skin and soft tissue
- Gait: including observational gait analysis (OGA)
- Functional level, including, but not limited to, activities of daily living (ADLs), bed mobility, sitting, transfers, and standing
- Equipment, including use of orthotics, appliances, and assistive devices, and environmental needs upon discharge

INSTRUMENTS/PROCEDURES

See References for sources.

Functional Level
- Barthel ADL index
- PULSES profile

Motor Function
- motor unit estimating methodology

Mobility
- goniometry

Special Tests to Which the Physical Threrapist May or May Not Have Access
- electromyography (EMG)
- muscle biopsy
- nerve conduction studies
- serologic tests

Strength
- Cybex testing
- manual muscle testing

PROBLEMS
- The client often reports a gradual pattern of fatigue that can be either generalized or localized but is often most pronounced in the afternoon.
- The client may report diminished mental alertness.

- The client typically reports muscle weakness, especially in those muscles previously weakened.
- The client may notice muscular atrophy.
- The client may describe the appearance of fasciculations, especially in recently weakened muscles.
- The client typically has muscle pain often described as aching or cramping.
- The client often has joint pain that is exacerbated by activity.
- The client may report intolerance to cold.
- The client's symptoms can interfere with ADLs such as walking, climbing stairs, and dressing.
- The client may have difficulty with breathing.
- The client may have difficulty with swallowing.

TREATMENT/MANAGEMENT
- Instruct client in lifestyle modifications such as energy conservation techniques and pacing activities with rest to reduce chronic overuse.
- Instruct in proper body mechanics.
- Assess and treat for any secondary musculoskeletal dysfunction.
- Prescribe orthotics for joints that are overstressed.
- Assess gait pattern, and perform gait training as indicated.
- Assess for partial or full-time use of wheelchair.
- Exercise: Promote activity as indicated. Prescribe supervised nonfatiguing exercise program if client is deconditioned due to disuse. Exercise should target muscles with greater than fair strength (3/5). Reduce overactivity if chronic overuse is exacerbating symptoms. Muscles with less than fair strength (3/5) should not be overtaxed.
- Provide sources of psychosocial support and counseling to cope with new changes in symptoms.

PRECAUTIONS/CONTRAINDICATIONS
- Carefully monitor any exercise program.
- Encourage client to balance low-intensity exercise with rest.

DESIRED OUTCOME/PROGNOSIS
- The client will function at optimal level.
- Therapy will provide optimal joint function.

Notes: One report says clients may see an increase in muscle strength through resistance exercise that is nonfatiguing. The report cautions, however, that muscles should be tested every 3 months to ensure that the muscles are not undergoing overwork weakness. The influence of chronic overuse on weakness and pain is not fully understood. No research was found to support conventional muscle-strengthening programs.

REFERENCES

Assessment

Agre JC, Rodriguez AA, Franke TM. Subjective recovery time after exhausting muscular activity in postpolio and control subjects. *Am J Phys Med Rehabil.* 1998;77:140–144.

DeLisa D. *Rehabilitation Medicine: Principle and Practice.* Philadelphia, Pa: JB Lippincott Co; 1998.

Grabois M, Garrison SJ, Hart KA, Lehmkuhl LD. *Physical Medicine and Rehabilitation: The Complete Approach.* Malden, Mass: Blackwell Science; 2000.

Grimby G, Stalberg E, Sandberg A, et al. An 8-year longitudinal study of muscle strength, muscle fiber size, and dynamic electromyogram in individuals with late polio. *Muscle and Nerve*. 1998;21:1428–1437.

Ivanyi B, Nelemans PJ, deJonjh R, et al. Muscle strength in postpolio patients: a prospective follow-up study. *Muscle and Nerve*. 1996;19:738–742.

Kilmer DD, McCrory MA, Wright NE, et al. Hand-held dynamometry reliability in persons with neuropathic weakness. *Arch Phys Med Rehabil*. 1997;78:1364–1368.

Klein MG, Whyte J, Keenan MA, et al. Changes in strength over time among polio survivors. *Arch Phys Med Rehabil*. 2000;81:1059–1064.

Nollet F, Beelen A. Strength assessment in postpolio syndrome: validity of a hand-held dynamometer in detecting change. *Arch Phys Med Rehabil*. 1999;80:1316–1323.

Nollet F, Beelen A, Prins MH, et al. Disablility and functional assessment in former patients with and without postpolio syndrome. *Arch Phys Med Rehabil*. 1999;80:136–143.

Patla AE, Clous SD. Visual assessment of human gait: reliability and validity. *Rehabil Res*. 1998;1:87–96.

Rothstein JM, Roy SH, Wolf SL. *The Rehabilitation Specialist's Handbook*. 2nd ed. Philadelphia, Pa: FA Davis Co; 1998.

Sine R, Liss SE, Rousch RE, et al. *Basic Rehabilitation Techniques: A Self-Instructional Guide*. 4th ed. Gaithersburg, Md: Aspen Publishers; 2000.

Treatment

Bartfeld H, Ma D. Recognizing post-polio syndrome. *Hosp Pract*. 1996;31:95–107.

Bond V. Spotlight in post-polio syndrome. *Physiotherapy Moves*. 2000;15:17.

Grabois M, Garrison SJ, Hart KA, Lehmkuhl LD. *Physical Medicine and Rehabilitation: The Complete Approach*. Malden, Mass: Blackwell Science; 2000.

Grimby G, Jonsson AT. Disability in poliomyelitis sequelae. *Phys Ther*. 1994;74:415–424.

Halstead LS, Grimby G, eds. *Post-Polio Syndrome*. Philadelphia, Pa: Hanley and Belfus; 1995.

Hamzat TK. Cardiovascular responses to exercise test in subjects with poliomyelitits: A pilot study. *S Afr J Physiotherapy*. 2000;56:39–42.

Jubelt B, Drucker J. Poliomyelitis and the post-polio syndrome. In: Younger DS, ed. *Motor Disorders*. Philadelphia, Pa: Lippincott Williams and Wilkins; 1999.

Kendall FP, McCreary EK, Provance PG. *Muscles: Testing and Function*. 4th ed. Baltimore, Md: Williams and Wilkins; 1993.

Mayo clinic. Post-polio clinic. New problems from an old disease. *Mayo Clin Health Lett*. 2001;19:6.

McComas AJ, Galea V, de Bruin H. Motor unit populations in healthy and diseased muscles. *Phys Ther*. 1993;73:868–877.

Peach PE. Late effects of poliomyelitis. In: Fletcher GF, Banja JD, Jann BB, Wolf SL. *Rehabilitation Medicine Contemporary Clinical Perspectives*. Philadelphia, Pa: Lea and Febiger; 1992:128–135.

Torjan DA, Cashman NR. Pathophysiology and diagnosis of post-polio syndrome. *Neurorehabil*. 1997;8:83–92.

Umphred DA, ed. *Neurological Rehabilitation*. 3rd ed. St. Louis, Mo: CV Mosby Co; 1995.

Walker JM. Recognizing postpolio syndrome. *Can Fam Physician*. 1995;41:1155–1157.

Multiple Sclerosis

DESCRIPTION

Multiple sclerosis (MS) is a gradually progressive disease of the central nervous system. MS is also known as *disseminated sclerosis* due to disseminated spots of demyelination in the brain and spinal cord. The neurological problems reported by clients with MS demonstrate considerable variability. Women are affected slightly more frequently than men, with the age of onset occurring between 20 and 40.

CAUSE

Etiology is unknown, but MS is thought to be caused by an immunologic defect. There is also evidence suggesting genetic susceptibility. Environment may influence incidence, as MS occurs more frequently in temperate climates.

ASSESSMENT

Notes: See APTA's Guide to Physical Therapist Practice. 2nd ed. *Physical Therapy.* 2001;81.

Cardiopulmonary Preferred Practice Patterns: B, F, G

Integumentary Preferred Practice Pattern: A

Neuromuscular Preferred Practice Pattern: C

AREAS

- History, including medications and metabolic status
- Pain
- Posture
- Pulmonary
- Cardiovascular, including endurance to activities
- Mobility, including active and passive range of motion (ROM)
- Strength
- Spasticity
- Neurological, including sensation
- Skin and soft tissue, including open wounds
- Gait: including observational gait analysis (OGA)
- Functional level, including, but not limited to, activities of daily living (ADLs), bed mobility, sitting, transfers, and standing
- Equipment, including use of orthotics, appliances, and assistive devices, and environmental needs upon discharge

INSTRUMENTS/PROCEDURES

See References for sources.

Balance
- Berg Balance Test

Functional Level/Disability
- Barthel index
- Environmental and Incapacity Status Scales
- Expanded Disability Status Scale (EDSS) (expansion of the Disability Status Scale)
- Frenchay Activities Index
- Functional Independence Measure (FIM)
- Functional Systems Scale (FSS)
- Hospital Anxiety and Depression Scale
- Jebsen Test of Hand Function (JTHF)

- Katz Index of ADLs
- Kurtzke Functional Systems Scale (FSS)
- Level of Rehabilitation Scale (LORS–II)
- Minimum Record of Disability (MRD)
- Motor Club Assessment (MCA) and the Amended Motor Club Assessment (AMCA)
- Northwick Park ADL Index (NPI)
- Nottingham Extended ADL Index
- PULSES profile
- Rand Medical Outcomes Study long and short form health status scales
- Rivermead Mobility Index
- Rivermead Visual Gait Assessment
- Sickness Impact Profile (SF-36)
- Quality-Adjusted Life Years (QALYs)

Mobility
- Timed Up and Go Test

Spasticity
- Wartenberg pendulum test
- Ashworth grading scale

PROBLEMS

Problems reported by clients with MS demonstrate considerable variability with periods of remission and periods of exacerbation.

- The client often reports persistent fatigue.
- The client often reports visual disturbances. Specific disorders of diplopia, optic neuritis, scotoma, and nystagmus are common.
- The client often has impaired bowel, bladder, and sexual functions. Specifically, reports of urinary incontinence, retention, or urgency are common, along with sexual dysfunction.
- The client often has muscle weakness that varies from mild to total paralysis (due to upper motor neuron [UMN] syndrome or disuse atrophy).
- The client typically reports altered sensations, such as a pins-and-needles sensation (paresthesia) or numbness. The client may report an electric shock-like sensation triggered when the neck is flexed (Lhermitte's sign).
- Position sense and vibratory sense may be reduced.
- The client may report hypersensitivity to a minor stimulus or an abnormal burning or painful sensation.
- There can be severe facial pain.
- The client often has spasticity that varies from mild to severe.
- The client may have intention tremors, varying in severity from mild to large involuntary movements, that typically interfere with functional activities.
- The client may demonstrate movement disorders like dysmetria, dysdiadochokinesia, and ataxia if the cerebellum is involved.
- The client may experience vestibular dysfunction such as balance impairment, dizziness, or vertigo.
- The client may demonstrate mental or behavioral impairment, usually ranging from mild to moderate disturbance of function.
- The client often has difficulty with coordination of speech and swallowing musculature.

Secondary Problems
- cardiovascular deconditioning
- decreased respiratory endurance
- impaired mobility secondary to contractures

- osteoporosis with resultant fractures
- heterotopic ossification
- decubitus ulcers

TREATMENT/MANAGEMENT

- Provide sensory retraining for a client with diminished sensation. Techniques may include vigorous rubbing, tapping, or use of alternate sensory systems to provide feedback. Eg, biofeedback can provide alternate visual or auditory feedback.
- Provide education, care, and protection of desensitized areas through proper skin care.
- Encourage client to change positions every 2 hours while in bed or every 15 minutes when in a wheelchair. Provide pressure-reducing assistive devices as needed.
- If a decubitus ulcer is present, provide cleansing and debridement of wound. Hydrotherapy and wound dressings are successfully used to augment medical management of antibiotic therapy.
- Instruct in postural retraining and correction, using orthotic devices as needed.
- Secondary musculoskeletal pain may necessitate the use of modalities along with exercise and education.
- Treat spasticity with use of therapeutic exercise, modalities, and positioning. Modalities can include cold therapy. Provide stretching and ROM on land or in water. Relaxation techniques, selected proprioceptive neuromuscular facilitation (PNF) techniques like rhythmic initiation, neurodevelopment key points of control, or other techniques can be used to reduce tone. Positioning should include the use of postures that reduce tone. Facilitate the antagonist of the spastic muscle.
- Functional electrical stimulation and biofeedback procedures can also be used to inhibit spasticity or treat lack of muscle tone.
- The client should receive passive ROM several times a day; some references suggest at least daily for immobilized joints. Teach client active and active-assistive ROM exercises.
- Consider use of splinting or casting to achieve optimal positioning.
- Consider use of manual passive stretching or prolonged static stretching if the contracture is severe.
- Exercise prescriptions will vary with each client's individual needs and can include resistive training with progressive resistance exercise or isokinetics. Tone reduction activities are more appropriate if spasticity overrides.
- Instruct client in energy conservation techniques. Offer a low-stimulation environment.
- Consider use of facilitation techniques such as PNF patterns, weights (with caution), Frenkl's exercises, stationary bike, and aquatic therapy to promote stability.
- Gait training: strengthen weakened areas, such as quadriceps; prescribe assistive devices and orthosis as needed, such as ankle-foot orthosis, rocker shoes, or modified Danish clogs, canes, crutches, or walkers.
- For functional impairments, prescribe adaptive equipment, eg, a wheelchair, with attention to proper pressure relief and devices, especially for toileting, eating, dressing, and communication activities.
- Use compensatory techniques for ataxia and dysmetria. Techniques include the use of arm weights or weights on walkers or cane to decrease ataxia.
- Instruct client in respiratory exercises. Consider a fitness training program for suitable clients, such as those who are less impaired.
- Direct client to group and individual support for psychological and social issues.

PRECAUTIONS/CONTRAINDICATIONS

- Avoid trauma to the skin.
- Transcutaneous electrical nerve stimulation (TENS) for pain relief with MS has produced varied results, with some clients experiencing an increase in symptoms.

- Avoid prolonged time in a static posture if the client has spasticity.
- For functional electrical stimulation to be considered, the client must have an intact reflex arc and intersegmental reciprocal relationship.
- Caution should be used when stretching muscles. Avoid overstretching.
- Clients with MS fatigue easily, so choose activities that can optimally achieve goals. It is contraindicated to exercise to fatigue.
- Avoid warm environments for exercise.

DESIRED OUTCOME/PROGNOSIS
- The client and family will be educated about the psychosocial aspects of MS and be provided support.
- The client will maintain or increase ROM.
- The client will have increased sensory awareness.
- The client will be educated on skin care.
- The client will increase muscular strength and motor control.
- The client will experience decreased spasticity.
- The client will increase functional independence.
- The client will ambulate independently with assistive devices as needed.

Note: The course that MS follows is unpredictable and variable.

REFERENCES

Assessment

DeLisa D. *Rehabilitation Medicine: Principle and Practice.* Philadelphia, Pa: JB Lippincott Co; 1998.

Grabois M, Garrison SJ, Hart KA, Lehmkuhl LD. *Physical Medicine and Rehabilitation: The Complete Approach.* Malden, Mass: Blackwell Science; 2000.

Patla AE, Clous SD. Visual assessment of human gait: reliability and validity. *Rehabil Res.* 1998;1:87–96.

Rothstein JM, Roy SH, Wolf SL. *The Rehabilitation Specialist's Handbook.* 2nd ed. Philadelphia, Pa: FA Davis Co; 1998.

Sine R, Liss SE, Rousch RE, et al. *Basic Rehabilitation Techniques: A Self-Instructional Guide.* 4th ed. Gaithersburg, Md: Aspen Publishers; 2000.

Treatment

Anonymous. The challenge of the elderly multiple sclerosis patient. *Focus Geriatr Care Rehabil.* 1996;10:1–18.

Bohannon RW. Physical rehabilitation in neurologic diseases. *Curr Opinion Neurol.* 1993;6:765–772.

Brosseau L, Philippe P, Methot G, Duquette P, Haraoui B. Drug abuse as a risk factor of multiple sclerosis: case-control analysis and a study of heterogeneity. *Neuroepidemiology.* 1993;12:1:6–14.

Brouwer B, Andrade VS. The effects of slow stroking on spasticity in patients with multiple sclerosis; a pilot study. *Physiotherapy Theor Pract.* 1995;11:13–21.

Buchanan RJ, Lewis KP. Services that nursing facilities should provide to residents with MS: a survey of health professionals. *Rehabil Nurs.* 1997;22:67–72.

Chiara T, Carlos J Jr, Martin D, et al. Cold effect on oxygen uptake, perceived exertion, and spasticity in patients with multiple sclerosis. *Arch Phys Med Rehabil.* 1998;79:523–528.

Costello E, Curtis CI, Sandel IB, et al. Exercise prescription for individuals with multiple sclerosis. *Neurol Rep.* 1996;20:24–30.

DeSouza LH, Ashburn A. Assessment of motor function in people with multiple sclerosis. *Physiotherapy Res Int.* 1996;98–111.

DiFabio RP, Soderberg J, Choi T, et al. Extended outpatient rehabilitation: its influence on symptom frequency, fatigue, and functional status for persons with progressive multiple sclerosis. *Arch Phys Med Rehabil.* 1998;9:141–146.

Edwards S. *Neurological Physiotherapy; A Problem-solving Approach.* New York, NY: Churchill Livingstone; 1996.

Fabio RP, Choi T, Soderberg J, et al. Health-related quality of life for patients with progressive multiple sclerosis: influence of rehabilitation. *Phys Ther.* 1997;77:1704–1716.

Fawcett J, Sidney JS, Hanson MJ, Riley-Lawless K. Use of alternative health therapies by people with multiple sclerosis: an exploratory study. *Holistic Nurs Pract.* 1994;8:2: 36–42.

Fell NO. Mental imagery and mental practice for an individual with multiple sclerosis and balance dysfunction. *Phys Ther Case Rep.* 2000;3:3–10.

Freeman JA. Improving mobililty and functional independence in persons with multiple sclerosis. *J Neurol.* 2001;248:255–259.

Freeman JA, Langdon DW, Hobart JC, et al. The impact of inpatient rehabilitation on progressive multiple sclerosis. *Ann Neurol.* 1997;42:236–244.

Frzovic D, Morris ME, Vowels L. Clinical tests of standing balance: performance of persons with multiple sclerosis. *Arch Phys Med Rehabil.* 2000;81:215–221.

Fuller KJ, Dawson K, Wiles CM. Physiotherapy in chronic multiple sclerosis: a controlled trial. *Clin Rehabil.* 1996;10:195–204.

Garland SJ, Lavoie BA, Brown WF. Motor control of the diaphragm in multiple sclerosis. *Muscle and Nerve.* 1996;19:654–656.

Grabois M, Garrison SJ, Hart KA, Lehmkuhl LD. *Physical Medicine and Rehabilitation: The Complete Approach.* Malden, Mass: Blackwell Science; 2000.

Johnson KP, Baringer JR. Current therapy of multiple sclerosis. *Hosp Pract.* 2001;36:21–29.

Jones L, Lewis Y, Harrison J, et al. The effectiveness of occupational therapy and physiotherapy in multiple sclerosis patients with ataxia of the upper limb and trunk. *Clin Rehabil.* 1996;10:277–282.

Jonsson A, Revnborg MH. Rehabilitation in multiple sclerosis. *Crit Rev Phys Rehabil Med.* 1998;10:75–100.

Kirsch NR, Myslinski MJ. The effect of a personally designed fitness program on the aerobic capacity and function for two individuals with multiple sclerosis. *Phys Ther Case Rep.* 1999;2:19–26.

Kraft GH. Rehabilitation principles for patients with multiple sclerosis. *J Spinal Cord Med.* 1998;21:117–120.

Kraft GH. Rehabilitation still the only way to improve function in multiple sclerosis. *Lancet.* 1999;354;2016–2017.

LaBan MM, Martin T, Pechur J, et al. Physical and occupational therapy in the treatment of patients with multiple sclerosis. *Phys Med Rehabil Clin North Am.* 1998;9:603–614.

Leslie GC, Muir C, Part N, Roberts RC. A comparison of the assessment of spasticity by the Wartenberg pendulum test and the Ashworth grading scale in patients with multiple sclerosis. *Clin Rehabil.* 1992;6:41–48.

Livesley E. Effects of electrical neuromuscular stimulation on functional performance in patients with multiple sclerosis. *Physiotherapy.* 1992;78:914–917.

Lord SE, Halligan PW, Wade DT. Visual gait analysis: the development of a clinical assessment and scale. *Clin Rehabil.* 1998;12:107–119.

Lord SE, Wade DT, Halligan PW. A comparison of two physiotherapy treatment approaches to improve walking in multiple sclerosis: a pilot randomized controlled study. *Clin Rehabil.* 1998;12:477–486.

Loudon JK, Cagle PE, Figoni SF, Nau KL, Klein RM. *Medicine and Science in Sports and Exercise.* 1998;30:1299–1303.

Lundmark P, Branholm IB. Relationship between occupation and life satisfaction in people with multiple sclerosis. *Disability Rehabil.* 1996;18:449–453.

Melia D. Spasticity. *Professional Nurse.* 1998;13:858–861.

Menendez P. Evaluation and prescription for wheelchairs and seating. In: Myers RS, ed. *Saunders Manual of Physical Therapy Practice.* Philadelphia, Pa: WB Saunders Co; 1995:419–425.

O'Sullivan SB, Schmitz TJ, eds. *Physical Rehabilitation: Assessment and Treatment.* Philadelphia, Pa: FA Davis Co; 1994.

Peterson C. Exercise in 94 degrees F water for a patient with multiple sclerosis. *Phys Ther.* 2001;81:1049–1058.

Rijken PM, Dekker J. Clinical experience of rehabilitation therapists with chronic diseases; a quantitative approach. *Clin Rehabil.* 1998;12:143–150.

Rodgers MM, Mulcar JA, King DL, et al. Gait characteristics of individuals with multiple sclerosis before and after a 6-month aerobic training program. *J Rehabil Res Dev.* 1999; 36:183–188.

Rosche J, Rub K, Niemann-Delius B, et al. Effects of physiotherapy on F-wave amplitudes in spasticity. *Electromyogr Clin Neurophysiol.* 1996;36:509–511.

Rousch SE. The satisfaction of patients with multiple sclerosis regarding services received from physical and occupational therapists. *Int J Rehabil Health.* 1999;1:155–166.

Schwid SR, Goodman AD, Mattson DH, et al. The measurement of ambulatory impairment in multiple sclerosis. *Neurol.* 1997;49:1419–1424.

Smeltzer SC, Lavietes MH, Cook SD. Expiratory training in multiple sclerosis. *Arch Phys Med Rehabil.* 1996;77:909–1012.

Stulfbergen AK. Physical activity and perceived health status in persons with multiple sclerosis. *J Neurosci Nur.* 1997;29:238–243.

Umphred DA. *Neurological Rehabilitation.* St. Louis, Mo: CV Mosby Co; 1995.

Van Sint Annaland E, Lord S. Vigorous exercise for multiple sclerosis: a case report. *New Zealand J Physiotherapy.* 1999;42–44.

Wainapel SF, Langer-Broas BJ, Patak RJ. Alternate four-point sweep-through gait—a technique for patients with combined neuromuscular and visual impairments: case reports. *Am J Phys Med Rehabil.* 1999;78:163–165.

White C. Therapists vital in MS. *Ther Weekly.* 1999;26:1.

Wiens ME, Reimer MA, Guyn HL. Music therapy as a treatment method for improving respiratory muscle strength in patients with advanced multiple sclerosis: a pilot study. *Rehabil Nurs.* 1999;24:74–80.

Wiles CM, Newcombe RG, Fuller KJ, et al. Controlled randomized crossover trial of the effects of physiotherapy on mobility in chronic multiple sclerosis. *J Neurol Neurosurg Psychiatry.* 2001;70:174–179.

Parkinson's Disease

Also known as *paralysis agitans* and *shaking palsy*.

DESCRIPTION

Parkinson's disease is a gradually progressive degenerative disease of the central nervous system (CNS). It is characterized by tremor at rest, postural instability, ridigity, and bradykinesia. The mean age of onset is 57, but an earlier onset, even in childhood, is possible.

CAUSE

Parkinson's disease can be caused by a depletion of the pigmented neurons in the brain stem dopaminergic cell groups, such as the substantia nigra, which leads to a loss of dopamine. Dopamine loss or interference can also occur in the basal ganglia secondary to degenerative disease, metabolic conditions, medications, or toxins. Structural lesions, hematoma, or hydrocephalus can also lead to parkinsonism. Parkinson's disease can also be idiopathic.

ASSESSMENT

Note: See APTA's Guide to Physical Therapist Practice. 2nd ed. *Physical Therapy.* 2001;81.

Cardiopulmonary Preferred Practice Patterns: B, F, G

Integumentary Preferred Practice Pattern: A

Neuromuscular Preferred Practice Pattern: C

AREAS
- History, including medications and metabolic status
- Communication, including dysarthria
- Pain
- Posture
- Pulmonary
- Cardiovascular, including endurance to activities
- Mobility: active and passive range of motion (ROM)
- Motor control, including tone (resting and dynamic), rigidity, reflexes (tonic reflexes, righting reflexes, equilibrium responses), balance and postural reactions, and active movement control, including strength, coordination, patterned movement, and isolated movement
- Neurological, including sensation
- Skin and soft tissue, including edema or open wounds
- Gait: including observational gait analysis (OGA)
- Functional level, including, but not limited to, activities of daily living (ADLs), bed mobility, sitting, transfers, and standing
- Equipment, including use of orthotics, appliances, and assistive devices, and environmental needs upon discharge

INSTRUMENTS/PROCEDURES

See References for sources.

Functional Level
- Barthel index
- Functional Independence Measure (FIM)
- Katz Index of ADLs
- PULSES profile

- Hoehn and Yahr Stages
- Unified Parkinson's Disease Rating Scale (UPDRS)
- Parkinson's Disease Questionnaire (PDQ-39)
- Functional Status Questionnaire (FSQ)
- Posturo-Locomotor-Manual Test (PLM-Test)
- Box and Block test (BBT)
- Short Test of Mental Status (STMS)
- Webster Scale
- Clinical Stride Analyzer
- Parkinson's Disease Quality of Life questionnaire (PDQL)
- Sensory Integration and Praxis Test

Gait
- gait and balance examination
- stopwatch test

Mobility
- Timed Up and Go Test

Motor Control
1. balance
   - Berg Balance Test
   - gait and balance examination
2. rigidity
   - isokinetic dynamometry
   - joint angular stiffness (torque to joint-angle ratio) as an index of rigidity
   - relaxed oscillation test

Special Tests to Which the Physical Therapist May or May Not Have Access
- Motion analysis
- Isostation B-200 for ROM, isometric torque, and isoinertial performance.
- electromyography (EMG)

PROBLEMS
- The client typically has trouble balancing when standing, walking, or turning. Falls are common. There may be an absence of equilibrium and righting responses and diminished associated reaction.
- The client often has a delay in initiating movement, or akinesia, and demonstrates a decreased speed of execution of movement, or bradykinesia. This bradykinesia can lead to a severe freezing of movement.
- The client frequently complains of rigidity, either a jerky, "cogwheel" type or a constant, "lead pipe" type.
- The client may demonstrate tremor, especially with a "pill-rolling" motion of the hand. Tremors can also appear in the tongue, lips, jaw, and feet.
- The client often complains of fatigue.
- The client may be unable to perform 2 or more simultaneous movements.
- The hypokinesia, or poverty of movement, common to clients usually leads to a deviated gait pattern that is slow and shuffling. Festination— an abnormal increase in walking speed in order to avoid falling forward—is typical.
- A mask-like facial expression is common.
- The client may have impaired swallowing.
- The client often has dysarthria, or impaired speech.
- The client may have orthostatic hypotension and low blood pressure.
- The client may demonstrate dementia.
- Perceptual motor deficits may appear.
- The client may experience a sensory loss or abnormal sensation. Autonomic dysfunction may also occur. Basal ganglia deficits include the following problems:

poor dual task performance, poor execution of complex movement sequences, diminished ability to adapt gait pattern to varied environmental demands, especially regulation of stride length.
- The deconditioning common to clients can lead to musculoskeletal problems such as kyphosis, osteoporosis, muscular atrophy, and decreased ROM, leading to contracture. Other musculoskeletal abnormalities, such as scoliosis, can limit postural control.
- Circulatory changes such as edema and decubitus ulcers can often occur.

TREATMENT/MANAGEMENT
- Provide education related to the disorder to the client and family.
- Prescribe appropriate exercise—such as walking or bicycling—for cardiovascular conditioning.
- Provide activities that are progressively more complex—such as weight shifting on a mat and then on a gymnastic ball—to promote balance.
- Instruct client in exercises for mobility that promote functional movement patterns. Activities should stress postural control and can engage multiple body segments simultaneously, such as patterns found in proprioceptive neuromuscular facilitation (PNF).
- Many advocate using a task-specific approach to ADLs using alternative movement strategies. Three important skill domains include bed-related (getting in and out of and turning in bed), chair-related (sit to stand) and walking-related (initiation and termination of gait and turning).
- May use verbal instructional sets to normalize gait variables. (See Berhman.)
- Treatment plans should consider the following factors: degree of basal ganglia dysfunction, impact of medication, age-related changes, falls, and gait performance.
- Gait training techniques used may include:
  1. high stepping with alternating dorsiflexion of ankle with support
  2. weight shifting
  3. cues on floor for step length or width
  4. blocks on floor to promote floor clearance
  5. wooden support in hand of both client and therapist to promote reciprocal arm swing
  6. music to promote rhythm
  7. weights or orthotic support for balance
  8. PNF patterns for coordination
  9. use of treadmill to provide multisensory and mechanical input
- Encourage group support activities.
- Teach client ROM exercises that can be performed several times a day and continue with home ROM exercise program, with or without adaptive equipment.
- Utilize gentle rocking and rhythmic techniques to promote relaxation, and teach self-care relaxation techniques such as Jacobsen's progressive relaxation.
- Instruct client in deep-breathing respiratory exercises.
- Provide training in ADLs, and prescribe assistive devices as indicated.
- Explore the use of complex response speeds, directions, and amplitudes in varied environmental situations to elicit the ability to adapt.
- Vary timing and intensity of stimuli, especially auditory or visual, given before movement to stimulate change in client's motor response.

PRECAUTIONS/CONTRAINDICATIONS
- No excessive stretching or painful stretching activities.
- Remember when planning ROM activities, that the client with Parkinson's disease may also have undiagnosed osteoporosis.
- High levels of resistance are contraindicated for clients with increased tone.

DESIRED OUTCOME/PROGNOSIS

- The client will have functional ROM.
- The client will not develop contractures.
- The client will demonstrate correct posture.
- The client will be aware of safety factors related to impaired balance reactions.
- The client will ambulate with a functional gait pattern.
- The client will maintain or improve respiratory capacity.
- The client will maintain or improve speech function.
- The client will improve energy level and cardiovascular endurance.
- The client will maintain or improve independence in ADLs.
- The client and family will be assisted in psychological adjustment to a chronic illness.

Notes: Neuromuscular control of the ankle is critical to functional gait.

Comella et al found significant improvement in clients undergoing a program of regular exercise (3 times a week for 60 minutes) but gains were lost when clients stopped exercising.

REFERENCES

Assessment

Bain PG, Findley LJ, Atchinson P, et al. Assessing tremor severity. *J Neurol Neurosurg Psychiatry.* 1993;56:868–873.

Berg K, Maki B, Williams JI, et al. Clinical and laboratory measures of postural balance in an elderly population. *Arch Phys Med Rehabil.* 1992;73:1073–1083.

Bowes SG, Charlett A, Dobbs RJ, et al. Gait in relation to aging and idiopathic parkinsonism. *Scand J Rehabil Med.* 1992;24:181–186.

DeLisa D. *Rehabilitation Medicine: Principle and Practice.* Philadelphia, Pa: JB Lippincott Co; 1998.

Grabois M, Garrison SJ, Hart KA, Lehmkuhl LD. *Physical Medicine and Rehabilitation: The Complete Approach.* Malden, Mass: Blackwell Science; 2000.

Morris S, Norris ME, Iansek R. Reliability of measurements obtained with the Timed "Up and Go" test in people with Parkinson's disease. *Phys Ther.* 2001;81:810–818.

Oatis CA. The use of a mechanical model to describe the stiffness and damping characteristics of the knee joint in healthy adults. *Phys Ther.* 1993;73:740–749.

O'Sullivan SB, Schmitz TJ, eds. *Physical Rehabilitation: Assessment and Treatment.* Philadelphia, Pa: FA Davis Co; 1994.

Patla AE, Clous SD. Visual assessment of human gait: reliability and validity. *Rehabil Res.* 1998;1:87–96.

Rothstein JM, Roy SH, Wolf SL. *The Rehabilitation Specialist's Handbook.* 2nd ed. Philadelphia, Pa: FA Davis Co; 1998.

Sine R, Liss SE, Rousch RE, et al. *Basic Rehabilitation Techniques: A Self-Instructional Guide.* 4th ed. Gaithersburg, Md: Aspen Publishers; 2000.

Smithson FM, Morris ME, Lansek R. Performance on clinical tests of balance in Parkinson's disease. *Phys Ther.* 1998;78:577–585.

Traub MM, Rothwell JC, Marsden CD. Anticipatory postural reflexes in Parkinson's disease and other akinetic-rigid syndromes and in cerebellar ataxia. In: Lister MJ, ed. *Contemporary Management of Motor Control Problems: Proceedings of the II STEP Conference.* Fredricksburg, Va: Foundation for Physical Therapy; 1991:195–208.

Treatment

American Physical Therapy Association. Guide to physical therapist practice. 2nd ed. *Phys Ther.* 2001;81.

Behrman A. Parkinson's disease. *Neurol Rep.* 1997;107–139.

Behrman A. Therapeutic interventions for individuals with Parkinson's disease. *Neurol Rep.* 1997;21:107–108.

Berhman AL, Cauraugh JH, Light KE. Practice as an intervention to improve speeded motor performance and motor learning in Parkinson's disease. *J Neurol Sci.* 2000;174:127–136.

Berhman AL, Teiterlbaum P, Cauraugh JH. Verbal instructional sets to normalize the temporal and spatial gait variables in Parkinson's disease. *J Neurol Neurosurg Psychiatry.* 1998;65:580–582.

Black KJ, Racette B, Perlmutter JS. Preventing contractures (correction of contractions) in neuroleptic malignant syndrome and dystonia. *Am J Psychiatry.* 1998;155:1298–1299.

Bohannon RW. Physical rehabilitation in neurologic disease. *Current Opinion Neurol.* 1993;6:765–772.

Bridgewater KJ, Sharpe MH. Trunk muscle performance in early Parkinson's disease. *Phys Ther.* 1998;78:566–576.

Burford K. The physiotherapist's role in Parkinson's disease. *Geriatr Nurs Home Care.* 1988;8:1:14–16.

Chan J, Lee J, Neubert C. Physiotherapy intervention in Parkinsonian gait. *NZ J Physiotherapy.* 1993;21:1:23–28.

Chong RK, Barbas J, Garrison K. Does balance control deficit account for walking difficulty in Parkinson's disease? *Int J Clin Pract.* 2001;55:411–412.

Chong RK, Horak FB. Sensory organization for balance: specific deficits in Alzheimers but not in Parkinson's disease. *J Gerontol.* Series A, Biological Sciences and Medical Sciences. 1999;54:M129–135.

Chong RK, Horak FB, Woollacott MH. Parkinson's disease impairs the ability to change set quickly. *J Neurol Sci.* 2000;175:57–70.

Chong RK, Horak FB, Frank J, et al. Sensory organization for balance; specific deficits in Alzheimers but not in Parkinson's disease. *J Gerontol.* Series A, Biological Sciences and Medical Sciences. 1999;54:M122–128.

Chong RK, Jones CL, Horak FB. Postural set for balance control is normal in Alzheimers but not in Parkinson's disease. *J Gerontol.* Series A, Biological Sciences and Medical Sciences. 1999;54:M129–135.

Cicccone CD. Free-radical toxicity and antioxidant medications in Parkinson's disease. *Phys Ther.* 1998;78:313–319.

Comella CI, Stebbins GT, Brown-Toms N, et al. Physical therapy and Parkinson's disease: a controlled clinic trial. *Neurol.* 1994;44:376–378.

Dam M, Tonin P, Casson S, Bracco F, et al. Effects of conventional and sensory-enhanced physiotherapy on disability of Parkinson's disease patients. *Adv Neurol.* 1996;69:551–555.

De Boer AG, Springers MA, Speelman HD, et al. Predictors of health care use in patients with Parkinson's disease: a longitudinal study. *Movement Disord.* 1999;14:772–779.

De Goede CJ. The effects of physical therapy in Parkinson's disease: a research synthesis. *Arch Phys Med Rehabil.* 2001;82:509–515.

Fahn S. Medical treatment of Parkinson's disease. *J Neurol.* 1998;25 (II suppl 3):P15–24.

Formisano R, Pratesi L, Modarelli FT, Bonifati V, Meco G. Rehabilitation and Parkinson's disease. *Scand J Rehabil Med.* 1992;24:3:157–160.

Glendinning DS, Enoka RM. Motor unit behaviour in Parkinson's disease. *Phys Ther.* 1994; 74:61–70.

Grabois M, Garrison SJ, Hart KA, Lehmkuhl LD. *Physical Medicine and Rehabilitation: The Complete Approach.* Malden, Mass: Blackwell Science; 2000.

Grill S. Postural instability in Parkinson's disease. *Md Med J.* 1999;48:179–181.

Henneberg A. Additional therapies in Parkinson's disease patients: useful tools for the improvement of the quality of life or senseless loss of resources? *J Neurol.* 1998;245 suppl 1:S23–27.

Hildick-Smith M. Pragmatic physical therapy in Parkinson's disease: any scientific basis? *Adv Neurol.* 1999;80:561–564.

Hingten CM, Siemers E. The treatment of Parkinson's disease: current concepts and rationale. *Compr Ther.* 1998;2:560–566.

Homberg V. Motor training in the therapy of Parkinson's disease. *Neurol.* 1993;43:12(suppl 6):45–46.

Horak FB, et al. Patients with Parkinson's disease perseverate postural adjustments for compensatory stepping. *Neurol Rep.* 1998;22:180–181.

Jobst EE, Melnick ME, Byl NN, et al. Sensory perception in Parkinson's disease. *Arch Neurol.* 1997;54:450–454.

Kamsma YPT, Brouwer WH, Lakke JPW. Training of compensational strategies for impaired gross motor skills in Parkinson's disease. *Physiotherapy Theory Pract.* 1995;11:209–229.

Katsikitis M, Pilowsky I. A controlled study of facial mobility treatment in Parkinson's disease. *J Psychosom Res.* 1996;40:387–396.

Kokko S, Paltamaa J, Ahola E, et al. The assessment of functional ability in patients with Parkinson's disease: the PLM test and three clinical tests. *Physiotherapy Res Int.* 1997; 2:29–45.

Lewis S. Team Parkinson's. *Ther Weekly.* 2000;26:16.

Lindsey B. Hourly monitoring system for patients with Parkinson's disease. *Neurol Rep.* 1995;19:30–33.

Mackay-Lyons M. Variability in spatiotemporal gait characteristics over the course of the L-dopa cycle in people with advanced Parkinson's disease. *Phys Ther.* 1998;78:1083–1094.

Mackay-Lyons M, Turnbull G. Physical therapy in Parkinson's disease. *Neurol.* 1995;45: 1:205.

Melnick ME, Dowling GA, Aminoff MJ, et al. Effect of pallidotomy on postural control and motor function in Parkinson's disease. *Arch Neurol.* 1999;56:1361–1365.

Miyai I, Fujimoto Y, Ueda Y, et al. Treadmill training with body weight support: its effect on Parkinson's disease. *Arch Phys Med Rehabil.* 2000;81:849–852.

Montgomery Jr EB. Bradykinesia and akinesia of parkinsonism: implications for physical therapy. *Neurol Rep.* 1995;19:23–29.

Morris M, Huxham F, McGinley J. Strategies to prevent falls in people with Parkinson's disease. *Physiotherapy Singapore.* 1999;2:135–141.

Morris M, Huxham F, McGinley J. Gait and geriatrics down under. *Rehab Manage Int.* 1998;8:23–24.

Morris M, Iansek R. An interprofessional team approach to rehabilitation in Parkinson's disease. *Europ J Phys Med Rehabil.* 1997;7:166–170.

Morris ME. Movement disorders in people with Parkinson's Disease: a model for physical therapy. *Phys Ther.* 2000;80:578–597.

Morris ME, Iansek R. Gait disorders in Parkinson's disease: a framework for physical therapy practice. *Neurolog Rep.* 1997;21:125–31.

Morris ME, Matyas TA, Iansek R, et al. Temporal stability of gait in Parkinson's disease. *Phys Ther.* 1996;76:763–780.

Ng DC. Parkinson's disease. Diagnosis and treatment. *West J Med.* 1996;165:234–240.

Nieuwboer A, Feys P, De Weerdt W, et al. Clinical problem solving. Is using a cue the clue to the treatment of freezing in Parkinson's disease. *Physiotherapy Res Int.* 1997;2:125–134.

Onla-or S, Winstein CJ. Function of the direct and indirect pathways of the basal ganglia motor loop: evidence from reciprocal aiming movements in Parkinson's disease. *Brain Res Cogn Brain Res.* 2001;10:329–332.

Pacchetti C, Mancini F, Aglieri R, et al. Active music therapy in Parkinson's disease: an integrative method for motor and emotional rehabilitation. *Psychosom Med.* 2000; 62:386–393.

Protas EJ, Stanley RK, Jankovic J, MacNeill B. Cardiovascular and metabolic responses to upper and lower extremity exercise in men with idiopathic Parkinson's disease. *Phys Ther.* 1996;76:34–40.

Rijken PM, Dekker J. Clinical experience of rehabilitation therapists with chronic diseases: a quantitative approach. *Clin Rehabil.* 1998;12:143–150.

Rogers MW. Control of posture and balance during voluntary movements in Parkinson's disease. In: Duncan PW, ed. *Balance.* Alexandria, Va: American Physical Therapy Association; 1990:79–86.

Rogers MW. Motor control problems in Parkinson's disease. In: Lister MJ, ed. *Contemporary Management of Motor Control Problems: Proceedings of the II STEP Conference.* Fredricksburg, Va: Foundation for Physical Therapy; 1991:195–208.

Schenkman M. Selegiline and PT intervention in early Parkinson's disease. *PT-Magazine Phys Ther.* 1998;6:50–61.

Schenkman M, Cutson TM, Kuchibhatia M, et al. Reliability of impairment and physical performance measures for persons with Parkinson's disease. *Phys Ther.* 1997;77:19–27.

Schenkman M, Morey M, Kuchibhatia M. Spinal flexibility and balance control among community-dwelling adults with and without Parkinson's disease. *J Gerontol.* Series A, Biological Sciences and Medical Sciences. 2000;55:M441–445.

Schenkman ML, Clark K, Xie T, et al. Spinal movement and performance of a standing reach task in participants with and without Parkinson's disease. *Phys Ther.* 2001;81:1400–1411.

Sine R, Liss SE, Rousch RE, et al. *Basic Rehabilitation Techniques: A Self-Instructional Guide.* 4th ed. Gaithersburg, Md: Aspen Publishers; 2000.

Stanley RK, Protas EJ, Jankovic J. Exercise performance in those having Parkinson's disease and healthy normals. *Med Sci Sports Exerc.* 1999;31:761–766.

Thompson AJ, Playford ED. Rehabilitation for patients with Parkinson's disease. *Lancet.* 2001;357:410–411.

Umphred DA. *Neurol Rehabil.* St. Louis, Mo: CV Mosby Co; 1995.

Viliani T, Pasquetti P, Magnolfi S, et al. Effects of physical training on straightening-up processes in patients with Parkinson's Disease. *Disability Rehabil.* 1999;21:68–73.

Weissenborn S. The effect of using a two-step verbal cue to a visual target above eye level on the Parkinsonian gait: a case study. *Physiotherapy.* 1993;79:26–31.

Yekutiel MP. Patients' fall records as an aid in designing and assessing therapy in Parkinsonism. *Disability Rehabil*. 1993;15:4:189–193.

Young R. Update on Parkinson's disease. *Am Fam Phys*. 1999;59:2155–2167.

Balance

Bohannon R. Standing balance and function over the course of acute rehabilitation. *Arch Phys Med Rehabil*. 1995;76:994–996.

Chen H, Ashton-Miller J, Alexander N, et al. Effects of age and available response time on ability to stop over an obstacle. *J Gerontol*. 1994;49:M227–233.

DiFabio R, Seay R. Use of the "fast evaluation of mobility, balance, and fear" in elderly community dwellers: validity and reliability. *Phys Ther*. 1997;77:904–917.

Feltner M, MacRae P, McNitt-Gray J. Quantitative gait assessment as a predictor of prospective and retrospective falls in community-dwelling women. *Arch Phys Med Rehabil*. 1994;75:447–453.

Graham D, Newton RA. *Physiotherapy Res Int*. 1999;4:293–301.

Haarda N, Chiu V, Damron-Rodriques J, et al. Screening for balance and mobility impairment in elderly individuals living in residential care facilities. *Phys Ther*. 1995;75:462–469.

Jeka J. Light touch contact as a balance aid. *Phys Ther*. 1997;77:476–487.

Lord S, Castell S. Effect of exercise on balance, strength and reaction time in older people. *Aust J Physiotherapy*. 1994;40:83–88.

Lord SR, Ward JA, Williams P. Effect of water exercise on balance and related factors in older people. *Aust J Physiotherapy*. 1993;42:1110–1117.

Maki B, Holliday P, Topper A. A prospective study of postural balance and risk of falling in an ambulatory and independent elderly population. *J Geriatr*. 1994;49:M72–M84.

Maki B, McIlroy W. The role of limb movement in maintaining upright stance: the "change-in-support" strategy. *Phys Ther*. 1997;77:488–507.

Winter D. *ABCs of Balance during Standing and Walking*. Waterloos, Ontario: Waterloo Biomechanics; 1995.

Woollacott M, Tang P. Balance control during walking in the older adult: research and its implications. *Phys Ther*. 1997;646–660.

Peripheral Nerve Injury

DESCRIPTION

Peripheral nerve injury leads to sensory and motor loss at the involved site. Peripheral nerve injuries can be divided into three categories:

- *Neuropraxia* is a transient paralysis and sensory loss at a point of localized blockage. There may be nerve conduction above and below the lesion. Motor function may be more affected than sensory function.
- *Axonotmesis* results from Wallerian degeneration below the level of injury. However, the Schwann nerve sheath is left intact. After Wallerian degeneration, axons regrow to corresponding end organs. Deficit depends on the number of axons affected.
- *Neurotmesis* is a total disruption of axon and nerve sheath, with no conduction below the level of the lesion.

335

CAUSE

- Neuropraxia is caused by a crushing injury or by compression disorders.
- Axonotmesis is caused by stretch or compression of the axon. It may be a progressive result of chronic neuropraxia.
- Neurotmesis is caused by a cut separating the axon and epineurium that eliminates conduction.

ASSESSMENT

Note: See APTA's Guide to Physical Therapist Practice. 2nd ed. *Physical Therapy.* 2001;81.

Neuromuscular Preferred Practice Pattern: G

AREAS

- History, including medications and metabolic status
- Pain
- Motor function, including nerve conduction testing until day 21, strength duration curve after the 21st day
- Strength
- Neurological, including sensation, proprioception, temperature, touch, and two-point discrimination
- Skin and soft tissue
- Mobility: range of motion (ROM)
- Functional level
- Equipment, including appliances and assistive devices, and environmental needs upon discharge

INSTRUMENTS/PROCEDURES

See References for sources.

Functional Level
- Functional Independence Measure
- Katz Index of ADLs
- Mood Adjective Check List (MACL)
- Sickness Impact Profile (SIP)

Special Tests to Which the Physical Therapist May or May Not Have Access
- modality tests and quantitative assessment
- motor unit estimating methodology

Strength
- manual muscle testing

PROBLEMS

GENERAL PROBLEMS

- The client may have paralysis with no tone.
- The client often has muscular atrophy.
- There may be contracture of uninvolved muscle groups.
- There is often loss of sensation and proprioception.
- There may be localized inability to sweat.
- The client may have localized hair loss.
- The client may have poor wound healing.
- The client's skin will often demonstrate change in temperature.
- The client's nails are often brittle.

SPECIFIC NERVE LESIONS

Axillary Nerve Lesion
- There is often atrophy or a flattening of the shoulder area.
- The client typically complains of an inability to abduct or elevate the arm.

Median Nerve
- There is often an "ape-hand" or "monkey" deformity, with the thumb lying on the same plane as the hand.
- There is thenar eminence atrophy.
- There is a loss of the ability to use indicating gesture; flexion of index finger along with partial inability to flex middle finger.
- There is a loss of precision grip.
- There is often a loss of proprioception on the radial aspect of the hand.

Ulnar Nerve
- The hand assumes a clawing position, with hyperextension of fourth and fifth metacarpophalangeal joints and interphalangeal joint flexion.
- There is fifth-finger abduction.
- There is atrophy of the hypothenar eminence and interossei.
- The client complains of a weakened power grip.
- There is loss of finger precision movements.

Radial Nerve Injury
- There is atrophy of forearm extensor muscles.
- There is wrist drop.
- The client reports inability to put objects on a flat surface.
- The client complains of loss of flexor grip.

Common Peroneal Nerve
- The client has foot drop.
- There is a high-stepping gait.
- There is equinovarus foot positioning.

TREATMENT/MANAGEMENT
- Stimulate circulation with massage, elevation, and general exercise.
- Perform ROM activities as indicated with passive, active-assistive, and active movements.
- Stimulate strength in both affected and unaffected musculature with balance activities, active exercise, resistive exercise, aquatic therapy, and neuromuscular facilitation techniques. Motor training can be used post tendon transfer.
- Provide sensory reeducation or desensitization.
- Promote functional training.
- Prescribe splints as indicated. Usually the affected area is immobilized for 3 to 4 weeks. In general, a static splint is used to provide stability, whereas a dynamic splint is used to enhance mobility. A cock-up splint, with or without an outrigger, is used for a radial nerve injury. A thumb opponens splint is used for a median nerve injury. A dorsal-based splint is used for an ulnar nerve injury.
- With neurotomesis, surgical repair is necessary for healing. During weeks 1 to 3 postsurgically, maintain circulation and promote activity in unaffected areas. During weeks 3 to 8 postsurgically, perform ROM within prescribed limits and increase strength in unaffected musculature.

PRECAUTIONS/CONTRAINDICATIONS
- When using a splint, be especially alert for possible skin breakdown if sensation is impaired.

DESIRED OUTCOME/PROGNOSIS

NERVE REGENERATION

- Identify extent of loss of return and functional ability.
- The client will maintain or improve ROM.
- The client will maintain or increase circulation.
- The client will increase strength.
- Provide sensory reeducation.
- The client will improve in function.

Notes: In cases of neuropraxia, the client will usually recover in 6 weeks.

In cases of axonotmesis, recovery is usually good, but time depends on lesion location and length between injury site and receptors or muscle.

In cases of neurotmesis, recovery is variable. Recovery of function depends on axon recovery.

REFERENCES

Assessment

DeLisa D. *Rehabilitation Medicine: Principle and Practice.* Philadelphia, Pa: JB Lippincott Co; 1998.

Grabois M, Garrison SJ, Hart KA, Lehmkuhl LD. *Physical Medicine and Rehabilitation: The Complete Approach.* Malden, Mass: Blackwell Science; 2000.

Kendall FP, McCreary EK, Provance PG. *Muscles: Testing and Function.* 4th ed. Baltimore, Md: Williams and Wilkins; 1993.

McComas AJ, Galea V, de Bruin H. Motor unit populations in healthy and diseased muscles. *Phys Ther.* 1993;73:868–877.

O'Sullivan SB, Schmitz TJ, eds. *Physical Rehabilitation: Assessment and Treatment.* Philadelphia, Pa: FA Davis Co; 1994.

Patla AE, Clous SD. Visual assessment of human gait: reliability and validity. *Rehabil Res.* 1998;1:87–96.

Rothstein JM, Roy SH, Wolf SL. *The Rehabilitation Specialist's Handbook.* 2nd ed. Philadelphia, Pa: FA Davis Co; 1998.

Sine R, Liss SE, Rousch RE, et al. *Basic Rehabilitation Techniques: A Self-Instructional Guide.* 4th ed. Gaithersburg, Md: Aspen Publishers; 2000.

Wadsworth CT. Elbow, forearm, wrist, and hand. In: Myers R, ed. *Saunders Manual for Physical Therapy Practice.* Philadelphia, Pa: WB Saunders Co; 1995:911.

Treatment

Brandsma JW. Manual muscle strength testing and dynamometry for bilateral ulnar neuropraxia. *J Hand Ther.* 1995;8:191–194.

Doucette SA, Goble EM. The effect of exercise on patellar tracking in lateral patellar compression syndrome. *Am J Sports Med.* 1992;20:434–440.

Grabois M, Garrison SJ, Hart KA, Lehmkuhl LD. *Physical Medicine and Rehabilitation: The Complete Approach.* Malden, Mass: Blackwell Science; 2000.

Hsieh L, Liaw E, Cheng H, et al. Bilateral femoral neuropathy after vaginal hysterectomy. *Arch Phys Med Rehabil.* 1998;79:1018–1021.

Klingman RE. The pseudoradicular syndrome: a case report implicating double crush mechanisms in peripheral nerve tissue of the lower extremity. *J Man Manipulative Ther.* 1999;7:81–91.

Lake DA, Burns BL. Treatment of meralgia paresthetica using soft tissue mobilization. *Phys Ther Case Rep.* 1999;2:152–156.

Laska T, Hannig K. Physical therapy spinal accessory nerve injury complicated by adhesive capsulitis. *Phys Ther.* 2001;81:936–944.

Lorin S, Sivak M, Nierman DM. Critical illness polyneuropathy: what to look for in at-risk patients. *J Crit Illness.* 1998;608–612.

Manon-Espaillat R, Mandel S. Diagnostic algorithms for neuromuscular diseases. *Clin Podiatr Med Surg.* 1999;16:67–79.

McDaniel J, Khodadadi F. Pronator teres syndrome. *Top Clin Chiropractic.* 1999;6:51–55.

Persson LCG, Carlsson C, Carlsson JY. Long-lasting cervical radicular pain managed with surgery, physiotherapy, or a cervical collar: a prospective, randomized study. *Spine.* 1997;22:751–758.

Ramos LE, Zell JP. Rehabilitation program for children with brachial plexus and peripheral nerve injury. *Seminars in Pediatric Neurology.* 2000;7:52–57.

Silliman JF, Dean MT. Neurovascular injuries to the shoulder complex. *J Orthop Sports Phys Ther.* 1993;18:442–448.

Slade JF III, Mahoney JD, Dailinger JE, et al. Wrist and hand injuries in musicians: management and prevention: proper form, warm-up, and avoidance of sudden changes reduces injury. *J Musculoskeletal Med.* 1999;16:542–550.

Wadsworth CT. Elbow, forearm, wrist, and hand. In: Myers RS, ed. *Saunders Manual for Physical Therapy Practice.* Philadelphia, Pa: WB Saunders Co; 1995.

Warwick L, Seradge H. Early versus late range of motion following cubital tunnel surgery. *J Hand Ther.* 1995;8:245–248.

Reflex Sympathetic Dystrophy

Also known as *complex regional pain syndrome-type I* (CRPS) (sympathetic dystrophy) and *complex regional pain–type II* (causalgia), *sympathetically maintained pain, shoulder hand syndrome, post-traumatic dystrophy, post-traumatic neuralgia, Sudeck's atrophy,* and *minor causalgia.*

DESCRIPTION

Reflex sympathetic dystrophy (RSD) is a neurovascular syndrome in which pain accompanies autonomic changes and/or dystrophic changes in skin and bone and can lead to contracture in an extremity. The pain with RSD exceeds the level expected by initial injury or disease. Pain may start immediately, in hours, or weeks after the initial event. RSD is three times more common in women than in men and usually afflicts clients age 35 to 60. Three stages appear with RSD: acute, dystrophic, and atrophic.

CAUSE

Etiology is unknown. Predisposing factors may include surgery, trauma (especially shoulder injury or injury to the lower extremity), lesions, neurological disorders, or neuropathy. Possible causes also include a defect between sympathetic efferent fibers and sensory afferent fibers, which leads to a cycle of additional sympathetic outflow and increased pain sensation.

ASSESSMENT

Note: See APTA's Guide to Physical Therapist Practice. 2nd ed. *Physical Therapy.* 2001;81.

Musculoskeletal Preferred Practice Patterns: A, D

Neuromuscular Preferred Practice Pattern: G

Integumentary Preferred Practice Pattern: B

AREAS
- History
- Pain
- Posture
- Skin and soft tissue, including edema, and any dystrophic changes such as skin atrophy or hair loss
- Mobility, including active range of motion (ROM)
- Strength
- Functional level, including activities of daily living (ADLs)

INSTRUMENTS/PROCEDURES

See References for sources.

Pain
- Dartmouth Pain Questionnaire
- Impairment-level Sum Score (ISS)
- Sickness Impact Profile
- McGill Pain Questionnaire
- Modified Greentest
- Multidisciplinary Pain Inventory
- Radboud Dexterity test
- Radboud Skills Questionnaire
- visual analog scale

Special Tests to Which the Physical Therapist May or May Not Have Access
- three-phase bone scan

PROBLEMS
- The client often complains initially of a burning pain; later it may be described as aching or crushing pain.
- In the upper extremity, the client typically has changes in the hand that include edema and a mottled, slightly cyanotic appearance of the hand in the early stages. This is later replaced by warmth, reddening, and dryness of skin.
- In later stages, the client often experiences atrophy, contracture, and trophic skin changes. The client normally has pain with motion and capsular restriction of all or most upper extremity joints in differing degrees.
- The client may have edema of the lower extremity if injured in this area.
- The client often has dyesthesias, with pain and hypersensitivity to slight touch.
- After about 9 months, the client may experience a decrease in pain, but joint ankylosis, severe osteoporosis, and functional loss can occur.

TREATMENT/MANAGEMENT
- Educate client about skin protection.
- Work within pain-free range to increase ROM of shoulder and hand or, where indicated, use joint mobilization, muscle inhibition techniques, and soft tissue stretching.
- Begin movement with passive ROM, progressing to active assistive and on to active movement.
- Encourage independence in movement. Encourage active muscle contraction via isotonic and isometric exercise.

- Use light weight-bearing activities. Begin progressive schedule of compression and traction with weight bearing on affected extremity. One suggested schedule starts with 3 to 5 minutes three times daily. Add traction, such as carrying a weight in the hand, for 10 minutes three times daily. Increase compression and traction forces as indicated.
- Set up a home program for ROM, ADLs, and general conditioning.
- Consider use of ice for pain.
- Consider use of intermittent pneumatic compression or elevation and elastic compression for edema.
- Alter feedback loop by encouraging hypostimulation with relaxation techniques and biofeedback, or try hyperstimulation with environmental changes such as contrast baths or spray-and-stretch techniques.
- Consider transcutaneous electrical nerve stimulation (TENS), using conventional mode first. You may need to try a variety of treatment parameters with electrode placement and setting parameters.
- Modalities may also include contrast baths, massage, electrical stimulation, and thermography.
- Work with attending physician on rehabilitation plan following nerve block.
- Consider use of spinal manual therapy to impact the sympathetic nervous system.
- Consider use of splints to limit motions and pain in a resting hand position.

PRECAUTIONS/CONTRAINDICATIONS

- Exercise caution when using physical agents and modalities due to trophic changes.

DESIRED OUTCOME/PROGNOSIS

- The client will have an increase in circulation.
- The client will have a decrease in pain.

Notes: The areas involved will be desensitized in order to promote autonomic homeostasis.

Preventative measures include frequent active exercise of uninvolved joints with elevation of extremity as well.

Condition may resolve spontaneously but can linger for months or even years.

Early assessment and treatment are critical to break the pain cycle of RSD. Prognosis is improved if treatment begins at least 6 months from onset.

Pain associated with RSD is a definitive, physically driven pain, as opposed to cases of chronic pain, in which the pain is often poorly localized.

REFERENCES

Assessment

Cammack S, Eisenberg MG, eds. *Key Words in Physical Rehabilitation: A Guide to Contemporary Usage.* New York, NY: Springer Publishing Co; 1995.

DeLisa D. *Rehabilitation Medicine: Principle and Practice.* Philadelphia, Pa: JB Lippincott Co; 1998.

Grabois M, Garrison SJ, Hart KA, Lehmkuhl LD. *Physical Medicine and Rehabilitation: The Complete Approach.* Malden, Mass: Blackwell Science; 2000.

Headley BJ. Chronic pain management. In: O'Sullivan SB, Schmitz TJ, eds. *Physical Rehabilitation.* 3rd ed. Philadelphia, Pa: FA Davis Co; 1994:577–602.

O'Sullivan SB, Schmitz TJ, eds. *Physical Rehabilitation: Assessment and Treatment.* Philadelphia, Pa: FA Davis Co; 1994.

Patla AE, Clous SD. Visual assessment of human gait: reliability and validity. *Rehabil Res.* 1998;1:87–96.

Rothstein JM, Roy SH, Wolf SL. *The Rehabilitation Specialist's Handbook.* 2nd ed. Philadelphia, Pa: FA Davis Co; 1998.

Saidoff DC, McDonough AL. *Critical Pathways in Therapeutic Intervention.* Philadelphia, Pa: CV Mosby Co; 2002.

Sine R, Liss SE, Rousch RE, et al. *Basic Rehabilitation Techniques: A Self-Instructional Guide.* 4th ed. Gaithersburg, Md: Aspen Publishers; 2000.

Treatment

American Physical Therapy Association. Guide to physical therapist practice. 2nd ed. *Phys Ther.* 2001;81.

Arlet J, Mazieres B. Medical treatment of reflex sympathetic dystrophy. *Hand Clin.* 1997; 13:477–483.

Bengtson K. Physical modalities for complex regional pain syndrome. *Hand Clin.* 1997;443–454.

Bianchi S, Abdelwahib IF, Garcia J. Partial transient osteoporosis of the hand. *Skeletal Radiol.* 1999;28:324–329.

Bilkey AJ. Screening for psychological disorders. In: Boissonnault WG, ed. *Examination in Physical Therapy Practice.* New York, NY: Churchill Livingstone; 1991:250.

Birklein F, Riedl B, Sieweke N, et al. Neurological findings in complex regional pain syndromes—analysis of 145 cases. *Acta Neurologica Scandinavica.* 2000;101:262–269.

Bodur H, Gunduz OH, Yucel M. Reflex sympathetic dystrophy arising in a patient with familial Mediterranean fever. *Rheumatol In.* 1999;19:69–70.

Braverman DL, Kern HB, Nagler W. Recurrent spontaneous hemarthrosis associated with reflex sympathetic dystrophy. *Arch Phys Med Rehabil.* 1998;79:339–342.

Bryan BK, Kohnke EN. Therapy after skeletal fixation in the hand and wrist. *Hand Clin.* 1997;13:761–776.

Bushnell TG, Cobo-Castro T. Complex regional pain syndrome: becoming more or less complex? *Man Ther.* 1999;4:221–228.

Chenoll GG, Villaverde EC, Cortes MAO, et al. Reflex sympathetic dystrophy in children. *Rehabilitacion.* 1996;30:220–223.

Cooney WP. Somatic versus sympathetic mediated chronic limb pain. Experience and treatment options. *Hand Clin.* 1997;13:355–361.

Dowling K. Acupuncturists learn points on the treatment of RSI. *Physiotherapy Frontline.* 1996;2:12.

Faria SH, Flannery JC. Reflex sympathetic dystrophy syndrome: an update. *J Vascular Nurs.* 1998;16:25–30.

Fealy MJ, Ladd AL. Reflex sympathetic dystrophy: early diagnosis and active treatment. *J Musculoskeletal Med.* 1996;13:29–32.

Gellman H. Reflex sympathetic dystrophy: alternative modalitites for pain management. *Instructional Course Lect.* 2000;49:549–557.

Gersch MR. Reflex sympathetic dystrophy syndrome: a model for the multidisciplinary management of patients with pain. *Phys Ther Pract.* 1993;2:3:34–44.

Gobelet C, Waldburger M, Meier JL. The effect of adding calcitonin to physical treatment on reflex sympathetic dystrophy. *Pain.* 1992;48:171–175.

Grabois M, Garrison SJ, Hart KA, Lehmkuhl LD. *Physical Medicine and Rehabilitation: The Complete Approach.* Malden, Mass: Blackwell Science; 2000.

Hardy MA, Hardy SGP. Reflex sympathetic dystrophy: the clinician's perspective. *J Hand Ther.* 10:137–150.

Headley BJ. Chronic pain management. In: O'Sullivan SB, Schmitz TJ, eds. *Phys Rehabil.* 3rd ed. Philadelphia, Pa: FA Davis Co; 1994:577–602.

Hertling D, Kessler RM. *Management of Common Musculoskeletal Disorders.* 3rd ed. Philadelphia, Pa: JB Lippincott Co; 1996.

Hood-White R, Gainor J. Reflex sympathetic dystrophy in an 8-year-old: successful treatment by physical therapy. *Orthop.* 1997;20:73–74.

Kasdan ML, Johnson AL. Reflex sympathetic dystrophy. *Occup Med.* 1998;13:521–531.

Kemler MA, Barendse GA, van Kleef M, et al. Spinal cord stimulation in patients with chronic reflex sympathetic dystrophy. *N Engl J Med.* 2000;343:618–624.

Kemler MA, Reulen JP, Barendse GA. Impact of spinal cord stimulation on sensory characteristics in complex regional pain syndrome type I: a randomized trial. *Anesthesiol.* 2001;95:72–80.

Kemler MA, Rijks CP, de Vet HC. Which patients with chronic reflex sympathetic dystrophy are most likely to benefit from physical therapy? *J Manipulative Physiol Ther.* 2001; 24:272–278.

Kingery WS. A critical review of controlled clinical trials for peripheral neuropathic pain and complex regional pain syndromes. *Pain.* 1997;73:123–139.

Kisner C, Colby LA. *Therapeutic Exercise: Foundations and Techniques.* 3rd ed. Philadelphia, Pa: FA Davis Co; 1996.

Ku A, Lachmann E, Tunkel R, et al. Upper limb reflex sympathetic dystrophy associated with occult malignancy. *Arch Phys Med Rehabil.* 1996;77:726–728.

Lampen-Smith RA. Complex regional pain syndrome I (RSD) and the physiotherapeutic intervention. *NZ J Physiotherapy.* 1997;25:19–23.

Lindenfeld TN, Bach BR JR, Wojtys EM. Reflex sympathetic dystrophy and pain dysfunction in the lower extremity. *Instructional Course Lect.* 1997;46:261–268.

Lopez RF. Reflex sympathetic dystrophy. Timely diagnosis and treatment can prevent severe contractures. *Postgraduate Med.* 1997;101:185–190.

MacFarlane BV, Wright A, O'Callaghan J, et al. Chronic neuropathic pain and its control by drugs. *Pharmacol Ther.* 1997;75:1–19.

Maneksha FR, Mirza H, Popprs PJ. Complex regional pain syndrome (CPRS) with resistance to local anesthetic block: a case report. *J Clin Anesth.* 2000;12:67–71.

Murray CS, Cohen A, Perkins T, et al. Morbidity in reflex sympathetic dystrophy. *Arch Dis Childhood.* 2000;82:231–233.

Oerlemans HM, Goris JA, de Boo T, et al. Do physical therapy and occupational therapy reduce the impairment percentage in reflex sympathetic dystrophy? *Am J Phys Med Rehabil.* 1999;78:533–539.

Oerlemans HM, Oostendorp RA, de Boo T. Pain and reduced mobility in complex regional pain syndrome I: outcome of a prospective randomized controlled clinical trial of adjuvant physical therapy versus occupational therapy. *Pain.* 1999;83:77–83.

Oerlemans HM, Oostendorp RAB, de Boo T, et al. Adjuvant physical therapy versus occupational therapy in patients with reflex sympathetic dystrophy complex regional pain syndrome type I. *Arch Phys Med Rehabil.* 2000;81:49–56.

Pandita D, Danielson BD, Potti A. Complex regional pain syndrome type-I: a rare complication of arteriovenous graft placement. *J Rheumatol.* 1999;26:2254–2256.

Pittman DM, Belgrade MJ. Complex regional pain syndrome. *Am Fam Phys.* 1997;56:2265–2270.

Poncelet C, Perdu M, Levy-Weil F, et al. Reflex sympathetic dystrophy in pregnancy: nine cases and a review of the literature. *Eur J Obstet Gynecol Reprod Biol.* 1999;86:55–63.

Severens JL, Oerlemans HM, Weegels AJP, et al. Cost-effectiveness analysis of adjuvant physical or occupational therapy for patients with reflex sympathetic dystrophy. *Arch Phys Med Rehabil.* 1999;80:1038–1043.

Soucacos PN, Diznitsas LA, Beris AE, et al. Clinical criteria and treatment of segmental versus upper extremity reflex sympathetic dystrophy. *Acta Orhtopaedica Belgica.* 1998; 64:314–321.

Viel E, Ripart J, Pelissier J, et al. Management of reflex sympathetic dystrophy. *Ann Med Int* (Paris). 1999;150:205–210.

Wadsworth CT. Elbow, forearm, wrist, and hand. In: Myers RS, ed. *Saunders Manual of Physical Therapy Practice.* Philadelphia, Pa: WB Saunders Co; 1995:887–888.

Wu CT, Ho ST, Tsai CS, et al. Repeated lumbar sympathetic blockade for complex regional pain syndromes type I—a case report. *Acta Anaesthesiologica Sinica.* 1998;36:155–158.

Zuurmond WW, Langendijk PN, Bezemer PD, et al. Treatment of acute reflex sympathetic dystrophy with DMSO 50% in a fatty cream. *Acta Anaesthesiologica Scandinavica.* 1996;40:364–367.

Zyluk A. Results of the treatment of posttraumatic reflex sympathetic dystrophy of the upper extremity with regional intravenous blocks of methylprednisolone and lidocaine. *Acta Orthopaedica Belgica.* 1998;64:452–456.

Zyluk A. The reasons for poor response to treatment of posttraumatic reflex sympathetic dystrophy. *Acta Orthopaedica Belgica.* 1998;64:309–313.

Stroke

Also known as *cerebrovascular accident* or *cerebrovascular disease*.

DESCRIPTION

Cerebrovascular disease leads to vascular injury of the brain due to interruption of cerebral circulation followed by neurologic disability. Cerebrovascular disease can be divided into four main types: arteriovenous malformation, cerebral insufficiency (ischemia), hemorrhage, and infarction.

Stroke usually refers to an ischemic lesion. A stroke in evolution refers to an enlarging infarction with neurological deficits that increase over a period of 24 to 48 hours. A completed stroke refers to an infarction of brain tissue of abrupt onset followed by neurological defects of variable outcome but stable symptoms.

CAUSE

A stroke can occur in conjunction with other diseases, but cerebrovascular disease is usually due to hypertension, atherosclerosis, or both. The mechanisms involved in causing the stroke include embolism, hemorrhage secondary to trauma or aneurysm, and thrombus. Major risk factors for cerebrovascular disease include diabetes, heart disease, high blood pressure, cigarette smoking, and transient ischemic attacks (TIAs). A TIA is a sudden, brief dysfunction of the arterial system. Secondary risk factors include elevated cholesterol and lipid levels, excessive alcohol consumption, obesity, and physical inactivity.

ASSESSMENT

Note: See APTA's Guide to Physical Therapist Practice. 2nd ed. *Physical Therapy.* 2001;81.

Musculoskeletal Preferred Practice Patterns: B, G

Neuromuscular Preferred Practice Patterns: B, G

AREAS

- History, including medications and metabolic status
- Psychosocial, including depression and family support
- Vision
- Communication, including aphasia
- Cognition
- Pain
- Posture, including sitting, standing, and supine positions and any asymmetry
- Cardiovascular, including blood pressure, heart rate, endurance, and any vascular compromise
- Pulmonary, if indicated
- Urogenital, including incontinence
- Skin and soft tissue, including edema or pressure sores
- Mobility, including active and passive range of motion (ROM)
- Joint integrity, including any shoulder subluxation
- Motor control, including tone (resting and dynamic); reflexes (tonic reflexes, righting reflexes, equilibrium responses); balance and postural reactions; hemiplegia and active movement control components, such as strength, coordination, patterned movement, and isolated movement
- Neurological, including proprioception, sensation, DTRs, Babinski, and clonus; kinesthesia, level of consciousness (if indicated)
- Functional level, including activities of daily living (ADLs), bed mobility, sitting, transfers, standing, and use of wheelchair
- Gait including potential for body weight support ambulation.
- Equipment, including use of orthotics, appliances, and assistive devices, and environmental assessment of needs upon discharge
- Health status

INSTRUMENTS/PROCEDURES

See References for sources.

Note: References with an asterisk are the preferred standard instruments for patient assessment in stroke.

Balance
- Berg Balance Test*
- adaptability measures
- balance response to external displacement
- balance response to volitional movement
- sway excursion
- verticality measures
- Clinical Test for Sensory Interaction on Balance (CTSIB)
- functional reach
- postural control evaluation
- Timed Up and Go Test
- Tinetti test

Cognition
- Activity Index
- Folstein Mini-Mental State Examination*
- Neurobehavioural Cognition Status Exam (NCSE)*

Communication
- Boston Diagnostic Aphasia Examination*
- Boston Naming test
- Communicative Abilities in Daily Living test
- Functional Communication Profile
- Promoting Aphasic's Communicative Effectiveness (PACE)
- Minnesota Test for Differential Diagnosis of Aphasia
- Porch Index of Communicative Ability (PICA)*
- Token test
- Western Aphasia Battery*

Disability
- Chedoke-McMaster Stroke Assessment (Chedoke), to be used in conjunction with Uniform Data System for Medical Rehabilitation (UDS)
- Functional Autonomy Measurement System (SMAF)
- Rankin Scale* and modified Rankin Scale
- NIH Stroke Scale*
- World Health Organization International Classification of Impairment, Disability and Handicap Functional Level
- Action Research Arm test
- Acute Care Index for Function
- ADLs: Activity Index
- Barthel index
- Frenchay Activities Index*
- Functional Index Measure (FIM; a component of Uniformed Data System for Medical Rehabilitation)*
- Katz Index of ADLs
- Kenny Self-Care Evaluation
- Klein-Bell Activities Scale
- Level of Rehabilitation Scale (LORS-II)-revision of LORS-I
- Motor Activity Log (MAL)
- Patient Evaluation Conference System (PECS); a modification of PECS is the Clinical Outcome Variable Scale
- PGC Instrumental Activities of Daily Living*
- PULSES profile
- Rehabiliation Activities Profile
- Rivermeade ADL Assessment

Geriatric assessments
- Lawton's Activities of Daily Living Scale
- Older Americans Resources & Services (OARS) Multidimensional Functional Assessment Questionnaire
- Functional Life Scale
- Philadelphia Geriatric Center Multilevel Assessment Instrument
- Stroke Impairment Assessment Set (SIAS)

Gait
- Functional Ambulation Profile (FAP)
- gait analysis
- Gait Assessment Rating Sheet (GARS)
- Tinetti test
- Scandinavian Stroke Scale
- TELER

Health Status
- Medical Outcomes Study (MOS) 36-Item Short-Form Health Survey*
- Sickness Impact Profile (SIP)*

Mobility
- goniometry
- Rivermeade Mobility Index*
- Timed Up and Go Test

Motor Control and Muscular Performance
1. General
   - Activity Index
   - Fugl-Meyer scale
   - manual muscle testing
   - Motoricity Index Score*
   - Motor Assessment Scale*
   - Modified Motor Assessment Scale (MMAS)
   - Medical Research Council six-point scale
2. Hemiplegia
   - Bobath and modified Bobath methods of assessment of postural and movement patterns
   - Brunnstrom method of assessment
   - Fugl-Meyer Assessment (FMA; expansion of Brunnstrom)*
3. Tone
   - Ashworth Scale of Muscle Spasticity
   - isokinetic dynamometer
   - myometer

Neurological
- Canadian Neurological Scale*
- Glasgow Coma Scale*
- two-point discrimination

Psychosocial
1. depression
   - Beck Depression Inventory (BDI)*
   - Center for Epidemiologic Studies-Depression (CES-D)*
   - Geriatric Depression Scale (GDS)*
   - Hamilton Depression Scale*
2. family support
   - Family Assessment Device (FAD)*

Vision
- visual scanning test

PROBLEMS

PSYCHOSOCIAL
- The client may have poststroke mood disorder, especially depression (more with left-hemisphere injury), emotional lability, irritability, confusion, and, if multiple infarcts have occurred, dementia.

VISION
- Visual defects, such as loss of depth perception and homonymous hemiannopsia, or visual field defect, commonly accompany hemiplegia. There may also be forced gaze deviation.

347

COMMUNICATION
- The client may have communication impairment. Aphasia, or acquired communication disorder, is often associated with left hemispheric lesion (right hemiplegia).
- The client may also have dysarthria, or impairment of speech production.

COGNITION
- The client may have cognitive deficits. Deficits can affect orientation, attention span, ability to process information, conceptualizing ability, memory, and activity tolerance.
- The client may demonstrate perceptual deficits. These include distorted body image, unilateral neglect, and visuospatial distortions like topographical disorientation.

PAIN
- Knee pain can accompany any hyperextension with gait.
- The client often has shoulder subluxation and pain. Reflex sympathetic dystrophy may accompany the pain (see Precautions).

CARDIOVASCULAR
- The client with cardiac disease may also demonstrate cardiac decompensation, along with deconditioning and limited exercise tolerance.
- Deep-venous thrombosis and pulmonary embolism may occur if the client is immobilized.

UROGENITAL
- The client may have bladder and bowel dysfunction.

SKIN
- There may be edema and pain.

MOBILITY
- The client may have decreased ROM and joint contractures.
- The client often has impaired mobility influenced by motor programming deficits. Functional ability impairment leads to difficulty with rolling, sitting, standing, gait.

MOTOR CONTROL
- The client will typically have paresis or weakness.
- The client may have impairment of motor power. Hypotonicity is initially common and replaced by hypertonicity, hyperreflexia, and mass patterns of movement.
- The client may have weak or absent muscle strength.
- The client may have ataxia, or incoordination.
- The client may have apraxia, or inability to perform purposive movements, usually associated with left hemispheric lesion (see Table 10.2).

NEUROLOGICAL
- The client often has sensory impairment, without total loss, on hemiplegic side.
- The client may have symptoms of crossed anesthesia, defined as ipsilateral facial impairments with contralateral trunk and limb deficits, usually associated with brain stem lesions.
- The client may have proprioceptive loss. There may also be loss of superficial touch, along with pain and altered temperature sensation.
- The client may lose combined sensations such as two-point discrimination.
- Initial contralateral sensory loss may be followed by burning pain on the hemiplegic side, called *thalamic syndrome*.

TABLE 10.2
Comparison of Left and Right Hemiplegia

Right Hemiplegia	Left Hemiplegia
Verbal communication difficulties, such as receptive or expressive global aphasia	Visual, perceptual deficits
	Left visual field deficit
Right visual field deficit	Distractable
Decreased computation (mathematical skills)	Denial of problem with the left side of the body
Left/right confusion	Impulsive behavior
Deficits in memory	Dressing apraxia
Depression	Difficulty crossing midline of body
Motorapraxia	

Source: Quintana. Evaluation of Perception and Cognition. In: Trombly CA, Radomsky MV, eds. *Occupational Therapy for Physical Dysfunction.* 4th ed. Lippincott Williams and Wilkins; 2002:204.

TREATMENT/MANAGEMENT

TREATMENT APPROACHES

Recent theories and principles have led to revised treatment approaches for clients with neurological deficits. The main approaches used include the compensatory approach, the muscle reeducation approach, the neurotherapeutic facilitation approach, and the contemporary task-oriented approach (also called motor control/motor learning). Many therapists use an integrated approach using any or all of these various approaches depending on the individual needs of the client. General treatment considerations are listed here; see References for detailed treatment plans.

Compensatory Approach
- Focus on improving function instead of individual impairment by structuring task to be performed in a predictable environment.

Muscle Reeducation Approach
- Focus on individual muscle isolation of muscle action.
- Avoid secondary impairments.
- Teach client to avoid compensatory movement patterns.
- Teach functional activities.
- Use orthopedic supports as indicated.
- Increase strength of intact motor units.

Neurotherapeutic Facilitation Approach
- Provide proprioceptive input to facilitate normal movement patterns.
- Normalize tone.
- Break up abnormal synergies.
- Inhibit primitive reflexes and any abnormal tone.
- Prevent learning of abnormal movement patterns.
- Therapist provides hands-on sensory feedback to correct movement patterns.

Contemporary Task-Oriented Approach
- Teach client motor problem-solving skills appropriate to context needed.
- Explore effective compensation.
- Practice functional activities in varied environmental conditions, and vary the tasks performed.

- Encourage client to achieve task goals through problem solving and error detection. Allow client to make mistakes and analyze outcome.
- Use developmental sequence activities only in a manner appropriate to client's age and activity.
- Feedback should be task specific and designed to discourage over-dependency of the client on the therapist.
- Posturing of extremities focuses on maintaining the necessary muscle length needed for ADLs using passive ROM or serial casting.

GENERAL CONSIDERATIONS IN THE ACUTE STAGE

Positioning
- Prevent hip and knee contractures when client is on bed rest.
- Use egg-crate mattress for pressure relief.
- Client should be turned every 2 to 3 hours in early stage if on prolonged bed rest.
- Assume upright posture as soon as possible and when client is stable.
- Avoid pulling on weakened extremity.
- Protect hemiplegic shoulder from downward displacement through a scapular position of slight protraction and upward rotation.
- Arrange room to maximize the client's awareness of the hemiplegic side.

ROM
- Perform full ROM in all areas of deficit. Upper extremity motions should include external rotation of the arm and scapular mobilization and upward rotation during shoulder elevation activities.
- Assess for temporary use of sling.
- Consider use of neurotherapeutic facilitation to promote joint stability.
- Consider use of inflated pressure splint to promote optimal positioning and sensory reeducation.

Mobility
- Encourage early mobilization, after the client is medically stable, to prevent secondary impairments like psychological problems, decreasing ROM, contracture and deformity, deep-venous thrombosis, pain, shoulder dysfunction, and deconditioning.
- Encourage use of both sides of the body.
- Encourage client to participate actively in movement as soon as possible.
- Concentrate on functional activities like rolling, sitting up, bridging, standing, and transfers.
- Consider use of extremity movement patterns to improve rolling.
- Encourage weight-bearing activity on the hemiplegic side.
- Upright activities should promote stability, followed by controlled mobility and then dynamic balance challenges.
- Promote normalization of chewing, expressive, respiratory, and swallowing functions.

GENERAL CONSIDERATIONS DURING THE POSTACUTE STAGE

Provide education about the disease and rehabilitation program for client and family. Offer counseling in the areas of need, including recreational, psychological, sexual, and vocational counseling. Provide discharge planning.

Motor Control
- Stress function that is meaningful to client.
- Incorporate bilateral activities when possible.
- Mental rehearsal of activities may be indicated.

- Encourage movement patterns that are out of synergy, and permit completion of functional tasks.
- Inhibit unwanted muscle activity.
- Select postures that promote desired motion, and reduce any unwanted excess in tone or interference from reflexes. Progress to more challenging postures.
- Activate muscles in a variety of patterns and situations.
- Emphasize a balanced interaction between agonists and antagonists.
- Use stimuli to facilitate hypotonia; exteroceptive, proprioceptive, and reflex stimulation techniques may be considered.
- Continue static control and balance activities begun in the acute stage.
- Promote control of upper extremity and lower extremity.
- Initiate gait training early. Consider use of assistive device.
- Identifiy and correct specific movement deficits.
- Advanced gait training emphasizes selective movement control combined with normal timing. Practice gait activities in varied directions and on surfaces. Dynamic EMG can be used to guide hand placement during gait training and to decrease spasticity.
- Practice elevation activities.
- Consider use of an orthosis, most often an ankle-foot orthosis.
- Control knee problems by adjustment of ankle position.
- Continue functional training in ADLs.
- Establish cardiovascular conditioning program for those who are candidates.
- Consider use of isokinetic training to stimulate improved lower extremity reciprocal movement during gait activities.
- Consider use of neuromuscular electrical stimulation (NMES) to facilitate voluntary motor control or functional electrical stimulation (FES) to reestablish normal joint alignment.
- Consider use of biofeedback to improve motor function.

Sensory Loss
- Encourage use of affected side.
- Present repeated sensory stimuli, such as stretch, stroking, deep and superficial pressure, along with weight bearing.
- Utilize localization of touch.
- Consider electrical stimulation to activate sensorimotor response.
- Avoid adverse effects with excessive intensity.
- Consider use of pressure splints or in severe cases, intermittent pressure therapy.
- Educate client on issue of anesthetic limbs.
- Consider forced non-use of unaffected limb.

PRECAUTIONS/CONTRAINDICATIONS
- Overhead pulleys are generally contraindicated for self ROM to avoid shoulder impingement or rotator cuff injury.
- Monitor circulation when using sling, especially figure-eight harness-type sling. Sling is often contraindicated with spasticity.
- Watch for depression, and refer for psychological/psychiatric support as indicated. Client may need medical treatment for depression.
- Generally, it is advisable to arrange the room to maximize the client's awareness of the hemiplegic side, but this strategy is contraindicated with clients who have unilateral neglect or anosognosia because this may actually stimulate withdrawal.

DESIRED OUTCOME/PROGNOSIS
- The client will be aware of and use the hemiplegic side.
- The client will be functionally mobile.
- The client will be independent with ADLs.

- The client will have adequate cardiopulmonary endurance.
- The client will maintain ROM and prevent deformity.
- The client will regain oromotor function.
- The client will have postural control, balance, and control of elective movements.
- The client will engage in socialization activities.
- Secondary complications will be prevented.

Notes: Clinical trials support an early initiation of physical therapy for more favorable outcomes.

Studies report improved functional outcome and increased independence after physical therapy, but no single optimal approach has been identified. Approximately 75% to 85% of clients are discharged back home.

Clients who generally do not respond well to rehabilitation efforts include those with the following problems:

- diminished alertness and ability to learn
- severe anosognosia
- severe medical complications
- severe language impairment

Approximately 30% of stroke victims die in the acute phase. Of those who survive, approximately 30% to 40% are left with severe disability.

Early diagnosis of reflex sympathetic dystrophy (RSD) is critical to optimal outcome. Watch for swelling and tenderness of hand and fingers and accompanying shoulder pain. The skin may appear red and glossy and be warm to touch, with fingernails appearing white or opaque. In later stages of the problem, the skin turns cool, cyanotic, and contracted.

The first 6 weeks to 2 months is generally the period of optimal spontaneous recovery for speech abilities.

Clients with thalamic syndrome generally have a poor functional outcome.

Functional outcomes are difficult to predict and recovery factors are multifactorial (eg, comorbidity, family supports, financial resources, motivation and rehabilitation potential).

REFERENCES

Assessment

Berg K, Maki B, Williams JI, et al. Clinical and laboratory measures of postural balance in an elderly population. *Arch Phys Med Rehabil.* 1992;73:1073–1083.

Bohannon RW, Learey KM, Cooper J. Independence in floor-to-stand transfers soon after stroke. *Topics Geriatr Rehabil.* 1995;11:1:6–9.

Cammack S, Eisenberg MG, eds. *Key Words in Physical Rehabilitation: A Guide to Contemporary Usage.* New York, NY: Springer Publishing Co; 1995.

Collen FM, Wade DT, Robb GF, Bradshaw CM. The Rivermeade Mobility Index: a further development of the Rivermeade Motor Assessment. *Int Disability Stud.* 1991;13:50–54.

Cromwell S. Balance instability. In: Myers RS, ed. *Saunders Manual of Physical Therapy Practice.* Philadelphia, Pa: WB Saunders Co; 1995:376.

DeLisa D. *Rehabilitation Medicine: Principle and Practice.* Philadelphia, Pa: JB Lippincott Co; 1998.

Dickstein R, Hocherman S, Amdor G, Pillar T. Reaction and movement times in patients with hemiparesis for unilateral and bilateral elbow flexion. *Phys Ther.* 1993;73:374–380.

DiFabio RP, Badke MB. Relationship of sensory organization to balance function in patients with hemiplegia. *Phys Ther.* 1990;70:542–548.

DiFabio RP, Badke MB. Stance duration under sensory conflict conditions in patients with hemiplegia. *Arch Phys Med Rehabil.* 1991;72:292–295.

Dodd KJ, Morris ME, Wrigley TV. Clinical analysis of lateral pelvic displacement disorders in stroke. *Physiotherapy Singapore.* 2000;3:98–105.

Duncan PW, Goldstein LB, Matchar D, et al. Measurement of motor recovery after stroke: outcome assessment and sample size requirements. *Stroke.* 1992;23:1084–1089.

Duncan PW, Weiner DK, Chandler J, Studenski S. Assessing the influence of sensory interaction of balance. *J Gerontol.* 1990;45:M192–M197.

Dvir Z, Panturin E. Measurement of spasticity and associated reactions in stroke patients before and after physiotherapeutic intervention. *Clin Rehabil.* 1993;7:1:15–21.

Flores AM. Objective measurement of standing balance. *Neurol Rep.* 1992;16:1:17–21.

Goldie PA, Matyas TA, Spencer KL, McGinley RB. Postural control in standing following stroke: test-retest reliability of some quantitative clinical tests. *Phys Ther.* 1990;70:234–243.

Gowland C, Stratford P, Ward M, Moreland J, Torresin W. Measuring physical impairment and disability with the Chedoke-McMaster Stroke Assessment. *Stroke.* 1993;24:1:58–61.

Grabois M, Garrison SJ, Hart KA, Lehmkuhl LD. *Physical Medicine and Rehabilitation: The Complete Approach.* Malden, Mass: Blackwell Science; 2000.

Hamilton BB, Granger CV. Disability outcomes following inpatient rehabilitation for stroke. *Phys Ther.* 1994;74:494–503.

Jones F. The accuracy of predicting functional recovery in patients following a stroke, by physiotherapists and patients. *Physiotherapy Res Int.* 1998;3:244–256.

Keating JL, Parks C, Mackenzie M. Measurements of ankle dorsiflexion in stroke subjects obtained using standardized dorsiflexion force. *Aust J Physiotherapy.* 2000;46:203–213.

Kendall FP, McCreary EK, Provance PG. *Muscles: Testing and Function.* 4th ed. Baltimore, Md: Williams and Wilkins; 1993.

Lennon S. Using standardized scales to document outcome in stroke rehabilitation. *Physiotherapy.* 1995;81:200–202.

Lincoln N, Edmans JA. A re-validation of the Rivermeade ADL scale for elderly patients with stroke. *Age and Aging.* 1990;19:19–24.

Livesley E. The intra-observer reliablity of the hand-held myometer in the measurement of isotonic muscle strength in chronic spasticity. *Physiotherapy.* 1992;78:918–921.

O'Sullivan SB, Schmitz TJ, eds. *Physical Rehabilitation: Assessment and Treatment.* Philadelphia, Pa: FA Davis Co; 1994.

Pathokinesiology Service Observational Gait Analysis. Downey, Ca: Rancho Los Amigos Medical Center; 1993.

Patla AE, Clous SD. Visual assessment of human gait: reliability and validity. *Rehabil Res.* 1998;1:87–96.

Perry J. *Gait Analysis: Normal and Pathological Function.* Thorofare, NJ: Slack; 1992.

Podsiadlo D, Richardson S. The timed "up and go": a test of basic functional mobility for frail elderly persons. *J Am Geriatr Soc.* 1991;39:142–148.

Rogers MW, Hedman LD, Pai Y. Kinetic analysis of dynamic transitions in stance support accompanying voluntary leg flexion movements in hemiparetic adults. *Arch Phys Med Rehabil.* 1993;74:19–25.

Rosecrance JC, Giuliani CA. Kinematic analysis of lower-limb movement during ergometer pedaling in hemiplegic and nonhemiplegic subjects. *Phys Ther.* 1991;71:334–343.

Rothstein JM, Roy SH, Wolf SL. *The Rehabilitation Specialist's Handbook.* 2nd ed. Philadelphia, Pa: FA Davis Co; 1998.

Sanford J, Moreland J, Swanson LR, Stratford PW, Gowland C. Reliability of the Fugl-Meyer Assessment for testing motor performance in patients following stroke. *Phys Ther.* 1993;73:447–454.

Sartor-Glittenberg C, Powers R. Quantitative measurement of kinesthesia following cerebral vascular accident. *Physiotherapy Can.* 1993;45:179–186.

Sine R, Liss SE, Rousch RE, et al. *Basic Rehabilitation Techniques: A Self-Instructional Guide.* 4th ed. Gaithersburg, Md: Aspen Publishers; 2000.

Stanko E, Goldie P, Nayler M. Development of a new mobility scale for people living in the community after stroke: content validity. *Aust J Physiotherapy.* 2001;47:201–209.

Stevenson TJ. Detecting change in patients with stroke using the Berg Balance Scale. *Aust J Physiotherapy.* 2001;47:29–38.

Thornton H, Jackson D, Turner-Stokes L. Accuracy of predication of walking for young stroke patients by use of the FIM. *Physiotherapy Res In.* 2001;6:1–14.

Tousignant M, Arsenoult H, Corriveau P. Clinical evaluation of patient following stroke: Proposed stroke patient taxonomy based on cluster analysis. *Physiotherapy Theory Pract.* 2000;16:81–93.

Tripp EJ, Harris SR. Test-retest reliability of isokinetic knee extension and flexion torque measurements in persons with spastic hemiparesis. *Phys Ther.* 1991;71:390–396.

Wade DT, Collen FM, Robb GP, Warlow CP. Physiotherapy intervention late after stroke and mobility. *Br Med J.* 1992;304:609–613.

Wagenaar RC, Beek WJ. Hemiplegic gait: a kinematic analysis using walking speed as a basis. *J Biomech.* 1992;25:1007–1015.

Wagenaar RC, vanWieringen PC, Netelenbos JB, et al. The transfer of scanning training effects in visual inattention after stroke: five single-case studies. *Disability Rehabil.* 1992;14:51–60.

Ware JE, Sherbourne CD. The MOS 36-Item Short-Form Health Survey (SF-36): I. Conceptual framework and item selection. *Med Care.* 1992;30:473–483.

Williams BK, Galea MP, Winter AT. What is the functional outcome for the upper limb after stroke? *Aust J Physiotherapy.* 2001;47:19–27.

Wolfson L, Whipple R, Amerman P, Tobin JN. Gait assessment in the elderly: a gait abnormality rating scale and its relation to falls. *J Gerontol.* 1990;45:1:M12–M19.

Treatment

Andrews AW. Effect of physical therapy intervention on muscle strength and functional limitations in a patient with chronic stroke. *Phys Ther Case Rep.* 2000;3:17–21.

Andrews AW, Bohannon RW. Distribution of muscle strength impairments following stroke. *Clin Rehabil.* 2000;14:79–87.

Aruin AS, Hanke T, Chaudhuri G, et al. Compelled weightbearing in persons with hemiparesis following stroke: the effect of a lift insert and goal-directed balance exercise. *J Rehabil Res Dev.* 2000;37:65–72.

Ballinger C, Ashburn A, Low J, et al. Unpacking the black box of therapy—a pilot study to describe occupational therapy and physiotherapy interventions for people with stroke. *Clin Rehabil.* 1999;13:301–309.

Baskett JJ, Broad JB, Reekie G, et al. Shared responsibility for ongoing rehabilitation: a new approach to home-based therapy after stroke. *Clin Rehabil.* 1999;13:23–33.

Bate PJ, Matyas TA. Negative transfer of training following brief practice of elbow tracking movements with electromyographic feedback from spastic antagonists. *Arch Phys Med Rehabil.* 1992;73:1050–1058.

Berg KO, Maki BE, Williams JI, et al. Clinical and laboratory measures of postural balance in an elderly population. *Arch Phys Med Rehabil.* 1992;73:1073–1080.

Bernhardt J, Bate, Matyas TA. Accuracy of observational kinematic assessment of upper-limb movements. *Phys Ther.* 1998;78:259–270.

Blanton S, Wolf SL. An application of upper-extremity constraint-induced movement therapy in a patient with subacute stroke. *Phys Ther.* 1999;79:847–853.

Bogataj U, Gros N, Klijajic M, et al. The rehabilitation of gait in patients with hemiplegia: a comparison between conventional therapy and multi-channel functional electrical stimulation therapy. *Phys Ther.* 1995;75:490–502.

Bogle Thorbahn LD, Newton RA. Use of the Berg Balance Test to predict falls in the elderly. *Phys Ther.* 1996;76:576–585.

Bohannon RW. Physical rehabilitation in neurologic disease. *Curr Opinion Neurol.* 1993; 6:765–772.

Bohannon RW. Strength associated motor deficits following stroke. *Percep Motor Skills.* 1997;84:393–394.

Brosseau L, Philippe P, Potvin L, et al. Post-stroke inpatient rehabilitation. I. Predicting length of stay. *Am J Phys Rehabil.* 1996;75:422–430.

Brown DA, Kautz SA. Speed-dependent reductions of force output in people with poststroke hemiparesis. *Phys Ther.* 1999;79:919–930.

Daley K, Mayo N, Wood-Dauphinee S. Reliability of scores on the Stroke Rehabilitation Assessment of Movement (STREAM) measure. *Phys Ther.* 1999;79:8–19.

Daly JJ, Ruff RL. Electrically induced recovery of gait components for older patients with chronic stroke. *Am J Phys Med Rehabil.* 2000;79:349–360.

Davidson I, Waters K. Physiotherapists working with stroke patients: a national survey. *Physiotherapy.* 2000;86:69–80.

De Weerdt W, Nuyens G, Feys H, et al. Group physiotherapy improves time use by patients with stroke in rehabilitation. *Aust J Physiotherapy.* 2001;47:53–61.

De Weerdt W, Selz B, Nuyens G, et al. Time use of stroke patients in an intensive rehabilitation unit: a comparison between a Belgian and a Swiss setting. *Disability Rehabil.* 2000; 22:181–186.

Dickstein R, Abulaffio N. Postural sway of the affected and nonaffected pelvis and leg in stance of hemiparetic patients. *Arch Phys Med Rehabil.* 2000;81:364–367.

Dickstein R, Sheffi S, Ben Haim Z, et al. Activation of flexor and extensor trunk muscles in hemiparesis. *Am J Phys Med Rehabil.* 2000;79:228–234.

DiFabio RP, Seay R. Use of the "fast evaluation of mobility balances and fear" in elderly community dwellers: validity and reliability. *Phys Ther.* 1997;77:904–917.

Dowswell G, Dowswell T, Lawler J, et al. Post-stroke physiotherapy in context. *Br J Ther Rehabil.* 2001;8:446–453.

Dowswell G, Forster A, Young J, et al. The development of a collaborative stroke training programme for nurses. *J Clin Nurs.* 1999;8:743–752.

Duncan PW. Stroke: physical therapy assessment and treatment. In: Lister MJ, ed. *Contemporary Management of Motor Control Problems: Proceedings of the II STEP Conference.* Alexandria, Va: Foundation for Physical Therapy; 1991:209–218.

Dursun E, Hamamci N, Donmez S. Angular biofeedback device for sitting balance for stroke patients. *Stroke.* 1996;27:1354–1357.

Engardt M, Olsson E. Body weight-bearing while rising and sitting down in patients with stroke. *Scand J Rehabil Med.* 1992;24:67–74.

Engardt M, Ribbe T, Olsson E. Vertical ground reaction force feedback to enhance stroke patients' symmetrical body-weight distribution while rising/sitting down. *Scand J Rehabil Med.* 1993;25:41–48.

Faghri PD, Rodger MM, Glaser RM, et al. The effects of functional electrical stimulation on shoulder subluxation, arm function recovery, and shoulder pain in hemiplegic stroke patients. *Arch Phys Med Rehabil.* 1994;75:73–79.

Feeney DM. From laboratory to clinic: noradrenergic enhancement of physical therapy for stroke or trauma patients. *Adv Neurol.* 1997;73:383–394.

Finn AM, Horgan NF. The scope for rehabilitation in severely disabled stroke patients. *Disability Rehabil.* 2000;22:196–198.

Fisher BE, Winstein CJ, Velicki MR. Deficits in compensatory trajectory adjustments after unilateral sensorimotor stroke. *Exp Brain Res.* 2000;132:328–344.

Fishman MN, Colby LA, Sachs LA, Nichols DS. Comparison of upper-extremity balance tasks and force platform testing in persons with hemiparesis. *Phys Ther.* 1997;77:1052–1062.

Flick C. Stroke rehabilitation 4: stroke outcome and psychosocial consequences. *Arch Phys Med Rehabil.* 1999;80:521–526.

Fletcher GF, Banja JD, Jann BB, Wolf SL, eds. *Rehabilitation Medicine: Contemporary Clinical Perspectives.* Philadelphia, Pa: Lea and Febiger; 1992.

Forster A, Dowswell G, Young J, et al. Effects of a physiotherapist-led stroke training programme for nurses. Effects of a physiotherapist-led training programme on attitudes of nurses caring for patients after stroke. *Clin Rehabil.* 1999;13:113–122.

Freburger JK. Analysis of the relationship between the utilization of physical therapy services and outcomes for patients with acute stroke. *Phys Ther.* 1999;79:906–918.

Garland SJ, Stevenson TJ, Ivanova T. Postural responses to unilateral arm pertubation in young, elderly, and hemiplegic subjects. *Arch Phys Med Rehabil.* 1997;78:1072–1077.

Gibbon B. An Investigation of interprofessional collaboration in stroke rehabilitation team conferences. *J Clin Nurs.* 1999;8:246–252.

Gil-Body KM, Papat RA, Parker SW, et al. Rehabilitation of balance in two patients with cerebellar dysfunction. *Phys Ther.* 1997;77:534–552.

Giuliani CA. Understanding AHCPR Clinical Practice Guideline No. 16: post-stroke rehabilitation. *PT-Magazine of Physical Therapy.* 1995;3:10:51–83.

Goldie Pam Matyas TA, Evans OM. Defiict and change in gait velocity during rehabilitation after stroke. *Arch Phys Med Rehabil.* 1996;77:1074–1084.

Gowland C, deBruin H, Basmajian JV, et al. Agonist and antagonist activity during voluntary upper-limb movement in patients with stroke. *Phys Ther.* 1992;72:624–633.

Grabois M, Garrison SJ, Hart KA, Lehmkuhl LD. *Physical Medicine and Rehabilitation: The Complete Approach.* Malden, Mass: Blackwell Science; 2000.

Granger CV, Cotter AC, Hamilton RB, Fielder RC. Functional assessment scales: a study of persons after stroke. *Arch Phys Med Rehabil.* 1993;74:133–138.

Gresham GE, Duncan PW, Stason WB, et al. Post-Stroke Rehabilitation: Assessment, Referral, and Patient Management. *Clin Pract Guideline.* Rockville, Md: US Dept of Health and Human Services, Agency for Health Care Policy and Research; 1995. AHCPR Pub. No 95-0663, Quick Reference Guide for Clinicians, No. 16.

Hale LA, Eales CJ. Consulting the South African Experts in Physiotherapeutic Stroke Rehabilitation. *S Afr J Physiotherapy.* 2001;32–40.

Hesse S, Uhlenbrock D, Sarkodie-Gyan T. Gait pattern of severely disabled hemiparetic subjects on a new controlles gait trainer as compared to assisted treadmill walking with partial body weight support. *Clin Rehabil.* 1999;13:401–410.

Hochstenbach J, Mulder T. Neuropsychology and the relearning of motor skills following stroke. *Int J Rehabil Res.* 1999;22:11–19.

Horgan NF, Finn AM. Motor recovery following stroke: a basis for evaluation. *Disability Rehabil*. 1997;19:64–70.

Hui Chan CW, Levin MF. Stretch reflex latencies in spastic hemiparetic subjects are prolonged after transcutaneous electrical nerve stimulation. *Can J Neurol Sci*. 1993;20:2:97–106.

Hummelsheim H, Eickof C. Repetitive sensorimotor training for arm and hand in a patient with locked-in syndrome. *Scand J Rehabil Med*. 1999;31:250–256.

Indredavik B, Bakke F, Slordahl SA, et al. Treatment in a combined acute and rehabilitation stroke unit: which aspects are most important? *Stroke*. 1999;30:917–923.

Jones F. The accuracy of predicting functional recovery in patients following a stroke, by physiotherapists and patients. *Physiotherapy Res Int*. 1998;244–256.

Katrak P, Bowring G, Conroy P, et al. Predicting upper limb recovery after stroke: the place of early shoulder and hand movement. *Arch Phys Med Rehabil*. 1998;79:758–761.

Krebs HI, Hogan N, Volpe BT, et al. Overview of clinical trials with MIT-MANUS: a robot-aided neuro-rehabilitaiton facility. *Tech Health Care*. 1999;7:419–423.

Kristeins AE, Black-Schaffer RM, Richard RL. Stroke rehabilitation. 3. Rehabilitation Management. *Arch Phys Med Rehabil*. 1999;80:517–520.

Kurabayashi H, Kubota K, Machida I, et al. Effects of physical therapy on immunological parameters in patients with cerebrovascular diseases. *J Med*. 1996;27:171–175.

Kurabayashi H, Machida I, Handa H, et al. Effects of physical therapy on cytokines and two color analysis-lymphocyte subsets in patients with cerebrovascular diseases. *J Med*. 1999;30:31–37.

Kwakkel G, van Dijk GM, Wagenaar RC. Accuracy of physical and occupational therapists' early predictions of recovery after severe middle cerebral artery stroke. *Clin Rehabil*. 2000;14:28–41.

Kwakkel G, Wagenaar RC, Koelman TW, et al. Effects of intensity of rehabilitation after stroke. A research synthesis. *Stroke*. 1997;28:1550–1556.

Kwakkel G, Wagenaar RC, Twisk JW, et al. Intensity of leg and arm training after primary middle-cerebral-artery stroke: a randomized trial. *Lancet*. 1999;354:191–196.

Langhorne P, Wagenaar R, Partridge C. Physiotherapy after stroke: more is better? *Physiotherapy Res Int*. 1996;1:75–88.

Laufer Y, Dickstein R, Chefez Y, et al. The effect of treadmill training of the ambulation of stroke survivors in the early stages of rehabilitation: a randomized study. *J Rehabil Res Dev*. 2001;38:69–78.

Laufer Y, Dickstein R, Resnik S, et al. Weight-bearing shifts of hemiparetic and healthy adults upon stepping on stairs of various heights. *Clin Rehabil*. 2000;14:125–129.

Lennon S. Gait re-education based on the Bobath concept in two patients with hemiplegia following stroke. *Phys Ther*. 2001;81:924–935.

Lettings A, Mol A. Clinical specificity and the non-generalitites of science. On innovation strategies for neurological physical therapy. *Theor Med Bioeth*. 1999;20:517–535.

Liepert J, Bauder H, Wolfgang HR, et al. Treatment-induced cortical reorganization after stroke in humans. *Stroke*. 2000;31:1210–1216.

Lin FM, Sabbahi M. Correlation of spasticity with hyperactive stretch reflexes and motor dysfunction in hemiplegia. *Arch Phys Med Rehabil*. 1999;80:526–530.

Lincoln NB, Parry RH, Vass CD. Randomized, controlled trial to evaluate increased intensity of physiotherapy treatment of arm function after stroke. *Stroke*. 1999;30:573–579.

Lindstorm B, Gerdle B, Forsgren L. Repeated maximum reciprocal knee movements in patients with minimal overt symptoms after ischaemic stroke: an evaluation of mechanical performance and EMG. *Scand J Rehabil Med*. 1998;30:47–54.

Liu M, Tsuji T, Tsujiuchi K, et al. Comorbidities is stroke patients as assessed with a newly developed comorbidity scale. *Am J Phys Med Rehabil.* 1999;78:416–424.

Maki BE, McIlroy WE. The role of limb movements in maintaining upright stance: the "change in support" strategy. *Phys Ther.* 1997;77:488–507.

Malouin F, Potvin M, Prevost J, et al. Use of an intensive task-oriented gait training program in a series of patients with acute cerebrovascular accidents. *Phys Ther.* 1992;72:781–793.

Mayer M, Grulichova J, Bazala J. Some manoeuvres for releasing the hypertonus of spastic and shortened muscles. *Acta Univ Palacki Olomuc Fac Med.* 1999;142:85–87.

McCulloch K. Standardized assessment tools for traumatic brain injury in physical therapy. 1998. *Neurol Rep.* 22:114–125.

Mercier C, Bourbonnais D, Bilodeau S, et al. Description of a new motor re-education programme for the paretic lower limb aimed at improving the mobility of stroke patients. *Clin Rehabil.* 1999;13:199–206.

Miyai I, Suzuki T, Kang J, Volpe BT. Improved functional outcome in patients with hemorrhagic stroke in putamen and thalamus compared with those with stroke restricted to the putamen or thalamus. *Stroke.* 2000;31:1365–1369.

Moreland J, Thomson MA. Efficacy of electromyographic biofeedback compared with conventional physical therapy for upper-extremity function in patients following stroke: a research overview and meta-analysis. *Phys Ther.* 1994;74:534–547.

Morris ME, Matyas TA, Bach TM, Goldie PA. Electrogoniometric feedback; its effect on genu recurvatum in stroke. *Arch Phys Med Rehabil.* 1992;73:1147–1154.

Mozzoni MP, Bailey JS. Improving training methods in brain injury rehabilitation. *J Head Trauma Rehabil.* 1996;11:1–17.

Mueller K, Cornwall M, McPoil JT, et al. Effect of a tone-inhibiting dynamic ankle-foot orthosis on the foot-loading pattern of a hemiplegic adult: a preliminary study. *J Prosthet Orthot.* 1992;4:2:86–92.

Nichols DS. Balance retraining after stroke using force platform biofeedback. *Phys Ther.* 1997;77:553–558.

Olney SJ, Griffin MP, McBride ID. Multivariate examination of data for gait analysis of persons with stroke. *Phys Ther.* 1998;78:814–828.

On AY, Kirazli Y, Kismali B, et al. Mechanisms of action of phenol block and botulinus toxin Type A in relieving spasticity: electrophysiologic investigation and follow-up. *Am J Phys Rehabil.* Jul–Aug 1999;*78*(4):344–349.

O'Sullivan SB. Stroke. In: O'Sullivan SB, Schmitz TJ, eds. *Physical Rehabilitation: Assessment and Treatment.* 3rd ed. Philadelphia, Pa: FA Davis Co; 1994:327–373.

Parry RH, Lincoln NB, Vass CD. Effect of severity of arm impairment on response to additional physiotherapy early after stroke. *Clin Rehabil.* 1999;13:187–198.

Partridge C, Mackenzie M, Edwards S, et al. Is dosage of physiotherapy a critical factor in deciding patterns of recovery from stroke; a pragmatic randomized controlled trial. *Physiotherapy Res Int.* 2000;5:230–240.

Pohl PS, Winstein CJ. Practice effects on the less-affected upper extremity after stroke. *Arch Phys Med Rehabil.* 1999;80:668–675.

Price SJ, Reding MJ. Physical therapy philosophies and strategies. In: Good DC, Couch JR, eds. *Handbook of Neurorehabilitation.* New York, NY: Marcel Dekker Inc; 1994:181–197.

Rice-Oxley M, Turner-Stokes L. Effectiveness of brain injury rehabilitation. 1999;13 suppl 1:7–24.

Richards CL, Malouin F, Dean C. Gait in stroke: assessment and rehabilitation. *Clin Geriatr Med.* 1999;15:833–855.

Richards CL, Malouin F, Wood-Dauphinee S, et al. Task-specific physical therapy for optimization of gait-recovery in acute stroke patients. *Arch Phys Med Rehabil.* 1993; 74:612–620.

Riddoch MJ, Humphreys GW, Bateman A. Cognitive deficits following stroke. *Physiotherapy.* 1995;81:465–473.

Riddoch MJ, Humphreys GW, Bateman A. Stroke: issues in recovery and rehabilitation. *Physiotherapy.* 1995;81:689–695.

Robichaud JA, Agostinucci J, Vander-Linden DW. Effect of air-splint application on soleus muscle motorneuron reflex excitability in nondisabled subjects and subjects with cerebrovascular accidents. *Phys Ther.* 1992;72:176–185.

Rodriquez AA, Black PO, Kile KA, et al. Gait training efficacy using a home-based practice model in chronic hemiplegia. *Arch Phys Med Rehabil.* 1996;77:801–805.

Rogers MW, Hedman LD, Pai YC. Kinetic analysis of dynamic transitions in stance support. *Arch Phys Med Rehabil.* 1993;74:19–25.

Sackley C. Long-term therapy for all stroke patients. *Physiotherapy.* 2001;87:54.

Sackley CM, Baguley BI, Gent S, Hodgson P. The use of a balance performance monitor in the treatment of weight-bearing and weight-transference problems after stroke. *Physiotherapy.* 1992;78:907–913.

Said CM, Goldie PA, Patla AE, et al. Obstacle crossing in subjects with stroke. *Arch Phys Med Rehabil.* 1999;80:1054–1059.

Sandstrom R, Mokler PJ, Hoppe KM. Discharge destination and motor function outcome in severe stroke as measured by the functional independence measure/function-related group classification system. *Arch Phys Med Rehabil.* 1998;79:762–765.

Shumway-Cook A, Woolacott M. *Motor Control: Theory and Practical Application.* Baltimore, Md: Williams and Wilkins; 1995.

Shutter L, Whyte J. Increased intensity of physiotherapy after stroke. *Stroke.* 1999;30: 2242–2243.

Sine R, Liss SE, Rousch RE, et al. *Basic Rehabilitation Techniques: A Self-Instructional Guide.* 4th ed. Gaithersburg, Md: Aspen Publishers; 2000.

Smith GV, Silver KH, Goldberg AP, et al. "Task-oriented" exercise improves hamstring strength and spastic reflexes in chronic stroke patients. *Stroke.* 1999;30:2112–2118.

Snels IA, Beckerman H, Lankhorst GJ, et al. Treatment of hemiplegic shoulder pain in the Netherlands: results of a national survey. *Clin Rehabil.* 2000;14:20–27.

Sonde L, Gip C, Fernaeus SE, Nilsson CG, et al. Stimulation with low frequency transcutaneous electric nerve stimulation increases motor function of the post-stroke paretic arm. *Scand J Rehabil Med.* 1998;30:95–99.

Stark SC. Physiotherapy and botulinum toxin in spasticity management. *Br J Ther Rehabil.* 2001;8:386–392.

Stevenson TJ, Garland SJ. Standing balance during internally produced perturbations in subjects with hemiplegia: validation of the balance scale. *Arch Phys Med Rehabil.* 1996; 77:656–662.

Sullivan PE, Markos PD. *Clinical Decision Making in Therapeutic Exercise.* Norwalk, Conn: Appleton & Lange; 1994.

Sunderland A, Tinson DJ, Bradley EL, Fletcher D. Enhanced physical therapy improves recovery of arm function after stroke. *J Neurol Neurosurg Psychiatry.* 1992;5:530–537.

Suzuki K, Mamada Y, Handa T, et al. Relationsip between stride length and walking rate in gait training forpartic stroke. *Am J Phys Med Rehabil.* 1999;78:147–152.

Taub E, Wolf SL. Constraint induced movement techniques to facilitate upper extremity use in stroke patients. *Topics in Stroke Rehabilitation.* 1997;3:38–61.

Taylor D, Luxford B, Lawson H. Effect of neuromuscular electrical stimulation on joint range of motion in hemiplegia: a single case study. *NZ J Physiotherapy*. 2000;28:17–22.

Thaut MH, McIntosh GC, Rice RR. Rhythmic facilitation of gait training in hemiparetic stroke rehabilitation. *J Neurolog Sci*. 1997;151:207–212.

Tolfts A, Stiller K. Do patients with traumatic brain injury benefit from physiotherapy? *Physiotherapy Theory Pract*. 1997;13:197–206.

Tyson SF. Trunk kinematics in hemiplegic gait and the effect of walking aids. *Clin Rehabil*. 1999;13:295–300.

Umphred D. *Neurological Rehabilitation*. 3rd ed. St Louis, Mo: CV Mosby Co; 1995.

van der Lee JH, Wagenaar RC, Lankhorst GJ, et al. Forced use of the upper extremity in chronic stroke patients: results form a single-blind randomized clinical trial. *Stroke*. 1999;30:2369–2375.

van de Weg FB, Kuik DJ, Lankhorst GJ. Post-stroke depression and functional outcome: a cohort study investigating the influence of depression on functional recovery from stroke. *Clin Rehabil*. 1999;268–272.

Velicki MR, Winstein CJ, Pohl PS. Impaired direction and extent specification of aimed arm movements in humans with stroke-related brain damage. *Exp Brain Res*. 2000;130:362–374.

Wade DT, Collen FM, Robb GF, Warlow CP. Physiotherapy intervention late after stroke and mobility. *Br Med J*. 1992;304:609–613.

Walker C, Brouwer BJ, Culham EG. Use of visual feedback in retaining balance following acute stroke. *Phys Ther*. 2000;80:886–895.

Wang RY. Effect of proprioceptive neuromuscular facilitation on the gait of patients with hemiplegia of long and short duration. *Phys Ther*. 1994;74:1108–1115.

Wang RY, Chan RC, Tsai MW. Effects of thoraco-lumbar electric sensory stimulation on knee extensor spasticity of persons who survived cerebrovascular accident. *J Rehabil Res Dev*. 2000;37:73–79.

Weingarden HP, Zeilig G, Heruti R, et al. Hybrid functional electrical stimulation orthosis system for the upper limb: effects on spasticity in chronic stable hemiplegia. *Am J Phys Med Rehabil*. 1998;276–281.

Werner RA, Kessler S. Effectiveness of an intensive outpatient rehabilitation program for postacute stroke patients. *Am J Phys Med Rehabil*. 1996;75:114–120.

Wikander B, Ekelund P, Milsom I. An evaluation of multidisciplinary intervention goverened by functional independence measure (FIMSM) in incontinent stroke patients. *Scand J Rehabil Med*. 1998;30:15–21.

Winstein CJ, Merians AS, Sullivan KJ. Motor learning after unilateral brain damage. *Neuropsychologia*. 1999;37:975–987.

Winward CE, Halligan PW, Wade DT. Current practice and clinical relevance of somatosensory assessment after stroke. *Clin Rehabil*. 1999;13:48–55.

Wittwer JE, Goldie P, Matyas TA, et al. Quantification of physiotherapy treatment time in stroke rehabilitation—criterion-related validity. *Aust J Physiotherapy*. 2000;46:291–298.

Wolf SL, Catlin PA, Gage K, et al. Establishing the reliability and validity of measurements of walking time using the Emory Functional Ambulation Profile. *Phys Ther*. 1999;79:1122–1133.

Wolf SL, Segal RL, Catlin PA, et al. Determining consistency of elbow joint threshold angle in elbow flexor muscles with spastic hypertonia. *Phys Ther*. 1996;586–600.

Worthington A, Willims C, Young K, et al. Re-training gait components for walking in the context of abulia. *Physiotherapy Theory Pract*. 1997;13:247–256.

Young J, Forster A. Day hospital and home physiotherapy for stroke patients: a comparative cost-effectiveness study. *J Royal College of Physicians of London.* 1993;27:252–258.

Balance

Bohannon R. Standing balance and function over the course of acute rehabilitation. *Arch Phys Med Rehabil.* 1995;76:994–996.

Chen H, Ashton-Miller J, Alexander N, et al. Effects of age and available response time on ability to stop over an obstacle. *J Gerontol.* 1994;49:M227–233.

DiFabio R, Seay R. Use of the "fast evaluation of mobility, balance, and fear" in elderly community dwellers: validity and reliability. *Phys Ther.* 1997;77:904–917.

Feltner M, MacRae P, McNitt-Gray J. Quantitative gait assessment as a predictor of prospective and retrospective falls in community-dwelling women. *Arch Phys Med Rehabil.* 1994;75:447–453.

Geiger RA, Allen JB, O'Keefe J, et al. Balance and mobility following stroke: effects of physical therapy interventions with and without biofeedback/forceplate training. *Phys Ther.* 2001;81:995–1005.

Graham D, Newton RA. Relationship between balance abilities and mobility aids in elderly at discharge from an acute care setting. *Physiotherapy Res Int.* 1999;4:293–301.

Haarda N, Chiu V, Damron-Rodriques J, et al. Screening for balance and mobility impairment in elderly individuals living in residential care facilities. *Phys Ther.* 1995;75:462–469.

Hellstrom K, Nilsson L, Fugl-Meyer AR. Relationship of confidence in task performance with balance and motor function after stroke. *Physiotherapy Theory Pract.* 2001;17: 55–66.

Jeka J. Light touch contact as a balance aid. *Phys Ther.* 1997;77:476–487.

Lord S, Castell S. Effect of exercise on balance, strength and reaction time in older people. *Aust J Physiotherapy.* 1994;40:83–88.

Lord SR, Ward JA, Williams P. Effect of water exercise on balance and related factors in older people. *Aust J Physiotherapy.* 1993;42:1110–1117.

Maki B, Holliday P, Topper A. A prospective study of postural balance and risk of falling in an ambulatory and independent elderly population. *J Geriatr.* 1994;49:M72–M84.

Maki B, McIlroy W. The role of limb movement in maintaining upright stance: the "change-in-support" strategy. *Phys Ther.* 1997;77:488–507.

Winter D. *ABCs of Balance During Standing and Walking.* Waterloo, Ontario, Canada: Waterloo Biomechanics; 1995.

Woollacott M, Tang P. Balance control during walking in the older adult: research and its implications. *Phys Ther.* 1997;646–660.

Thoracic Outlet Syndrome

Also known as *neurovascular compression syndromes of the shoulder girdle, scalenus anticus syndrome,* and *cervical rib syndrome.*

DESCRIPTION

Thoracic outlet syndrome (TOS) is a combination of symptoms noted by pain and paresthesias that usually appear gradually in the neck, shoulder, arm, or hand and possibly in the anterior chest wall. Some clients experience severe vascular-autonomic changes in the hand. Age of onset is typically between 35 and 55, with the condition occurring more frequently in women.

CAUSE

Etiology is uncertain. Thoracic outlet syndrome can be due to compression of the neurovascular bundle that includes the brachial plexus, axilliary artery, and the subclavian vessels. The presence of a cervical rib, an abnormal first thoracic rib, or abnormal insertion of the scalene muscle can lead to narrowing of the thoracic outlet where the compression occurs.

ASSESSMENT

Note: See APTA's Guide to Physical Therapist Practice. 2nd ed. *Physical Therapy.* 2001;81.

Musculoskeletal Preferred Practice Pattern: F

Neuromuscular Preferred Practice Pattern: D

AREAS
- History
- Pain
- Posture
- Joint integrity
- Skin and soft tissue
- Mobility, including active and passive range of motion (ROM) and accessory motion
- Arterial compression
- Strength, including grip strength
- Functional level, including activities of daily living (ADLs)

INSTRUMENTS/PROCEDURES

See References for sources.

Arterial Compression
- Adson's test
- Allen maneuver
- costoclavicular test
- Halstead maneuver
- hyperabduction test
- Roo's test (EAST)

Special Tests to Which the Physical Therapist May or May Not Have Access
- nerve conduction studies for carpal tunnel syndrome
- dexterity and coordination tests
- x-rays
- magnetic resonance imaging (MRI)
- arteriograms and venograms
- plethysmography
- tests for cervical nerve root involvement

Strength
- manual muscle testing

PROBLEMS
- The client often reports that using arms overhead leads to fatigue.
- The client often reports a feeling of arm falling asleep or "pins-and-needles" sensation.
- The symptoms are often aggravated by sleeping with arms overhead.
- Pain typically begins distally and progresses proximally.
- The pain and paresthesia lead to functional limitations.
- There may be cold sensitivity at a later stage.

TREATMENT/MANAGEMENT
- Instruct client in postural correction.
- Suggest modification of work and sleep postures.
- Teach scapular stabilization exercises.
- Consider modalities as indicated.
- Consider mobilization of first cervical rib and clavicle.
- Stretch scalenes, pectoralis minor, or other involved musculature.
- Instruct in self-stretches.
- Avoid repetitive movements.

PRECAUTIONS
- Presence of cyanosis in one or more fingers can indicate presence of emboli, and the therapist should refer the client to a doctor.

DESIRED OUTCOME/PROGNOSIS
- The client will experience a decrease in pressure on involved structures.
- Therapy will promote proper upright posture.

Note: Condition often takes weeks or even months to resolve. Compliance with a home program is critical.

REFERENCES

Assessment

Daniels L, Worthingham C. *Muscle Testing Techniques of Manual Examination.* 6th ed. Philadelphia, Pa: WB Saunders Co; 1995.

DeLisa D. *Rehabilitation Medicine: Principle and Practice.* Philadelphia, Pa: JB Lippincott Co; 1998.

Grabois M, Garrison SJ, Hart KA, Lehmkuhl LD. *Physical Medicine and Rehabilitation: The Complete Approach.* Malden, Mass: Blackwell Science; 2000.

Kendall FP, McCreary EK, Provance PG. *Muscles: Testing and Function.* 4th ed. Baltimore, Md: Williams and Wilkins; 1993.

O'Sullivan SB, Schmitz TJ, eds. *Physical Rehabilitation: Assessment and Treatment.* Philadelphia, Pa: FA Davis Co; 1994.

Patla AE, Clous SD. Visual assessment of human gait: reliability and validity. *Rehabil Res.* 1998;1:87–96.

Rothstein JM, Roy SH, Wolf SL. *The Rehabilitation Specialist's Handbook.* 2nd ed. Philadelphia, Pa: FA Davis Co; 1998.

Sine R, Liss SE, Rousch RE, et al. *Basic Rehabilitation Techniques: A Self-Instructional Guide.* 4th ed. Gaithersburg, Md: Aspen Publishers; 2000.

Tomberlin JP, Saunders HD. *Evaluation, Treatment and Prevention of Musculoskeletal Disorders. Vol 2: Extremities.* Chaska, Minn: The Saunders Group; 1994.

Treatment

Aligne C, Barral X. Rehabilitation of patients with thoracic outlet syndrome. *Ann Vascular Surg.* 1992;6:381–389.

Atasoy E. Thoracic outlet compression syndrome. *Orthop Clin N Am.* 1996;27:265–303.

Athanassiadi K, Kalavrouziotis G, Karydakis K, et al. Treatment of thoracic outlet syndrome: long-term results. *World J Surg.* 2001;25:553–557.

Baker CL Jr, Liu SH. Neurovascular injuries to the shoulder. *J Orthop Sports Phys Ther.* 1993;18:360–364.

Grabois M, Garrison SJ, Hart KA, Lehmkuhl LD. *Physical Medicine and Rehabilitation: The Complete Approach.* Malden, Mass: Blackwell Science; 2000.

Hama H, Matsusue Y, Ito H, Yamamuro T. Thoracic outlet syndrome associated with an anomalous coracoclavicular joint: a case report. *J Bone Joint Surg.* 1993;75A:1368–1369.

Kamkar A, Irrgang JJ, Whitney SL. Nonoperative management of secondary shoulder impingment syndrome. *J Orthop Sports Phys Ther.* 1993;17:212–224.

Kenny RA, Traynor GB, Withington D, Keegan DJ. Thoracic outlet syndrome: a useful exercise treatment option. *Am J Surg.* 1993;165:282–284.

Langley P. Scapular instability associated with brachial plexus irritation: a proposed causative relationship with treatment implications. *J Hand Ther.* 1997;10:35–40.

Levoska S, Keinanen-Kiukaanniemi S. Active or passive physiotherapy for occupational cervicobrachial disorders: a comparison of two treatment methods with a 1-year follow-up. *Arch Phys Med Rehabil.* 1993;74:425–430.

Novak CB. Conservative management of thoracic outlet syndrome. *Semin Thorac Cardiovasc Surg.* 1996;8:201–207.

Novak CB, Collins ED, Mackinnon SE. Outcome following conservative management of thoracic outlet syndrome. *J Hand Surg.* 1995;20A:542–548.

Poole GV, Thomas KR. Thoracic outlet syndrome reconsidered. *Am Surg.* 1996;62:287–291.

Rayan GM. Thoracic outlet syndrome. *J Shoulder Elbow Surg.* 198;7:440–451.

Silliman JF, Dean MT. Neurovascular injuries to the shoulder complex. *J Orthop Sports Phys Ther.* 1993;18:442–448.

Talmage DM, Lemke C. Thoracic outlet syndrome: how has it changed over the centuries? *Top Clin Chiropractic.* 1999;6:39–50.

Walsh MT. Therapist management of thoracic outlet syndrome. *J Hand Ther.* 1994;7:131–144.

Vestibular and Balance Disorders

ICD-9-CM Codes:

386 Vertiginous syndromes and other disorders of vestibular system

386.0 Ménière's disease

386.11 Benign paroxysmal positional vertigo

386.12 Vestibular neuronitis

386.2 Vertigo of central origin

386.3 Labyrinthitis

386.4 Labyrinthine fistual

386.5 Labyrinthine dysfunction

386.50 Labyrinthine dysfunction, unspecified

386.53 Hyoactive labyrinth, unilateral

386.54 Hypoactive labyrinth, bilateral

386.8 Other disorders of labyrinth

386.9 Unspecified vertiginous sydromes and labyrinthine disorders

APTA Practice Guidelines: 5B, 5D

DESCRIPTION

Vestibular and balance disorders refer to impairments of the vestibular system and related central structures involving visual and somatosensory (proprioceptual and kinesthetic) systems that cause vertigo, disequilibrium, and secondary gait and balance problems. The most common vestibular impairment is *benign paroxysmal positional vertigo* (BPPV), also known as *benign position vertigo, positional vertigo,* or *benign positional nystagmus.* Other common vestibular disorders are *chronic labyrinthitis,* also known as *chronic vestibulopathy, chronic vestibular neuronitis,* or *unilateral vestibular hypofunction.* Clients may also be seen with less common problems such as Ménière's disease, bilateral vestibular hypofunction, or bilateral vestibular weakness; or following resection of an acoustic neuroma or after head trauma that causes labyrinthine concussion, which can be part of a post-concussion syndrome. Common central or multisystem disorders are disequilibrium of aging, Parkinson's disease, and other central disorders that often affect balance.

The human vestibular system is composed of three components: a peripheral sensory apparatus, a central process, and a mechanism for motor control. The peripheral apparatus consists of motor sensors—specifically the vestibular nucleus and cerebellum—that provide information about head angular velocity, linear acceleration, and orientation of the head in relation to the gravitational axis. The central nervous sytem processes signals from the motion sensors and combines them with other sensory information to estimate head orientation. The output of the vestibular system goes to the ocular muscles and spinal cord via two reflexes, the vestibulo-ocular reflex (VOR) and the vestibulospinal reflex (VSR). The VOR generates eye movements that facilitate clear vision while the head is in motion. The VSR generates compensatory body movement to maintain head and postural stability (Hain, et al, 2001, p. 3).

The vestibular system provides three primary functions: 1) stabilizes visual images on the fovea of the retina during head movement to allow clear vision; 2) maintains postural stability, especially during movement of the head, and 3) provides information used for spatial orientation (Schubert & Herdman, 2000, p. 822). When the VSR is not functioning correctly, head motion may cause the person to lean or fall to one side. When the VOR is not functioning correctly, the result is a sensation of dizziness because the eyes continue to move after the head has stopped moving. Lesions of the vestibular system cause impaired balance and related gait ataxia, disorientation manifested as vertigo, ie, the illusion of spinning or falling, blurred vision due to decreased accuracy of the vestibulo-ocular reflex, and increased autonomic responses during gait and head movements. Clients complain of falling, staggering vertigo, and nausea. They may also have hearing loss, muscle weakness, other musculoskeletal problems, and cardiac or respiratory symptoms.

CLASSIFICATION BY DIAGNOSIS

(Beers & Berkow, 1999; Fetter, 2000)

1. *Peripheral vestibular disorders:* involve the peripheral vestibular organ or cranial nerve VIII.
   - *Benign paroxysmal positional vertigo* (BPPV): Also known as *benign position vertigo, position vertigo, positional vertigo,* or *benign positional nystagmus.*
     - Violent vertigo lasting less than 30 seconds and induced by certain head positions (Beers & Berkow, p. 679).
     - Vertigo due to the otoconia in the semicircular canals being displaced from the utricle (Schubert & Herdman, p. 841).
   - *Vestibular neuronitis* (acute, recurrent, and chronic): A benign disorder characterized by the sudden onset of severe vertigo that is persistent at first, then paroxysmal (Beers & Berkow, 1999, p. 678).
   - *Labyrinthitis:* Inflammation of the inner ear by bacteria that is characterized by severe vertigo and nystagmus. Purulent labyrinthitis invariably results in

complete hearing loss and is often followed by facial paralysis (Beers & Berkow, 1999, p. 680).

- *Ménière's disease:* A disorder characterized by recurrent prostrating vertigo, sensory hearing loss, tinnitus, and a feeling of fullness in the ear associated with generalized dilation of the membranous labyrinth (Beers & Berkow, 1999, p. 678).
- *Herpes Zoster Oticus:* Also known as *Ramsay Hunt's Syndrome, viral neuronitis, ganglionitis,* and *Geniculate Herpes.* Invasion of the 8th nerve ganglia and the geniculate ganglion of the facial nerve by the herpes zoster virus, producing severe ear pain, hearing loss, vertigo, and paralysis of the facial nerve (Beers & Berkow, 1999, p. 679).
- *Drug-Induced Toxicity:* Drugs can affect both the auditory and vestibular portion of the inner ear. Drugs that affect the vestibular portion include streptomycin, viomycin, gentamicin, and tobramycin. High doses of salicylates produce tinnitus (Beers & Berkow, 1999, p. 682).
- *Perilymphatic fistula:* A rupture of the oval or round windows, using an opening between the middle and inner ear (Schubert & Herdman, p. 842).
- *Acoustic neuroma:* Also known as *acoustic schwannomas, acoustic neurinomas, 8th nerve tumors,* and *benign tumor of the vestibulocochlear cranial nerve.* As the tumor grows larger, it projects from the internal auditory meatus into the cerebellopontine angle and begins to compress the cerebellum and brain stem (Beers & Berkow, 1999, p. 683).
- *Vestibular paroxysmia.* Also known as *disabling positional vertigo.* Neurovascular cross-compression of the root entry zone of the vestibular nerve can elicit disabling positional vertigo. The compression can cause local demyelinization of the root zone of the eighth nerve (Fetter, 2000, p. 98).

2. *Central vestibular disorders* involve a vestibular pathway located in the central nervous system.
   - Cervical vertigo including central positional nystagmus and malignant positional vertigo
   - Head injury or traumatic brain injury
   - Brain tumors: meningiomas growing in the area of the temporal lobe can cause pressure on the vestibular mechanism (Allison & Fuller, 2001, p.618).
   - Migraine headaches
   - Panic and anxiety symptoms with dizziness
   - Cerebellar disorders—ataxia, degeneration
   - Neurological disorders: Multiple sclerosis, Parkinson's disease
   - Vascular events: transient ischemic attacks including anterior inferior communicating artery (AICA) ischemia and posterior inferior communicating artery (PICA) ischemia

3. *Multisensory Disequilibrium and Older Adults with Vestibular Loss*
   - Eye disorders: macular degeneration, cataracts, glaucoma
   - Neuropathies: associated with diabetes, HIV infection
   - Arthritis: rheumatoid
   - Connective tissues: lupus

CLASSIFICATION BY IMPAIRMENT AND LIMITATION

(Herdman, 2000; Schubert & Herdman, 2001; Whitney & Rossi, 2000)

1. *Peripheral Causes of Dizziness*
   - Unilateral vestibular dysfunction (unilateral vestibular lesion): Meniere's disease, acoustic neuroma, acute vestibular neuronitis
   - Chronic unilateral vestibular paresis, loss, or uncompensated loss
   - Benign paroxysmal position vertigo

- Bilateral vestibular loss (bilateral vestibular lesion)
- Multisensory dysequilibrium and older adults with vestibular loss
- Vestibular hypofunction
- Complete vestibular loss
- Motion sensitivity

2. *Central Causes of Dizziness*
(Furman & Whitney, 2000; Whitney & Rossi, 2000)
   - Cervical vertigo
   - Trauma (head injury, head trauma, traumatic brain injury, temporal bone fracture)
   - Panic and anxiety symptoms with dizziness
   - Cerebellar disorders
   - Cerebellar degeneration
   - Multiple Sclerosis
   - Vascular events
   - Central vestibular lesion (central vestibular dysfunction)
   - Mal de Debarquement
   - Migraine
   - Brain-stem stroke and verte-brobasilar insufficiency

Note: Vestibular and balance disorders can also be classified by duration based on how long the symptoms last (seconds, minutes, hours, or days).

DEFINITIONS

- Balance (Human): the ability to maintain equilibrium or the ability to maintain the center of gravity (COG) over the base of support (BOS). Balance requires the ability to maintain a position, to stabilize during voluntary activity, and to react to external perturbations. (Brody, p. 112)
- Balance impairment or balance dysfunction: difficulty in maintaining equilibrium or inability to maintain the center of gravity over the base of support. (See: definition of balance)
- Base of support (BOS): the area of the single contact between the body and support surface or, if there is more than one contact with the support surface, the area enclosing all the contacts with the support surface. (Pollock, et al)
- Center of gravity (COG): the point through which the vector of total body weight passes. (Pollock, et al)
- Disequilibrium: subjective sensation that a person is off balance, which typically occurs in acute and chronic vestibular lesions but may occur in nonvestibular problems such as decreased somatosensation or weakness in the lower extremities. (Schubert & Herdman, p. 825)
- Line of gravity: a vertical line running through the center of gravity.
- Postural control: the act of maintaining, achieving, or restoring the line of gravity within the base of support which results in a state of balance during any posture or activity. (Pollock, et al) Involves the vestibular, visual, and somatosensory systems. (Brody, p. 113)
- Postural stability: the ability to maintain the COG within the stability limits. (Brody, p. 112)
- Postural sway: the normal, continuous shifting of the body's COG over the BOS. (Brody, p. 112)
- Stability (Human): the inherent ability of a person to maintain, achieve, or restore a specific state of balance and not to fall. The inherent ability refers to the motor and sensory systems and to the physical properties of the person. (Pollock, et al)
- Stability limits or limits of stability: the boundaries of space or spatial area in which the individual can maintain equilibrium without changing the BOS. (Brody, p. 112)
- Vertigo (dizziness): an abnormal sensation of rotary movement associated with difficulty in balance, gait, and navigation of the environment. (Beers & Berkow, 1999, p. 665) Vertigo may be caused by a variety of factors in addition to

vestibular disorders including various drugs, low blood pressure, cardiac rhythm disorders, and migraine.
- Vestibular function: pertaining to the sense of balance.
- Vestibular dysfunction: pertaining to problems with the sense of balance.

CAUSE

In general, there are three categories of causes: biomechanical, motor and sensory. BPPV is caused by displacement of otoconia (microscopic calcium carbonate crystals) from the otoliths to the semicircular canals within the labyrinth, and is due to age-related changes, head trauma, or viral infection. Chronic labyrinthitis, bilateral vestibular weakness, and vestibular neuronitis are caused by viral infection, connective tissue disorders, or perhaps vascular changes. The etiology of Ménière's disease and acoustic neuroma are unknown. Disequilibrium of aging is due to generalized age-related sensory loss, combined with general weakness and effects of other central problems.

Balance impairment can be caused by injury to or disease of any of the structures involved in balance (eyes, inner ear, peripheral receptors, spinal cord, cerebellum, basal ganglia, and cerebrum) by disrupting the reception, organization, and transfer of information in the stages of sensory input, sensory information processing, and motor output generation. Examples of cause include increased pressure on structures due to tumors, hemorrhage or blockage due to stroke, lesions due to Huntington's disease, plaques due to multiple sclerosis, loss of basal ganglia function such as in Parkinson's disease and others.

Vestibular disorders may occur independently or in conjuction with neurological disease or injury. The causes are varied and include infections, vascular disease, neoplasia, trauma, metabolic disorders, toxic drugs, and diseases of unknown etiology. (Allison & Fuller, 2001, p. 617)

ASSESSMENT

AREAS

- Neck, trunk, limb, and foot range of motion
- Muscle strength
- Endurance
- Vestibular functioning: vertigo, dizziness
- Standing balance and sway
- Dynamic balance
- Posture and postural alignment
- Gait
- Mobility skills
- Visual tracking
- Visual field
- Visual acuity
- Lower extremity sensation
- Activities of daily living (ADLs)
- Quality of life

INSTRUMENTS/PROCEDURES

Quiet Standing
- motor control test
- nudge/push
- one-legged stance test (OLST) or single-leg stance test
- postural stress test
- postural sway: sway magnetometry
- potentiometric displacement transducer
- Romberg or timed Romberg test
- sharpened Romberg/tandem Romberg
- static and dynamic force platforms

Active Standing
- functional reach test: assesses upper extremity balance focusing on postural adjustments that anticipate upper extremity movement
- limits of stability

Sensory Manipulation
- Clinical Test of Sensory Interaction and Balance (Foam and Dome Test)
- Dynamic Platform Posturography test
- Equitest/Sensory Organization test (Computerized Dynamic Posturography)
- Fukuda Stepping test
- Mechanical ataxia meters
- Motion Sensitivity Quotient
- Nystagmus
- Oculomotor tests
- Semicircular Canal Function
- Sensory Organization test (SOT)
- Vertiginous Positions
- Visual Acuity
- Visual-Vestibular Interaction

Balance
- Berg Balance Scale
- Dynamic Gait Index
- Gait Assessment Rating Scale (GARS)
- Timed Up and Go Test
- Tinetti Performance Oriented Assessment of Balance
- Tinetti Performance Oriented Assessment of Gait
- visual analog scale

Combination Test Batteries
- Barthel index
- Fregley-Graybiel Ataxia Test Battery
- Fugl-Meyer Sensorimotor Assessment of Balance performance
- Postural Dyscontrol test
- Speechley's Physical Therapy Checklist

Function Performance or Quality of Life
- Activities of Daily Living Scales (ADL Scales)
- Activities-Specific Balance Confidence test
- Disability Index
- Dizziness Handicap Inventory
- Functional Disability Scale
- Home Safety Checklist for Detection of Fall Hazards
- Instrumental Activities Scale
- Medical Outcomes Study
- Motion Sensitivity Quotient
- Physical Activity Scale

Semicircular Canal Function
- Hallpike-Dix maneuver – Use to test for benign paroxysmal position vertigo. The head is turned to one side and patient is moved from a sitting into a supine position with the head hanging over the end of the table.
- The client is observed for nystagmus, and complaints of vertigo are noted. (Whitney & Herdman, 2000, p. 345)

Vertigo
- qualitative scales of vertigo, eg, from 1 to 3 or 1 to 5

Other
- obstacle course
- physical performance test

PROBLEMS
- Client may have vertigo—the illusion of self-motion: spinning or falling
- Client may have oscillopsia—the illusion of motion in the surrounding visual environment
- Client may report feelings of disequilibrium, especially with head movement
- Client may report falls or fear of falling, especially in dim light
- Client may report nausea or queasy stomach
- Client may have muscle weakness

- Client may have limitations in range of motion
- Client may report lightheadedness, sometimes described as a "floating" sensation
- Client may have blurred vision with head movement
- Client may have nystagmus
- Client may have difficulty with visual tracking
- Client may demonstrate visual field loss
- Client may have loss of spatial orientation
- Client may report difficulty dealing with heights, open spaces, and crowds of people
- Client may have optokinetic or visual motion sensitivity

TREATMENT/MANAGEMENT

Vestibular rehabilitation is a comprehensive approach to assessing and treating symptoms of vestibular system pathology. The overall goal of assessment is to document the patient's functional problems, and the many sensory, motor, and cognitive limitations contributing to loss of functional independence. (Shumway-Cook, 2000, p. 478)

Treatment may involve one session to instruct the client in a home program of exercises tailored to meet the client's needs or may involve therapy of 3 to 6 months depending on the diagnosis and length of time the client has had symptoms.

GENERAL
- Provide or instruct client in balance-retraining exercises to improve balance on various surfaces (flat, moving, uneven) with eyes open and closed and different head positions
- Provide or instruct client in eye-head exercises to decrease dizziness during changes in head position
- Provide or instruct client in VOR training and exercises to improve gaze stabilization
- Provide or instruct client in habituation exercises to decrease dizziness during changes in body position
- Provide or instruct client in general conditioning/reconditioning and fitness exercises

BPPV
- Classic treatment was developed by Cawthorne and Cooksey, who describe a series of exercises beginning in supine, progressing to sitting, and then to standing. They start with gentle relaxation movements of the head and shoulders, then advance to eye and head movements with gradual increase in speed. The exercises are performed in a group setting where possible and games are added when appropriate. This is known as the Cawthorne-Cooksey exercise program. (See Herdman, 2000, p. 398.)
- Perform the canalith repositioning maneuver, also known as Epley's maneuver or the Epley maneuver; Brandt and Daroff exercises; or liberatory maneuver, also known as Semont's maneuver or the Semont maneuver. Together these are known as particle repositioning maneuvers to return the otoconia to the vestibule. Use mobilization tables to alter body position for clients with limited cervical range of motion. Canalith repositioning uses sequential head positions that cause the free-floating crystals to move through the long handle of the posterior canal and fall back into the utricle where they belong. (Denham & Wolf, p. 93) Examples of the techniques appear in Schuberg & Herdman, 2000, p. 833–834. After the maneuver, the client must adhere to a series of precautions, including sleeping only at a 45-degree angle for 2 days, avoiding flexion or extension of the neck, and refraining from sleeping on the affected side for 5 days. (Denham & Wolf, p. 93)

- Instruct the client on how to perform the Brandt and Daroff exercises for habitation and to move the otoconia in a nonspecific pattern. The Brandt-Daroff exercises involve having the client sit on a flat surface and move quickly into the side-lying position on the affected side. The client stays in that position until the vertigo stops plus an additional 30 seconds. The client then sits up and again waits for the vertigo to stop. The client then repeats the movement on the opposite side, stays in this position for 30 seconds, and sits up. The process is repeated 10 to 20 times, 3 times a day until the client has 2 days in a row with no vertigo. (Herdman & Tusa, p. 466)
- Instruct client in gaze stabilization exercise. Client looks at a 1-inch letter an arm's length away while moving the head from side to side for 2 minutes. Once the client is able to keep the letter in focus, the exercise is made more difficult by having the client move the head faster, by moving the letter closer or farther away, by changing the background of the letter from a solid to a complex pattern, and by having the client perform the exercise while walking. (Denham & Wolf, p. 94)

UNILATERAL VESTIBULAR HYPOFUNCTION AND MENIERE'S DISEASE
- Use vestibular habituation exercises, ie, repetitive head movement exercises.
- Use gaze stabilization exercises to restore gaze stability during head movements.
- Provide a general strengthening program to increase or improve conditioning.
- Give instruction in home safety to reduce hazards and increase sources of external stability.
- Balance exercises.
- Gait training.

UNILATERAL VESTIBULAR DYSFUNCTION
- Provide exercises to enhance the gain of the vestibulo-ocular reflex (VOR) that involve visual-vestibular interaction such as ×1 viewing and ×2 viewing.
- Provide exercises to improve postural control in static stability such as activities with eyes open, eyes closed, and on different types of surfaces.
- Provide exercises to improve postural control in dynamic stability such as walking with progressively difficult head movements. An example of a balance exercise program is provided in Schubert & Herdman, 2000, p. 837.
- Provide exercises to improve tolerance to movements of the head and body that can prevent deficits in range of motion and encourage habituation. Habituation exercises allow the abnormal sensory input to be integrated into the new global pattern of information. (Whitney & Rossi, p. 661)
- Instruct client on home exercise program.
- Instruct client in fall prevention.

CHRONIC UNILATERAL VESTIBULAR LOSS AND UNCOMPENSATED LOSS
- Provide gaze stabilization exercises.
- Provide static postural control exercise.
- Provide dynamic postural control exercises, including a walking program.
- Provide habituation exercises.
- Instruct client in fall prevention.
- Instruct client on how to manage the symptoms of dizziness and imbalance.
- Inform client that symptoms may increase before they improve and improvement may take about 6 weeks to occur. (Whitney & Rossi, p. 662)

BILATERAL VESTIBULAR LOSS
- Provide exercises to enhance gaze stability through visual vestibular activities and enhancement of the cervical ocular reflex (COR). Different velocities should be considered as client may be unable to compensate at velocities greater than 1 or 2 Hz. It is estimated that the COR contributes up to 25% of the compensatory eye movement in clients with bilateral vestibular loss.

- Instruct client to avoid operating heavy machinery and driving until coordination, balance, and gaze stabilization have occurred. Client may need to pass a driving test.
- Instruct client not to swim underwater since orientation in space and ability to locate the surface may be impaired.
- Instruct client in fall prevention. Client may need to use canes for additional proprioceptive input. Stress proper lighting to enhance visual input.

Note: Habitation exercises are NOT indicated for those with substantial, bilaterally symmetrical vestibular loss. (Whitney & Rossi, p. 663)

MULTISENSORY DISEQUILIBRIUM/OLDER ADULTS WITH VESTIBULAR LOSS
- Consider a home assessment to address environmental hazards in addition to standard instruction on fall prevention. Stress the importance of good lighting to enhance visual cues.
- Encourage client to wear supportive but thin-soled shoes to improve sensory input.
- Encourage strengthening and conditioning activities. Provide a program of exercises, if needed.
- Assist client in identifying assistive devices that may be helpful.
- Work with the physician to determine if prescription drugs may be contributing to dizziness or falls.

BALANCE IMPAIRMENTS DUE TO CENTRAL NERVOUS SYSTEM DISORDER (BRODY)
- Begin with muscle strengthening, joint mobility, and pain management first. If any of these are problems, then reassess for balance impairment.
- *Static and dynamic balance exercises:* increase or improve sitting balance, trunk stability, and weight distribution beginning with a stable surface and moving to an unstable surface. Chairs or tables can provide a stable surface while rehabilitation/therapeutic balls, foam rollers, foam surfaces, chairs, or a minitrampoline can provide uneven surfaces. Examples of exercises might include sitting on a stable surface while catching a ball tossed from different directions, sitting on a therapy ball while catching a ball tossed from different directions, and wearing foam rollers in a bilateral stance to practice weight shifting while catching a ball tossed from different directions. Tai Chi exercises have also been used.
- *Walking exercises:* improve gross motor coordination and balance by walking on lines drawn on the floor, walking on balance beams.
- *Postural training:* improve postural awareness through increased feedback. Begin with static postures such as half kneeling, tall kneeling, and standing; progress to standing heel to toe or a single-leg stance. Dynamic movement can be superimposed by adding an activity. Equipment may include a supportive chair, therapeutic ball, form roll, firm floor, foam pad, balance board, or therapy pool. Trunk rotations combined with changes in head position provide a variety of exercises or use of PNF techniques such as chop and lift may be applied. Force platforms or scales can be used to work on weight distribution. Practicing before a mirror may be useful.
- Mental imagery and mental practice have been used for clients with limited endurance (Fell, 2000). The environment for balance training depends on the individual. For older individuals exercises should take place in a safe environment under supervision such as a clinic or in the home if postural awareness is needed. For athletes or active individuals with musculoskeletal causes for balance impairment, balance activities may be carried out at home, a health club, or pool. Safety should always be stressed whether the exercises are supervised or carried out independently.
- Sequence of exercises should progress from simple to complex, involving changes in mode (equipment), posture, and movement, from stable surface to unstable, eyes

open to eyes closed, arms at side for sway exercises to arms folded across chest, simple sway within sitting or standing balance to perturbations that require postural readjustment such as stepping forward, and minilunges with minimal knee bend to deep lunges with near 90 degrees of knee flexion.

- *Frequency, intensity, and duration:* Frequency depends on the client's overall condition and the goals for balance training. Practice increases the likelihood of habit formation. Intensity is not prescribed because there is no external resistance or load to apply. Duration is determined by level of fatigue. Client should stop when level of performance is less than initial performance.
- *Client education:* Safety should always be stressed. Assistive devices can increase the BOS, thus increasing safety. The home should be evaluated for potential loss of balance. Loose rugs, slippery floors or bathtubs, uneven doorways or thresholds, and stairs with railings are examples of hazards. Footwear should be assessed to determine if the shoes can slip on the foot or on the floor and if the shoes tend to stick to the floor; all can increase potential for falls. The client should be educated regarding the limits of balance skills including such factors as time, distance, time of day, and type of environment. Client should be taught strategies for maximizing balance in situations which may challenge balance skills such as changes in lighting conditions, increased noise, and crowds of people. Examples might include taking an assistive device, using a friend's arm for balance, planning a path where stable objects are available to provide external assistance, or asking for assistance from an employee or other customer.

CERVICAL VERTIGO
- Vibration on the client's calves may improve anterior-posterior or medial lateral sway.
- Improve faculty alignment of the cervical spine.
- Correct muscle imbalances that may exist in the cervical area.
- Improve neck kinesthesia and range of motion with eye-head exercises.

HEAD INJURY: MANAGEMENT DEPENDS ON THE SPECIFIC INJURY OR DYSFUNCTION

PANIC AND ANXIETY SYMPTOMS WITH DIZZINESS
- Provide balance and habituation exercises that address the client's specific complaints.
- Provide client education about balance disorders and how to control symptoms.

CEREBELLAR DISORDERS
- Provide an individualized exercise program based on the symptoms presented. (see Burton JM, Gill-Body KM, et al)

MULTIPLE SCLEROSIS: NO SPECIFIC MANAGEMENT TECHNIQUES GIVEN

VASCULAR EVENTS: NO SPECIFIC MANAGEMENT TECHNIQUES GIVEN

PRECAUTIONS/CONTRAINDICATIONS

PRECAUTIONS
- Safety is always important. Exercises should be selected which are within the client's skill level based on initial and ongoing assessment, and should be supervised if there is likelihood of falling. The environment should be structured with safety in mind. Eliminate obstacles or unsafe objects and provide addition stabilization such as a gait belt, hand contacts, parallel bars, or other stable external objects for the client to hold on to or grab.

- Exercises should be specific for the deficits the client presents to promote compliance. Do not give an exhaustive list of many exercises.
- Performing canalith repositioning maneuvers correctly requires advanced training. Do not perform such maneuvers without training because the condition could be aggravated.
- Osteoporotic changes in the spine: be aware that exercises involving rotation or sudden changes in position could cause vertebral fractures.
- History of falling: a client with a history of falls should be closely supervised until the nature or cause of the falls is remediated or level of safe performance is well understood by the client.
- Trunk and/or lower extremity weakness: increases likelihood of falling due to lack of proprioceptive and kinesthetic feedback.
- Numbness in feet: increases likelihood of falling due to decrease in sensory feedback.
- Significant visual impairment: increases likelihood of falling due to decrease in sensory feedback.
- Sudden loss of hearing: suggests auditory involvement.
- Increased feeling of pressure or fullness to the point of discomfort in one or both ears.
- Severe ringing (tinnitus) in one or both ears.
- Observe post-surgical client for discharge of fluid from the ears or nose which may indicate a cerebrospinal fluid leak.
- A client with an acute neck injury may not be able to tolerate canalith repositioning treatment or gaze stability exercises. (Schubert & Herdman, p. 839)

CONTRAINDICATIONS
- Unstable cervical spine: increased potential for vertebral fractures even when conservative exercises are performed.
- Acute and severe vertigo: may be due to an acute infection or toxin, which should be treated medically.
- Acute nausea or vomiting: may be due to an acute infection or toxin which should be treated medically.

DESIRED OUTCOME/PROGNOSIS

Outcome depends both on the type of vestibular disorder and the degree of involvement. Following are some general outcomes and some that are specific to a disorder:
- Client reports none or decreased vertigo.
- Client is able to prevent falls.
- Client has improved balance and postural control.
- Client has a functional gait and is walking.
- For client with BPPV, the otoconia has been replaced into the vestibule.
- For client with BPPV, daily activity involving head motion is possible.
- For client with unilateral vestibular dysfunction there is improved stability of gaze during head movement.
- For client with unilateral vestibular dysfunction, there is decreased sensitivity to motion.
- Client with bilateral vestibular lesion demonstrates a knowledge of activities that may be more difficult to perform due to the disorder.
- Client with central vestibular dysfunction demonstrates knowledge of compensatory strategies to assist in gaze stability.

REFERENCES

Activities-Specific Balance Confidence Scale (ABC)

Powell LE, Myers AM. The activities-specific balance confidence (ABC) scale. *J Gerontol.* 1995;50A(1):M18–M34. Copy of form in Herdman, 2000, p. 822.

Berg Balance Test

Berg KO, Wood-Dauphinee SL, Williams JT, Gayton D. Measuring balance in the elderly: preliminary development of an instrument. *Physiotherapy Can.* 1989;41:304–311. Copy of form in Whitney, 2000, p. 528 and Herdman, 2000, pp. 482–485 or 518–521.

Brandt-Daroff Exercises

Brandt T, Daroff RB. Physical therapy for benign paroxysmal positional vertigo. *Arch Otolaryngology.* 1980;106:484–485.

Clinical Test of Sensory Interaction and Balance

Shumway-Cook A, Horak FB. Assessing the influence of sensory interaction on balance. *Phys Ther.* 1986;66:1548–1550.

Cawthorne-Cocksey Exercises

Cawthorne T. The physiological basis for head exercises. *J Chartered Society of Physiotherapy.* 1944;30:106–107.

Cawthorne T. Vestibular injuries. *Proceedings of the Royal Society of Medicine.* 1946; 39:170–173.

Cocksey FS. Rehabilitation in vestibular injuries. *Proceedings of the Royal Society of Medicine.* 1946;39:273–278.

Dynamic Gait Index (DGI)

Shumway-Cook A, Woollacott M. Assessment and treatment of the patient with mobility disorders. In: Shumway-Cook A, Woollacott M, eds. *Motor Control: Theory and Practical Applications.* Baltimore, Md: Williams and Wilkins; 1995:315–318. Form in Herdman, 2000, pp 357–358.

Dizziness Handicap Inventory

Jacobson GP, Newman CW. The development of the Dizziness Handicap Inventory. *Arch Otolaryngology Head Neck Surg.* 1990:116;424–427. Form in Schubert & Herdman, p. 826 and Herdman, 2000, p. 371–372.

Dynamic Platform Posturography Test

Cass SP, Borello-France D, Durman JM. A practical workup for vertigo. *Am J Otology* 1996:17:581–593.

Epley Maneuver

Epley JM. The canalith repositioning procedure: for treatment of benign paroxysmal positional vertigo. *Otolaryngol Head Neck Surg.* 1992;107:399–404.

Fall Risk Index

Tinetti ME, Williams TF, Mayewski R. Fall risk index for elderly patients based on the number of chronic disabilities. *Am J Med.* 1986;80:429–434.

Fast Evaluation of Mobility, Balance, and Fear

Arroyo JF, Herrmann F, Saber H. Fast evaluation test for mobility, balance, and fear: a new strategy for the screening of elderly fallers. *Arthritis Rheum.* 1994;37:S416. (Abstract). Form in Di Fabio & Seay, p. 916–917. Modified form in Herdman, 2000, p. 523–525.

Fregley-Graybiel Ataxia Test Battery

Fregley AR, Graybiel A. An ataxia test battery not requiring rails. *Aerospace Med.* 1982; 39:277–282.

Fugl-Meyer Physical Performance Battery

Fugl-Meyer AR, Jasko L, Leyman L, Olsson S, Steglind S. The post-stroke hemiplegic patient: A method for evaluation of physical performance. *Scand J Rehabil Med.* 1975;7: 13–31.

Fukuda's Stepping Test (FST)

Fukuda T. The stepping test: two phases of the labyrinthine reflex. *Acta Otolaryngol* 1959;50:95–108.

Functional Disability Scale (FDS)

Telian SA, Shepard NT, Smith-Wheelock M, Kemink JL. Habituation therapy for chronic vestibular dysfunction: Preliminary results. *Otolaryng Head Neck Surg.* 1990;103: 89–95.

Functional Obstacle Course (FOC)

Means KM, Rodell DE, O'Sullivan PS. Use of an obstacle course to assess balance and mobility in the elderly. *Am J Phys Med Rehabil.* 1996;75:88–95.

Functional Reach Test (FRT)

Duncan PW, Weiner DK, Chandler J, Studenski S. Functional reach: A new clinical measure of balance. *J Gerontol.* 1990;45:M192–M197.

Get Up and Go Test

Mathias S, Nayak ULS, Issacs B. Balance in elderly patients: the "Get up and Go" test. *Arch Phys Med Rehabil.* 1986;67:387–389.

Hallpike-Dix Maneuver

Herdman S. Treatment of benign paroxysmal positional vertigo. *Phys Ther.* 1990;70:381–388.

Home Safety Checklist for Detection of Fall Hazards

U.S. National Safety Council. *Home Safety Checklist for Detection of Fall Hazards.* Itasca, Ill: American Association for Retired Persons; 1982.

Modified Falls Efficacy Scale

Hill KD, Schqarz JA, Kalogeropoulos AJ, Gibson SJ. Fear of falling revised. *Arch Phys Med Rehabil.* 1996;77:1024–1029.

Motion Sensitivity Quotient

Smith-Wheelock M. Shepard NT, Telian SA. Physical therapy program for vestibular rehabilitation. *Am J Otology* 1991;12:218–225. Protocol form also printed in Schubert & Herdman, p. 827, and in Herdman, 2000, p. 400.

Motor Control Test

Nashner L. Evaluation of postural stability, movement, and control. In: Hasson S, ed. *Clinical exercise physiology.* Philadelphia, Pa: CV Mosby Co; 1994.

One-Legged Stance

Briggs RC, Gossman MR, Birch R, Brews JE, Shaddeau SA. Balance performance among non-institutionalised elderly women. *Phys Ther.* 1989;69:748–756.

Physical Performance Test

Reuben DB, Siu AL. An objective measure of physical function of elderly outpatients. *J Am Geriatr Soc.* 1990;38:1105–1112.

Performance-Oriented Mobility Assessment—Balance and Gait

Tinetti ME. Performance-oriented assessment of mobility problems in elderly patients. *J Am Geriatr Soc.* 1986;34:119–126.

Postural Stress Test (PST)

Wolfson LI, Whipple R, Amerman P, Kleinberg A. Stressing the postural response—a quantitative method for testing balance. *J Am Geriatr Soc.* 1986;34:845–850.

Reach Test

Goldie AM. Skill acquisition. In Carr JH, Shepherd RB, Godron J, Gentile AM, Held JM, eds. *Found Phys Ther—Movement Sci.* London, England: Heinemann Physiotherapy; 1987:93–154.

Semont Maneuver

Semont A, Freys G, Vitte E. Curing the BPPV with a Liberatory maneuver. *Adv Otorhinolaryngol.* 1988;42:290–295.

Sensory Organization Test

Anacher SL, Di Fabio RS. Influence of sensory inputs on standing balance in community-dwelling elders with recent history of falling. *Phys Ther.* 1992;72(8):575–583.

Sensory-Oriented Mobility Assessment Instrument (SOMAI)

Tang P-F, Moore S, Woollacott MH. Correlation between two clinical balance measures in older adults: functional mobility and sensory organization test. *J Gerontol: Med Sci.* 1996;53A:M140–M146.

Shoulder Tap Test

Pastor M, Day B, Marsden C. Vestibular induced postural responses in Parkinson's disease. *Brain.* 1993;116:1177–1182.

Single Leg Stance Test

Gehlsen GM, Whaley MH. Falls in the elderly: Part II. Balance, strength and flexibility. *Arch Phys Med Rehabil.* 1990;71:739–741.

Step Test

Hill KD, Bernhardt J, McGann AM, Maltesse D, Berkovits D. A new test of dynamic standing balance for stroke patients: reliability, validity and comparison with health elderly. *Physiotherapy Can.* 1996;48:257–263.

Timed Standing

Bohannon RW, Larkin PA, Cook AC, Gear JA, Singer J. Decrease in timed balance test scores with ageing. *Phys Ther.* 1984;64:1067–1070.

Tinetti Balance Test

See Performance-oriented mobility assessment.

Timed "Up and Go" Test (TUG)

Podsciadlo D, Richardson S. The Timed "Up and Go": A test of basic functional mobility for frail elderly persons. *J Amer Geriotr Soc.* 1991;39:142–148.

REFERENCES

Allison L, Fuller K. Balance and vestibular disorders. In: Umphred DA, ed. *Neurological Rehabilitation.* 4th ed. St. Louis, Mo: CV Mosby Co; 2001:616–660.

Blatt PH, Georgakakis GA, Herdman SJ, Clendaniel RA, Tusa RJ. The effect of the canalith repositioning maneuver on resolving postural instability in patients with benign paroxysmal positional vertigo. *Am J Otol.* 2000;21:356–363.

Bogle Thorbahn LD, Newton RA. Use of the Berg Balance Test to predict falls in the elderly. *Phys Ther.* 1996;76:576–585.

Bohannon RW. Observations of balance among elderly patients referred to physical therapy in an acute care hospital. *Physiotherapy Theory Pract.* 1999;15(3):185–189.

Borello-France D, Whitney SL. Physical therapy management of a patient with bilateral peripheral vestibular loss: a case report. *Neurology Rep.* 1996;20(3):54–60.

Brauer S, Burns Y, Galley P. Lateral reach: a clinical measure of medio-lateral postural stability. *Physiotherapy Res Int.* 1999;4(2):81–88.

Brody LT. Balance impairment. In: Hall CM, Brody TB, eds. *Therapeutic exercise: Moving Toward Function*. Philadelphia, Pa: Lippincott Williams and Wilkins; 1999:112–127.

Brown KE, Whitney SL, Wrisley DM, Furman JM. Physical therapy outcomes for persons with bilateral vestibular loss. *Laryngoscope*. 2001;111(10):1812–1817.

Browne JE, O'Hare NJ. Review of the different methods for assessing standing balance. *Physiotherapy*. 2001;87(9):489–495.

Burton JM. Physical therapy management of a patient with central vestibular disfunction: a case report. *Neurol Rep*. 1996;20(3):61–62. [Published erratum appears in Neurology Reports 1996;20(4):21.]

Campbell AJ, Robertson MC, Garder MM, Norton RN, Tilyard MW, Buchner DM. Randomized controlled trail of a general practice programme of home based exercise to prevent falls in elderly women. *BMJ*. 1997;315:1065–1069.

Cass SP, Borello-France D, Furman JM. Function outcome of vestibular rehabilitation in patients with abnormal sensory-organization testing. *Am J Otol*. 1997;17(4):581–594.

Clendaniel RA. Outcome measures for assessment of treatment of the dizzy and balance disorder patient. *Otolaryngol Clin North Am*. 2000;33:519–533.

Clendaniel RA, Tucci, DL. Vestibular rehabilitation strategies in Meniere's disease. *Otolaryngol Clin North Am*. 1997;30:1145–1158.

Cowand JL, Wrisley DM, Walker M, Strasnich B, Jacobson JT. Efficacy of vestibular rehabilitation. *Otolaryngol Head Neck Surg*. 1998;118:49–54.

Denham T, Wolf A. Vestibular rehabilitation. *Rehab Manage* 1997;10(3):93–94, 144.

DiFabio RP, Seay R. Use of the "fast evaluation of mobility balance and fear" in elderly community dwellers: validity and reliability. *Phys Ther*. 1997;77:904–917.

Enloe LJ, Shields RK. Evaluation of health-related quality of life in individuals with vestibular disease using disease-specific and general outcome measures. *Phys Ther*. 1997;77:890–903.

Fell, NT. Mental imagery and mental practice for an individual with multiple sclerosis and balance dysfunction. *Phys Ther Case Rep*. 2000;3(2):3–10.

Fishman MN, Colby LA, Sachs LA, Nichols DS. Comparison of upper-extremity balance tasks and force platform testing in persons with hemiparesis. *Phys Ther*. 1997;77:1052–1062.

Ford G, Marsden J. Physical exercise regimes—practical aspects. In Luxon LM, Davies RA, eds. *Handbook of Vestibular Rehabilitation*. San Diego, Calif: Singular Publishing Group; 1997:101–115.

Ford-Smith D. The individual treatment of a patient with benign paroxysmal positional vertigo. *Phys Ther*. 1997;77(8):848–855.

Furman JM, Whitney SL. Central causes of dizziness. *Phys Ther*. 2000;80(2):179–187.

Gill-Body KM, Popat RA, Parker SW, Krebs DE. Rehabilitation of balance in two patients with cerebellar disfunction. *Phys Ther*. 1997;77(5):534–552.

Giorgetti MM, Harris BA, Jette A. Reliability of clinical balance outcome measures in the elderly. *Physiotherapy Res Int*. 1998;3(4):274–283.

Haas BM, Burden AM. Validity of weight distribution and sway measurements of the Balance Performance Monitor. *Physiotherapy Res Int*. 2000;5(1):19–32.

Haas BM, Whitmarsh TE. Inter-and intra-tester reliability of the Balance Performance Monitor in a non-patient population. *Physiotherapy Res Int*. 1998;3(2):135–147.

Hain TC, Fuller, L. Weil L, Kotsias J. Effects of t'ai chi on balance. *Arch Otolaryngol—Head Neck Surg*. 1999;125:1191–1195.

Hain TC, Helminski JO, Reis IL, Uddin MK. Vibration does not improve results of the canalith repositioning procedures. *Arch Otolaryngol—Head Neck Surg.* 2000;126: 617–622.

Hain TC, Ramaswamy TS, Hillman MA. Anatomy and physiology of the normal vestibular system. In: Herdman SJ, ed. *Vestibular Rehabilitation.* 2nd ed. Philadelphia, Pa: FA Davis Co; 2000:3–24.

Herdman SJ. Balance rehabilitation: Background, techniques and usefulness. In: Jacobson GP, Newman CW, Kartush JM, eds. *Handbook of Balance Function Testing.* St. Louis, Mo: Mosby Year Book; 1993:392–406.

Herdman SJ. Vestibular rehabilitation. In: Baloh RW, Halmagyi GM, eds. *Disord Vestibular Syst.* New York, NY: Oxford University Press; 1996:583–597.

Herdman SJ. Advances in the treatment of vestibular disorders. *Phys Ther.* 1997;77(6):602–618.

Herdman SJ. Role of vestibular adaptation in vestibular rehabilitation. *Otolaryngol Head Neck Surg.* 1998;119(1):49–54.

Herdman SJ. Physical therapy diagnosis for vestibular disorders. In: Herdman SJ, ed. *Vestibular Rehabilitation.* 2nd ed. Philadelphia, Pa: FA Davis Co; 2000:566–573.

Herdman SJ, Blatt PJ, Schubert MC. Vestibular rehabilitation of patients with vestibular hypofunction or with benign parozysmal positional vertigo. *Curr Opinions Neurol.* 2000;13(1):39–43.

Herdman SJ, Blatt P, Schubert MC, Tusa RJ. Falls in patients with vestibular deficits. *Am J Otol.* 2000;21(6):847–851.

Herdman SJ, Schubert MC, Tusa RJ. Role of central programming in dynamic visual acuity with vestibular loss. *Arch Head Neck Surg.* 2001;127(10):1205–1210.

Herdman SJ, Schubert MC, Tusa RJ. Strategies or balance rehabilitation: fall risk and treatment. *Ann NY Acad Sci.* 2001;942:394–412.

Herdman SJ, Tusa RJ. Complications of the canalith repositioning procedure. *Arch Otolaryngol Head Neck Surg.* 1996;122:281–286.

Herdman SJ, Tusa RJ. Assessment and treatment of patients with benign paroxysmal positional vertigo. In: Herdman SJ, ed. *Vestibular Rehabilitation.* 2nd ed. Philadelphia, Pa: FA Davis Co; 2000:451–475.

Herdman SJ, Tusa RJ, Blatt P, Suzuki A, Venuto PJ, Roberts D. Computerized dynamic visual acuity test in the assessment of vestibular deficits. *Am J Otol.* 1998;19(6): 790–796.

Horak FB, Henry SM, Shumway-Cook A. Postural perturbations: new insights for the treatment of balance disorders. *Phys Ther.* 1997;77:517–533.

Horak FB, Shupert C. Role of the vestibular system in postural control. In: Herdman SJ, ed. *Vestibular Rehabilitation.* 2nd ed. Philadelphia, Pa: FA Davis Co; 2000:25–51.

Hu MH, Woollacott MH. Balance evaluation, training and rehabilitation of frail fallers. *Rev Clin Gerontol.* 1996;685–90.

Humphreis RL, Baguley DM, Peerman S, Mitchell TE, Moffat DA. Clinical outcomes of vestibular rehabilitation. *Physiotherapy.* 2001;87:368–373.

Huxham FE, Goldie PA, Patla AE. Theoretical considerations in balance assessment. *Aust J Physiotherapy.* 2001;47(2):89–100.

Jacob RG, Whitney SL, Detweiler-Shostak G, Furman JM. Vestibular rehabilitation for patients with agoraphobia and vestibular dysfunction: A pilot study. *J Anxiety Disord.* 2001;15(1–2):131–146.

Kalsi-Ryan S, Verrier M. An organizational framework for the measurement of posture and balance in stroke. *Physiotherapy Can.* 1998;50(2):109–111.

Karlberg M, Magnusson M, Malmstrone E, Melander A, Moriz U. Postural and symptomatic improvement after physiotherapy in patients with dizziness of suspected cervical origin. *Arch Phys Med Rehabil.* 1996;77(9):874–882.

Keshner EA. Postural abnormalities in vestibular disorders. In: Herdman SJ, ed. *Vestibular Rehabilitation.* 2nd ed. Philadelphia, Pa: FA Davis Co; 2000:52–76.

Lindmark B, Lagerstrom C, Naessen T, Larsen H, Persson I. Performance in functional balance tests during menopausal hormone replacement: a double-blind placebo-controlled study. *Physiotherapy Res Int.* 1999;4(1):43–54.

Mackenzie M. A simplified measure of balance by functional reach. *Physiotherapy Res Int.* 1999;4(3):233–236.

Mann GC, Whitney SL, Redfern MS, Borello-France DF, Furman JM. Functional reach and single leg stance in patients with peripheral vestibular disorders. *J Vestibular Res.* 1996; 6:343–353.

Melnick ME, Oremland B. Movement dysfunction associated with cerebellar problems. In: Umphred DA, ed. *Neurol Rehabil.* 4th ed. St Louis, Mo: CV Mosby Co; 2001:717–740.

Monsell EM, Furman JM, Herdman SJ, Konrad HR, Shepard NT. Computerized dynamic platform posturography. *Otolaryngol Head Neck Surg.* 1997;117(4):394–398.

Murphy J. Balance assessment heightened through thorough testing. *Adv Phys Ther.* 1996; June 10;22–23,29.

Pollock AS, Burward BR, Rowe PJ, Paul JP. What is balance? *Clin Rehabil.* 2000;14:402–408.

Protas EJ, Wang C-Y, Harris C. Usefulness of an individualized balance and gait intervention programme based on the problem-oriented assessment of mobility in nursing home residents. *Disability Rehabil.* 2001;23(5):192–198.

Ragnarsdóttir M. The concept of balance. *Physiotherapy.* 1996;82(6):368–375.

Reynolds JP. Balance strategies: 2000 and beyond. *PT Magazine Phys Ther.* 1997;5(6): 24–31.

Rine RM, Schubert MC, Balkany TJ. Visual-vestibular habilitation and balance training for motion sickness. *Phys Ther.* 1999;79(10):949–957.

Rubenstein LZ, Josephson KR, Trueblood PR, Yeung K, Harker JO, Robbins AS. The reliability and validity of an obstacle course as a measure of gait and balance in older adults. *Aging.* 1997;9:127–135.

Rutley RF. Relaxation for patients with peripheral vestibular disorders. In: Luxon LM, Davies RA, eds. *Handbook of Vestibular Rehabilitation.* San Diego, Calif: Singular Publishing Group; 1997:116–124.

Schubert MC, Herdman SJ. Vestibular rehabilitation. In: O'Sullivan SB, Schmitz TJ. *Phys Rehabil Assess Treatment.* 4th ed. Philadelphia, Pa: FA Davis Co; 2001:821–843.

Schubert MC, Herdman SJ, Tusa RJ. Functional measure of gaze stability in patients with vestibular hypofunction. *Ann NY Acad Sci.* 2001;942:490491.

Stevenson TJ, Garland SJ. Standing balance during internally produced perturbations in subjects with hemiplegia; validation of the balance scale. *Arch Phys Med Rehabil.* 1996;77(7):656–662.

Turano KA, Dagnelie G, Herdman SJ. Visual stabilization of posture in persons with central visual field loss. *Invest Ophthalmol Visual Sci.* 1996;37(8):1483–1493.

Tusa RJ, Grant MP, Buettner UW, Herdman SJ, Zee DS. The contribution of the vertical semicircular canals to high-velocity horizontal vestibulo-ocular reflex (VOR) in normal subjects and patients with unilateral vestibular nerve section. *Acta Otolaryngol.* 1996;116(4):507–512.

Wegener L, Kisner C, Nichols D. Static and dynamic balance responses in persons with bilateral knee osteoarthritis. *J Orthop Sports Phys Ther.* 1997;25:13–18.

Whitney SL. Differential diagnosis of dizziness in the older adult. In: Kauffman TL, ed. *Geriatr Rehabil Man*. New York, NY: Churchill Livingstone; 1999:327–338.

Whitney SL. Efficacy of vestibular rehabilitation. *Otolaryngol Clin North Am*. 2000;33:659–672.

Whitney SL. Management of the elderly person with vestibular dysfunction. In: Herdman SJ, ed. *Vestibular Rehabilitation*. 2nd ed. Philadelphia, Pa: FA Davis Co; 2000:510–533.

Whitney SL, Borello-France D. Bilateral vestibular disease: An overview. *Neurol Rep*. 1996; 20:41–45.

Whitney SL, Herdman SJ. Physical therapy assessment of vestibular hypofunction. In Herdman SJ, ed. *Vestibular Rehabilitation*. Philadelphia, Pa: FA Davis Co; 2000;333–372.

Whitney SL, Hudak MT, Marchetti GF. The activities-specific balance confidence scale and the dizziness handicap inventory: a comparison. *J Vestibular Res*. 1999;9:253–259.

Whitney SL, Hudak MT, Marchetti GF. The dynamic gait index relates to self-reported fall history in individual with vestibular dysfunction. *J Vestibular Res*. 2000;10(2):99–105.

Whitney SL, Poole JL, Cass SP. A review of balance instruments for older adults. *Am J Occup Ther*. 1998;52:666–671.

Whitney SL, Wrisley DM, Brown KE, Furman JM. Physical Therapy for migraine-related vestibulopathy and vestibular dysfunction with history of migraine. *Laryngoscope*. 2000;110(9):1528–1534.

Wrisley DM, Spartan PJ, Whitney SL, Furman JM. Cervicogenic dizziness: a review of diagnosis and treatment. *J Orthop Sports Phys Ther*. 2000;30(12):755–766.

Ye MT, Herdman SJ, Tusa RJ. Oscillopsia and pseudonystagmus in kidney transplant patient. *Am J Ophthalmol*. 1999;128(6):768–770.

Zimbelman JL, Stoecker J, Haberkamp TJ. Outcomes in vestibular rehabilitation. *Phys Ther Case Rep*. 1999;2(6):232–240.

Zimbelman JL, Walton TM. Case in point. Vestibular rehabilitation for a patient with persistent Mal de Debarquement. *Phys Ther Case Rep*. 1999;1(4):129–38. [Includes commentary by Clendaniel R.]

Chapter 11

Oncology

Breast Cancer

DESCRIPTION

Cancer is a *cellular malignancy* characterized by the loss of the usual controls. This allows unrestricted cellular proliferation that can invade normal tissues as well as metastasize to other sites. If left untreated, this uncontrolled spread of abnormal cells can lead to death.

Around 180,000 women in the United States are diagnosed with breast cancer each year. Medical treatment for breast cancer varies depending on the diagnosis. Systemic treatments—such as chemotherapy and hormone therapy—may control cancer cells throughout the body. Localized treatments include radiation and surgery. Surgery, however, is the most common choice for treating breast cancer.

CAUSE

Breast cancer is influenced by the following risk factors:

- for women: age, breast disease, family history, and reproductive history
- for men: age, cancer therapy, genetic predisposition, gynecomastia, and Klinefelter's syndrome

ASSESSMENT

Note: See APTA's Guide to Physical Therapist Practice. 2nd ed. *Physical Therapy.* 2001;81.

Musculoskeletal Preferred Practice Patterns: D, I

Integumentary Preferred Practice Pattern: A

AREAS

- History, including hand dominance and type of surgery, particularly breast reconstruction
- Psychosocial
- Chest wall: swelling, appearance in general
- Pain
- Posture
- Cardiopulmonary screen, including peripheral pulses, vital signs during activity, respiration
- Mobility: active range of motion (ROM), including neck, shoulder, and upper extremities
- Skin and soft tissue: color changes, edema, and scar, including any adhesions
- Neurological, including sensation
- Strength, especially upper quarter region, with emphasis on thorax and shoulder
- Balance
- Functional level, including activities of daily living (ADLs)

INSTRUMENTS/PROCEDURES

See References for sources.

Functional Level
- Katz Index of ADLs
- Barthel ADL index
- Functional Independence Measure

Physical Performance Status Scales
- American Joint Committee on Cancer Performance Status Scale
- Eastern Cooperative Oncology Group Performance Status Scale

- Karnofsky Performance Status Scale
- World Health Organization Performance Status Scale

Pain
- finger dynameter
- pain intensity number scale
- visual analog scale

Skin and Soft Tissue
1. edema
    - circumferential measurements
    - volumetrics

Special Tests to Which the Physical Therapist May or May Not Have Access
- biopsy
- bone scan
- breast exam
- bronchoscopy
- colonoscopy
- diaphanoscopy
- hormone receptor tests
- imaging techniques
- mammography
- needle aspiration
- radiograph, magnetic resonance imaging (MRI) or computed tomography scan (CT)
- sigmoidoscopy
- sputum cytology
- urinalysis and stool guaiac

PROBLEMS
- The client may develop lymphedema.
- The client often has pain.
- The client may have spasm in the posterior cervical region and shoulder girdle.
- The client may have neurological symptoms, such as hyperesthesia, paresthesia, throbbing pain, phantom breast sensations, weakness, and skin trophic changes that are secondary to nerve damage during surgery, radiotherapy, or chemotherapy.
- The client may have weakness, especially in the involved upper extremity.
- The client may develop contracture secondary to immobilization of upper extremity.
- The client may have sensory loss with radiating pain or aching.
- The client may develop postural asymmetry.
- The client may have difficulty with psychological adjustment to body image and sexual functioning.
- The client may have menopausal symptoms such as hot flashes, interrupted periods, or vaginal dryness due to hormone therapy.

TREATMENT/MANAGEMENT

LYMPHEDEMA TREATMENT
- Design treatment to meet individual needs.
- Lymphedema prevention involves arm mobilization, shoulder strengthening, prevention and treatment of upper extremity edema, and education on arm function.
- Consider use of manual lymph drainage, elevation, compression, and retrograde massage with a good skin conditioner.
- Consider use of complex physical therapy: a combination of skin hygiene, lymphatic massage, compression bandaging and garment, and specific exercises to supplement massage.
- Modalities for edema include intermittent compression, massage, taping, exercise, continual elevation, and elastic gradient support garments or bandages.
- The use of pumps is under debate. One suggested pumping program consists of mechanical pumping, 1 to 3 days for 8 to 10 hours per day, and then fitting client

with a custom compression garment. Switch to progressively smaller garments every 4 to 6 weeks.

POST-SURGICAL TREATMENT
- The client should receive pain medication shortly before treatment.
- Instruct the client in positioning. If the client is on bed rest, the arm may be in slight shoulder abduction and flexion, with distal elevation and support.
- Encourage active movement of the hand, wrist, forearm, and elbow.
- Begin with passive and active assistive ROM activities for the shoulder without harming healing of suture area, until the surgical drains are removed. Internal and external rotation to tolerance and 40–45 degrees of flexion and abduction until the 4th day as tolerated. Future advance should be based on surgical protocols and client tolerance. Overhead pully may assist with ROM.
- Educate the client to avoid holding affected arm in flexed protective posture against body.
- On day 4 or 5 postsurgery, begin active exercises. Include neck ROM, shoulder shrugs, shoulder rotation, flexion and abduction to tolerance, and protraction and retraction of scapula. Use unaffected arm to assist as needed. Progress to isometric exercise and resistive elastic band as tolerated.
- Modalities for pain, relaxation, or edema include cold packs, mechanical compression, and massage (not with bone tumor).
- Initiate stretching activities. Neuropathic symptoms may be relieved by stretching adhesions and increasing ROM.
- Instruct the client to watch for signs of edema: increased fullness in arm; change in color (usually more reddened); increase in skin temperature. Circumferential changes greater than 2 cm should be reported. See Table 11.1 for specific instructions.
- Use orthotic and assistive devices as indicated for ADLs.
- Prescribe exercise program with emphasis on strength, flexibility, and endurance. Types of exercise may include shoulder shrugging, ROM for cervical spine and shoulder with shoulder circle exercise, and exercises for spinal extensor musculature and upper extremity strength. Manual isotonic resistance exercise may be initiated with physician consultation, usually on the 4th day postsurgery.
- Consider use of joint mobilization for glenohumeral joint and scapulothoracic joint.
- Emphasize postural instruction.
- Provide gait training if indicated.
- Clients who are at increased risk of pathological fractures—those with bone metastases—should be instructed in prevention of falls and consider use of prophylactic orthotics.

PRECAUTIONS/CONTRAINDICATIONS

Note: See Pfalzer, *Physical Agents and the Patient with Cancer*, in Treatment references.
- Heat and cold modalities are contraindicated in the area of the axilla if it was irradiated.
- Tissue should not blanch when stretched.
- Modify exercise as indicated if client also has bone metastases or osteoporosis.
- Generally, exercise can be unrestricted if platelet counts are above 30,000 to 50,000.
- Non-resistive activities can be considered if platelet counts are above 10,000 to 20,000.
- Usually, active therapy is contraindicated if platelet counts are below 10,000.
- Exercise is contraindicated with fever above 104 degrees F.

TABLE 11.1
Skin Care Tips To Avoid Lymphedema

**For the breast cancer patient who is at risk of
lymphedema or who has developed lymphedema:**

Do	Do keep the edemic or "at risk" arm very clean. Use lotion after bathing. When drying, be gentle, but thorough.
	Avoid vigorous, repetitive movements against resistance with the affected arm.
	Avoid heavy lifting with the affected arm.
	Avoid extreme temperature changes. Do keep the arm protected from the sun.
	Avoid any type of trauma, such as insect bites or cat scratches.
	Do wear gloves while doing work that could result in even a minor injury.
	Avoid cutting your cuticles when manicuring your nails.
	If you have lymphedema, wear a well-fitted compression sleeve, especially when traveling.
	Patients with large breasts should wear light breast prostheses and a well-fitted bra that is not too tight and has no wire support.
	Warning: If you notice a rash, blistering, redness, increase of temperature, or fever, see your physician immediately. An inflammation or infection in the affected arm could be the beginning of lymphedema or a worsening of lymphedema.
	Maintain your ideal weight. Lymphedema is a high-protein edema, but eating too little protein will not reduce the protein element in the lymph fluid; rather, this will weaken the connective tissue and worsen the condition. The diet should contain protein that is easily digested, such as a chicken and fish.
	Avoid smoking and alcoholic beverages.
Don't	Don't ignore any slight increase of swelling in the arm, hand, fingers, or chest wall (consult with your doctor immediately).
	Don't allow an injection of a blood drawing in the affected arm(s).
	Don't have blood pressure checked in the affected arm.
	Don't wear tight jewelry or elastic bands around affected fingers or arm(s).
	Although exercise is important, don't overtire an at-risk arm; if it starts to ache, lie down and elevate it. Recommended exercises: walking, swimming, light aerobics, bike riding, and specially designated ballet or yoga. (Do not lift more than 12 lb.)

Source: Reprinted with permission from S Thiadens, National Lymphedema Network; Skin Care Tips to Avoid Lymphedema, in Pauls J: *Therapeutic Approaches to Women's Health: A Program of Exercise and Education.* Gaithersburg, Md: Aspen Publishers; 1995:7-1:26.

- Exercise typically includes ROM, aerobic activity, light resistive with 2–4 pounds, and deep breathing.
- Clients with hepatic veno-occlusive disease should avoid supine exercise or abdominal exercise.
- Take precautions with graft versus hose disease.
- Cardiotoxic agents can affect physical performance.
- If exercise creates extreme fatigue it was probably too intense.

DESIRED OUTCOME/PROGNOSIS
- The client will prevent lymphedema formation.
- The client will prevent postural deficits.

- The client will prevent contractures.
- The client will improve symmetry in posture.
- The client will protect skin and monitor own status.
- The client will be independent in ADLs.
- The client will have a decrease in pain and symptoms.
- The client will have an increased ability to cope with the diagnosis.
- The client will have a well-healed wound site.
- The client will have adaptive equipment, such as a prosthesis, if needed.

Notes: In general, if cancer is detected at an early stage, it is often curable. One study reports that early intervention offers a significant increase in return to normal function post mastectomy with no increased incidence of postoperative complications or increase in hospital stay.

One study reports a highly significant decrease in edema post use of complex PT. Sensory loss with radiating pain or aching usually diminishes within 6 months to a year.

One aerobic conditioning program reported 40% improvement in functional capacity after 10 weeks of aerobic training 3 times per week.

REFERENCES

Assessment

Adcock JL. Rehabilitation of the breast cancer patient. In: McGarvery CL, ed. *Physical Theraphy for the Cancer Patient: Clinics in Physical Therapy.* New York, NY: Churchill Livingstone; 1990;67–84.

American Physical Therapy Association. Guide to physical therapist practice. 2nd ed. *Phys Ther.* 2001;81.

Gerber L, Lampert M, Wood C, et al. Comparison of pain, motion, and edema after modified radical mastectomy vs local excision with axillary dissection and radiation. *Breast Cancer Res Treatment.* 1992;21:139–145.

Goodman C, Synder T. *Differential Diagnosis in Physical Therapy.* 2nd ed. Philadelphia, Pa: WB Saunders Co; 2000.

Konecne SM. Postsurgery breast cancer inpatient program. *Clin Manage Phys Ther.* 1992; 12:4:42–49.

Pfalzer LA. Oncology: examination, diagnosis, and treatment. Medical and surgical considerations. In: Myers RS, ed. *Saunders Manual of Physical Therapy Practice.* Philadelphia, Pa: WB Saunders Co; 1995;65–147.

Pfalzer LA. Oncology: examination, diagnosis, and treatment. Physical therapy considerations. In: Myers RS, ed. *Saunders Manual of Physical Therapy Practice.* Philadelphia, Pa: WB Saunders Co; 1995:149–190.

Treatment

Balzarini A, Pirovano C, Diazzi G, et al. Ultrasound therapy of chronic arm lymphedema after surgical treatment of breast cancer. *Lymphology.* 1993;26:128–134.

Body JJ, Lossignol D, Ronson A. The concept of rehabilitation of cancer patients. *Curr Opinions Oncol.* 1997;9:332–340.

Campbell KL, Harris SR. Physical activity in the primary prevention of estrogen-related cancers. *Physiotherapy Can.* 2000;52:198–207.

Croarkin E. Osteopenia in the patient with cancer. *Phys Ther.* 1999;79:196–201.

Dean JT, Davidson G. Trismus after radiation therapy. *Clin Manage Phys Ther.* 1992; 12:4:70–76.

Frankiel M. The physical therapist and post-mastectomy rehabilitation. *J Obstet Gynecol Phys Ther.* 1992;16:1:9–11.

Friedenreich CM, Curneya KS. Exercise as rehabilitation for cancer patients. *Clin J Sports Med.* 1996;6:237–244.

Frymark SL. Taking control. Cancer rehabilitation allows patients to increase the quality of their lives and reclaim independence. *Rehabil Manage.* 1998;11:80–86.

Grabois M, Garrison SJ, Hart KA, Lehmkuhl LD. *Physical Medicine and Rehabilitation: The Complete Approach.* Malden, Mass: Blackwell Science; 2000.

Gudas SA. Directives in cancer rehabilitation. *Clin Manage Phys Ther.* 1992;12:4:32–36.

Hack TF, Cohen L, Katz J, et al. Physical and psychological morbidity after axillary lymph node dissection for breast cancer. *J Clin Oncol.* 1999;17:143–149.

Hamburgh RR. Principles of cancer treatment. *Clin Manage Phys Ther.* 1992;12:4:37–41.

Hanson KP, Demin EV, Blinov NN, et al. Supportive care in cancer patients in St. Petersburg. *Support Care Cancer.* 1996;4:160–162.

Hladiuk M, Huchcroft S, Temple W, Schnurr BE. Arm function after axillary dissection for breast cancer: a pilot study to provide parameter estimates. *J Surg Oncol.* 1992; 50:1:47–52.

Hock K. Ambulatory oncology program. *Clin Manage Phys Ther.* 1992;12:4:87–91.

Impello RF, Crane J. Clinical profiles. Musculoskeletal intervention for postmastectomy complications. *Phys Ther Case Rep.* 2000;3:22–24.

Johansson K, Ingvar C, Albertsson M, et al. Arm lymphoedema, shoulder mobility and muscle strength after breast cancer treatment – a prospective 2-year study. *Adv Physiotherapy.* 2001;3:55–66.

Kelley SM, Jull GA. Breast surgery and neural tissue mechanosensitivity. *Aust J Physiotherapy.* 1998;44:31–37.

Konecne SM. Postsurgery breast cancer inpatient program. *Clin Manage Phys Ther.* 1992;12:4:42–49.

Ku A, Lachmann E, Tunkel R, et al. Upper Limb reflex sympathetic dystrophy associated with occult malignancy. *Arch Phys Med Rehabil.* 1996;77:726–728.

Lee MM, Lin SS, Wrensch, et al. Alternative therapies used by women with breast cancer in four ethnic populations. *J Natl Cancer Inst.* 2000;92:42–47.

Liu S, Tunkel R, Lachmann E, et al. Paraneoplastic cerbellar degeneration as the first evidence of cancer: a case report. *Arch Phys Med Rehabil.* 2000;81:834–836.

Mackey KM, Sparling JW. Experiences of older women with cancer receiving hospice care: significance for physical therapy. *Phys Ther.* 2000;80:459–468.

Marcant D, Rapin CH. Role of the physiotherapist in palliative care. *J Pain Manage.* 1993;8: 2:68–71.

Mason M. The treatment of lymphoedema by complex physical therapy. *Aust J Phys Ther.* 1993;39:1:41–45.

Michael TH. Do physiotherapists have a role in palliative care? *Physiotherapy Res Int.* 2001; 6:v–vi.

Miller LT. Postsurgery breast cancer outpatient program. *Clin Manage Phys Ther.* 1992; 12:4:50–56.

Myers RS, ed. *Saunders Manual of Physical Therapy Practice.* Philadelphia, Pa: WB Saunders Co; 1995.

Pauls J. Mastectomy. In: Pauls J, ed. *Therapeutic Approaches to Women's Health: A Program of Exercise and Education.* Gaithersburg, Md: Aspen Publishers; 1995.

Peabody TD, Gibbs CP, Simon MA. Evaluation and staging of musculoskeletal neoplasms. *J Bone Joint Surg Am.* 1998;80:1204–1218.

Pfalzer L. Physical agents and the patient with cancer. *Clin Manage Phys Ther.* 1992; 12:4:83–86.

Pfalzer L, Walter J. Facts and fiction: cancer in the 1990's. *Clin Manage Phys Ther.* 1992; 12:4:26–31.

Phillips LL. Managing the pain of bone metastases in the home environment. *Am J Hospice Palliative Care.* 1998;8:32–42.

Pomerantz E. Speaking with and listening to the breast cancer patient. *J Obstet Gynecol Phys Ther.* 1992;16:1:12–13.

Rashleigh L. Physiotherapy and palliative oncology. *Aust J Physiotherapy.* 1996;42:307–312.

Sabers SR, Kokal JE, Girardi JC, et al. Evaluation of consultation-based rehabilitation for hospitalized cancer patients with functional impairment. *Mayo Clin Proc.* 1999;74:855–861.

Sicard-Rosenbaum L, Danoff J. Cancer and ultrasound: a warning letter. *Phys Ther.* 1993;73: 404–406.

Sliwa JA, Marciniak C. Physical rehabilitation of the cancer patient. *Cancer Treatment Res.* 1999;100:75–89.

Smith WB, Gracely RH, Safer MA. The meaning of pain: cancer patients' rating and recall of pain intensity and affect. *Pain.* 1998;78:123–129.

Snyder R. Physical therapy in terminal illness. *Clin Manage Phys Ther.* 1992;12:4:96–100.

Tool JL. Physical therapy in the care of patients with a diagnosis of cancer. *Clin Manage Phys Ther.* 1992;12:4:96–100.

Watchie J. Cardiopulmonary complications of cancer. *Clin Manage Phys Ther.* 1992;12:4: 92–95.

Woods EN. Reaching out to patients with breast cancer. *Clin Manage Phys Ther.* 1992;12:4: 58–63.

Yoshioka H. Rehabilitation for the terminal cancer patient. *Am J Phys Med Rehabil.* 1994; 73:199–206.

Lymphedema

Balzarini A, Pirovano C, Diazzi G, et al. Ultrasound therapy of chronic arm lymphedema after surgical treatment of breast cancer. *Lymphol.* 1993;26:128–134.

Carson CJ, Coverly K, Lasker-Hertz S. The incidence of co-morbidities in the treatment of lymphedema. *J Oncol Manage.* 1999;8:13–17.

Casley-Smith JR, Casley-Smith JR. Modern treatment of lymphoedema. 1. Complex physical therapy: the first 200 Australian limbs. *Aust J Dermatol.* 1992;33:2:61–68.

Foldi E. Prevention of dermatolymphangioadenitis by combined physiotherapy of the swollen arm after treatment for breast cancer. *Lymphology.* 1996;29:48–49.

Foldi E. Treatment of lymphedema and patient rehabilitation. *Anticancer Res.* 1998;18: 2211–2212.

Frymark SL. Taking control. Cancer rehabilitation allows patients to increase the quality of their lives and reclaim independence. *Rehabil Manage.* 1998;11:80–86.

Gerber L, Lampert M, Wood C, et al. Comparison of pain, motion, and edema after modified radical mastectomy vs local excision with axillary dissection and radiation. *Breast Cancer Res Treatment.* 1992;21:139–145.

Harris SR, Hugi MR, Olivotto IA. Clinical practice guidelines for the care and treatment of breast cancer: 11. Lymphedema. *CMAJ.* 2001;164:191–199.

Hull MM. Lymphedema in women treated for breast cancer. *Semin Oncol Nurs.* 2000; 16:226–237.

Johansson K, Albertsson M, Ingvar C, et al. Effects of compression bandaging with or without manual lymph drainage treatment in patients with postoperative arm lymphedema. *Lymphology.* 1999;32:103–110.

Kasseroller R. Sodium selenite as prophylaxis against erysipelas in secondary lymphedema. *Anticancer Res.* 1998;18:2227–2230.

Mark B. Lymphedema: etiology and management techniques. *J Obstet Gynecol Phys Ther.* 1994;18:2:5–8.

Mark B, Feltman B. Case studies in the management of post-mastectomy lymphedema. *J Obstetr Gynecol Phys Ther.* 1994;18:3:5–9.

Mason M. Spotlight on lymphoedema. *Physiotherapy Moves.* 2000;16:17.

Matthews KL, Smith JG. Effectiveness of modified Complex Physical Therapy for lymphoedema. *Aust J Physiotherapy.* 1996;42:323–328.

Megens A, Harris SR. Physical therapist management of lymphedema following treatment for breast cancer: a critical review of its effectiveness. *Phys Ther.* 1998;78:1302–1311.

Morgan RG, Casley-Smith JR, Mason MR, Casley-Smith JR. Complex physical therapy for the lymphoedematous arm. *J Hand Surg.* 1992;17B:437–441.

Mortimer PS. Therapy approaches for lymphedema. *Angiology.* 1997;48:87–91.

Norman S, Miller LT, Erikson HB, et al. Development and validation of a telephone questionnaire to characterize lymphedema in women treated for breast cancer. *Phys Ther.* 2001;81:1192–1205.

Rinehart-Ayres ME. Conservative approaches to lymphedema treatment. *Cancer.* 1998;83: 2828–2832.

Rockson SG, Miller LT, Senie R, et al. American Cancer Society Lymphedema workshop. Workgroup III: Diagnosis and management of lymphedema. *Cancer.* 1998;83:2828–2832.

Szuba A, Cooke JP, Yousuf S, et al. Decongestive lymphatic therapy for patients with cancer-related or primary lymphedema. *Am J Med.* 2000;109:296–300.

Wozniewski M, Jasinski R, Pilch U, et al. Complex physical therapy for lympoedema of the limbs. *Physiotherapy.* 2001;87:252–256.

Head and Neck Cancer

DESCRIPTION

Cancer is a *cellular malignancy* characterized by the loss of the usual controls. This allows unrestricted cellular proliferation that can invade normal tissues as well as metastasize to other sites. If left untreated, this uncontrolled spread of abnormal cells can lead to death.

Cancers of the head and neck are cancers that affect the upper aerodigestive tract. The most common sites for these cancers are the larynx, oral cavity, pharynx, and salivary glands. The lips, nose, sinuses, and ears may also be affected. Reportedly, 80% of head and neck cancers originate in the mucosa of the aerodigestive tract.

The squamous cell carcinoma is the most common type of malignant neoplasm of the head and neck region.

CAUSE

Cancers of the head and neck are often caused by tobacco and alcohol abuse. Nasopharyngeal cancer is also linked to Epstein-Barr virus.

ASSESSMENT

Note: See APTA's Guide to Physical Therapist Practice. 2nd ed. *Physical Therapy.* 2001;81.

Musculoskeletal Preferred Practice Patterns: D, I

Integumentary Preferred Practice Pattern: A

AREAS

- History
- Psychosocial factors
- Pain
- Posture
- Skin and soft tissue, including wound assessment, color, and edema
- Pulmonary as indicated
- Mobility, including active and passive range of motion (ROM), especially in head, neck, and shoulder area
- Strength
- Neurological, including sensation
- Functional level

INSTRUMENTS/PROCEDURES

See References for sources.

Functional Level
- Karnofsky Performance Status Scale
- Performance Status Scale for Head and Neck Cancer Patients
- Katz Index of ADLs
- Barthel ADL index
- Functional Independence Measure

Physical Performance Status Scales

- American Joint Committee on Cancer Performance Status Scale
- Eastern Cooperative Oncology Group Performance Status Scale
- Karnofsky Performance Status Scale
- World Health Organization Performance Status Scale

Pain
- finger dynameter
- pain intensity number scale
- visual analog scale

Special Tests to Which the Physical Therapist May or May Not Have Access
- bone scan
- bronchoscopy
- colonoscopy
- radiograph, magnetic resonance imaging (MRI)
- or computed tomography scan (CT)
- sigmoidoscopy
- sputum cytology
- urinalysis and stool guaiac

PROBLEMS
- The client often has diminished or lost functionality in the area of the head, neck, and shoulder due to the radical or modified dissection of muscle, nerve, vessels, and lymphatic groups.
- The client may have pain in the shoulder.
- The client typically has trapezius muscle dysfunction or paralysis.
- The scapula may be medially rotated and laterally deviated.

- The client may have clavicle subluxation.
- The client may have scapular fixation that limits active motion to 130 degrees flexion and 90 degrees abduction.
- The client may have diminished sensation in the upper extremities.

TREATMENT/MANAGEMENT
- The therapist should be part of a team approach to rehabilitation.
- Educate area musculature to substitute in shoulder motions of elevation, retraction, and stabilization during flexion and abduction.
- Instruct the client in an exercise program that can be followed on an outpatient or home care basis, to be adapted to individual needs. This may include chin retraction, cervical flexion, rotation, sidebending, circumduction, upper extremity flexion, and pendulum exercises. Shoulder exercises include stregthening of the scapular stabilizers (serratus anterior, rhomboids, levator scapula) and stretching of the protractors. Avoid internal rotation.
- If there is TMJ involvement, motion can be increased with active stretching exercises or mechanical stretching with tongues blade, and continuous passive motion (CPM) devices.
- Consider use of functional electrical stimulation if there is a neurapraxic lesion.
- Educate the client about potential dangers due to sensory deficits, especially extreme temperatures.
- Respiratory treatment may include cough instruction, pursed lip breathing, and energy conservation techniques.
- Address issues of social and psychological impact if facial disfigurement is involved.

PRECAUTIONS/CONTRAINDICATIONS
- Until the wound is properly healed, the client should be well supported on the affected shoulder and neck area to avoid unnecessary trapezius muscle stretching.
- Exercise program should be delayed in the client with fistula formation, delayed wound healing, or carotid rupture.
- Neck exercise is contraindicated if there is a risk of carotid rupture.
- Generally, exercise can be unrestricted if platelet counts are above 30,000 to 50,000.
- Non-resistive activities can be considered if platelet counts are above 10,000 to 20,000.
- Often, active therapy is contraindicated if platelet counts are below 10,000.
- Exercise is contraindicated with fever above 104 degrees F.
- Exercise usually includes ROM, aerobic activity, light resistive with 2–4 pounds and deep breathing.
- Clients with hepatic veno-occlusive disease should avoid supine exercise or abdominal excise.
- Take precautions with graft versus hose disease.
- Cardiotoxic agents can affect physical performance.
- If exercise creates extreme fatigue it was likely too intense.
- Use physical agents and modalities with caution.

Note: In general, heat modalities are contraindicated.

DESIRED OUTCOME/PROGNOSIS
- The client will increase ROM in neck and shoulder areas to within normal limits.
- The client will increase the strength of the neck and affected arm to the highest capacity possible and will maintain scapular alignment.
- The client will maintain shoulder alignment and prevent postural problems.

Notes: A grade of "good" is commonly reached in shoulder musculature. Usually the wound is healed enough in 10 to 14 days to permit initiation of an exercise program. No one muscle group can completely compensate for the loss of trapezius musculature.

REFERENCES

Assessment

American Physical Therapy Association. Guide to physical therapist practice. 2nd ed. *Phys Ther.* 2001;81.

Pfalzer LA. Oncology: examination, diagnosis, and treatment. Medical and surgical considerations. In: Myers RS, ed. *Saunders Manual of Physical Therapy Practice.* Philadelphia, Pa: WB Saunders Co; 1995:65–147.

Pfalzer LA. Oncology: examination, diagnosis, and treatment. Physical therapy considerations. In: Myers RS, ed. *Saunders Manual of Physical Therapy Practice.* Philadelphia, Pa: WB Saunders Co; 1995:149–190.

Roberts WL. Rehabilitation of the head and neck cancer patient. In: McGarvery CL, ed. *Physical Therapy for the Cancer Patient: Clinics in Physical Therapy.* New York, NY: Churchill Livingstone; 1990:47–65. Adapted from Snow JB.

Yoshioka H. Rehabilitation for the terminal cancer patient. *Am J Phys Med Rehabil.* 1994; 73:199–206.

Treatment

Body JJ, Lossignol D, Ronson A. The concept of rehabilitation of cancer patients. *Curr Opinions Oncol.* 1997;9:332–340.

Bussieres A, Cassidy JD, Dzus A. Spinal cord astrocytoma presenting as torticollis and scoliosis. *J Manipulative Physiol Ther.* 1994;17:113–118.

Croarkin E. Osteopenia in the patient with cancer. *Phys Ther.* 1999;79:196–201.

Dean JT, Davidson G. Trismus after radiation therapy. *Clin Manage Phys Ther.* 1992; 12:4:70–76.

Delisa JA, Miller RM, Melnick RR, et al. Rehabilitation of the cancer patient. In: Gudas SA. Directives in cancer rehabilitation. *Clin Manage Phys Ther.* 1992;12:4:32–36.

Friedenreich CM, Curneya KS. Exercise as rehabilitation for cancer patients. *Clin J Sports Med.* 1996;6:237–244.

Frymark SL. Taking control. Cancer rehabilitation allows patients to increase the quality of their lives and reclaim independence. *Rehabil Manage.* 1998;11:80–86.

Futran ND, Trotti A, Gwede C, et al. Pentoxifylline in the treatment of radiation-related soft tissue injury: preliminary observations. *Laryngoscope.* 1997;107:391–395.

Grabois M, Garrison SJ, Hart KA, Lehmkuhl LD. *Physical Medicine and Rehabilitation: The Complete Approach.* Malden, Mass: Blackwell Science; 2000.

Hamburgh RR. Principles of cancer treatment. *Clin Manage Phys Ther.* 1992;12:4:37–41.

Hock K. Ambulatory oncology program. *Clin Manage Phys Ther.* 1992;12:4:87–91.

Kriss TC, Kriss VM. Neck pain. Primary care work-up of acute and chronic symptoms. *Geriatr.* 2000;55:47–57.

Marcant D, Rapin CH. Role of the physiotherapist in palliative care. *J Pain Symptom Manage.* 1993;8:2:68–71.

Michael TH. Do physiotherapists have a role in palliative care? *Physiotherapy Res Int.* 2001;6:v–vi.

Peabody TD, Gibbs CP, Simon MA. Evaluation and staging of musculoskeletal neoplasms. *J Bone Joint Surg Am.* 1998;80:1204–1218.

Pfalzer L. Physical agents and the patient with cancer. *Clin Manage Phys Ther.* 1992; 12:4:83–86.

Pfalzer L, Walter J. Facts and fiction: cancer in the 1990's. *Clin Manage Phys Ther.* 1992; 12:4:26–31.

Phillips LL. Managing the pain of bone metastases in the home environment. *Am J Hospice Palliative Care.* 1998;8:32–42.

Rashleigh L. Physiotherapy and palliative oncology. *Aust J Physiotherapy.* 1996;42:307–312.

Ridder T. Orofacial physiotherapy after radiotherapy in the head and neck region. *Cranio.* 1993;11:242–244.

Sabers SR, Kokal JE, Girardi JC, et al. Evaluation of consultation-based rehabilitation for hospitalized cancer patients with functional impairment. *Mayo Clin Proc.* 1999;74:855–861.

Sicard-Rosenbaum L, Danoff J. Cancer and ultrasound: a warning letter. *Phys Ther.* 1993;73:404–406.

Sliwa JA, Marciniak C. Physical rehabilitation of the cancer patient. *Cancer Treatment Res.* 1999;100:75–89.

Smith WB, Gracely RH, Safer MA. The meaning of pain: cancer patients' rating and recall of pain intensity and affect. *Pain.* 1998;78:123–129.

Snyder R. Coping: you and your patient with cancer. *Clin Manage Phys Ther.* 1992;12:4:64–69.

Snyder R. Physical therapy in terminal illness. *Clin Manage Phys Ther.* 1992;12:4:96–100.

Tool JL. Physical therapy in the care of patients with a diagnosis of cancer. *Clin Manage Phys Ther.* 1992;12:4:96–100.

Watchie J. Cardiopulmonary complications of cancer. *Clin Manage Phys Ther.* 1992; 12:4:92–95.

Yoshioka H. Rehabilitation for the terminal cancer patient. *Am J Phys Med Rehabil.* 1994; 73:199–206.

Leukemia

DESCRIPTION

Leukemia is defined as a *malignant neoplasm* of the blood-forming tissues. This disorder leads to production of abnormal white blood cells in the blood and bone marrow. Leukemia is designated as acute or chronic depending on cellular maturity. Acute leukemia is mainly undifferentiated cell groups, and chronic leukemias are further developed cell populations. There are four major types of leukemia: *acute lymphoblastic leukemia* (ALL), *acute myelogenous leukemia* (AML), *chronic myelogenous leukemia* (CML), and *chronic lymphocytic leukemia* (CLL).

CAUSE

The cause of leukemia is not clearly defined. Two viruses have been identified, the Epstein-Barr virus and the human acute leukemia/lymphoma virus. Exposure to some chemical and ionizing radiation has also been associated with an increased risk of leukemia. Other factors include immunological and genetic disorders.

ASSESSMENT

Note: See APTA's Guide to Physical Therapist Practice. 2nd ed. *Physical Therapy.* 2001;81.

Musculoskeletal Preferred Practice Pattern: D

AREAS

- History
- Psychosocial
- Pain
- Posture
- Cardiopulmonary, including endurance
- Musculoskeletal, including joint integrity
- Strength
- Mobility, including range of motion (ROM)
- Neurological
- Genitourinary
- Skin, including color, edema, and any wounds
- Functional level, including activities of daily living (ADLs)

INSTRUMENTS/PROCEDURES

Functional Level
- Katz Index of ADLs
- Barthel ADL index
- Functional Independence Measure

Physical Performance Status Scales

- American Joint Committee on Cancer Performance Status Scale
- Eastern Cooperative Oncology Group Performance Status Scale
- Karnofsky Performance Status Scale
- World Health Organization Performance Status Scale

Pain
- finger dynameter
- pain intensity number scale
- visual analog scale

Special Tests to Which the Physical Therapist May or May Not Have Access
- bone scan
- bronchoscopy
- colonoscopy
- sigmoidoscopy
- sputum cytology
- radiograph, magnetic resonance imaging (MRI) or computed tomography scan (CT)
- urinalysis and stool guaiac

PROBLEMS

ACUTE SYMPTOMS
- The client often has joint pain.
- There can be cyanosis.
- The client may have frequent infections.
- There is a tendency to bleed or bruise easily.
- There can be enlarged lymph nodes, spleen, testicles, and liver.
- There can be headache, diplopia, cranial nerve palsy, papilledema, or mental changes.

Due to prolonged hospitalization:

- The client typically has loss of strength and endurance.
- Osteoporosis can develop secondary to bed rest.
- The client may have activity restriction secondary to nausea and vomiting.

TREATMENT/MANAGEMENT
- Adjust treatment to accommodate diagnosis, age, and course of treatment for cancer. The client may be undergoing chemotherapy or radiation treatment that can affect physical therapy treatment.
- Provide preventive care to counteract problems triggered by prolonged hospitalization.
- Educate the client about an exercise program of active exercise and walking.
- For clients with neuropathies, consider splinting, stretching exercise, and orthosis such as ankle or foot to prevent contractures and maintain function.

PHYSICAL THERAPY TREATMENT IN CONJUNCTION WITH BONE MARROW TRANSPLANTATION (BMT)
- Provide comprehensive exercise program. Include upper extremity, weight bearing, back extension, ambulation, and proximal musculature strengthening.
- Add ROM, balance, strengthening, endurance, and progressive ambulation activities as indicated.

PRECAUTIONS/CONTRAINDICATIONS

IN CONJUNCTION WITH CHEMOTHERAPY
- Side effects of chemotherapy can include lowered blood counts, nausea, vomiting, loss of hair, adult respiratory distress syndrome, cardiotoxic effects, peripheral neuropathies, proximal muscle weakness, aseptic necrosis of hips or shoulder joint, joint pain, neuropsychologic effects, and encephalopathy.
- Monitor vital signs closely during exercise and activity.
- Low white cell count can mean that the client is at an increased risk for infection.
- Low platelet count may place the client at increased risk for bleeding and may contraindicate resistive exercise.
- Clients with low blood volume may be able to tolerate only gentle bedside exercise.

IN CONJUNCTION WITH BMT
- BMT may lead to the side effects of impaired renal, cardiovascular, or neuromuscular function, increased risk for lung infection, hepatic veno-occlusive disease, mucositis, and graft-versus-host disease (GVHD).
- The treatment of GVHD with the use of steroids in high doses increases risk of aseptic necrosis, osteoporosis, and steroid myopathies.

GENERAL HEMATOLOGIC GUIDELINES
- Avoid resistive exercise when platelet counts are below 50,000/mm3.
- Avoid all activity when platelet counts are below 20,000/mm3 or hematocrit is below 25%, hemoglobin is below 8 mg/dl, or white blood cells are below 500/mm3.
- Exercise should be mild when hemoglobin is as low as 8 to 10 mg/dl.
- Other factors that affect tolerance to activity include dialysis, intubation, prolonged bed rest, and presence of any intracranial bleeding.

DESIRED OUTCOME/PROGNOSIS
- Neuropathies secondary to chemotherapy usually resolve spontaneously after 1 to 2 years with support provided by treatment mentioned earlier.

REFERENCES

Assessment

American Physical Therapy Association. Guide to physical therapist practice. 2nd ed. *Phys Ther.* 2001;81.

Gerber L, Lampert M, Wood C, et al. Comparison of pain, motion, and edema after modified radical mastectomy vs local excision with axillary dissection and radiation. *Breast Cancer Res Treatment.* 1992;21:139–145.

Pfalzer LA. Oncology: examination, diagnosis, and treatment. Medical and surgical considerations. In: Myers RS, ed. *Saunders Manual of Physical Therapy Practice.* Philadelphia, Pa: WB Saunders Co; 1995:65–147.

Pfalzer LA. Oncology: examination, diagnosis, and treatment. Physical therapy considerations. In: Myers RS, ed. *Saunders Manual of Physical Therapy Practice.* Philadelphia, Pa: WB Saunders Co; 1995:149–190.

Yoshioka H. Rehabilitation for the terminal cancer patient. *Am J Phys Med Rehabil.* 1994;73: 199–206.

Treatment

Body JJ, Lossignol D, Ronson A. The concept of rehabilitation of cancer patients. *Curr Opinions Oncol.* 1997;9:332–340.

Croarkin E. Osteopenia in the patient with cancer. *Phys Ther.* 1999;79:196–201.

Dean JT, Davidson G. Trismus after radiation therapy. *Clin Manage Phys Ther.* 1992;12: 4:70–76.

Friedenreich CM, Curneya KS. Exercise as rehabilitation for cancer patients. *Clin J Sports Med.* 1996;6:237–244.

Frymark SL. Taking control. Cancer rehabilitation allows patients to increase the quality of their lives and reclaim independence. *Rehabil Manage.* 1998;11:80–86.

Grabois M, Garrison SJ, Hart KA, Lehmkuhl LD. *Physical Medicine and Rehabilitation: The Complete Approach.* Malden, Mass: Blackwell Science; 2000.

Gudas SA. Directives in cancer rehabilitation. *Clin Manage Phys Ther.* 1992;12:4:32–36.

Hamburgh RR. Principles of cancer treatment. *Clin Manage Phys Ther.* 1992;12:4:37–41.

Hock K. Ambulatory oncology program. *Clin Manage Phys Ther.* 1992;12:4:87–91.

Marcant D, Rapin CH. Role of the physiotherapist in palliative care. *J Pain Symptom Manage.* 1993;8:2:68–71.

Michael TH. Do physiotherapists have a role in palliative care? *Physiotherapy Res Int.* 2001;6:v–vi.

Peabody TD, Gibbs CP, Simon MA. Evaluation and staging of musculoskeletal neoplasms. *J Bone Joint Surg Am.* 1998;80:1204–1218.

Pfalzer L. Physical agents and the patient with cancer. *Clin Manage Phys Ther.* 1992; 12:4:83–86.

Pfalzer L, Walter J. Facts and fiction: cancer in the 1990's. *Clin Manage Phys Ther.* 1992; 12:4:26–31.

Phillips LL. Managing the pain of bone metastases in the home environment. *Am J Hospice Palliative Care.* 1998;8:32–42.

Rashleigh L. Physiotherapy and palliative oncology. *Aust J Physiotherapy.* 1996;42:307–312.

Sabers SR, Kokal JE, Girardi JC, et al. Evaluation of consultation-based rehabilitation for hospitalized cancer patients with functional impairment. *Mayo Clin Proc.* 1999;74:855–861.

Sayre RS, Marcoux BC. Exercise and autologous bone marrow transplants. *Clin Manage Phys Ther.* 1992;12:4:78–82.

Sicard-Rosenbaum L, Danoff J. Cancer and ultrasound: a warning letter. *Phys Ther.* 1993; 73:404–406.

Sliwa JA, Marciniak C. Physical rehabilitation of the cancer patient. *Cancer Treatment Res.* 1999; 100:75–89.

Smith WB, Gracely RH, Safer MA. The meaning of pain: cancer patients' rating and recall of pain intensity and affect. *Pain.* 1998;78:123–129.

Snyder R. Coping: you and your patient with cancer. *Clin Manage Phys Ther.* 1992;12:4: 64–69.

Snyder R. Physical therapy in terminal illness. *Clin Manage Phys Ther.* 1992;12:4:96–100.

Tool JL. Physical therapy in the care of patients with a diagnosis of cancer. *Clin Manage Phys Ther.* 1992;12:4:96–100.

Watchie J. Cardiopulmonary complications of cancer. *Clin Manage Phys Ther.* 1992;12:4: 92–95.

Yoshioka H. Rehabilitation for the terminal cancer patient. *Am J Phys Med Rehabil.* 1994; 73:199–206.

Zoerink-Baker M. The adult leukemias and physical therapy considerations. *Rehabil Oncol.* 1998;16:19–21.

Lung Cancer

DESCRIPTION

Cancer is a *cellular malignancy* characterized by the loss of the usual controls. This allows unrestricted cellular proliferation that can invade normal tissues as well as metastasize to other sites. If left untreated, this uncontrolled spread of abnormal cells can lead to death.

Lung cancer usually begins in the epithelium of the bronchial and bronchioalveolar surfaces as well as in the bronchial mucous glands. Lung cancer is the most common cause of death from cancer.

CAUSE

The main cause of lung cancer is cigarette smoking. Other factors include exposure to chemicals such as chromium, arsenic, and nickel, as well as to compounds such as asbestos dust, chloromethyl ethers, and vinyl chloride.

ASSESSMENT

Note: See APTA's Guide to Physical Therapist Practice. 2nd ed. *Physical Therapy.* 2001;81.

Cardiopulmonary Preferred Practice Patterns: A, B

AREAS

A client tolerance assessment should be performed preoperatively.

- History
- Psychosocial, including family and social support, employment history, and history of exposure to carcinogenic agents

- Pain
- Posture
- Strength, including trunk and abdominal musculature
- Mobility, including active range of motion (ROM)
- Functional level
- Pulmonary, including rate, rhythm, and pattern of respiration; chest mobility; structure of thorax; degree of dyspnea, cough productivity and effectiveness; type and amount of sputum; breath sounds
- Cardiovascular, including endurance

INSTRUMENTS/PROCEDURES

See References for sources.

Functional Level
- Katz Index of ADLs
- Barthel ADL index
- Functional Independence Measure

Physical Performance Status Scales

- American Joint Committee on Cancer Performance Status Scale
- Eastern Cooperative Oncology Group Performance Status Scale
- Karnofsky Performance Status Scale
- World Health Organization Performance Status Scale

Pain
- finger dynameter
- pain intensity number scale
- visual analog scale

Special Tests to Which the Physical Therapist May or May Not Have Access
- arterial blood gases
- blood chemistry
- bone scan
- computed tomography (CT) scan
- electrocardiogram
- magnetic resonance imaging (MRI)
- mediastinoscopy
- pulmonary function test
- x-rays

PROBLEMS

Problems associated with the postsurgical client are as follows:
- The client often has an ineffective and unproductive cough.
- The client typically has a decreased chest expansion.
- The client often has a poor breathing ratio.
- The client may have decreased trunk mobility.
- There may be a decreased tolerance for ambulation.

TREATMENT/MANAGEMENT

Physical therapy intervention in the client with lung cancer usually relates to recovery from surgery, although the client may also undergo chemotherapy and/or radiation therapy.

PREOPERATIVE INSTRUCTION
- Instruct the client in manual assistive and independent coughing techniques to be performed every 30 minutes and with every position change (ideally 20 minutes post change). Teach independent coughing, utilizing huffing techniques.
- Teach proper breathing techniques, including diaphragmatic, pursed-lip, and segmental breathing techniques. Instruct in active and isometric lower extremity exercises and postural considerations.

POSTOPERATIVE EXERCISE PROGRAM

- The breathing exercise program begins post extubation with diaphragmatic, pursed-lip, and segmental patterns. Begin in supine position, and progress to sitting and then standing as tolerated by the client. Encourage maximal chest expansion. May need to use transcutaneous electrical nerve stimulation (TENS) for analgesia.
- Progressive ambulation may begin on day 2 with assistance as needed.
- Begin trunk mobility exercises after chest tubes are removed. Include flexion, extension, lateral flexion, and rotation exercises.
- Stress continued awareness of posture.
- Continue emphasis on chest expansion, trunk mobility, and endurance for ambulation. Address the need for pain management, as indicated.
- Follow progression of exercise program, including a home self-care program.
- Pain management may include the use of modalities.

PRECAUTIONS/CONTRAINDICATIONS

- Coughing with knees and hips flexed can help avoid overstressing abdominal musculature.
- Generally, exercise can be unrestricted if platelet counts are above 30,000 to 50,000.
- Non-resistive activities can be considered if platelet counts are above 10,000 to 20,000.
- Usually, active therapy is contraindicated if platelet counts are below 10,000.
- Exercise is also contraindicated with fever above 104 degrees F.
- Exercise usually includes ROM, aerobic activity, light resistive with 2–4 pounds and deep breathing.
- Clients with hepatic veno-occlusive disease should avoid supine exercise or abdominal exercise.
- Take precautions with graft versus hose disease.
- Cardiotoxic agents can affect physical performance.
- If exercise creates extreme fatigue it was likely too intense.

DESIRED OUTCOME/PROGNOSIS

- The client will demonstrate an effective and productive cough.
- The client will resume preoperative chest expansion in the proportion appropriate to the amount of lung resection.
- The client will demonstrate appropriate breathing pattern and ratio.
- The client will resume preoperative level of trunk mobility.
- The client will tolerate ambulation of at least 1,000 feet with no dyspnea.
- The client will be able to manage pain.

REFERENCES

Assessment

American Physical Therapy Association. Guide to physical therapist practice. 2nd ed. *Phys Ther.* 2001;81.

Pfalzer LA. Oncology: examination, diagnosis, and treatment. Medical and surgical considerations. In: Myers RS, ed. *Saunders Manual of Physical Therapy Practice.* Philadelphia, Pa: WB Saunders Co; 1995:65–147.

Pfalzer LA. Oncology: examination, diagnosis, and treatment. Physical therapy considerations. In: Myers RS, ed. *Saunders Manual of Physical Therapy Practice.* Philadelphia, Pa: WB Saunders Co; 1995:149–190.

Yoshioka H. Rehabilitation for the terminal cancer patient. *Am J Phys Med Rehabil.* 1994;73:199–206.

Treatment

Anonymous. Like a breath of fresh air. *Physiotherapy Frontline.* 1999;5:18.

Body JJ, Lossignol D, Ronson A. The concept of rehabilitation of cancer patients. *Curr Opinions Oncol.* 1997;9:332–340.

Croarkin E. Osteopenia in the patient with cancer. *Phys Ther.* 1999;79:196–201.

Dean JT, Davidson G. Trismus after radiation therapy. *Clin Manage Phys Ther.* 1992; 12:4:70–76.

Friedenreich CM, Curneya KS. Exercise as rehabilitation for cancer patients. *Clin J Sports Med.* 1996;6:237–244.

Frymark SL. Taking control. Cancer rehabilitation allows patients to increase the quality of their lives and reclaim independence. *Rehabil Manage.* 1998;11:80–86.

Gudas SA. Directives in cancer rehabilitation. *Clin Manage Phys Ther.* 1992;12:4:32–36.

Grabois M, Garrison SJ, Hart KA, Lehmkuhl LD. *Physical Medicine and Rehabilitation: The Complete Approach.* Malden, Mass: Blackwell Science; 2000.

Hamburgh RR. Principles of cancer treatment. *Clin Manage Phys Ther.* 1992;12:4:37–41.

Hock K. Ambulatory oncology program. *Clin Manage Phys Ther.* 1992;12:4:87–91.

Liu S, Tunkel R, Lachmann E, et al. Paraneoplastic cerebellar degeneration as the first evidence of cancer: a case report. *Arch Phys Med.*

Marcant D, Rapin CH. Role of the physiotherapist in palliative care. *J Pain Symptom Manage.* 1993;8:2:68–71.

Michael TH. Do physiotherapists have a role in palliative care? *Physiotherapy Res Int.* 2001;6:v–vi.

Peabody TD, Gibbs CP, Simon MA. Evaluation and staging of musculoskeletal neoplasms. *J Bone Joint Surg Am.* 1998;80:1204–1218.

Pfalzer L. Physical agents and the patient with cancer. *Clin Manage Phys Ther.* 1992; 12:4:83–86.

Pfalzer L, Walter J. Facts and fiction: cancer in the 1990's. *Clin Manage Phys Ther.* 1992; 12:4:26–31.

Phillips LL. Managing the pain of bone metastases in the home environment. *Am J Hospice Palliative Care.* 1998;8:32–42.

Rashleigh L. Physiotherapy and palliative oncology. *Aust J Physiotherapy.* 1996;42:307–312.

Sabers SR, Kokal JE, Girardi JC, et al. Evaluation of consultation-based rehabilitation for hospitalized cancer patients with functional impairment. *Mayo Clin Proc.* 1999;74:855–861.

Sicard-Rosenbaum L, Danoff J. Cancer and ultrasound: a warning letter. *Phys Ther.* 1993;73:404–406.

Sliwa JA, Marciniak C. Physical rehabilitation of the cancer patient. *Cancer Treatment Res.* 1999;100:75–89.

Smith WB, Gracely RH, Safer MA. The meaning of pain: cancer patients' rating and recall of pain intensity and affect. *Pain.* 1998;78:123–129.

Snyder R. Coping: you and your patient with cancer. *Clin Manage Phys Ther.* 1992;12:4:64–69.

Snyder R. Physical therapy in terminal illness. *Clin Manage Phys Ther.* 1992;12:4:96–100.

Tool JL. Physical therapy in the care of patients with a diagnosis of cancer. *Clin Manage Phys Ther*. 1992;12:4:96–100.

Watchie J. Cardiopulmonary complications of cancer. *Clin Manage Phys Ther*. 1992; 12:4:92–95.

Yoshioka H. Rehabilitation for the terminal cancer patient. *Am J Phys Med Rehabil*. 1994; 73:199–206.

Soft Tissue Sarcoma

DESCRIPTION

Cancer is a *cellular malignancy* characterized by the loss of the usual controls. This allows unrestricted cellular proliferation that can invade normal tissues as well as metastasize to other sites.

Soft tissue sarcoma is a malignant tumor that begins in the soft connective tissue area. There are 30 types of sarcomas. These are usually named after the cell of origin, such as *liposarcoma,* arising from adipose tissue. The types of soft tissue sarcomas include *fibrosarcomas, malignant fibrous histiocytomas, synovial sarcomas, rhabdomyosarcomas, liposarcomas,* and *leiomyosarcomas.*

CAUSE

Risk factors for soft tissue sarcoma include exposure to phenoxyacetic acids, vinyl chloride, and high doses of radiation; rare genetic defects; certain inherited diseases, such as von Rechlinghausen's disease; and a retrovirus in the case of Kaposi's sarcoma.

ASSESSMENT

Note: See APTA's Guide to Physical Therapist Practice. 2nd ed. *Physical Therapy.* 2001;81.

Musculoskeletal Preferred Practice Patterns: D, I

Integumentary Preferred Practice Pattern: A

AREAS

- History
- Psychosocial
- Pain
- Posture
- Cardiopulmonary, including endurance
- Musculoskeletal, including joint integrity
- Strength
- Mobility, including active range of motion (ROM)
- Neurological
- Genitourinary
- Skin, including color, edema, and open wounds
- Functional level: including activities of daily living (ADLs)

INSTRUMENTS/PROCEDURES

See References for sources.

Functional Level
- Katz Index of ADLs
- Barthel ADL index
- Functional Independence Measure

Physical Performance Status Scales

- American Joint Committee on Cancer Performance Status Scale
- Eastern Cooperative Oncology Group Performance Status Scale
- Karnofsky Performance Status Scale
- World Health Organization Performance Status Scale

Pain

- finger dynameter
- pain intensity number scale
- visual analog scale

Special Tests to Which the Physical Therapist May or May Not Have Access

- urinalysis and stool guaiac
- radiograph, magnetic resonance imaging (MRI) or computed tomography scan (CT)
- bone scan
- sputum cytology
- colonoscopy
- sigmoidoscopy
- bronchoscopy

PROBLEMS

PROBLEMS RELATED TO SIDE EFFECTS OF CANCER MEDICAL TREATMENT PROTOCOLS

- The client may have nausea, vomiting, alopecia, cardiomyopathy, peripheral neuropathy (mixed sensorimotor), mucositis, myelosuppression, delayed healing, decreased endurance, amenorrhea, and sexual dysfunction.

COMPLICATIONS DUE TO PREOPERATIVE RADIATION

- There may be a predisposition to fracture of long bones due to devascularization and delayed healing.
- Often, there are radiation reactions of dermatitis or erythema. There may be fibrosis of connective tissue, leading to joint contracture.
- The client may have edema, pain, and decreased function due to bone necrosis, endarteritis, and decreased elasticity of lymphatic channels. The client may have edema in the lower extremities.
- If the glenoid complex is intact, the upper extremity is likely normal. Glenoid removal leads to decreased arm ROM, especially beyond 90 degrees.
- Usually there is pain and fatigue.

PROBLEMS POST BUTTOCK RESECTION

- Client may complain of pain at the incision site.
- The client may have difficulty climbing stairs.
- The client may have altered sexual function.
- The client may have altered bowel habits.
- The client historically has an altered body image.

PROBLEM IN SOFT TISSUE SARCOMA OF THE THIGH

- The client may develop pain.
- The client may have joint dysfunction.
- The client may have drainage at the site of excision.
- The client may develop chronic lymphedema.
- The client may have altered sexual function.

PROBLEMS POST MEDIAL EXCISION

- The client often has pain.
- The client may have edema.

- There may be excision of the hamstring muscle.
- The client may have stiffness after prolonged sitting.

TREATMENT/MANAGEMENT
- Provide whirlpool/debridement for burns or open wound.
- Encourage an active exercise program.

FOR LIMB-SPARING TREATMENT
- Rehabilitation should begin at diagnosis and continue for life.
- Make assistive devices available, such as over-the-bed trapezes for bed mobility, seating cushioning, and grab bars for safety.
- Consider transcutaneous electrical nerve stimulation (TENS) for pain.
- Instruct the client in use of support hose for lower extremity edema.

POST BUTTOCK RESECTION
- Strengthen remaining hip musculature.
- Supply seat cushion or other assistive devices.
- Consider a prosthetic buttock device.

INTERNAL HEMIPELVECTOMY
- Provide shoe lifts immediately after bed rest restrictions are removed (often not for 3–6 weeks post surgery).
- Provide gait training using partial weight bearing with crutches. The client may be on crutches for 6 months or until sufficient bone union occurs.
- Exercise distal musculature and upper extremities with active exercise.

SOFT TISSUE SARCOMA OF THE THIGH
- The client stays in bed with a knee immobilizer until more activity is allowed. Ankle motion can be performed at this time.
- When ambulation has been approved, begin with partial weight bearing with splint. Consider use of ankle-foot orthosis at about 2 weeks postsurgery.
- As drainage diminishes and drainage tubing is removed, therapy can become more aggressive, with ambulation and exercise.
- Apply splint to knee and foot as needed to protect the wound.

SARCOMA OF THE MEDIAL THIGH, RESULTING IN EXCISION OF THE ADDUCTOR MUSCLES
- Activities are typically minimal.
- Support stockings are indicated for upright activities.
- Instruct the client in proper care of skin and positioning to diminish edema and precautions to prevent injury leading to infection.

PRECAUTIONS/CONTRAINDICATIONS

If ambulation occurs without the brace (after removal of the quadriceps muscle), the joint may hyperextend the knee, and there may be a subsequent increase in lumbar lordosis, with an increased risk of falling, loss of balance, and back pain.

- Generally, exercise may be unrestricted if platelet counts are above 30,000 to 50,000.
- Nonresistive activities can be considered if platelet counts are above 10,000 to 20,000.
- Usually, active therapy is contraindicated if platelet counts are below 10,000.
- Exercise is also contraindicated with fever above 104 degrees F.
- Exercise usually includes ROM, aerobic activity, light resistive with 2–4 pounds and deep breathing.

- Clients with hepatic veno-occlusive disease should avoid supine exercise or abdominal exercise.
- Take precautions with graft versus hose disease.
- Cardiotoxic agents can affect physical performance.
- If exercise creates extreme fatigue it was likely too intense.

DESIRED OUTCOME/PROGNOSIS
- The client will experience a reduction in pain.
- The client will control edema formation.
- The client will prevent infection.
- The client will achieve a maximum level of function.

Notes: Change can occur up to 6 months after cancer treatment. Most of the side effects are reversible over time. Active stretching may reverse muscle fibrosis. Chronic changes may be irreversible.

REFERENCES

Assessment

American Physical Therapy Association. Guide to physical therapist practice. 2nd ed. *Phys Ther.* 2001;81.

Pfalzer LA. Oncology: examination, diagnosis, and treatment. Medical and surgical considerations. In: Myers RS, ed. *Saunders Manual of Physical Therapy Practice.* Philadelphia, Pa: WB Saunders Co; 1995:65–147.

Pfalzer LA. Oncology: examination, diagnosis, and treatment. Physical therapy considerations. In: Myers RS, ed. *Saunders Manual of Physical Therapy Practice.* Philadelphia, Pa: WB Saunders Co; 1995:149–190.

Yoshioka H. Rehabilitation for the terminal cancer patient. *Am J Phys Med Rehabil.* 1994; 73:199–206.

Treatment

Agency for Health Care Policy and Research. *Management of cancer pain guideline panel. Management of cancer pain. Clinical practice guideline no. 9.* U.S. Department of Health and Human Services. AHCPR Pub. No. 94–0592, 1994:75–88.

Body JJ, Lossignol D, Ronson A. The concept of rehabilitation of cancer patients. *Curr Opinions Oncol.* 1997;9:332–340.

Croarkin E. Osteopenia in the patient with cancer. *Phys Ther.* 1999;79:196–201.

Dean JT, Davidson G. Trismus after radiation therapy. *Clin Manage Phys Ther.* 1992;12: 4:70–76.

Delisa JA, Miller RM, Melnick RR, et al. Rehabilitation of the cancer patient. In: Friedenreich CM, Curneya KS. Exercise as rehabilitation for cancer patients. *Clin J Sports Med.* 1996;6:237–244.

Frymark SL. Taking control. Cancer rehabilitation allows patients to increase the quality of their lives and reclaim independence. *Rehabil Manage.* 1998;11:80–86.

Gerber LH. Rehabilitation management for women with breast cancer: maximizing functional outcomes. In: Harris JR, Lippman MG, Morrow M, et al, eds. *Disease of the Breast.* Philadelphia, Pa: Lippincott-Raven, 1996;939–947.

Grabois M, Garrison SJ, Hart KA, Lehmkuhl LD. *Physical Medicine and Rehabilitation: The Complete Approach.* Malden, Mass: Blackwell Science; 2000.

Gudas SA. Directives in cancer rehabilitation. *Clin Manage Phys Ther.* 1992;12:4:32–36.

Hamburgh RR. Principles of cancer treatment. *Clin Manage Phys Ther.* 1992;12:4:37–41.

Hock K. Ambulatory oncology program. *Clin Manage Phys Ther.* 1992;12:4:87–91.

Marcant D, Rapin CH. Role of the physiotherapist in palliative care. *J Pain Symptom Manage.* 1993;8:2:68–71.

Peabody TD, Gibbs CP, Simon MA. Evaluation and staging of musculoskeletal neoplasms. *J Bone Joint Surg Am.* 1998;80:1204–1218.

Pfalzer L. Physical agents and the patient with cancer. *Clin Manage Phys Ther.* 1992; 12:4:83–86.

Pfalzer L, Walter J. Facts and fiction: cancer in the 1990's. *Clin Manage Phys Ther.* 1992; 12:4:26–31.

Phillips LL. Managing the pain of bone metastases in the home environment. *Am J Hospice Palliative Care.* 1998;8:32–42.

Rashleigh L. Physiotherapy and palliative oncology. *Aust J Physiotherapy* 1996;42:307–312.

Sabers SR, Kokal JE, Girardi JC, et al. Evaluation of consultation-based rehabilitation for hospitalized cancer patients with functional impairment. *Mayo Clin Proc.* 1999;74:855–861.

Sicard-Rosenbaum L, Danoff J. Cancer and ultrasound: a warning letter. *Phys Ther.* 1993; 73:404–406.

Sliwa JA, Marciniak C. Physical rehabilitation of the cancer patient. *Cancer Treatment Res.* 1999;100:75–89.

Smith WB, Gracely RH, Safer MA. The meaning of pain: cancer patients' rating and recall of pain intensity and affect. *Pain.* 1998;78:123–129.

Snyder R. Coping: you and your patient with cancer. *Clin Manage Phys Ther.* 1992;12:4:64–69.

Snyder R. Physical therapy in terminal illness. *Clin Manage Phys Ther.* 1992;12:4:96–100.

Tool JL. Physical therapy in the care of patients with a diagnosis of cancer. *Clin Manage Phys Ther.* 1992;12:4:96–100.

Watchie J. Cardiopulmonary complications of cancer. *Clin Manage Phys Ther.* 1992;12:4:92–95.

Yoshioka H. Rehabilitation for the terminal cancer patient. *Am J Phys Med Rehabil.* 1994; 73:199–206.

Chapter 12
Pediatric Disorders

Arthrogryposis Multiplex Congenita

Also known as *multiple congenital contractures.*

ICD-9-CM Code: 754.89 Other specified nonteratogenic anomalies, Other
APTA Guide Patterns: 4B, 4D

DESCRIPTION

A syndrome complex characterized by multiple joint contractures (especially of the upper limbs and neck) without other serious congenital abnormalities and with relative normal intelligence. Arthrogryposis is prenatal fixation of joints in a flexed (ie, contracted) position (Beers & Berkow, 1999, p. 2221). Various forms of arthrogryposis include amyoplasia (43%, the "classic arthrogryposis"); a contracture syndrome (35%); distal arthrogryposis (7%); a neuromuscular syndrome (7%); congenital anomalies (6%); and chromosomal abnormalities (2%) (Donohoe & Bleakney, 2000, p. 303). Characteristic features include featureless extremities that are often cylindrical in shape with absent skin creases; rigid joint with significant contractures; dislocation of joint, especially the hips; atrophy or absence of muscle groups; and intact sensation, although deep tendon reflexes may be diminished or absent (Stanger, 1999, p. 401). Body parts affected in order of prevalence are foot (67%), hip (50%), wrist (43%), knee (41%), elbow (30%), and shoulder (4%) (Donohoe & Bleakney, 2000, p. 303). The disorder is nonprogressive but the long-term sequelae can be very disabling especially in the areas of mobility and activities of daily living (ADLs).

CAUSE

Joint development occurs in the second month of gestation, and disorders that impair in utero movement (eg, uterine malformation, multiple gestations, oligohydramnios) can result in arthrogryposis. Arthrogryposis multiplex congenita (AMC), anterior horn cell disease, and maternal myasthenia gravis have been proposed as causes of the associated amyoplasia. AMC is not genetic, although genetic disorders such as trisomy 18 and spina bifida have an increased incidence of arthrogryposis (Beers & Berkow, 1999, p. 2221). Distal arthrogryposis is inherited as an autosomal dominant trait; Type 1 maps to chromosome 9. The source of neuropathic arthrogryposis is found on chromosome 5. Possible causes for other types may include hyperthermia during the first trimester, prenatal viral infection, and vascular compromise (Donohoe & Bleakney, 2000, p. 303). Incidence is 1 in 3,000 births but may be higher in North, Central, and South America and in Europe.

ASSESSMENT

AREAS
- Range of motion (ROM)
- Muscle strength
- Developmental motor milestones: rolling, prone tolerance, sitting control, scooting, creeping, crawling, transitional movements, standing tolerance, and upright mobility
- Need for assistive or supportive devices

INSTRUMENTS/PROCEDURES
- Goniometry
- For muscle strength use observation of movement and palpation of muscle contractions
- Alberta Infant Motor Scale (AIMS) (Piper & Darrah, 1994)
- Bayley Scales of Infant Development–II (BSID–II) (Bayley, 1993)

- Peabody Developmental Motor Scales–2nd Edition (PDMS–2) (Folio & Fewell, 1999)
- Pediatric Evaluation of Disability Inventory (PEDI) (Haley et al, 1992)

PROBLEMS

- Contractures are typically symmetrical.
- Two types of resting posture abnormalities. In one, the child has flexed and dislocated hips, extended knees, clubfeet (equinovarous), internally rotated shoulders, flexed elbows, and flexed and ulnarly deviated wrists. In the other type, the child has abducted and externally rotated hips, flexed knees, clubfeet, internally rotated shoulders, extended elbows, and flexed and ulnarly deviated wrists. In the first type parents may refer to the legs as "jackknifed" and in the second as "frog-like." Hand position in second type may be described as "waiter's tip" position.
- Movement in the joints is "wooden" or "marionette-like."
- Muscle strength imbalance of oppositional muscles: stronger muscles are often shortened.
- Limited functional mobility skills: rolling, creeping, transitional movements, and transfers.
- Decreased endurance.
- Ambulation speed may be slower than peers.
- Motor milestones may be delayed or skipped.
- May have fine motor difficulty which interfere with writing speed and formation of letters.
- May have scoliosis.
- May have respiratory problems.
- May have abdominal hernias.
- May have congenital heart disease.
- May have dimpling of skin over joints.
- May have absent or decreased finger creases.

TREATMENT/MANAGEMENT

A team approach that includes the family or caregivers is recommended.

INFANT

- Improve positioning by placing infant in as normal alignment as possible beginning shortly after birth. A wide Velcro band strap around the thighs will keep the legs in a more neutral alignment. Knee splints and AFOs using molded thermoplastics can facilitate positioning the leg, ankle, and foot. Cock-up wrist splints can be used for hand: a dorsal cock-up with palmar arch in neutral position and slight stretch into wrist extension for day and a dorsal cock-up with a pan to allow finger stretching at night. Elbow splints may also require 2 types: flexion for day to facilitate feeding and extension at night. Neck and trunk supports may be to maintain the head and trunk in a better position. Foam wedges or rolls can be used to position in supine, prone, or sitting positions. Standing frame can be used for an upright posture.
- Improve range of motion shortly after birth using passive range of motion or stretching exercises of all joints exhibiting limitation. Stretching should be done gently and held at the end range for only a few repetitions rather than many quick repetitions. Stretching should be done 2 or 3 times daily. Combine stretching exercises with other activities such as diaper changes, changing clothes, and bathing.
- Consider using a splint or cast to maintain the stretch and range of motion. Splints offer the advantage of being removable for bathing and active exercise, but casting ensures a more prolonged stretch with forces distributed over a wider area. (Graubert, Chaplin, & Jaffe, 1998, p. 89)

- Consider use of serial casting for foot deformities, knee flexion contracture, and wrist flexion contractures. Splints are more often used for hands and wrist.
- Maintain surgical correction of contractures by splinting, using strengthening exercises, and active function movement.
- Maximize strength through play activities.
- Upper extremity intervention should have the goal of optimum function and independence with self-care skills that include flexion and extension of the elbows. If flexion and extension are not possible then one elbow should be flexed for feeding activities and the other extended for reaching and toileting activities.
- Facilitate development of mobility skills. Rolling may be difficult to accomplish due to lower extremity contractures. Some children may learn to scoot on the belly or back first. Sitting is possible but getting to the sitting position may be difficult. After sitting is achieved, floor mobility should be encouraged. Creeping on hands and knees may be difficult and scooting on the bottom may be preferred. Pulling to standing may be limited by lower extremity contractures.
- Enhance general sensorimotor development. Gross motor skills should be monitored closely to determine if they are progressing normally. Watch for the development of head and trunk control. If these do not develop, facilitate by positioning. Also watch for compensatory movement such as scooting in supine position because of weak flexors. Recommend infant be placed in prone position frequently during the day to increase flexor strength. For additional suggestions see Graubert, Chaplin, & Jaffe (1998) in References.
- Preambulation activities should begin before 1 year of age if the child is developmentally ready.
- Educate family and caregivers in proper handling and positioning, stretching techniques, and avoidance of harmful activities so they are comfortable and knowledgeable about the infant.
- Check out carrier and carseat to determine what supportive material is needed. A foam seat insert should be considered for better positioning during transportation.

TODDLER
- Facilitate development of maximum level of independence with mobility and self-care skills. Assistive and orthotic devices are often needed. Safety devices such as grab bars may also be needed. Position is important, especially for upper extremity activities where lack of elbow and shoulder flexion and wrist extension are present.
- Ambulation should be encouraged until proven impossible or impractical. Ankle splints (AFOs), long leg splints (KAFOs), and adapted walkers may be useful.
- Upper extremity skills should focus on feeding and dressing activities. Overhead supports for arms, built-up handles, universal cuff, dressing frame, and adapted clothing may be useful.
- Maintain acquired ROM and continue to increase ROM, if possible. For lower extremity, continue stretching exercises and splints at night. Add standing frame time to daily routine. For upper extremity, use static splints at night and dynamic during the day. Work with the occupational therapist.
- Strengthening exercise should be accomplished through age-appropriate activities when possible. For lower extremities, knee standing may be useful before standing. If knees do not flex to 90 degrees use a wedge. For upper extremities therapy, putting krinkle blocks and magnet blocks together may be useful. An adapted writing device may be needed to facilitate coloring, painting, and drawing activities. Swimming is a useful recreational activity. Adapted bicycles may be helpful.

SCHOOL AGE
- Consider use of adaptive and rehabilitation equipment to compensate for difficulties such as speed of ambulation or fine motor problems.

- Facilitate independence in the school setting and interaction with peers. Ambulation may be assisted with a rolling walker or the addition of a manual or powered chair for longer distances. Computer access can facilitate completion of assignments. A mouth stick may be needed to use the keyboard or a word prediction program may be preferred. Work with the occupational therapist or assistive technology specialist.
- Continue ROM exercises and splinting.
- Continue to encourage muscle strengthening through play and recreational activities.
- Continue to facilitate performance of ADLs through use of assistive devices.
- Home modification for better accessibility may be considered. Ramps at entrances, rails on stairs, and changes in floor coverings are examples.

TEENAGE YEARS

- Teenagers should be given as much responsibility for their actions and decisions as they are able to manage. Their interests and concerns should be considered and respected. Generally, a teenager will not have a regular program of physical therapy but will be seen periodically for updates.
- A self-stretching program should be learned. Splints are generally not used to maintain ROM but may be used to improve function such as walking.
- Encourage strengthening through participation in swimming, bicycling, and walking.
- Encourage good health habits, especially eating a well-balanced diet to avoid excess weight, which may decrease independence in transfers and walking.
- Encourage independence in self care and ADLs. Stress safety in performing activities around the house, at school, and in the community.
- Facilitate ordering of any special equipment that may be needed for ambulation.
- Assist in evaluating access to community resources including use of public transportation and driving.

GENERAL

- Increase passive ROM through positioning, casting, and splinting.
- Improve functional-active ROM by use of vigorous stretching activities.
- Maintain ROM with splints.
- Increase strength to achieve functional skill.
- Increase muscle strength to provide for transition and mobility skills.
- Prevent contractures through vigorous stretching activities.
- Promote attainment of developmental motor milestones.
- Recommend or provide adapted or rehabilitation equipment.
- Encourage attainment of ability to participate in inclusive activities at home, school, and in the community through use of developmentally appropriate games and activities.
- Provide education to the family or caregiver.

PRECAUTIONS/CONTRAINDICATIONS

- Small children do not generally tolerate vigorous stretching exercises well; it is counterproductive to stretch if the infant is upset or tense (Graubert, Chaplin, & Jaffe, 1998, p. 88).
- Stretching an infant with AMC can be emotionally exhausting to parents and caregivers because of their concern for "hurting" the child. Therapist needs to be sensitive to the concern and acknowledge it when it occurs.
- Gains made by vigorous stretching may not be maintained over time and surgery may be required to correct the contractures.

- Forceful aggressive stretching of a rigid joint can result in damage to the joint capsule and surrounding soft tissue.

DESIRED OUTCOME/PROGNOSIS
- Child has attained maximum functional range of motion and muscle strength.
- Child has mobility skills and is able to ambulate independently or with equipment.
- Child is able to perform self-care skills independently or with assistive devices.
- Child is able to attend school and participate in school activities.
- Child is able to interact with peers and participate in community activities.
- Child has been provided with adapted equipment and assistive devices as needed or appropriate.
- Child's family understands and is able to manage child's special needs for therapy, equipment, and devices, if needed.

REFERENCES

Axt MW, Niethard FU, Doderlein L, Weber M. Principles of treatment of the upper extremity in arthrogryposis multiplex congenita type I. *J Pediatr Orthop B*. 1997;3(6):179–185.

Beers MH, Berkow R, eds. *The Merck Manual of Diagnosis and Therapy*. Whitehouse Station, NJ: Merck Research Laboratories; 1999:2221–2222.

Donohoe M, Bleakney DA. Arthrogryposis multiplex congenita. In: Campbell SK, ed. *Phys Ther Child*. 2nd ed. Philadelphia, Pa: WB Saunders Co; 2000:302–319.

Graubert CS, Chaplin DL, Jaffe KM. Physical and occupational therapy. In Staheli LT, Hall JG, Jaffe KM, Paholke DO, eds. *Arthrogryposis: A Text Atlas*. Cambridge, Mass: Cambridge University Press; 1998;87–113.

Murray C, Fixsen JA. Management of knee deformity in classical arthrogryposis multiplex congenita (amyophasia congenita). *J Pediatr Orthop B*. 1997;6(3):186–191.

Ratliffe KT. Developmental orthopedic disorders—The child with arthrogryposis multiplex congenita. In: Ratliffe KT, ed. *Clinical Pediatric Physical Therapy: A Guide for the Physical Therapy Team*. St. Louis, Mo: CV Mosby Co; 1998;117–119.

Sala DA, Rosental DL, Grant AD. Clinical concerns. Early treatment of an infant with severe arthrogryposis. *Phys Occup Ther Pediatr*. 1996;16(3):73–89.

Stanger, M. Orthopedic management—arthrogryposis multiplex congenita. In: Tecklin JS, ed. *Pediatr Phys Ther*. 3rd ed. Philadelphia, Pa: Lippincott Williams and Wilkins; 1999: 401–403.

Asthma

ICD-9-CM Code: 493 Asthma.
APTA Guide Patterns: 6B, 6C, 6E, 6G, 6H, 6I

DESCRIPTION

A pulmonary disease characterized by reversible airway obstruction, airway inflammation, and increased airway responsiveness to a variety of stimuli (Beers & Berkow, 1999, p. 556). Asthma is the most common chronic respiratory illness in children and is the only treatable chronic condition in the Western world that is increasing in prevalence. (Ratliffe, 1998, p. 392)

TYPES OF TRIGGERS OR IRRITANTS

(Ratliffe, p. 392)

- Allergies: outcome allergens (pollen, molds); indoor allergens (house dust, feathers, molds, pets); foods (milk, soy, eggs)
- Emotions: emotional responses triggering deep breathing such as laughing, crying, yelling, anger, frustration, anxiety
- Exercise: Running and team sports
- Infections: Respiratory infection (bacterial and viral), colds, sinus infections
- Irritants: Cigarette smoke, air pollution, strong odors, aerosol sprays, paint fumes
- Weather: Cold air, weather allowing proliferation of molds or pollens

CAUSE

In the USA, about 12 million persons have asthma. From 1982 to 1992, the prevalence of asthma increased from 34.7 to 49.4 per 1000. The death rate increased 40% from 13.4 to 18.8 per million; it was 5 times higher for blacks than for whites. Asthma is the leading cause of hospitalization for children and the number one chronic condition causing school absenteeism (Beers & Berkow, 1999, p. 557). Prevalence is between 5% and 10% of all children. More boys than girls are affected. More children of black ethnicity are affected. Children in urban areas are more affected. More children living in the Western states are affected (Ratliffe, 1998, p. 393).

ASSESSMENT

AREAS

- Ability to speak
- Breath sounds
- Breathing patterns
- Heart rate
- Level of alertness
- Muscle strength
- Posture
- Psychological state
- Range of motion (ROM), especially the shoulder girdle
- Respiratory rate
- Skin color
- Thorax index
- Use of accessory muscles to breathe

INSTRUMENTS/PROCEDURES

- auscultation to locate where bronchial secretions have accumulated and if areas of the lungs are poorly ventilated
- flow meters
- forced vital capacity
- measurement of thorax made during inspiration and expiration
- peak expiratory flow rate (PEFR)
- posture grid
- spirometer

PROBLEMS

- Child is hypersensitive to irritants including infection; cold temperatures; differences in humidity; exercise; irritants such as tobacco, smoke, or pollution; and allergens.
- Child's muscles that control airway diameter contract, causing decreased airway diameter.
- The child's mucous membranes become inflamed and swell, causing a further decrease in airway diameter.
- Child's mucus production increases, causing blockages of some airway passages.
- Child experiences ventilation or perfusion inequality leading to arterial hypoxemia.

- Child may have more frequent coughing, frequent respiratory infections, coughing after exercise or crying, coughing at night, chest tightness, shortness of breath, irritability, or wheezing.
- Child may be absent from school more frequently than average.
- Child may be taken to the emergency room more frequently than average.
- Child may have more difficulty with academic skill acquisition due to absences.
- Child may be overprotected by parents.

TREATMENT/MANAGEMENT

Treatment usually involves a team approach including the physician, physical therapist, teachers, and family. Treatment involves four factors: avoidance of trigger factors, prophylactic medication, allergy injections, and a team approach.

- Educate parents to monitor pulmonary functions at home.
- Educate parents to prevent acute episodes through monitoring the environment, activities, and exercise in which the child participates.
- Instruct parents in drainage positions and manual techniques that can be used at home.
- Develop an exercise program to increase level of fitness: swimming is recommended since it is most likely to be tolerated.
- Assist child in learning to control exercise-inducted asthma and increase endurance. A controlled training program might include free running, treadmill running, bicycle ergometry, and swimming.
- Consider teaching the child breathing training combined with Jacobson's relaxation techniques such as deep diaphragmatic breathing to improve respiratory patterns. Initiate deep, slow breathing at a slow rate. A maximal effect can result in decreased airway function.
- Use relaxation techniques to reduce anxiety and physical stress.
- Teach child to decrease use of accessory muscles during an acute episode once the residual volume diminishes and expiratory flow improves.
- Encourage nasal breathing since warm, humidified air provides an easy, cost-free method of reducing the bronchospasm that follows stressful exercise.
- Provide bronchial hygiene as needed to clear secretions.
- Provide breathing retraining as needed.
- Provide bronchial drainage as needed.
- Provide vibration as needed.
- Provide suctioning as needed.

PRECAUTIONS/CONTRAINDICATIONS

- Asthma may occur in children with neurodevelopmental or orthopedic problems that must be considered when designing an exercise program.
- Children with asthma must be monitored for signs of asthma attacks.
- Record secretion volume, color, consistency, and vital signs before, during, and after treatment.
- There is little rationale for physical therapy in a child with status asthmaticus or intractable acute asthma, because the child is unable to cooperate in therapy (Tecklin, 1999, p. 547).

DESIRED OUTCOME/PROGNOSIS

- Child is able to breathe without airway constriction.
- Child and parents are knowledgeable about irritants that cause asthma attacks and have learned to take steps to reduce the number and severity of the attacks.
- Child and parents are able to monitor pulmonary functions.
- Child and parents know what to do when an attack occurs, including approaches which may reduce the severity of the attacks.

- Parents know how to facilitate pulmonary drainage.
- Child has an exercise program which is performed daily.
- Child is able to participate in daily life activities at home, in school, and in the community.

REFERENCES

Beers MH, Berkow R, eds. *The Merck Manual of Diagnosis and Therapy*. Whitehouse Station, NJ: Merck Research Laboratories; 1999.

Emtner M, Hedin A, Stalenheim G. Asthmatic patients' views of a comprehensive asthma rehabilitation programme: a three-year follow-up. *Physiotherapy Res Int*. 1998;3(3): 175–193.

Magee CL. Asthma. In: Campbell SK, ed. *Physical Therapy for Children*. 2nd ed. Philadelphia, Pa: WB Saunders Co; 2000:764–785.

Ratliffe KT. Medical disorders—Respiratory disorders of childhood: asthma. In: Ratliffe KT. *Clinical Pediatric Physical Therapy: A Guide for the Physical Therapy Team*. St. Louis, Mo: CV Mosby Co; 1998:392–395.

Tecklin JS. Pulmonary disorders in infants and children and their physical therapy management—Asthma. In: Tecklin JS, ed. *Pediatric Physical Therapy*. 3rd ed. Philadelphia, Pa: Lippincott Williams and Wilkins; 1999:545–549.

Wallis C, Prasad A. Who needs chest physiotherapy? Moving from anecdote to evidence. *Arch Dis Child*. 1999;80:393–397.

Atelectasis

Also known as *collapsed lung*.

ICD-9-CM Code: 518.0 Pulmonary collapse
APTA Guide Pattern: 6J

DESCRIPTION

A shrunken, airless state affecting all or part of a lung (Beers & Berkow, 1999, p. 590). Primary atelectasis occurs in the neonate as a result of pulmonary immaturity or at any age due to inadequate respiratory effort. Secondary atelectasis occurs when gas in a lung segment is reabsorbed without subsequent refilling of that segment (Tecklin, 1999, p. 538).

CAUSE

Cause of primary atelectasis is pulmonary immaturity. Causes of secondary atelectasis include bronchial obstruction, abnormal pressure on the lung tissue, and removal of pulmonary surfactant by disease or trauma. Common causes of airway obstruction are mucus or other debris including meconium, amniotic content, foreign bodies, and aspirated gastrointestinal contents. Common causes of lung compression are enlarged heart or great vessels, congenital or acquired lung cysts, diaphragmatic hernia and congenital lobar emphysema (Tecklin, 1999, p. 538).

ASSESSMENT

AREAS
- Airway obstruction
- Breathing patterns
- Diaphragm and accessory muscle movement

- Gas exchange
- Lung and breathing sounds
- Respiratory rate
- Rib and chest expansion
- Secretions

INSTRUMENTS/PROCEDURES
- Review patient's chart to understand pathophysiology and identify type.
- Review roentgenographic findings to identify position of the atelectasis. Palpation may also help because an airless lung has a dull percussion. Although auscultatory finds vary, most frequently there is a diminution of breath sounds in the involved area. Complete obstruction may result in no breath sounds but in patchy or incomplete atelectasis; crackles may be heard.
- Observe patient's chest and breathing. Large atelectasis narrows the rib interspace and decreases excursion of the involved hemothorax.
- Observe muscular pattern of respiration: diaphragmatic versus accessory.
- Observe patient's respiratory rate.
- Palpate to determine if a shift of the trachea has occurred toward the atelectasis owing to volume loss of the lung.

PROBLEMS
- Extent of the atelectasis
- Location of the atelectasis
- Mobility: Has the child been on bed rest for an extended period of time?
- Pain: Can the child take a deep breath and cough effectively?
- Cough: Can the child cough and have sufficient strength or neurologic competence?

TREATMENT/MANAGEMENT
- Bronchial drainage
- Percussion
- Vibration
- Depth breathing
- Maximal inspiratory efforts
- Electrical stimulation of the thorax with direct current
- Prevention

PRECAUTIONS/CONTRAINDICATIONS
- Secondary type requires bronchial hygiene procedures.

DESIRED OUTCOME/PROGNOSIS
- Child has normal breathing pattern.
- Child has expected gas exchange.
- Child has normal lung sounds.
- Child is using diaphragm but not accessory muscles for normal breathing.
- Child has expected respiratory rate for age and development.
- Child has bilateral rib and chest expansion.
- Child does not have excessive secretions.

REFERENCES

Beers MH, Berkow R, eds. *The Merck Manual of Diagnosis and Therapy*. Whitehouse Station, NJ: Merck Research Laboratories; 1999.

Tecklin JS. Pulmonary disorders in infants and children and their physical therapy management—Atelectasis. In: Tecklin JS, ed. *Pediatric Physical Therapy*. 3rd ed. Philadelphia, Pa: Lippincott Williams and Wilkins; 1999:538–540.

Wallis, C. Who needs chest physiotherapy? Moving from anecdote to evidence. *Arch Dis Child*. 1999;80:393–397.

Autistic Spectrum Disorder

Also called *early infantile autism, childhood autism, Kanner's autism, Kanner's syndrome, autism, autistic disorder,* and *infantile psychosis.* Associated terms are *pervasive developmental disorder* and *Asperger's syndrome.*

ICD-9-CM Code: 299.0 Infantile autism
APTA Guide Pattern: 5A

DESCRIPTION

The essential features of Autistic Spectrum Disorder are the presence of markedly abnormal or impaired development in social interaction and communication and a markedly restricted repertoire of activity and interests. Manifestations of the disorder vary greatly depending on the development level and chronological age of the individual (DSM–IV, p. 66). Autism was first described by Leo Kanner in 1943.

A syndrome of early childhood characterized by abnormal social relationships; language disorder with impaired understanding, echolalia, and pronominal reversal (eg, particularly using "you" instead of "I" or "me" when referring to one's self); rituals and compulsive phenomena (ie, an insistence on the preservation of sameness); and uneven intellectual development with mental retardation in most cases (Beers & Berkow, 1999, p. 2420)

Autistic disorder is classified as a Pervasive Developmental Disorder in the DSM–IV along with Asperger's syndrome, which is similar to Autistic disorder except that verbal skills are usually more advanced and the outcome for near-normal behavior is better, especially with appropriate accommodations and educational methodology. Asperger's syndrome was first described by Hans Asperger in 1944.

CAUSE

The exact cause is unknown. CT scans have isolated a subgroup of autistic children with enlarged ventricles and magnetic resonance imaging (MRI) has recently identified a subgroup of autistic adults with hypoplasia of the cerebellar vermis. Individual cases of autism have been associated with the congenital rubella syndrome, cytomegalic infusion disease, phenylketonuria, and the fragile X syndrome (*Merck Manual,* 1999, p. 2420).

For many years the cause was assumed to be psychological due to a traumatic event, regulation, or poor bonding with the child's mother. Parents were blamed for the disorder because they were too rigid and emotionally distant. The child was viewed as normal but withdrawn. This theory is no longer accepted. Autistic disorder is a neurobiological disorder and not a psychological one (Ratliffe, 1998, p. 325).

Autism is 2 to 4 times more common in boys than girls. The concordance rate is significantly greater in monozygotic than dizygotic twins, indicating the importance of genetic factors. The syndrome is defined by its behavior manifestations (Beers & Berkow, 1999, p. 2420).

ASSESSMENT

AREAS
- Range of motion (ROM)
- Muscle strength
- Muscle tone
- Reflexes and reactions
- Posture
- Functional skills
- Activities of daily living (ADLs)
- Need for adaptive equipment
- Recreation and leisure skills

INSTRUMENTS/PROCEDURES

No specific instruments identified.

PROBLEMS

- Often has deficits in gross motor skills.
- Often has stereotypical movements such as hand flicking in front of the eyes, head banging, spinning, rocking, or complex whole-body movements.
- Often has one or more preoccupations with parts of objects or the specific actions of objects such as: spinning wheels of toy cars, lining up toys precisely in a row, sniffing or smelling objects, feeling the texture of objects repetitively, or carrying around an unusual object such as a piece of string, dust bunnies, or cigarette butts.
- Often exhibits distress tantrum over minute changes in environment such as a picture being moved a few inches on the wall, indicative of poor coping skills.
- Often has a narrow range of interests which become obsessions for a certain length of time.
- Often has speech and language differences such as echolalic speech or appears to be deaf to voice commands.
- Often has poor social skills such as not mixing with other children, standing apart from other children, poor eye contact, and inappropriate laughing or giggling.
- Often is behind in academic skills although may be at grade level in math and spelling.
- May have delays in gross motor skill acquisition such as climbing stairs, jumping, or running.
- May be clumsy.
- May have poor balance.
- May have decreased strength in specific body areas such as trunk and hips.
- May lose range of motion in some joints such as the ankles.
- May have poor aerobic fitness.

TREATMENT/MANAGEMENT

- Develop gross motor skills in individual or group session which address the specific skill area.
- Increase strength using exercises such as pelvic bridges, curl-ups, and creeping on hands and knees.
- Improve or maintain ROM through stretching exercises and selected tasks such as walking up and down stairs.
- Improve or maintain aerobic fitness through selected activities such as Special Olympics, hiking, baseball, and therapeutic horseback riding.
- Improve performance of ADLs through recommendations of adaptive equipment, teaching techniques such as hand over hand, or modifications of the environment.
- Support academic progress by recommending adaptive equipment or modifications to the environment.
- Therapist should set limits on certain behaviors or give particular consequences for certain behaviors.
- Therapist should encourage behaviors which are acceptable by rewarding child.
- Therapist should speak clearly, keep instructions simple, and be patient.
- Therapist should make sure child is facing therapist before talking to give visual and auditory cues that the child is being addressed.
- Therapist should structure the therapy session the same way each day to facilitate coping skills.
- Therapist should prepare the child for changes in routine and be prepared to handle adverse behaviors.
- Therapist should involve the child in social situations, even if the child is reluctant to be included.

PRECAUTIONS/CONTRAINDICATIONS
- If child has seizures, precautions such as wearing a helmet may be necessary.
- If self-injurious behavior occurs such as head banging or biting the hand, precautions to limit opportunities for such behavior should be instituted.

DESIRED OUTCOME/PROGNOSIS
- Most persons with autism will require assisted living either at home with parents or in group homes.
- Child is able to perform gross motor skills that are age appropriate.
- Child achieves and maintains normal muscle strength and tone.
- Child achieves and maintains normal ROM.
- Child's posture and balance are improved.
- Child's aerobic fitness is maintained.
- Child is able to perform ADLS with adapted equipment or modified teaching techniques as needed.
- Child is able to participate in all school activities with adapted equipment or modified teaching techniques as needed.
- Child is able to participate in recreational and leisure activities which may include activities designed for persons with disabilities.

REFERENCES

American Psychiatric Association. *Diagnostic and Statistical Manual of Mental Disorders.* 4th ed. Washington, DC: American Psychiatric Association; 1994.

Beers MH, Berkow R, eds. *The Merck Manual of Diagnosis and Therapy.* Whitehouse Station, NJ: Merck Research Laboratories; 1999.

Ratliffe KT. Sensory, processing, and cognitive disorders—Luke, a boy with autism. In: Ratliffe KT. *Clinical Pediatric Physical Therapy: A Guide for the Physical Therapy Team.* St. Louis, Mo: CV Mosby Co; 1998:313–320.

Ratliffe KT. Sensory, processing, and cognitive disorders of childhood—The child with a pervasive developmental disorder. In: Ratliffe KT. *Clinical Pediatric Physical Therapy: A Guide for the Physical Therapy Team.* St. Louis, Mo: CV Mosby Co; 1998:324–327.

Balance Dysfunction in Children

Also known as *balance disorder.*

ICD-9-CM Code: 781.9 Other symptoms involving nervous and musculoskeletal systems, Abnormal posture

APTA Guide Pattern: 4B

DESCRIPTION

Balance dysfunction involves difficulty or an inability to maintain a functional posture, both statically and dynamically, through motor actions that distribute weight evenly around the body's center of gravity. *Static balance* is the ability to maintain a posture such as balancing while standing or sitting, and *dynamic balance* is the ability to maintain postural control during movements such as reaching for an object or walking on various surfaces (Habib & Westcott, 1998, p. 101). *Postural control* is the ability to maintain equilibrium in a gravitational field by keeping or returning the center of mass (COM) over its base of support

(BOS) (Westcott, Murray, & Pence, 1998, p. 48). *Postural sway* or postural stability is the constant small corrective deviations from the vertical during standing (Habib & Westcott, 1998, p. 101). *Balancing* is the process by which postural stability is maintained (Westcott, Lowes, & Richardson, 1997, p. 630). *Orientation* is the ability to maintain an appropriate relationship between the body segments and between the body and the environment for a task (Howle, 1999, p. 39).

Various factors influence postural and balance abilities in children, including prior postural experiences, age, gender, environmental affordances, task constraints, and biological competence (Habib & Westcott, 1998, p. 101). Balance depends on inputs from visual, somatosensory (ie, proprioceptive, cutaneous, and joint receptors), vestibular systems, and on the ability of the central nervous system to interpret the relative importance of each input (Howle, 1999, p. 39). *Sensory organization* is the ability to select from among redundant sensory inputs to identify the sensory system that is providing the most accurate input for maintaining postural stability (Westcott, Lowes, Richardson, 1997, p. 635). Reports by various investigators suggest that the critical period for the development of postural control is between the ages of 3 and 7 years (Rine et al, 1996, p. 56). The postural control system is viewed as an important component of motor control that enables an individual to orient in space and as necessary for optimal motor development and performance (Rine et al, 1998, p. 16). *Protective reactions* involve the ability to break the fall if stability limits are exceeded when the COM of the body is displaced outside the BOS (Howle, 1999, p. 39).

There are two major theoretical perspectives. The first is based on the reflex/hierarchical theories of motor control, which propose that balance and stability are the result of using reflexes and automatic reactions that are organized hierarchically within the individual's nervous system to stabilize the body against gravity. Balance response is controlled by the highest center of the brain: the cerebral cortex (Westcott, Murray, & Pence, 1998, pp. 48–49). Clinically, postural control is described in terms of balance and equilibrium reactions, which include a progression from reliance on protective extension, to tilt reactions, and finally to postural fixation (Rine et al, 1996, p. 59).

The second set of theories based on the systems model suggests that balance stability is the result of the interaction of the individual and environment in a goal-oriented system to maintain the COM within certain stability limits. In the systems-based theories, all the different systems (neurological, sensory and motor, biomechanical, muscular and skeletal, motivational, emotions and needs, etc.) work together for the end goal with no fixed director within the brain. Thus, any system may be the director for maintaining postural control, depending on the external conditions in the environment and the internal conditions within the person (Westcott, Murray, & Pence, 1998, pp. 48–49).

CAUSE

Balance dysfunction in children may be caused by several disorders or diseases including at-risk infants, brain tumors, cerebral palsy, developmental delay, genetic disorders, hearing impairment, infections involving the central nervous system, learning disorders, myelomeningocele, muscular dystrophy, orthopedic impairments, scoliosis, spinal cord injury, traumatic brain injury, and visual impairment.

ASSESSMENT

AREAS
- Static balance: sitting, standing
- Dynamic balance
- Motor coordination
- Muscle strength
- Postural sway
- Range of motion (ROM): active
- Sensory systems: vision, vestibular, proprioception

INSTRUMENTS/PROCEDURES

Assessment instruments include those which measure sensory organization and conflict, motor coordination, developmental skills, functional skills, and activities of daily living (ADLS).

- Alberta Infant Motor Scale (AIMS) (Piper & Darrah, 1994)
- Bayley Scales of Infant Development–II (BSID–II) (Bayley, 1993)
- Bruininks-Oseretsky Test of Motor Proficiency (BOTMP) (Bruininks, 1978)
- Childhood Health Assessment Questionnaire (Singh et al, 1994)
- Clinical Observation of Motor and Postural Skills, 2nd ed. (COMPS) (Wilson et al, 2000)
- DeGangi-Berk Test of Sensory Integration (DeGangi & Berk, 1983)
- Functional Reach Test (Duncan PW, 1990)
- Functional Standing Test (Triolo et al, 1992)
- Gross Motor Function Measure, 2nd ed. (GMFM) (Russell et al, 1993)
- Hawaii Early Learning Profile (HELP) (Parks, 1999)
- Juvenile Arthritis Status Index (JASI) (Wright et al, 1992)
- Miller Assessment of Preschoolers (MAP) (Miller, 1988)
- Movement Assessment of Infants (MAI) (Chandler, Andrews, & Swanson, 1980)
- Peabody Developmental Motor Scales, 2nd ed. (PDMS–2) (Folio & Fewell, 1999)
- Pediatric Clinical Test of Sensory Interaction for Balance (P–CTSIB) (Crowe et al, 1990)
- Pediatric Evaluation of Disability Inventory (PEDI) (Haley et al, 1992)
- Sensory Integration and Praxis Test (SIPT) (Ayres, 1989)
- Smart Balance Master System: NeuroCom International, Clackamas, OR, USA
- Southern California Postrotary Nystagmus Test (PRNT) (Ayres, 1975)
- Test of Sensory Functions in Infants (TSFI) (DeGangi & Greenspan, 1989)
- Timed Up and Go (TUG) (Podsciadlo & Richardson, 1991)
- force platform (nonstandardized)
- goniometry
- manual muscle testing and dynamometry
- past pointing
- Romberg test
- tandem walking
- tiltboard perturbations (nonstandardized)
- vestibulo-ocular reflex (VOR) testing

PROBLEMS

- May exhibit clumsiness.
- May exhibit motor incoordination.
- May fall frequently compared to other children.
- May be unable to stand or have difficulty standing on one leg (single-leg stance with eyes open and with eyes closed).
- May be unable to or have difficulty with kicking, jumping, skipping, or hopping.
- May have difficulty walking a balance beam.
- May appear to have dysfunction in the development and integration of body righting reactions.
- May demonstrate inadequate inhibition of primitive reflexes.
- May demonstrate failure to develop adaptive equilibrium reactions.
- May have increased postural sway.
- May demonstrate increased reliance on vision for maintenance of standing balance.
- May demonstrate persistence of developmentally immature patterns of equilibrium response.

- May have difficulty maintaining sitting or standing balance

TREATMENT/MANAGEMENT

In the hierarchically based theories, a typical treatment would involve passive weight shifting to disturb the center of mass and thus elicit equilibrium reactions, or active weight shift by rocking in a repetitive manner to encourage equilibrium responses and practice in balancing. In systems-based theories, shifting of weight should be done actively, not passively, and should be incorporated into a functional activity rather than practiced in isolation (Westcott, Murray, & Pence, 1998, p. 49). Techniques can also be divided into feedforward and feedback. Feedforward activities challenge the client to achieve the necessary postural set prior to performing a movement task or functional activity. Feedback activities require adjustment after the task or functional activity has begun.

TECHNIQUES FOR MODERATE TO SEVERE BALANCE DYSFUNCTION
(Westcott, Murray, & Pence, 1998, pp. 52–53)

- Use active functional activities.
- Use perturbation of the support surface.
- Use gait assistive devices.
- Use ankle/foot orthotic devices.
- Use strengthening exercises.
- Use positioning devices.
- Use perturbance of the body.
- Use vestibular stimulation.
- Use sports activities.
- Use ROM exercises.

Techniques rarely or never used for moderate to severe balance dysfunction were electrical stimulation, biofeedback, maneuvering on a narrow surface, and practice on a narrow base of support.

TECHNIQUES FOR MILD BALANCE DYSFUNCTION
(Westcott, Murray, & Pence, 1998, p. 53)

- Use active functional activities.
- Use activities that require a dynamic unilateral stance such as hopping.
- Use activities that require maneuvering on a narrow surface such as a balance beam.
- Use activities that require static unilateral stance such as standing on one leg while counting.
- Use sports activities.
- Use activities that perturb the support surface such as a vestibular or rocker board.
- Techniques rarely or never used for mild problems in balance dysfunction were electrical stimulation, positioning devices, and biofeedback.

PRECAUTIONS/CONTRAINDICATIONS
- Child should be cautioned to avoid ambulation in dark areas or on uneven surfaces until adequate balance skills have been acquired or adequate compensatory techniques have been incorporated.

DESIRED OUTCOME/PROGNOSIS
- Child is able to maintain static balance in sitting and standing tasks with orthotic or assistive devices, if needed.
- Child is able to maintain dynamic balance in movement activities with orthotic or assistive devices, if needed.
- Child has sufficient postural control to maintain the center of mass with the base of support during balancing activities.
- Child has learned compensatory techniques to avoid falls or injuries if balance dysfunction continues to exist.

REFERENCES

Deitz JC, Richardson P, Crowe TK, Westcott SL. Performance of children with learning disabilities and motor delays on the Pediatric Clinical Test of Sensory Interaction for Balance (P-CTSIB). *Phys Occup Ther Pediatr.* 1996;16(3):1–21.

Di Fabio RP, Foudriat BA. Responsiveness and reliability of a pediatric strategy score for balance. *Physiotherapy Res Int.* 1996;1(3):180–194.

Habib A, Westcott S. Assessment of anthropometric factors on balance tests in children. *Pediatr Phys Ther.* 1998;10(3):101–109.

Howle JMW. Cerebral palsy. In: Campbell SK. *Decision Making in Pediatric Neurologic Physical Therapy.* New York, NY: Churchill Livingstone; 1999:23–83.

Liano H-F, Mae P-J. Test-retest reliability of balance tests in children with cerebral palsy. *Dev Med Child Neurol.* 2001;43:180–186.

Martin S. *Pediatric Balance Program.* San Antonio, Tex: Therapy Skill Builders; 1998.

Rine RM. Evaluation and treatment of vestibular and postural control deficits in children. In: Herdman SJ. *Vestibular Rehabilitation.* Philadelphia, Pa: FA Davis Co; 2000:545–565.

Rine RM, Lindeblad S, Donovan P, Vergara K, Gostin J, Mattson K. Balance and motor skills in young children with sensorineural hearing impairment: A preliminary study. *Pediatr Phys Ther.* 1996;8(2):55–61.

Westcott SL, Lowes LP, Richardson PK. Evaluation of postural stability in children: current theories and assessment tools. *Phys Ther.* 1997;77(6):629–645.

Westcott SL, Murray KH, Pence K. Survey of preferences of pediatric physical therapists for assessment and treatment of balance dysfunction in children. *Pediatr Phys Ther.* 1998;10(2):48–61.

Brachial Plexus Injuries

Also known as *brachial plexus lesion.*

ICD-9-CM: 767.6 Injury to brachial plexus

APTA Guide Pattern: 5A

DESCRIPTION

Disorder of the brachial plexus causing a mixed motor and sensory disorder of the corresponding limb. The pattern does not fit the distribution of individual roots or nerves (Beers & Berkow, 1999, p. 1490).

Generally three types are recognized: *Erb's* or *upper-plexus type* involving C5 and C6, sometimes C7, *Klumpke's* or *lower-plexus type* involving C7, C8, and T1), and *whole-arm type* (C5-T1). Variation ranges from a mild edema affecting one or two roots to total avulsion of the entire plexus. Involvement is often unilateral.

In the upper-plexus type, the dysfunction typically involves the rhomboids, levator scapulae, serratus anterior, deltoid, supraspinatus, infraspinatus, biceps brachii, brachioradialis, brachialis, supinator, and long extensors of the wrist, fingers, and thumb. In the lower-plexus type, the dysfunction usually involves the intrinsic muscles of the hand and the extensors and flexors of the wrist and fingers. In the whole-arm type, altered movement patterns and soft tissue length changes are present due to the paralysis or weakness of certain muscles, unopposed activity of some muscles and the resultant muscle imbalance. The results are persistent movement substitutions, abnormal posturing of the arm, posterior displacement of the humeral epiphysis and posterior radial dislocation, and later skeletal deformity and poor bone growth.

Other complications may be present, including injury to the facial nerve causing facial paralysis, fracture of the clavicle or humerus, traction to the cervical cord causing upper motoneuron lesion, subluxation of the shoulder, torticollis, intrapartum asphyxia, and ipsilateral hemiparalysis of the diaphragm.

CAUSE

Most common cause is difficult birth. Factors include high birth weight, prolonged maternal labor, a sedated, hypotonic infant, a heavily sedated mother, traction in a breech presentation or rotation of the head in a cephalic presentation, difficult cesarean extraction, and abnormal uterine posture leading to a pressure neuropathy. The incidence ranges from 0.6 to 3 per 1,000 births which is a decline from reports of earlier years (Shephard, 1999, p. 235).

ASSESSMENT

AREAS
- Functional motor movement such as reaching to grasp an object
- Grip strength
- Range of motion of the upper extremity joints
- Reflexes and reactions
- Resting posture to observe for possible contractures
- Sensory response and awareness

INSTRUMENTS/PROCEDURES

Motor
- Videotaping range of motion under standardized conditions.
- Force transducer, a grip force dynamometer or rubber bulb connected to a manometer to measure grip strength.
- Observation of movement. Look for spontaneous movement and posture as the infant lies in a supine and a prone position followed by moving child around, cuddling and talking to child.
- Reflex and reaction testing—especially the Moro reflex—placing reaction of the hands, the Galant (trunk incurvation) reflex, neck-righting reaction, and downward parachute reaction.
- Palpation of muscles during active movement.
- EMG recording of muscle activation, especially done repeatedly every 6 to 8 weeks for as long as indicated.
- Use of a muscle chart to record activation such as 0 = absent, 1 = present, but lacking full range of movement and 2 = present throughout a full range of movement.
- In older children, the Nine Hole Peg Test (Kellor et al, 1971) may be used.

Sensory
- Pinprick recorded on a body chart
- O'Riain's wrinkle test; the fingers are immersed in water at 40 degrees C for 30 minutes. Normal skin wrinkles but denervated skin does not.
- In older children, 2-point discrimination with an esthesiometer may be used.

PROBLEMS
- Lack of or decreased spontaneous movement of the involved limb when compared to the uninvolved limb
- Altered movement and substitute patterns due to weakness or paralysis (sometimes called synkinetic movements or associated movements); may have shoulder elevation and slight abduction instead of shoulder depression and abduction in resting posture. In reaching to grasp, the pattern is wrist flexion and forearm

pronation with finger extension. Contractions of the biceps brachii and deltoid muscles may occur with inspiration.

- Soft tissue length changes and possible contractures especially in the elbow.
- In whole-plexus type, subluxation and dislocation of the glenohumeral joint may occur due to lack of muscle activity.
- Failure to reach for objects with the involved limb when placed in visual field.
- Learned non-use may occur if muscle paralysis is present, which results in delay in achieving certain motor milestones such as independent sitting, and an inability to perform two-handed actions.
- Lack of sensation in the involved limb.
- Scapula may adhere to the humerus, changing the dynamic ratio between the humerus and scapular to 1:1 instead of 6:1 during the first 30 degrees of abduction.
- Phrenic nerve paralysis, if present, will decrease movement of the ipsilateral thorax with resulting respiratory distress and cyanosis. May mimic diaphragmatic hernia except there is unilateral diaphragmatic elevation and atelectasis.

TREATMENT/MANAGEMENT

Allow hemorrhage and edema to resolve before beginning intervention on a newborn. Intervention should begin within the first 2 weeks of life.

GOALS ARE TO:
- Optimize conditions for recovery of motor function.
- Provide the environmental conditions and the motivation necessary to enable muscles to resume function as neural regeneration occurs.
- Train motor control by practicing actions such as reaching for objects.

IF THERE IS NO MOVEMENT, THE PURPOSES ARE TO:
- Simulate activity in muscles whose nerve supply is only temporarily disconnected.
- Enable muscles to be activated as soon as nerve regeneration has occurred.
- Prevent or minimize:
  - Soft tissue contracture by maintaining soft tissue length.
  - Disorganized movements of the shoulder and shoulder girdle.
  - Learned nonuse of the limb.
  - Use of adaptive or "trick" movement patterns, behavior or habits (substitutions, or pathologic motor stereotypes).
- Provide specificity of muscle stimulation as innervation is returning.
- Use functional movements and task-related motor control once affected muscles are reinnervated and able to contract.
- Provide guidance and feedback to ensure the infant uses the appropriate muscles for each movement attempted.
- Provide feedback and reinforcement for successful performance such as verbal comment, smiling, or general attitude of pleasure, even for small infants.
- Focus attention first on muscles which are essential for a specific movement such as reaching to grasp an object, which would require abductors, flexors, and lateral rotators of the shoulder; scapular rotators, retractors, and protractors; supinators of the forearm; wrist extensors and radial deviators; and palmar abductor of the thumb (Shepherd, p. 243).
- Training should begin using the best conditions for each muscle such as best leverage, best relationship of limb to gravity, start with movement using eccentric contract before concentric contraction, and use optimal alignment for required muscle action. To accomplish these objectives, the therapist must search for the presence of a muscle contraction, check different sectors of the movement range to determine where the movement occurs best, check different rela-

tionships of the limb to gravity to facilitate muscle action, and begin with eccentric activity. For example, attempting to elicit activity in the deltoid muscle by encouraging the infant to take his hand to his face would require the muscle to work both concentrically and as a fixator.

- Modify tasks to fit the muscle movement potential. For example, the wrist extensors may not be able to contract enough to extend the hand from a position of wrist flexion concentrically, but may be able to contract eccentrically from a position in which the extensors are already shortened. For an older child, if the deltoid is not strong enough to raise the arm from the side it may be able to hold the arm and lower it a few degrees from a horizontal position when the patient is in a sitting position or hold it in a vertical position when the patient is lying down.
- Suggestions for promoting reaching to grasp:
  - Attempt sitting the patient in a semireclined and supported posture in a chair.
  - Use an object that is easy to grasp and of irresistible appeal to the infant.
  - Move the object across the visual field at a distance of 5 to 7 inches rather than holding the object stationary.
  - As the infant matures, add games that require reaching and place the object so that shoulder flexion and external and forearm flexion are encouraged, while shoulder internal rotation and abduction and forearm pronation are discouraged.
- Provide object-mediated guidance to ensure that correct movement is obtained. First place the toy or object so that desired movement is likely to occur. Then provide guidance with therapist's or parent's hand, which may include holding the arm in desired position or placing the hand on the scapula, upper arm, or forearm to guide and maintain the desired position of the upper extremity. The objective is to avoid use of adaptive or substitute movements.
- Facilitate the stages of motor learning:
  - *Cognitive:* child tries to understand the overall idea of the task and what it demands.
  - *Associative:* continuous adjustment and reorganization of motor behavior in which components are tried and combined.
  - *Autonomous:* characterized by coordinated execution of the task requiring little cognitive control and less subject to distraction. Movement is stimulated only at the automatic level by play or by facilitation of movement.
- "Force" movement patterns as muscles regain the capacity to contract and generate movement. "Forced" use is typically done by constraining the uninvolved limb or by limiting the movement patterns which the infant can make because the therapist or parent is holding the arm and body in such a manner that certain movements are not possible.
- If movement disorganization has occurred, begin with shoulder girdle and shoulder actions. Stimulate the rhomboids and serratus anterior muscles to retract, protract, and rotate the scapula. Scapular retracts can be encouraged by shifting the infant's weight backward onto the hands. Serratus anterior action can be encouraged by having the infant take weight through the hands while the therapist stabilizes the scapula against the thoracic wall. The goal is a more normal relationship between protractors and retractors and between muscles which act as stabilizers and synergists.
- Encourage forearm supination by stabilizing the elbow and arm to prevent other movements and flex and elbow. For older children, beating a drum or placing hand over hand on a rod may be useful to promote both shoulder adduction and forearm supination.
- Biofeedback may be useful to reinforce the desired motor behavior.
- Electrical stimulation may be useful but needs to be used for several hours a day. Functional electrical stimulation is recommended over galvanic stimulation.

- Splinting or strapping can be used to prevent excessive use of unopposed or poorly opposed muscles until the child can be trained to contract the muscles needed for correct movement. The splint or strap needs to be worn during most of the day. An example is a small molded static splint designed to hold the thumb in palmar abduction or to hold the wrist in extension. A dynamic splint may be useful to promote wrist extension if there is C7 paralysis.
- If recovery does not occur, provide specific training to muscles after microsurgical repair or for surgery to transplant muscles or arthrodeses joints.
- If passive movement is used to prevent soft tissue contracture of the shoulder region, care should be taken to prevent joint damage whether performed by therapist or parent.
    Note: See Precautions. Splinting to prevent contractures is controversial because it may lead to "overmobility" of the glenohumeral joint which could contribute to abnormality or dislocation.
- If neglect of the arm or learned nonuse has occurred, "forced" use may be effective. Constrain the unaffected arm while providing intensive task-related training for short periods daily for about 6 months.
- Sensory unawareness can be remediated once the infant is old enough to play sensory games such as locating objects in sand or rice, localizing touch stimuli, and recognizing and naming objects while blindfolded. With older children, 2-point discrimination and stereognosis guessing games may be used.
- Provide parent or caregiver education for home exercise program.
- Provide parent or caregiver with suggestions for holding the infant to minimize substitute patterns such as holding the infant with the involved extremity against the parent's body to encourage shoulder flexion rather than abduction.

PRECAUTIONS/CONTRAINDICATIONS
- Therapist should be aware that what appears to be normally functioning muscles will become weak from disuse if other muscles normally used together in a movement pattern are involved (weak or paralyzed) in the brachial plexus injury.
- Be aware that the forced passive supination of the forearm when the pronators are contracted may result in dislocation of the radius.
- Use passive movement gently to avoid damage to an unprotected shoulder joint. Do not use forceful manipulation to prevent soft tissue contractures—especially scapulohumeral adhesions.
- Do not manually restrain the scapula when the humerus is moved beyond 30 degrees of motion because elevation of the arm without rotation of the scapula and lateral rotation at the glenohumeral joint can damage that joint by causing the humerus to impinge on the immobile acromion process.

DESIRED OUTCOME/PROGNOSIS
- Outcome is generally favorable with a 90% recovery rate. Best indicator of recovery by 12 months is extension of the elbow, wrist, thumb, and fingers at 3 months of age.
- Motor training should continue as long as recovery is still occurring, which is generally considered to be 2 years.
- Terminal goal is normal movement patterns for reaching to grasp and normal use of hands.

REFERENCES

Beers MH, Berkow R, eds. *The Merck Manual of Diagnosis and Therapy.* Whitehouse Station, NJ: Merck Research Laboratories; 1999.

Duclos L, Gilbert A. Obstetrical palsy: early treatment and secondary procedures. *Ann Acad Med Singapore.* 1995;24(6):841–845.

Leblebicioglu G, Leblebicioglu-Konu D, Tugay N, Atay OA, Gogus T. Obstetrical brachial plexus palsy: an analysis of 105 cases. *Turk J Pediatr.* 2001;43(3):181–189.

Norton ES. Developmental muscular torticollis and brachial plexus injury. In: Campbell SK, ed. *Physical Therapy for Children.* 2nd ed. Philadelphia, Pa: WB Saunders Co; 2000:282–301.

Ramon LE, Zell JP. Rehabilitation program for children with brachial plexus and peripheral nerve injury. *Seminars in Pediatric Neurology.* 2000:7(1):52–57.

Ratliffe KT. Other orthopedic disorders—Tyler, an infant with congenital torticollis and Erb's palsy. In Ratliffe KT. *Clinical Pediatric Physical Therapy: A Guide for the Physical Therapy Team.* St. Louis, Mo: CV Mosby Co; 1998:131–138.

Ratliffe KT. Other orthopedic disorders—The child with brachial plexus injury. In Ratliffe KT. *Clinical Pediatric Physical Therapy: A Guide for the Physical Therapy Team.* St. Louis, Mo: CV Mosby Co; 1998:137–139.

Saidoff DC, McDonough AL. Large and broad-shouldered infant with monoparetic arm after breech delivery. In: Saidoff DC, McDonough AL, eds. *Critical Pathways in Therapeutic Intervention: Extremities and Spine.* St. Louis, Mo: CV Mosby Co; 2002:203–220.

Shepherd RB. Brachial plexus injury. In: Campbell SK. *Decision Making in Pediatric Neurologic Physical Therapy.* New York, NY: Churchill Livingstone; 1999:235–259.

Bronchopulmonary Dysplasia

Also known as *BPD.*

ICD-9-CM Code: 770.7 Chronic respiratory disease arising in the perinatal period
APTA Patterns: 6C, 6F, 6J

DESCRIPTION

A chronic lung disorder causing persistent respiratory distress, characteristic x-ray changes with parenchymal streaks and hyperexpansion, and an ongoing need for mechanical ventilation at 36 weeks corrected gestational age in newborns who have been treated for respiratory distress from any cause with intermittent mandatory ventilation (Beers & Berkow, p. 2139). BPD was first described in 1967 and is the most common chronic lung disease in infants (Kelly, p. 715). Disorders associated with BPD include cerebral palsy and intraventricular hemorrhage.

CAUSE

Lung injury occurring from repeated overdistention of alveoli and alveolar ducts due to mechanical ventilation (volutrauma), high inspired O_2 concentrations, and endotracheal intubation. The disorder is more common among infants of early gestational age. BPD is often a sequela of respiratory distress syndrome (hyaline membrane disease) especially when pulmonary interstitial emphysema has occurred (Beers & Berkow, 1999, p. 2139).

ASSESSMENT

AREAS
- Balance
- Endurance
- Gross motor skills
- Oral motor skills
- Postural control
- Sensory hypersensitivity, especially oral

INSTRUMENTS/PROCEDURES

Bayley Scales of Infant Development–II (BSID–II) (Bayley, 1993)

PROBLEMS

- Child often has chronic respiratory problems.
- Child often has increased energy expenditure related to increased work of breathing.
- Child often has decreased endurance and fatigues quickly.
- Child may have delayed motor development.
- Child may have overall growth and developmental delays.
- Child may experience failure to thrive because of intolerance for feeding related to oral motor sensitivity, poor sucking ability, and decreased physical stamina.

TREATMENT/MANAGEMENT

Comprehensive management of BPD requires a team of professionals to manage nutritional, respiratory, pharmacologic, psychosocial, and developmental needs. Current management includes the use of high-frequency ventilators and surfactant replacement therapy.

- Provide opportunity to practice balance and postural control.
- Facilitate gross motor development.
- Increase endurance to motor activity.
- Improve oral motor skills.
- Decrease oral hypersensitivity.

PRECAUTIONS/CONTRAINDICATIONS

- Therapist should be knowledgeable about the equipment and its function. Do not change or rearrange equipment setup without permission.
- Watch for signs of limited fluid intake.
- Watch for signs of fatigue related to poor cardiorespiratory endurance. Do not push child past endurance level.
- Child is at high risk for chronic developmental disabilities.

DESIRED OUTCOME/PROGNOSIS

- Child has been weaned from ventilator or dependence has been decreased.
- Child has motor skills at age-appropriate level.
- Child has endurance that is age appropriate.
- Child has feeding skills at age-appropriate level.
- Child's overall development is at age-appropriate level.

REFERENCES

Beers MH, Berkow R, eds. *The Merck Manual of Diagnosis and Therapy.* Whitehouse Station, NJ: Merck Research Laboratories; 1999.

Burns YR, Gray PYH, O'Callaghan MJ. Bronchopulmonary dysplasia: a comparative study of motor development to two years of age. *Aust J Physiotherapy.* 1997;43(1):19–25.

Campbell, SK. The infant at risk for developmental disability—Risk related to bronchopulmonary dysplasia. In: Campbell SK, ed. *Decision Making in Pediatric Neurologic Physical Therapy.* New York, NY: Churchill Livingstone; 1999:271–272.

Kahn-D'Angelo L, Unanue RA. The special care nursery—Bronchopulmonary dysplasia. In: Campbell SK, ed. *Physical Therapy for Children.* 2nd ed. Philadelphia, Pa: WB Saunders Co; 2000:845–846.

Kelly MK. Children with ventilator dependence. In: Campbell SK, ed. *Physical Therapy for Children.* 2nd ed. Philadelphia, Pa: WB Saunders Co; 2000:715:719–720.

Burns

ICD-9-CM Codes: 941–945 Burns

APTA Guide Patterns: 6G, 7B, 7C, 7D, 7E

DESCRIPTION

Tissue injury caused by thermal, radiation, chemical, or electrical contact resulting in protein denaturation, burn wound edema, and loss of intravascular fluid volume due to increased vascular permeability (Beers & Berkow, 1999, p. 2434).

Burn-related injuries are a leading cause of death in children younger than 14 years of age. Burns are also a common mechanism of child abuse. In young children most burn injuries occur indoors whereas in adolescence most injuries occur outdoors (Moore, 2001, p. 813).

The same type of burn will result in a different burn depth depending of the age of the child and the location on the body. A young child has not yet fully developed the dermis and thus the heat of burn mechanism penetrates further into the body. Skin varies in thickness on the body surface. It is thickest on the back and palm of the hands. These areas will regenerate faster. Skin is thinnest on the inner arm surface (Moore, 2001, p. 813).

CLASSIFICATION OF BURNS

- Primary mechanism of injury: see Cause below
- Extent of injury: Percent of total body surface area burned
- Rule of nines: Considered unreliable in children younger than 15 years of age because it underestimates burned areas of head and neck areas and overestimates burned areas of the legs.
- Portion of total body surface: Method is adjusted for age groups. For example, head and neck of an infant are considered to be 20% of total body surface whereas in adults the head and neck are considered to be 9%.

DEPTH OF INJURY

- First-degree burns are red, very sensitive to touch, and usually moist. The surface markedly and widely blanches to light pressure; no blisters develop.
- Second-degree burns may or may not produce blisters. The bases of the blisters may be erythematous or whitish with a fibrinous exudate; they are sensitive to touch and blanch to pressure.
- Third-degree burns usually do not produce blisters. The burn's surface may be white and pliable; black, charred, and leathery; or bright red because of fixed Hemiglobin in the subdermal region. Pale third-degree burns may be mistaken for normal skin, but the subdermal vessels do not blanch to pressure. Third-degree burns are generally anesthetic or hypoesthetic. Hairs may be pulled easily from their follicles (Beers & Berkow, 1999, p. 2434).

THICKNESS OF EPIDERMIS AND DERMIS BURNED

- *Superficial* (First degree): superficial epidermis
- *Partial thickness, superficial* (Second degree): epidermis and small portion of dermis
- *Partial thickness, deep* (Second degree): epidermis and a deeper portion of the dermis
- *Full thickness* (Third degree): Total destruction of the epidermis and dermis, may involve deeper tissue such as fascia and tendons, muscle, bone, or subcutaneous fat. Full thickness burns are most common on digits, hands, feet, and over bony prominences including the iliac crest, patella, anterior tibia, and cranium (Moore, 2001, pp. 814–815).

See Table 12.1 for a summary of the classification of burns.

TABLE 12.1
Classification of Burns

Degree	Description
Superficial (first- degree)	epidermis layer is involved
Partial-thickness (second-degree)	
Superficial	outer level of the dermis is involved
Deep	much of the dermis is involved, and there may be alteration in hair follicles and sweat glands
Full-thickness (third-degree)	all of the dermis has been burned
Subdermal (fourth-degree)	All of the tissue from the epidermis to and through the subcutaneous tissue is destroyed. This may include muscle and bone.

CAUSE

Thermal burns may be due to any external heat source capable of raising the temperature of skin and deeper tissues to a level that causes cell death and protein coagulation or charring. The most common causes are flame, scalding liquids, and hot objects or gases contacting the skin. About 95% of burns are thermal injuries.

Radiation burns are most commonly due to prolonged exposure to the sun's ultraviolet radiation (sunburn) but may be due to prolonged or intense exposure to other sources of ultraviolet radiation (eg, from tanning beds) or to source of x-ray or other radiation. This type of burn is rare.

Chemical burns may be due to strong acids or alkalis, phenols, cresols, mustard gas, or phosphorus. All of these agents produce necrosis, which may extend slowing for several hours.

Electrical burns result from the generation of heat, which may reach 5000 degrees Celsius or 9032 degrees Fahrenheit. Because most of the resistance to electrical current occurs where the conductor contacts the skin, electrical burns usually affect the skin and subjacent tissues (Beers & Berkow, 1999, p. 2434).

Although most burns are accidental, about 9% may be the result of abuse from cigarettes, and forcible immersion in a scalding bath (Ratliffe, 1998, p. 296).

ASSESSMENT

AREAS

Postinjury Status
- Developmental status
- Educational level
- Existing medical conditions
- Pain
- Posture and activity that aggravate wound or scar
- Type of burn: evidence of bleeding, signs of infection, and exposed anatomic structures
- Wound issue status: epithelium, granulation, mobility, necrosis, slough, texture, and turgor

Postacute Stage
- Burn scars: scar mobility or pliability, sensation, turgor, texture, banding, and pigmentation
- Edema
- Functional ability
- Gait

- Joint contractures
- Muscle strength
- Pain
- Range of motion (ROM): especially joints adjacent to burned areas

Posthospital Stage
- Accessibility

INSTRUMENTS/PROCEDURES

No specific assessment instruments were identified.

PROBLEMS
- Child often has loss of movement in response to burns especially if the surface area is greater than 12%.
- Child often has pain.
- Child often has edema that may require escharotomy or incision through the burn to relieve pressure and permit circulation to be maintained.
- Child often needs to have necrotic tissue produced by the burn removed.
- Child may develop an infection.
- Child may have peripheral nerve involvement due to electrical injury, edema, metabolic abnormalities, or localized nerve compression or stretching.
- Child may have exposed tendons and joints.
- Child may develop heterotopic bone formation especially if the elbow area is burned.
- Child may develop contractures due to hypertrophic scarring and loss of muscle strength.
- Child may have an amputation.
- Child may exhibit a variety of signs of psychologic distress and depression related to burn care including regression, anxiety, decreased physical activity, withdrawal, behavior problems, decreased social interaction, and play.
- Child may experience continuing disability after discharge from the burn unit.

TREATMENT/MANAGEMENT

A multidisciplinary team is usually assembled to treat burn injuries and generally includes physicians, nursing personnel, occupational therapists, clinical nutritionists, social workers, psychologists, recreational therapists, school teachers, orthotists, and prosthetists in addition to physical therapists. Wounds may be closed by use of autographing, biologic dressing, biosynthetic dressing, artificial skin, or cultured skin.

GENERAL
- Prevent deformities.
- Prevent functional loss of skills.
- Optimize development skills.
- Provide instruction and education to family and child about disability associated with burns.

SPECIFIC
- Work with nursing staff to encourage frequent changes of position every 2 to 4 hours to reduce risk of decubitus and contracture, and facilitate the return of functional movement. Splints may be used to maintain positioning during

unsupervised periods and during sleep. Splint material should be pliable and lightweight. Low-heat thermoplastic material is usually preferred.

- Participate in providing adequate support in different positions to decrease edema.
- Participate in daily or twice daily dressing changes.
- Participate in wound management by providing hydrotherapy that includes non-submersion and submersion techniques. Nonsubmersion usually includes a shower head to allow water to run over the burn wounds while the patient is on a stretcher suspended over a tank or tub. Submersion involves submerging the patient or burned extremity in a tub, tank, or whirlpool that may or may not include water agitation.
- Participate in pain management. Behavior modification may be used including de-sensitization, modeling, operant conditioning, and environmental manipulation.
- Participate in immobilization of joints during period when skin graft is adhering to tissue. Splints are frequently used.
- Maintain or increase active ROM which is usually done in connection with dress-ing changes.
- ROM can be done 4 to 6 days after skin grafting has occurred. Splints may be used to maintain ROM. Splints may be worn 24 hours a day until child can be-come active. Then splints are worn at night.
- Provide stretching of healing skin. Usually gentle passive stretching can occur af-ter day 6 or 7.
- Participate in scar management techniques including use of presized or custom-fit elastic pressure garments, silicone elastomer face mask, and application of Coban or Ace bandages and inserts. Signs that pressure is successful include blanching of scar tissue, flattening of scar, increased softness, decreased edema, minimal blistering and no tingling or numbness. Pressure is typically applied 23 hours a day.
- Increase skin pliability and desensitization of burn areas using modalities such as continuous passive motion, fluidotherapy, and paraffin.
- Increase muscle strength using graded resistive exercises.
- Increase endurance.
- Encourage early ambulation. Lower extremities may require extra padding or foam-soled slippers on the feet and elastic bandages applied from toe to groin using a figure eight wrap technique to avoid venous stasis.
- Increase coordination and physical conditioning. Bicycling, dancing, and swim-ming may be used.
- Increase independence.
- Increase functional activities including play and self-care activities.
- Establish an exercise program to increase movement. The program must be customized to the child and needs to be creative. Computer-generated exercise programs may be one solution. Assistive devices may be helpful to make functional use of limited movements such as extended-length spoon to accommodate lack of elbow flexion and jaw exerciser to maintain stretch on the mouth.
- Facilitate the development of coping behavior.
- If contracture scar bands occur, conforming splints may be used over the volar surface of the neck, hand, wrist, elbow, posterior knee, or dorsum of the ankle and foot to oppose contracture formation. For extensor surfaces of the wrist, hand, the posterior elbow dynamic splints are most effective. For small children, serial casting may be an alternative—especially for the feet and ankles. Casting may be followed by paraffin, massage, ROM exercise, and splints.
- If disabilities continue after hospitalization, reduction of architectural barriers may be needed to facilitate mobility and independence.

PRECAUTIONS/CONTRAINDICATIONS

- Always tell the child in advance what to expect during therapy and encourage the child to assist and participate to the extent possible.
- Gauze should be wrapped distally to proximally on burned extremities.
- Two burned surfaces should not be allowed to touch each other. Each should be wrapped separately including fingers, toes, and ears to prevent webbing and facilitate active and functional movements.
- Skin grafts must be undisturbed to take to the underlying tissue. Joints must be immobilized until the skin graft has taken.
- Cultured skin grows into very fragile skin that is easily cut and bruised and lacks tensile strength. Problems may persist with cultured skin for up to 2 years post treatment.
- The exercise program should not compromise or dislodge lines and airways. Ambulation while the child is still intubated should be monitored closely.
- Pressure applications should be checked to determine when too much or too little pressure is being applied.
- If a splint is used, it should be checked at least once a day for problems such as pain, numbness, tingling, inflammation, or maceration of tissue from a poorly fitted splint or improper application of the splint. Problems with a splint should be corrected immediately to avoid further damage.

DESIRED OUTCOME/PROGNOSIS

Survival and outcome depend in part on the percentage of burned area. In children younger than 15 years of age, there is a 50% mortality rate if the burns are greater than 95% of total body surface area. Infants less than 12 months have a poorer outcome if there is a 30% or greater burned area compared to older children with the same amount of burned area. Health status, physical disability, disfigurement, vocation, and psychosocial function remain factors in outcome after burned areas have healed (Moore, 2001, pp. 813–814).

- Child has functional ROM in all joints.
- Child has muscle strength and endurance expected for age.
- Child has functional skills in self care and mobility which are age appropriate.
- Child has age-appropriate roles within the family, at play, and at school.
- Child participates in home, school, play, and community activities.

REFERENCES

Beers MH, Berkow R, eds. *The Merck Manual of Diagnosis and Therapy*. Whitehouse Station, NJ: Merck Research Laboratories; 1999.

de Linde LG. Rehabilitation of the child with burns. In: Tecklin JS, ed. *Pediatr Phys Ther*. 3rd ed. Philadelphia, Pa: Lippincott Williams and Wilkins; 1999:468–517.

Moore ML. The burn unit. In: Campbell SK, ed. *Phys Ther Child*. 2nd ed. Philadelphia, Pa: WB Saunders Co; 2000:813–839.

Ratliffe KT. Traumatic disorders—Noelle, a young child with severe burns. In: Ratliffe KT. *Clinical Pediatric Physical Therapy: A Guide for the Physical Therapy Team*. St. Louis, Mo: CV Mosby Co; 1998:275–278.

Ratliffe KT. Traumatic disorders—The child with a burn injury. In: Ratliffe KT. *Clinical Pediatric Physical Therapy: A Guide for the Physical Therapy Team*. St. Louis, Mo: CV Mosby Co; 1998:295–302.

Cancer and Pediatric Oncology

ICD-9-CM Codes:

- 171 Neoplasms of connective and other soft tissue, malignant
- 173 Neoplasms of skin, other malignant
- 191 Neoplasms of brain, malignant
- 192 Neoplasms of other and unspecified parts of nervous system, malignant
- 215 Neoplasms of connective and other soft tissues, benign,
- 216 Neoplasm of skin, benign
- 225 Neoplasm of brain and other parts of nervous system, benign
- 237 Neoplasm of uncertain behavior of endocrine glands
- 239 Neoplasms of unspecified nature

APTA Guide Patterns: 5B, 5C, 5D, 5F, 6F, 6G, 7B, 7C, 7D, 7E

DESCRIPTION

A proliferation of cells whose unique trait, loss of normal controls, results in unregulated growth, lack of differentiation, local tissue invasion, and metastasis (Beers & Berkow, 1999, p. 973). The most common types of cancers in children are leukemia (acute lymphoblastic leukemia [ALL], acute myelogenous leukemia [AML], and chronic myelogenous leukemia [CML]); brain and nervous system tumors (see list following); lymphomas (Hodgkins disease and non-Hodgkins lymphoma); kidney (nephroblastoma or Wilms' tumor); bone (osteosarcoma and Ewings sarcoma); and soft tissue tumors occurring in muscle (rhabdomyosarcoma), tendons, bursae, fascia, fibrous tissues, connective tissue, lymphatic or vascular tissues; and eye (retinoblastoma). Leukemia, brain tumors, nervous system tumors, and lymphomas account for over 70% of childhood cancers. The rate of childhood cancers has been increasing 1–2% per year in the past 2 decades but the survival rate is also increasing (Ratliffe, 1998, p. 404). The following are types of nervous system tumors in children (Ratliffe, 1998, p. 406):

- *Astrocytoma:* Two subtypes: Cerebellar and supratentorial. About 50% of childhood tumors are astrocytomas
- *Brain-stem Glioma:* About 15%
- *Craniopharyngioma:* Under 10%
- *Ependymoma:* Under 10%
- *Medulloblastoma:* About 15%
- *Neuroblastoma:* No data

CAUSE

There are many known causes but many unknown as well. Among the known are molecular abnormalities such as oncogenes and lack of tumor suppressor genes; chromosomal abnormalities; environmental factors such as viruses, parasites, chemical carcinogenesis, chronic irritation to skin; and several immunologic disorders (Beers & Berkow, 1999, pp. 975–977). However, the specific causes of pediatric cancers are largely unknown.

ASSESSMENT

AREAS

Musculoskeletal
- Muscle strength
- Pain
- Posture: monitor for lateral head tilt in children with brain tumors, scoliosis, kyphosis and leg length discrepancies
- Range of motion (ROM), especially cervical mobility in children with brain tumors and limb mobility in children where amputation is performed

Neurologic
- Balance and equilibrium
- Coordination
- Muscle tone
- Reflexes
- Sensory system: monitor for diplopia, field cuts, facial paralysis

Other
- Cardiovascular endurance
- Respiratory status
- Functional status: transfers, gait and mobility
- Developmental and gross motor skills
- Activities of daily living (ADLs) and self-help skills

INSTRUMENTS/PROCEDURES
- Functional Independence Measure for Children (WeeFIM) (Granger, Hamilton, & Kayton, 1989)
- Pediatric Evaluation of Disability Inventory (PEDI) (Haley, Coster, Ludlow, Haltiwanger, & Andrellos, 1992)

PROBLEMS
- Child may have weakness and poor endurance.
- Child may have contractures.
- Child may have a surgical amputation.
- Child may have pain.
- Child may have ataxia, clumsiness, and awkward gait.
- Child may have hemiparesis.
- Child may have high steppage due to peripheral neuropathy.
- Child may have vomiting, anorexia, diarrhea, and weight loss.
- Child may have irritability and fatigue.
- Child may have headaches or seizures.
- Child may have visual disturbances.

TREATMENT/MANAGEMENT

Typical medical interventions include surgery, irradiation, and chemotherapy. Bone marrow transplantation is used in some cases of leukemia that do not respond well to chemotherapy.

GENERAL
- Preventive: avoiding disabling sequelae
- Restorative: maximize motor return
- Supportive: promote greatest level of functional independence possible
- Palliative: Increase or maintain comfort and independence in children in terminal stage

SPECIFIC
- Improve general strength.
- Increase endurance.
- Provide pain management.
- Provide rehabilitation for amputation.
- Prevent or decrease effects of contractures: an ankle splint may be useful.
- Provide mobility including bed mobility and walking retraining.
- Increase ROM—passive and active—through play activities.
- Maintain functional skills through use of play activities.

PRECAUTIONS/CONTRAINDICATIONS
- Use caution in applying resistance to child with low platelet count (thrombocytopenia) to avoid bleeding into muscle or joint and bruising of skin.

DESIRED OUTCOME/PROGNOSIS

Prognosis and outcome depend on the type of cancer and the stage in which treatment begins. Survival rates have increased substantially since the 1960s when less than 20% of children with leukemia survived.

- Child has expected muscle strength for age as seen in age-appropriate play activities.
- Child has normal range of motion without contractures.
- Child does not experience pain or is able to manage the pain.
- Child has functional skills with or without prostheses or orthoses.
- Child is able to ambulate with or without prosthesis.
- Child participates in daily life, school, play, and community activities.

REFERENCES

Beers MH, Berkow R, eds. *The Merck Manual of Diagnosis and Therapy.* Whitehouse Station, NJ: Merck Research Laboratories; 1999.

Kerkering GA, Phillips WE. Brain injuries: Traumatic brain injuries, near-drowning, and brain tumors. In: Campbell SK, ed. *Physical Therapy for Children.* 2nd ed. Philadelphia, Pa: WB Saunders Co; 2000:597–620.

Morgan CR. Pediatric oncology. In: Tecklin JS, ed. *Pediatric Physical Therapy.* 3rd ed. Philadelphia, Pa: Lippincott Williams and Wilkins; 1999:352–377.

Ratliffe KT. Medical disorders—Caroline, a teenager recovering from cancer. In: Ratliffe KT. *Clinical Pediatric Physical Therapy: A Guide for the Physical Therapy Team.* St. Louis, Mo: CV Mosby Co; 1998:385–392.

Ratliffe KT. Medical disorders—Childhood cancers. In: Ratliffe KT. *Clinical Pediatric Physical Therapy: A Guide for the Physical Therapy Team.* St. Louis, Mo: CV Mosby Co; 1998:404–409.

Cerebral Palsy

ICD-9-CM Code 343: Cerebral Palsy
APTA Guide Patterns: 5A, 5B, 6F, 6G, 7A

DESCRIPTION

A term used broadly to describe a number of motor disorders characterized by impaired voluntary movement resulting from prenatal developmental abnormalities, or perinatal or postnatal central nervous system (CNS) damage occurring before age 5. The term cerebral palsy (CP) is not a diagnosis but identifies children with non-progressive spasticity, ataxia, or involuntary movements (Beers & Berkow, 1999, p. 2416).

CP is characterized by impairments of the neuromuscular, musculoskeletal, and sensory systems that are either the immediate result of the existing pathophysiology or are the indirect consequences developed to compensate for the underlying abnormality. The signs often appear to be progressive because the abnormality affects a changing organism in which a developing but abnormal central nervous system attempts to interact with and influence other maturing systems (Howle, p. 23).

CP is not a diagnosis but rather the description of the clinical sequelae resulting from a nonprogressive encephalopathy in an immature brain whose cause may be prenatal, perinatal, or postnatal. Several classifications have been developed to organize the complex nature of CP. Some are described below.

CLASSIFICATION BY TYPE OF IMPAIRMENT

The following classification was adopted in 1956 (Minear) by the American Academy for Cerebral Palsy (now the American Academy for Cerebral Palsy and Developmental Medicine).

- *Spasticity:* characterized by muscles that are perceived as stiff in which velocity-dependent resistance to passive movement produces increased muscle tone; selective control is limited, producing abnormal and limited movement synergies; the active range of motion is limited by coactiviation of muscle activity; and the timing of muscle activation and postural responses is abnormal. Spastic CP is the most common type with *spastic diplegia* as the most common subtype, followed by *spastic hemiplegia,* and *quadriplegia.* The spastic group comprised 75% of all children with CP and is caused by insult to the cortical sensorimotor areas of the brain.
- *Dyskinesia:* characterized by movements which are perceived to be uncontrolled and purposeless. This group includes athetosis, rigidity, and tremor. *Athetosis,* the most common subtype, accounts for 20% of CP cases. Athetosis involves involuntary movements which are poorly executed in timing, direction, and spatial characteristic; impairment of postural stability and abnormal coactivation of muscles that produce abnormal timing and coordination in reversal of motion; increased latency of onset of movement; and oral-motor dysfunction involved in feeding and speech production. In addition there may be hypotonia in infancy and asymmetrical postural alignment. *Rigidity* is characterized by continued resistance to movement throughout the range of motion in both the agonists and antagonists which is not velocity dependent. This type of hypertonicity is often called "lead pipe" rigidity because the tone is increased throughout the range during flexion and extension. *Tremor* is the less common type subtype. Dyskinesia is associated with impairment of the basal ganglia, their connections to the prefrontal and motor cortex, and the role of selective activation or suppression of complex movement sequences.
- *Ataxia:* characterized as impaired postural control of balance and impaired control in the timing of coordinated movement which represents less that 10% of CP cases. Ataxia results from deficits in the cerebellum but the specific symptoms depend on the area that is affected. Specific impairments include impaired postural alignment, anticipatory postural adjustment during movement, and abnormal postural stability. In addition there is usually hypotonia, impaired force and power production during voluntary movement, and impaired motor planning affecting sequencing of speech (dysarthria) and the rhythm and orderly progression for reciprocal gross (dysmetria and ataxia) and fine movements (dysdiadochokinesia).
- *Hypotonia:* characterized by diminished resting muscle tension, a decreased ability to generate voluntary muscle force, excessive joint flexibility, and postural instability. Hypotonia is often a transient stage in the evolution of spasticity and athetosis but is not related to a particular neural lesion. Infants with hypotonia are sometimes called "floppy" infants because their limbs and head seem to flop when not supported.

CLASSIFICATION BY TOPOGRAPHIC DISTRIBUTION
OF TONE, POSTURE, AND MOVEMENT
- *Diplegia:* all limbs involved but the lower body and legs more than the arms
- *Hemiplegia:* involves the arm and leg on one side of the body
- *Paraplegia:* involvement of both lower extremities
- *Quadriplegia:* involves the entire body, with equal or greater involvement of the arms and upper body

- *Double hemiplegia:* a type of quadriplegia in which one side of body is significantly more impaired than the other side (Howle, 1999, p. 25; Styer-Acevedo, 1998, p. 109)

CLASSIFICATION BY DEGREE OF MOTOR DISABILITY

- *Mild:* Describes children with sensorimotor impairments that lead to poorly coordinated and inefficient movement when compared to peers but whose functional limitations are found only in those most advanced gross motor skills used in daily life relative to the child's present chronological age. Such children do not require special assistance or equipment but may require extra time to complete age-appropriate tasks such as dressing, grooming, eating, writing, or crossing the street.
- *Moderate:* Characterized by sensorimotor impairments that produce functional limitation in whole-body functions such as walking, sitting, changing posture, hand use, and speech. Such children are unable to attain motor milestones within normal age limits. With modifications in amount of time, environment, equipment, task, or the addition of physical assistance, such children can participate in most age-appropriate activities.
- *Severe:* Characterized by sensorimotor impairments that produce social disability which restricts the child from performing activities necessary to fulfill normal life roles such as a student in a public school or citizen using public transportation. Activities of daily living (ADLs) cannot be performed because the child lacks balance or the inability to use arms and hands for skilled movements or both. Participation in play or family activities are deficient due to difficulties in communication. The quality of life of both the child and the family is seriously affected.
- *Profound:* Characterized by sensorimotor impairments that are so severe there is no useful or purposeful motor ability and therefore the child is unable to access community or society. Motor dysfunction is so severe the child is unable to change position or sit independently without special equipment, is unable to use arms and hands for feeding or self-care, and is unable to use speech for communication. All ADLs require the assistance of a caregiver and one or more pieces of technology, mobility aids, or special equipment. Health issues are serious complications.

GROSS MOTOR FUNCTION CLASSIFICATION SYSTEM

Note: Classification system marks ability at ages 2, 4, 6, and 12. Only the 2-year-old level is given here as an example of the system. These levels are adapted from Palisano et al (1997):

- *Level 1:* Walks without restrictions: limitations are present in more advanced motor skills. An infant in this category can move in and out of sitting, sit independently on the floor, manipulate objects with the hands before 18 months and is able to ambulate independently before age 2 without assistive devices.
- *Level 2:* Walks without assistive devices: limitations are present in walking outdoors and in the community. An infant in this category is able to maintain sitting position on the floor but needs to use hands to maintain balance, is able to commando or belly crawl, can pull to stand on furniture and begins to cruise before age 2.
- *Level 3:* Walks with assistive mobility devices; limitations are present in walking outdoors and in the community. An infant in this category is able to sit on the floor when the low back is supported, is able to roll and creep forward on the stomach by age 2.
- *Level 4:* Self mobility with limitations; children are transported or use power mobility outdoors and in the community. An infant in this category has head control but truncal support is needed for sitting and is able to roll independently by age 2.

- *Level 5:* Self mobility is severely limited, even with use of assistive technology. An infant in this category has limited voluntary control movement by age 2. The infant is unable to hold up the head or trunk against gravity and requires adult assistance to roll.

CLASSIFICATION BASED ON IMPAIRMENT TO BODY SYSTEMS
- *Single-system impairment:* involves primarily the muscular and skeletal system-generated actions such as insufficient force generation, spasticity, abnormal extensibility, and exaggerated or hyperactive reflexes in the muscular system and malalignments of the skeletal system.
- *Multisystem impairments:* involves the neuromuscular system-controlled actions such as selective control of muscle activity, poor regulation of activity in muscle groups in anticipation of postural changes and body movement and decreased ability to learn unique movements (Olney & Wright, 2001, pp. 536–537).

CAUSE

The cause is often hard to establish, but prematurity, in utero disorders, neonatal jaundice, birth trauma, and perinatal asphyxia play important roles. Birth trauma and perinatal asphyxia probably cause about 15% of cases. Spastic paraplegia is especially common after premature birth, spastic quadriparesis after perinatal asphyxia, and athetoid and dystonic forms after perinatal asphyxia or kernicterus. CNS trauma or severe systemic disease during early childhood (eg, meningitis, sepsis, dehydration) may also cause a CP syndrome (Beers & Berkow, 1999, p. 2416).

The prevalence is 2 per 1,000 births in industrialized countries but is higher in underdeveloped countries. The prevalence has not declined despite improvements in obstetric and perinatal care (Styer-Acevedo, 1998, p.108).

ASSESSMENT

AREAS
- Augmentative communication
- Anticipatory regulation of muscle groups
- Body alignment
- Developmental history: milestones for locomotion, sitting and standing, language and speech, self-help skills, hand use, and current developmental status
- Family and environmental characteristics: includes size of family and household; stability of family environment; cultural standards; family's understanding of disability and expectations for change or improvement; and internal and external resources such as financial, emotional, and intellectual support
- Feeding
- Force generation potential of muscles
- Functional skills
- Gait
- Grip strength
- Joint alignment
- Joint integrity: dislocation potential
- Medical history: prenatal history, problems in pregnancy such as premature birth; perinatal history such as medical complications, multiple birth, anoxia and birth trauma; postnatal course including length of hospital stay, seizures, feeding problems, irritability, and lack of or inappropriate responses
- Mobility and ambulation
- Motor control and motor learning
- Muscle tone
- Muscle strength: isometric, isotonic, endurance

- Postural control, stability, and balance
- Range of motion (ROM): slow, maintained, passive stretch and active
- Respiration
- Seating
- Selective control of muscle groups
- Sensory: includes vision and hearing; behavioral and physiologic characteristics such as orientation and attention, learning style and preferences, adaptability to personal and environmental demands, motivation and cooperation, temperament and emotional stability, and energy levels and endurance
- Spasticity: severity, distribution
- Weight bearing

INSTRUMENTS/PROCEDURES
- anthropometric measurements
- dynamometer
- ergometer
- goniometer
- Alberta Infant Motor Scale (AIMS) (Piper & Darrah, 1994)
- Assessment of Muscle Tone (see Howle, 1999, p. 37)
- Bayley Scales of Infant Development–II (BSID–II) (Bayley, 1993)
- Bruininks-Oseretsky Test of Motor Proficiency (BOTMP) (Bruninks, 1978)
- Canadian Occupational Performance Measure, 3rd ed. (COPM) (Law et al, 1998)
- Functional Independence Measure for Children (WeeFIM) (Granger et al, 1989)
- Gross Motor Function Measure, 2nd ed. (GMFM) (Russell et al, 1993)
- Gross Motor Performance Measure (GMPM) (Boyce et al, 1998)
- modified Ashworth scale (Bohannon & Smith, 1987)
- Movement Assessment of Infants (MAI) (Chandler et al, 1980)
- Peabody Developmental Motor Scales, 2nd ed. (PDMS–2) (Folio & Fewell, 1999)
- Pediatric Evaluation of Disability Inventory (PEDI) (Haley et al, 1992)
- School Function Assessment (SFA) (Coster et al, 1998)
- Sitting Assessment for Children with Neuromotor Dysfunction (SACND) (Reid, 1997)
- Sitting Assessment Scale (SAS) (Myhr & Wendt, 1991)
- Supported Walker Ambulation Performance Scale (SWAPS) (Malouin et al, 1997)
- Test of Infant Motor Performance (TIMP) (Campbell et al, 1993)
- Vineland Adaptive Behavior Scales–Revised (VABS) (Sparrow et al, 1984)
- Vulpe Assessment Battery, 2nd ed. (VAB) (Vulpe, 1994)

PROBLEMS
- Child often has abnormal alignment and distribution in weight bearing: femoral anteversion, femoral and tibial torsion.
- Child often has abnormal muscle tone: spasticity, alternating tone, clonus, hypotonia, abnormal extensibility.
- Child often has impaired balance and postural control.
- Child often has impaired motor control.
- Child often has insufficient force generation and impaired muscle strength.
- Child often has limitations in passive and active ROM.
- Child often has difficulty with mobility and ambulation.
- Child often has difficulty performing functional skills including self-care.
- Child may have joint restrictions or contractures.
- Child may have primitive reflexes that present past the age to which they should be integrated; some may be obligatory, exaggerated, or hyperactive.
- Child may not have developed postural reactions that should be present based on chronological age.

- Child may have poor selective control of muscle activity especially in reciprocal relationships between agonist and antagonist muscles during voluntary movement.
- Child may have poor regulation of activity in muscle groups called anticipatory regulation.
- Child may have decreased ability to learn unique movements.
- Child may have respiratory problems associated with abnormal motor system.
- Child may be difficult to feed or have difficulty eating due to influence of primitive reflexes, tactile defensiveness, and abnormal tone.
- Child may acquire secondary complications to existing impairments such as torticollis and scoliosis.
- Child may have mental retardation or learning disabilities (50–75%).
- Child may have speech and language disorders (25%).
- Child may have auditory impairments (25%).
- Child may have seizure disorders (25–30%).
- Child may have visual disorders (40–50%).
- Child may have problems with drooling (10%).
- Child and family may have social and psychological problems.
- Child may need orthoses, adaptive equipment, or assistive devices.

TREATMENT/MANAGEMENT

Treatment and management usually involves a team approach including medical personnel, educational personnel, family, and community agencies. Medical personnel may include physicians, nurses, nutritionists, occupational therapists, orthotics and prosthetics specialists, recreational therapists, social workers, as well as physical therapists. Educational personnel may include teachers, child-care specialists, psychologists, and speech-language pathologists.

Treatment is based on nine assumptions about normal and abnormal motor development and control. Two approaches have been widely used to treat CP. In North America, the neurodevelopmental treatment (NDT) approach by the Bobaths has been most popular. NDT is based on the assumption that the inhibiting of modifying abnormal reflex patterns and spasticity can improve movement. In Europe, the Vojta approach has been more popular. Vojta assumed that proprioceptive information coming from the trunk and extremities would activate the CNS and act as a guide toward normal motor ontogenesis by eliciting the necessary movement patterns.

Other approaches include Conductive Education developed by Peto that is based on the assumption that problems with motor dysfunction are actually problems of learning.

GENERAL
- Prevent secondary impairments including contractures and deformities.
- Improve alignment and postural control.
- Improve movement in areas of body most involved.
- Develop rotation around the longitudinal body axis with weight shift during transitions.
- Encourage initiation of movement with appropriate body part for the task.
- Increase the variety of movement patterns.
- Increase strength and endurance.
- Provide opportunities for age-appropriate skills needed for self-care and play.
- Educate parents regarding rationale for intervention.
- Educate family about disability to enable them to become advocates for their child.
- Educate family about the condition of CP to enable them to plan for the future.

INFANCY

- Educate family about disorder using instruction, books, computer-generated programs, or videotapes.
- Provide support to family in their acceptance of the child's disability including encouraging the parents to participate in parental support group.
- Assist parents in making decisions about managing their lives and the child's life.
- Foster collaborative goal-setting and programming strategies with the parents.
- Promote ongoing communication between families and service providers.
- Assist parents in making realistic goals for the child.
- Instruct parents and caregivers in handling and caring for the infant including positioning, carrying, feeding, and dressing techniques. For example, the infant should be carried, seated, and fed in a symmetric position that does not allow axial or trunk hyperextension and keeps the hips and knees flexed. Infant should be positioned to allow hands to be seen and practice midline play, reach for feet, or suck on fingers.
- Prevent secondary impairments and limitations by teaching parents to promote symmetry, limit abnormal posturing and movement, and facilitating function motor activity. Encourage a variety of movements and postures to promote senses, encourage use of positions that promote the full lengthening of spastic or hypoextensible muscles, and promote use of positions that facilitate functional voluntary movements of limbs.
- Facilitate optimal sensorimotor experiences and skills.
- Promote well-aligned postural stability.
- Facilitate emergence of motor skills such as reaching, rolling, sitting, crawling, transitional movements, standing, and pre-walking skills.
- Encourage movements that include trunk rotation, dissociation of body segments, weight shifting, weight bearing, and isolate movements using gross motor exercises and activities.
- Use equipment to facilitate attainment of functional positions such as sitting if child is unable to attain or maintain the position independently. Toys may also be used to attain activity that child is unable to perform, such as providing normal oral-motor sensory input.

PRESCHOOL

- Important goals for the child include locomotion, cognition, communication, fine motor skills, self-care, and social abilities. Therapy should be challenging and meaningful to the child and motor skills should be integrated into functional and cognitively directed learning.
- Facilitate achievement of independent mobility. If walking is not feasible, consider manual mobility, such as a tricycle or wheelchair, or powered mobility. If power mobility is considered, fine motor control, cognitive abilities, behavior, environment, visual and auditory abilities as well as financial resources should be considered.
- Continue promotion of gross motor skills through play activities. Encourage parents not to overprotect child during play time.
- Reduce impairments and prevent secondary effects of impairments.
- Facilitate optimal postural alignment and movement of the body through exercise.
- Increase force generation through activities that demand both concentric and eccentric muscle force such as transitional movements, ball gymnastics, games, and use of stairs.
- Contribute to the decisions on managing spasticity with botulinum toxin A (botox injections) or dorsal rhizotomy surgical to selectively cut dorsal nerve rootlets to the lower extremity muscles.

- Contribute to the decisions regarding orthopedic surgery, such as Achilles tendon lengthening.
- Maintain or increase muscle extensibility and joint mobility using manual stretching programs. *Note:* Research suggests a short program of 30–35 minutes reduced spasticity in plantar flexors but not dorsiflexors, and a prolonged stretch of 6 hours prevented muscle-body contracture but did not prevent shortening of the tendon (Onley & Wright, 2001, pp. 546–547). Casting for 3 weeks can be effective for hypoextensiblity if the imbalance is between the triceps surae and dorsiflexor muscles but not if the impairment is due to lack of muscle growth in relation to bone growth.
- Prevent contracture and deformity of lower extremity through use of ankle-foot orthoses (AFOs), solid or hinged, or by use of bivalved casts and therapist-fabricated splints.
- Use equipment to improve positioning as needed to facilitate function, travel, and sleep. Positions in sitting, standing, lying, and for play activities are most important. Seating includes use of strollers, wheelchairs, and car seats. Standing should include movement to provide intermittent loading and muscle strain.
- Use equipment to improve ambulation such as walkers and crutches.
- Work with families and other professionals to determine which goals should be stressed.

SCHOOL-AGE AND ADOLESCENCE
- Continue refinement and increase basic functional skills.
- Continue to provide independent mobility including use of manual and powered mobility. The adolescent may want to participate in driver training.
- Continue promotion of gross motor skills.
- Increase endurance to perform routine activities. Energy expenditure for some children with CP may be 3 times higher than those without CP. Orthoses such as an AFO can reduce energy demands.
- Prevent contractures from developing during periods when bones are growing faster than muscles leading to muscle imbalance and abnormal posturing.
- Maintain muscle extensibility and force generation. Use of ankle weights for 6 weeks may increase stride length and knee flexion (Onley & Wright, 2001, p. 553).
- Maintain joint integrity and mobility. Hypomobility may be treated with manual therapy techniques including joint mobilization.
- Reduce the effects of spasticity. Electrical stimulation may be helpful. Child may be able to reduce their responsiveness to a stretch reflex stimulus. Botulinum toxin A and casting are also helpful.
- Casting may be used to increase ROM by lengthening muscles or tendons.
- Maintain or increase physical fitness through an exercise program and participation in community activities such as horseback riding, swimming, skiing, sailing, canoeing, camping, kayaking, fishing, bungee jumping, yoga, and tai chi.
- Strive for goals that are developed jointly with the child or adolescent.
- Foster self-esteem and assertiveness by emphasizing the child's or adolescent's abilities.
- Recommend or provide environmental accommodations to facilitate accessibility such as ramps to buildings or washroom renovations. Computer-based systems may also be useful to reduce the physical demands on a child in the classroom.
- Assist child and family to make realistic decisions regarding education and social situations.
- Provide instruction to school personnel regarding positioning, lifting, and transferring the child. Other issues may include transportation evacuation and safety.
- Provide instruction to classmates about conditions such as CP and about disability.

- Participate in education about safety in the community including avoiding becoming a victim of crime. Attending a self-defense course should be encouraged and remind the child or adolescent not to carry large sums of money or valuables.

PRECAUTIONS/CONTRAINDICATIONS

- Avoid quick stretch reflex activity on spastic muscles.
- If child takes Baclofen orally, one side effect is drowsiness. A continuous infusion pump may be preferred to reduce the side effect.
- Carryover after use of biofeedback has been found to be limited and poorly generalized to real-life situations.
- Watch for signs of scoliosis in child and adolescent due to spasticity, abnormal extensibility of muscles, muscular imbalance, and decreased force generation.
- Spinal deformity can reduce respiratory status.
- If child or adolescent participates in sports, pay careful attention to the following: comprehensive injury prevention program such as strengthening, flexibility, aerobic and anaerobic training activities, and use of appropriate protective and orthotic equipment.
- Persons with disabilities are at risk of suffering abuse, including sexual abuse from caregivers, personal care attendants, transportation providers, residential care staff, and other disabled individuals. Therapist should be sensitive and receptive to clients who may choose to confide information and should know the proper procedures to follow if abuse is suspected.

DESIRED OUTCOME/PROGNOSIS

CP is a lifelong, pervasive condition even though the original lesion or damage does not change. However, the disabilities do change as the child grows and develops and the demands from the environment increase. Outcomes acceptable at one point in time are not sufficient at another and must be reviewed and revised. Prognosis depends on many interrelated factors, many of which are not under the therapist's control. Positive predictors of independence and employment include completion of high school, independence in mobility and travel, living in a small community, and a diagnosis of spasticity (Olney & Wright, 2001, p. 540). The statements below are general.

- Child has maximum force generation and strength.
- Child has functional ROM.
- Child has endurance to perform daily activities.
- Child has achieved gross motor skills with or without use of assistive technology.
- Child has independent mobility with or without assisted mobility devices.
- Child has functional skills within limits posed by the disability.
- Child demonstrates ability to use assistive technology as needed.
- Child participates in home, school, play, recreational, and community activities.
- Family is able to manage child's needs at home and community including use of assistive technology.
- School personnel are able to manage child's needs at school including use of assistive technology.

REFERENCES

Beers MH, Berkow R, eds. *The Merck Manual of Diagnosis and Therapy*. Whitehouse Station, NJ: Merck Research Laboratories; 1999.

Minear WI. A Classification of cerebral palsy. *Pediatr*. 1956;18:841.

Palisano R, Rosenbaum P, Walter S, et al. The development and reliability of a system to classify gross motor function in children with cerebral palsy. *Dev Med Child Neurol.* 1997; 39(4):214–223.

Bibliography

Almeida GL, Campbell SK, Girolami GL, Penn RD, Corcos DM. Case report. Multidimensional assessment of motor function in a child with cerebral palsy following intrathecal administration of baclofen. *Phys Ther.* 1997;77(7):751–764.

Barry MJ. Physical therapy interventions for patients with movement disorders due to cerebral palsy. *J Child Neurol.* 1996;11(suppl 1):S51–S61.

Beck S. Clinical perspective. Use of sensory level electrical stimulation in the physical therapy management of a child with cerebral palsy. *Pediatr Phys Ther.* 1997;9(3):137–138.

Bertoti DB, Stanger M, Betz RR, Akers J, Maynahom M, Mulcahey MJ. Percutaneous intramuscular functional electrical stimulation as an intervention choice for children with cerebral palsy. *Pediatr Phys Ther.* 1997;9(3):123–127.

Bjornson KF, Graubert CS, Buford VL, McLaughlin J. Validity of the Gross Motor Function Measure. *Pediatr Phys Ther.* 1998;10(2):43–47.

Bjornson KF, Graubert CS, McLaughlin JF, Kerfeld CK, Clark EM. Test-retest reliability of the Gross Motor Function Measure in children with cerebral palsy. *Phys Occup Ther Pediatr.* 1998;18(2):51–61.

Bower E, McLellan DL, Arney J, Campbell MJ. A randomised controlled trial of different intensities of physiotherapy and different goal-setting procedures in 44 children with cerebral palsy. *Dev Med Child Neurol.* 1996;38(3):226–237.

Burstein JR, Wright-Dredhsel ML, Wood A. Assistive technology. In: Dormans JP, Pellegrino L, eds. *Caring for Children with Cerebral Palsy: A Team Approach.* Baltimore, Md: Paul H. Brookes; 1998:371–390.

Butler PB. A preliminary report on the effectiveness of trunk targeting on achieving independent sitting balance in children with cerebral palsy. *Clin Rehabil.* 1998;12(4):281–293.

Cameron ME, Drummond SJ. Measurements to quantify improvement following a serial casting program for equinus deformity in children with cerebral palsy: a case study. *N Z J Physiotherapy.* 1998;26(1):28–32.

Carmick J. Clinical perspective. Guidelines for the clinical application of neuromuscular electrical stimulation (NMES) for children with cerebral palsy. *Pediatr Phys Ther.* 1997; 9(3):128–136.

Carmick J. Use of neuromuscular electrical stimulation and [corrected] dorsal wrist splint to improve the hand function of a children with spastic hemiparesis [published erratum appears in *Phys Ther.* 1997;77(8):859]. *Phys Ther.* 1997;77(6):661–671.

Comeaux P, Patterson N, Rubin M, Meiner R. Effect of neuromuscular electrical stimulation during gait in children with cerebral palsy. *Pediatr Phys Ther.* 1997;9(3):103–109.

Craig M. Physiotherapy management of cerebral palsy: current evidence and pilot analysis. *Phys Ther Rev.* 1999;4(4):215–228.

Curry JED. Promoting functional mobility. In: Dormans JP, Pellegrino L. *Caring for Children with Cerebral Palsy: A Team Approach.* Baltimore, Md: Paul H. Brookes; 1998:283–310.

Darrah J, Fan JSW, Chen LC, Nunweiler J, Watkins B. Review of the effectiveness of progressive resisted muscle strengthening in children with cerebral palsy: a clinical consensus exercise. *Pediatr Phys Ther.* 1997;9(1):12–17.

Darrach J, Wessel J, Nearingburg P, O'Connor M. Evaluation of a community fitness program for adolescents with cerebral palsy. *Pediatr Phys Ther*. 1999;11(1):18–23.

Duhaime A-C, Albinson-Scull S. Neurosurgical treatment of spasticity. In: Dormans JP, Pellegrino L, eds. *Caring for Children with Cerebral Palsy: A Team Approach*. Baltimore, Md: Paul H. Brookes; 1998:225–242.

Dumas HM, O'Neil ME, Fragala MA. Expert consensus on physical therapy intervention after Botulinum toxin A injection for children with cerebral palsy. *Pediatr Phys Ther*. 2001; 13(3):122–132.

Embrey DG, Adams LS. Clinical applications of procedural changes by experienced and novice pediatric physical therapists. *Pediatr Phys Ther*. 1996;8(3):122–132.

Embrey DG, Guthrie MR, White OR, Dietz J. Clinical decision making by experienced and inexperienced pediatric physical therapists for children with diplegic cerebral palsy. *Phys Ther*. 1996;76(1):20–33.

Embrey DG, Hylton N. Clinical applications of movement scripts by experienced and novice pediatric physical therapists. *Pediatr Phys Ther*. 1995;8(1):3–14.

Embrey DG, Nirider B. Clinical applications of psychosocial sensitivity by experienced and novice pediatric physical therapists. *Pediatr Phys Ther*. 1996;8(2):70–79.

Embrey DG, Yates L, Nirider, G, Hylton N, Adams LS. Recommendations for pediatric physical therapists: making clinical decisions for children with cerebral palsy . . . series of four articles. *Pediatr Phys Ther*. 1996;8(4):165–170.

Engsberg JR, Ross SA, Park TS. Changes in ankle spasticity and strength following selective dorsal rhizotony and physical therapy for spastic cerebral palsy. *J Neurosurg*. 1999; 91(5):727–732.

Farmer SE, Butler PB, Major RE. Targeted training for crouch posture in cerebral palsy: a case report. *Physiotherapy*. 1999;85(5):242–247.

Fetters L, Kluzik J. The effects of neurodevelopmental treatment versus practice on the reaching of children with spastic cerebral palsy. *Phys Ther*. 1995;76(4):346–358.

Fowler EG, Ho TW, Nwigwe AI, Dorey FJ. The effect of quadriceps femoris muscle strengthening exercises on spasticity in children with cerebral palsy. *Phys Ther*. 2001:81(6): 1215–1223.

Gudjonsdottir B, Mercer VS. Hip and spine in children with cerebral palsy: musculoskeletal development and clinical implications. *Pediatr Phys Ther*. 1997;9(4):179–185.

Haehl V, Giuliani C, Lewis C. Influence of hippotherapy on the kinematics and functional performance of children with cerebral palsy. *Pediatr Phys Ther*. 1999;11(2):89–101.

Haney NB. Muscle strengthening in children with cerebral palsy. *Phys Occup Ther Pediatr*. 1998;18(3/4):149–157.

Harris SR. The effectiveness of early intervention for children with cerebral palsy and related motor disabilities. In: Guralnick MJ. *The Effectiveness of Early Intervention*. Baltimore, Md: Paul H. Brookes; 1997:327–347.

Hartveld A, Hegarty J. Frequent weightshift practice with computerised feedback by cerebral palsied children—four single case experiments. *Physiotherapy*. 1996;82(10):573–580.

Holt KG, Ratliffe R, Jeng S. Head stability in walking in children with cerebral palsy and in children and adults without neurological impairment. *Phys Ther*. 1999;79(12):1153–1162.

Howle JMW. Cerebral palsy. In: Campbell SK, ed. *Decision Making in Pediatric Neurologic Physical Therapy*. New York, NY: Churchill Livingstone; 1999:23–83.

Jelsma J, Iliff P, Kelly L. Patterns of development exhibited by infants with cerebral palsy. *Pediatr Phys Ther*. 1999;11(1):2–11.

Johnson LM, Nelson MJ, McCormack CM, Mulligan HF. The effect of plantarflexor muscle strengthening on the gait and range of motion at the ankle in ambulant children with cerebral palsy: a pilot study. *NZ J Physiotherapy*. 1998:26(1):8–14.

Jonsdottir J, Fetter L, Kluzik J. Effects of physical therapy on postural control in children with cerebral palsy. *Pediatr Phys Ther*. 1997;9(2):68–75.

Kolobe THA, Palisano RJ, Stratford PW. Comparison of two outcome measures for infants with cerebral palsy and infants with motor delays. *Phys Ther*. 1998;78(10):1062–1072.

Law M, Darrah J, Pollock N, King G, Rosebaum P, Russel D, et al. Family-centered functional therapy for children with cerebral palsy: an emerging practice model. *Phys Occup Ther Pediatr*. 1998;18(1):83–102.

Leach J. Children undergoing treatment with botulinum toxin: the role for the physical therapists. *Muscle and Nerve Supplement*. 1997;6:S194–S207.

Lepage C, Noreau L, Bernard P. Association between characteristics of locomotion and accomplishment of life habits in children with cerebral palsy. *Phys Ther*. 1998;78(5):458–469.

MacPhail HEA, Edwards J, Golding J, Miller K, Mosier C, Zwiers T. Trunk postural reactions in children with and without cerebral palsy during therapeutic horseback riding. *Pediatr Phys Ther*. 1998;10(4):143–147.

Malaby L. Cerebral palsy: how PTs improve function through creativity. *HT Magazine for the Healthcare Traveling Professional*. 1997;4(5):18–25.

Malouin F, Richards CL, Menier C, Dumas F, Marcoux S. Supported Walker Ambulation Performance Scale (SWAPS): development of an outcome measure of locomotion status in children with cerebral palsy. *Pediatr Phys Ther*. 1997;9(2):48–53.

McAuliffe CA, Wenger RE, Schneider JW, Gaebler-Spira DJ. Usefulness of the Wee-Functional Independence Measure to detect functional change in children with cerebral palsy. *Pediatr Phys Ther*. 1998;10(1):23–28.

McKenzie M, Taylor L, Cummings GS, Andrews PD. Prevalence of muscle trigger points in children with cerebral palsy. *Phys Occup Ther Pediatr*. 1997;17(4):47–59.

McGee, Curry JED, Dormans JP. Postsurgical management of cerebral palsy. In: Dormans JP, Pellegrino L, eds. *Caring for Children with Cerebral Palsy: A Team Approach*. Baltimore, Md: Paul H. Brookes; 1998:193–224.

Montgomery PC. Predicting potential for ambulation in children with cerebral palsy. *Pediatr Phys Ther*. 1998;10(4):148–155.

Mulligan H, Climo K, Nanson C, Mauga P. Physiotherapy treatment intensity for a child with cerebral palsy: a single case study. *NZ J Physiotherapy*. 2000;28(2):6–12.

Murphy W. Clinical problem solving. AFOs and KFOs and surgery in cerebral palsy—what to use when? *Physiotherapy Res Int*. 1995;1(4):213–220.

Muthukumaraswamy GE. Abduction contractures in cerebral palsy children: two case studies. *NZ J Physiotherapy*. 1996;24(3):19.

Mweshi MM, Mpofu R. The perceptions of parents and caregivers on the causes of disabilities in children with cerebral palsy: a qualitative investigation. *S Afr J Physiotherapy*. 2001;57(2):28–31.

Nordmark E, Hagglung G, Jarnlo GB. Reliability of the Gross Motor Function Measure in cerebral palsy. *Scand J Rehabil Med*. 1997;29(1):25–28.

Nordmark E, Jarnlo GB, Hagglund G. Comparison of the Gross Motor Function Measure and Paediatric Evaluation of Disability Inventory in assessing motor function in children undergoing selective dorsal rhizotomy. *Dev Med Clin Neurol*. 2000;42(4):245–252.

Olney SJ, Wright MJ. Cerebral palsy. In: Campbell SK, ed. *Phys Ther Child*. 2nd ed. Philadelphia, Pa: WB Saunders Co; 2000:533–571.

Pape KE. Therapeutic electrical stimulation (TES) for the treatment of disuse muscle atrophy in cerebral palsy. *Pediatr Phys Ther*. 1997;9(3):110–112.

Radtka SA, Skinner SR, Dixon DM, Johanson ME. A comparison of gait with solid, dynamic, and no ankle-foot orthoses in children with spastic cerebral palsy. *Phys Ther*. 1997; 77(4):395–409.

Ratliffe KT. Cerebral palsy. In Ratliffe KT. *Clinical Pediatric Physical Therapy: A Guide for the Physical Therapy Team*. St. Louis, Mo: CV Mosby Co; 1998:163–217.

Richards CL, Malouin F, Dumas F, Marcoux S, Lepage C, Menier C. Early and intensive treadmill locomotor training for young children with cerebral palsy: a feasibility study. *Pediatr Phys Ther*. 1997;9(4):158–165.

Quint C, Toomey M. Powered saddle and pelvic mobility: an investigation into the effects on pelvic mobility of children with cerebral palsy of a powered saddle which imitates the MOV of a walking horse. *Physiotherapy*. 1998:84(8):376–384.

Scheinberg A, O'Flaherty S, Chaseling R, Dexter M. Continuous intrathecal baclofen infusion for children with cerebral palsy: a pilot study. *J Pediatr Child Health*. 2001:37(3): 283–288.

Shaw MI. Botulinum toxin in the treatment of spasticity in children with cerebral palsy. *Phys Occup Ther Pediatr*. 1997;17(4):65–75.

Stamer, M. *Posture and Movement of the Child with Cerebral Palsy*. San Antonio, Tex: Therapy Skill Builders; 2000.

Stanger M, Bertoti D. An overview of electric stimulation for the pediatric population. *Pediatr Phys Ther*. 1997;9(3):95–143.

Styer-Acevedo J. Physical therapy for the child with cerebral palsy. In: Tecklin JS, ed. *Pediatric Physical Therapy*. 3rd ed. Philadelphia, Pa: Lippincott Williams and Wilkins; 1999:107–162.

Trahan J, Malouin F. Changes in the gross motor function measure in children with different types of cerebral palsy: an eight-month follow-up study. *Pediatr Phys Ther*. 1999; 11(1):12–17.

Tyson S. Case report. The use of musculoskeletal techniques in adult cerebral palsy. *Physiotherapy Res Int*. 1998;3(4):292–295.

Valvano J, Newell KM. Practice of a precision isometric grip-force task by children with spastic cerebral palsy. *Dev Med Child Neurol*. 1998;40(7):464–473.

Vogtle LK, Morris DM, Denton BG. An aquatic program for adults with cerebral palsy living in group home. *Phys Ther Case Rep*. 1998;1(5):150–159.

Walker JS, Stanger M. Orthotic management. In: Dormans JP, Pellegrino L. *Caring for Children with Cerebral Palsy: A Team Approach*. Baltimore, Md: Paul H. Brookes; 1998: 391–438.

Wiepert SL, Lewis CL. Effects of a 6-week progressive exercise program on a child with right hemiparesis. *Phys Ther Case Rep*. 1998;1(1):21–26.

Wright FV, Belbin G, Slack M, Jutaie J. An evaluation of the David Hart Walker Orthosis: a new assistive device for children with cerebral palsy. *Physiotherapy Can*. 1999;51(4):280–291.

Wright FV, Liu G, Milne F. Reliability of the measurement of time-distance parameters of gait: a comparison in children with juvenile rheumatoid arthritis and children with cerebral palsy. *Physiotherapy Can*. 1999;51(3):191–200.

Young NL, Wright JG, Lam TP, Pajaratnum K, Stephens D, Wedge JH. Windswept hip deformity in spastic quadriplegic cerebral palsy. *Pediatr Phys Ther*. 1998;10(3):94–100.

Cognitive Disorders and Mental Retardation

ICD-9-CM Codes:
- 317 Mild mental retardation
- 318 Other specified mental retardation
- 318.0 Moderate mental retardation
- 318.1 Severe mental retardation
- 328.2 Profound mental retardation
- 319 Unspecified mental retardation

APTA Guide Pattern: 5A

DESCRIPTION

The American Association on Mental Retardation (AAMR) defines mental retardation as "substantial limitation in present functioning. It is characterized by significantly subaverage intellectual functioning, existing concurrently with related limitations in two or more of the following applicable adaptive skills areas: communication, self-care, home living, social skills, community use, self-direction; health and safety, functional academics, leisure , and work. Mental retardation manifests before age 18." (AAMR, 1992, p. 1)

The diagnostic criteria stated in the *Diagnostic and Statistical Manual of Mental Disorders* includes 1) significantly subaverage intellectual function: an IQ of approximately 70 or below on an individually administered IQ test (for infants, a clinical judgment of significantly subaverage intellectual functioning), 2) concurrent deficits or impairments in present adaptive functioning (ie, the person's effectiveness in meeting the standards expected for his or her age by his or her cultural group) in at least two of the following areas: communication, self-care, home living, social/interpersonal skills, use of community resources, self-direction, functional academic skills, work, leisure, health, and safety, and 3) onset before the age of 18 (American Psychiatric Association, 1995, p. 46). See Table 12.2.

About 50% of children with mental retardation have mild deficits, 30% have moderate retardation, 15% have severe retardation, and 5% are profoundly retarded (Ratliffe, 1998). A complex relationship exists between motor impairment and other domains such as spatial cognition and psychosocial development such as self-awareness. There may be links between independent mobility and the growth of some brain structures related to the ability to cope with the environment (McEwen, 2001, p. 509).

TABLE 12.2
Mental Retardation Classification

IQ Level	Retardation Level
From 50–55 to approximately 70	Mild
From 35–40 to approximately 50–55	Moderate
From 20–25 to approximately 35–40	Severe
Below approximately 20–25	Profound
Strong presumption of mental retardation but the client's intelligence is untestable by standardized testing	Mental retardation, Severity unspecified

Source: American Psychiatric Association; 1995.

CAUSE

According to the APA, etiological factors may be primarily biological, primarily psycho-social, or a combination of both. In approximately 30–40% of individuals no clear etiology can be determined despite evaluation efforts. Major predisposing factors include: heredity (approximately 5%), early alterations of embryonic development (approximately 30%), pregnancy and perinatal problems (approximately 10%), general medical conditions acquired in infancy or childhood (approximately 5%), and environmental influences and other mental disorders (approximately 10–20%) (APA, 1995, p. 43). Common biological causes include genetic defects such as Down syndrome and fragile X syndrome. Organic causes include maternal drug abuse, alcohol abuse, and viral infection. Perinatal causes includes asphyxia and birth trauma. Sociocultural causes include neglect and abuse, environmental deprivation, lack of education, lack of opportunity, and cultural differences (Ratliffe, 1998).

Some examples of disorders in which cognitive impairments are known to occur are cerebral palsy, cri-du-chat syndrome, cytomegalovirus infection, deLange syndrome, Down syndrome, fetal alcohol syndrome, fragile X syndrome, Hurler syndrome, Lesch-Nyhan syndrome, lissencephaly, Prader-Willi syndrome, Rett syndrome, and Williams syndrome (McEwen, 2001).

ASSESSMENT

The label of cognitive impairment or mental retardation requires administration and interpretation of a standardized, norm-referenced measure of intelligence usually by a psychologist or psychometrist. Physical therapists may assist by providing an optimal environment in which a child with motor impairment can give the best performance possible. Attention to positioning to enhance communication, eye contact, and hand use are examples. Determination of alternative response models may also be useful to the examiner. In addition, physical therapists may contribute by evaluating degree and type of motor impairment as part of the data used in determining placement of the child in school or eligibility for services. In infants, the physical therapist may be involved in test administration to assess cognitive abilities because many of the test items focus on an infant's sensorimotor development to determine cognitive performance.

AREAS

- Adaptive behavior
- Developmental milestones
- Endurance
- Functional skills
- Gross motor skills
- Joint flexibility
- Mobility skills
- Muscle strength and force production
- Muscle tone
- Postural control and balance
- Range of motion (ROM)
- Reflexes and reactions
- Self-help skills
- Need for assistive devices

INSTRUMENTS/PROCEDURES

Intelligence (typically not administered by a physical therapist)
- Columbia Mental Maturity Scale (Burgemeister et al, 1972)
- Fagan Text of Infant Intelligence (FTII) (Fagan & Shepherd, 1987)
- Kaufman Assessment Battery for Children (Kaufman & Kaufman, 1983)
- Raven's Progressive Matrices (Raven, 1958)
- Stanford-Binet Intelligence Scale (Terman & Merrill, 1973)
- Wechsler Intelligence Scale for Children (WISC-R) (Wechsler, 1974)

Adaptive Behavior (may be administered by a physical therapist)
- AAMR Adaptive Behavior Scales (Nihira et al, 1974)
- Battelle Developmental Inventory (Newborg et al, 1984)

- Canadian Occupational Performance Measure, 3rd ed. (COPM) (Law et al, 1994)
- Vineland Adaptive Behavior Scales, 2nd ed. (Sparrow et al, 1992)

PROBLEMS
- Child often has delays in acquisition of developmental skills including gross motor, fine motor, self-care, communication, and psychosocial skills.
- Child often has difficulty learning new tasks.
- Child often has difficulty generalizing learning from one situation to another.
- Child may have behavioral disorders.
- Child may have cardiopulmonary impairments such as congenital heart disease, pulmonary valvular stenosis, mitral stenosis, atrial septal defect, neonatal respiratory problems, recurrent upper respiratory tract infections, lung hypoplasia with pulmonary hypertension, heart murmur, mitral value prolapse, cardiac enlargement, hyperventilation and apnea.
- Child may have musculoskeletal impairments such as scoliosis, kyphosis, small status, small hands and feet, shot digits, joint hyperflexibility, ligamentous laxity, foot deformities, atlantoaxial instability, joint anomalies, hyperextensible joints, contractures, irregularly shaped bones, hip subluxation, and equinovarus deformities.
- Child may have neurologic impairments in areas such as force production, coordination, motor planning, postural control, postural reactions, balance, endurance, efficiency, hypotonia, hypertonia, spasticity, seizures, slow reaction time, feeding problems, visual motor deficits, ataxia, choreothestosis, dystonic, hyperkinesia, bradykinesia, stereotypic hand movements, drooling, and involuntary tongue movement.
- Child may have sensory deficits or dysfunctions.
- Child may have metabolic disorders.
- Child may have multiple system impairments.

TREATMENT/MANAGEMENT

Treatment and management are generally conducted using a team approach. The transdisciplinary model is recommended for children with severe and multiple disabilities. Typically, there is a primary service provider who spends the greatest amount of time with the child or has the skills necessary to address the largest number of the child's problems and needs. If service begins in infancy, the provider may be a parent or physical therapist. When the child begins school, a teacher may become the primary service provider. Other team members may include a special education teacher, school psychologist, occupational therapist, speech-language pathology, as well as the physical therapist. The team should determine which domains are most important: home, community, vocation, or recreation-leisure; determine the specific environments and subenvironments in which functions should be addressed; determine the activities needed to function in the subenvironment; and determine the skills needed to perform each activity. The "top-down" approach or hypothesis-oriented algorithm for clinicians (HOAC) are useful in planning for children with cognitive impairments. The team decides which functional outcomes should be addressed and identifies why the child can or cannot meet the desired outcome at the present time (McEwen, 2001).

Therapists should be aware of specific needs of the child that may affect delivery of physical therapy services, such as a behavioral management plan; likes and dislikes; family structure, and medical history. Often a child with mental retardation has related problems including blindness, deafness, severe behavioral challenges, or sensory defensiveness (Ratliffe, 1998). In addition, a child with cognitive impairments requires extra repetitions to learn, has difficulty generalizing (carryover) from one situation to another, and needs repeated practice to maintain skills. Learning "prerequisite" skills independently from the functional outcome in a simulated environment often is unsuccessful. Learning occurs best when the task is learned as a whole within the environment where performance is expected.

According to the APTA's *Guide*, physical therapists should provide (1) coordination, communication, and consultation; (2) student-related instruction; and (3) direct intervention.

- Educate family and other caregivers on management techniques for handling, carrying, and positioning child for daily care activities including diaper changes.
- Improve gross motor skills including mobility skills of the child, especially crawling, walking, and transfers.
- Provide consultation on use of one or more mobility devices such as crutches, strollers, and manual or electric wheelchairs for those who need assistance to achieve independent mobility. Studies suggest a child with normal intelligence can learn to use powered mobility at age 20 months (McEwen, 2001, p. 509). Children with cognitive impairments should also be capable of learning to use powered equipment sometime after that age depending on degree of cognitive impairment, experience with movement, and visual skills.
- Increase amount of time spent in upright, seated position. Recommend seating and other assistive positioning devices that can assist the child in interactions with the physical and social environment including variables such as hand function, switch activation, respiration, and communication with others. Upright positions can facilitate learning by increasing level of arousal, alertness, and interaction with teachers (McEwen, 2001, p. 510).
- Increase opportunity for exploration of various environments and manipulation of a variety of objects including toys and household items.
- Increase functional skills that facilitate participation in education such as hand skills.
- Decrease or prevent secondary impairments such as contractures.
- Provide consultation on selection and use of assistive technology that may be useful to the child in the classroom such as a computer, adapted seating, or standing frame.
- Provide consultation on selection and use of adapted equipment to facilitate participation in sports or other recreational activities.
- Provide consultation on environmental modifications to facilitate accessibility to the home, school, and community.
- Manage behavioral problems through behavioral programming. Positive reinforcement involves giving a reinforcer immediately after a behavior. Common positive reinforcers are food, stickers, praise, attention, or access to a favorite activity such as watching a video, playing a game, or listening to music. Shaping a behavior involves rewarding successive approximations of the desired behavior through instructions, models, cues, or physical prompts. Shaping makes use of antecedent events that are set up or determined in advance of the child's behavior. Backward chaining involves learning the last step in the sequence first, then the second to last, next the third to the last and so forth until the behavior is learned in total. Backward chaining provides a reward because the task is always completed and there is automatically a consequence.
- Participate in promoting effective communication through use of signs, communication boards, or electronic voice-output communication aids.
- Educate school personnel and other children about the child's abilities, disabilities, and how to help him or her participate in activities.
- For adolescents, participate in planning for vocational training and employment by providing information about the child's ability to perform job-related motor skills and assist in identifying jobs that are compatible with those skills.
- Participate in planning for independent living if adolescent is able to leave home or residential care if adolescent is unable to live at home.

PRECAUTIONS/CONTRAINDICATIONS
- Some children with mental retardation also have a seizure disorder.
- Some children with mental retardation have severe behavioral problems managed using a specific behavior plan which should be followed by the therapist during treatment to provide consistency by all adults with whom the child comes in contact.
- Cognitive impairment limits the ability to learn to use assistive technology, increases learning time, and safety is an important consideration.

DESIRED OUTCOME/PROGNOSIS

A child with mild or moderate mental retardation should attain advanced mobility skills and personal care skills. A child with severe mental retardation should attain basic mobility skills and elementary personal care skills. Most can live in group homes or with families unless there are associated disabilities that require specialized care. A child with profound mental retardation may not acquire basic mobility skills and can often perform only limited personal skills. They typically require supervised living arrangements in sheltered settings (APA, 1995).

- Child has independent means of mobility. Child with profound cognitive impairment may perform parts of mobility task such as increasing body movements used to activate switch on power chair.
- Child performs functional skills that are age appropriate. Child with profound cognitive impairment may perform parts of functional skills such as indicating a choice of food or activity.
- Child participates in home, community (eg, school, stores, and church), vocational, and recreation-leisure activities.

REFERENCES

American Association of Mental Retardation. *Mental Retardation: Definition, Classification and System of Supports*. 9th ed. Washington, DC: The Association; 1992:1.

American Psychiatric Association. *Diagnostic and Statistical Manual of Mental Disorders*. 4th ed. Washington, DC; 1995:39–46.

Lunnen KY. Children with multiple disabilities. In: Campbell SK. *Decision Making in Pediatric Neurologic Physical Therapy*. New York, NY: Churchill Livingstone; 1999:141–197.

McEwen IR. Children with cognitive impairments. In: Campbell SK, ed. *Physical Therapy for Children*. 2nd ed. Philadelphia, Pa: WB Saunders Co; 2000:502–532.

Ratliffe KT. Sensory, processing, and cognitive disorders of childhood—Children with mental retardation. In: Ratliffe KT. *Clinical Pediatric Physical Therapy: A Guide for the Physical Therapy Team*. St. Louis, Mo: CV Mosby Co; 1998:321–324.

Congenital and Acquired Limb Deficiencies and Amputations

Also known as *congenital limb deficiencies*.

ICD-9-CM Codes:
- 755 Other congenital anomalies of limbs
- 755.3 Reduction deformities of lower limb
- 897 Traumatic amputation of leg(s) complete or partial

APTA Guide Pattern: 4K

DESCRIPTION

Transverse or longitudinal limb deficiencies due to primary intrauterine growth inhibition or secondary intrauterine destruction of normal embryonic tissues. In transverse deficiencies, all elements beyond a certain level are absent, and the limb resembles an amputation stump. In longitudinal deficiencies, specific maldevelopments occur, eg, complete or partial absence of the radius, fibula, or tibia. Infants with transverse or longitudinal limb deficiencies may also have hypoplastic or bifid bones, synostoses, duplications, dislocations, or other body defects (Beers & Berkow, 1999, p. 2221).

CAUSE

The etiology of congenital amputation is often unclear, but teratogenic agents and amniotic bands are two known causes.

Causes of traumatic amputation vary according to age and geographic location. Accidents involving farm machinery, power tools and machinery, motor vehicle accidents, gunshot wounds, and railroad accidents are the leading causes of traumatic amputation in pediatrics. Lawn mowers and household accidents account for most amputations in the 1- to 4-year-old population, whereas vehicular accidents, gunshot wounds, power tools, and machinery are common causes of traumatic amputation in older children. Acquired amputations from both trauma and disease such as cancer account for about 40% of amputations in childhood, whereas congenital limb deficiencies account for 60% of childhood amputations. Young teenagers, ages 12 to 16, have the highest incidence of traumatic amputation (Stanger, 1998, p. 408–409).

ASSESSMENT

AREAS
- Development
- Environment in which the child needs to function
- Functional skills

INSTRUMENTS/PROCEDURES

No specific instruments were identified.

PROBLEMS
- Child is missing part or all of one or more bones in either the upper or lower extremities.
- Child may have lax or absent ligaments.
- Child may be missing specific muscles.
- Child may have soft tissue contractures.
- Child may have muscle weakness caused by the decreased lever arm or decreased length-to-strength ratio of the muscle.
- Child may have difficulty performing or be unable to perform functional skills.

TREATMENT/MANAGEMENT

Surgical management may include amputation to provide more stability and function, arthrodesis to fuse a joint for increased stability, rotation plasty to increase function, or tendon transfers to allow more functional use in the hand.

Treatment will usually involve a team management approach including the orthopedic physician, prosthetist, physical therapist, occupational therapist, teacher, family, and the child. Physical therapy services may be provided in the home, at school, or in an outpatient rehabilitation clinic.

GOALS
- Increase developmental skills.
- Increase functional skills.
- Decrease or reduce secondary impairments such as soft tissue contractures.

INFANT AND TODDLER
- Instruct caregivers on handling techniques.
- Instruct caregivers on techniques to promote normal development.
- Encourage symmetrical movements, weight bearing, and posture to counter the effects of the intrinsically asymmetrical limb deficiency.
- Encourage strength, coordination, and range of motion (ROM) by facilitating reaching with both upper extremities, rolling to both sides, pushing up to sit from both directions, turning and reaching to both sides in sitting and weight bearing through all extremities in a variety of positions.
- Encourage use of prosthesis to improve functional skills. Early introduction to a prosthesis increases the amount of motor development (Ratliffe, 1998, p. 107). An upper extremity prosthesis should be provided by age 8 months. A child with proximal femoral focal deficiency should be fitted with a preliminary lower extremity prosthesis by the time the child is developmentally ready to stand, ie, about 8–10 months.

PRESCHOOL AND EARLY SCHOOL-AGED CHILD
- Instruct caregivers in how to put on and take off the prosthesis and how to care for it. Instruct the child when he or she is able to assume responsibility. If the child is in school, the teacher should also know how to put on and take off the prosthesis.
- Instruct caregivers in how to care for and inspect the stump and on how to wrap the stump.
- Instruct caregivers on developmental activities to promote the use of the prosthesis by the child.
- Work with the teacher to help adapt the environment or activities in the school for child. Examples of adaptation may include raising or lowering the chair height to provide the optimal angle for writing and drawing, arranging the tables or desks into islands so the child using crutches does not need to negotiate individual tables or desks, or adapting circle games so the child using crutches can play.
- At about 15–18 months, a child with upper extremity deficiency should have a simple terminal device that will grasp and release objects. At 5 to 6 years a myoelectric upper extremity prosthesis can be considered. However the benefits and potential problems should be weighed carefully.
- At about 3 years of age, the child with a lower extremity limb deficiency is ready to operate a simple prosthetic knee. Begin by using a walker and progress to independent balance.
- Monitor the fit of the prosthetic device to reduce or avoid skin breakdown. If the limb deficiency is due to trauma, the stump must be monitored for edema.
- Monitor the ROM of related joints.
- Monitor strength of related muscles to encourage optimal functional skills.
- Promote appropriate movement transitions and mobility skills such as rolling, pulling to stand, and walking.
- Assist team members in promoting self-care skills, language, and communication skills.

SCHOOL-AGED CHILD AND ADOLESCENT
- Work with child and adolescent to solve problems that are experienced with various activities.

- Be aware that a child without upper extremities will learn to use feet, mouth, or chin for self-care skills and schoolwork even if an upper extremity prosthesis is available.
- Provide training in more advanced gait activities such as running, jumping, and skipping.
- An older child with a lower extremity limb deficiency may decide to use forearm crutches rather than a prosthesis. His or her wishes should be respected.
- Provide child with information about the Paralympics and support sports activity if child is interested.
- Assist adolescent's interest in learning to drive with adapted controls.

PRECAUTIONS/CONTRAINDICATIONS
- Always check the skin under the prosthesis for signs of pressure sores.
- Children younger than 6 should not be taught to use crutches.

DESIRED OUTCOME/PROGNOSIS
- Child can care for stump including checking the stump for redness or breakdown.
- Child can use prosthesis for lower or upper extremity functions.
- Child can perform functional skills with or without the prosthesis.
- Child can participate in home, school, recreational, and community activities.

REFERENCES

Beers MH, Berkow R, eds. *The Merck Manual of Diagnosis and Therapy.* Whitehouse Station, NJ: Merck Research Laboratories; 1999.

Ratliffe KT. Developmental orthopedic disorders—congenital limb deficiencies. In: Ratliffe KT. *Clinical Pediatric Physical Therapy: A Guide for the Physical Therapy Team.* St. Louis, Mo: CV Mosby Co; 1998:105–109.

Stanger M. Orthopedic management—amputations. In: Tecklin JS, ed. *Pediatric Physical Therapy.* 3rd ed. Philadelphia, Pa: Lippincott Williams and Wilkins; 1999:408–410.

Stanger M. Orthopedic management—congenital limb deficiencies. In: Tecklin JS, ed. *Pediatric Physical Therapy.* 3rd ed. Philadelphia, Pa: Lippincott Williams and Wilkins; 1999: 387–394.

Stranger M. Limb deficiencies and amputations. In: Campbell SK, ed. *Physical Therapy for Children.* 2nd ed. Philadelphia, Pa: WB Saunders Co; 2000:370–397. In: Campbell SK, ed. *Physical Therapy for Children.* 2nd ed. Philadelphia, Pa: WB Saunders Co; 2000: 406–411.

Congenital Heart Disease

ICD-9-CM Codes:
- 427 Cardiac dysrhythmias
- 425 Cardiomyopathy
- 747 Other congenital anomalies of circulatory system

APTA Guide Patterns: 5B, 5G, 6D, 6E

DESCRIPTION

Anatomic defects of the heart and great vessels produced at various stages of fetal development and present at birth (Beers & Berkow, 1999, p. 2198).

CLASSIFICATION
- *Acyanotic congenital heart diseases:* Blood is adequately saturated with oxygen but poorly distributed to the body.
- *Patent ductus arteriosus:* Failure of the ductus to close shortly after birth allows blood to go to the lungs for gas exchange. The function during fetal life is to shunt blood from the pulmonary artery to the descending aorta and away from the lungs, which do not participate in gas exchange during fetal life. After birth, the hemodynamic abnormality results in poorly oxygenated blood.
- *Atrial septal defect:* Abnormal communication between the atria, which results in a left-to-right shunt of blood at the site of abnormality in the atria.
- *Ventricular septal defect:* Hemodynamic changes from ventricular septal defects are a left-to-right shunt at the site of the abnormal communication between the ventricles.
- *Cyanotic congenital heart diseases:* Poorly oxygenated saturation of the blood.
- *Tetralogy of Fallot:* Defects include ventricular septal defect, pulmonary artery stenosis, right ventricular hypertrophy, and an aorta that overrides the interventricular septum. Hemodynamic abnormalities include a right-to-left shunt into the ascending aorta resulting in inadequate oxygenation, which results in cyanosis and associated dyspnea and syncopal episodes.
- *Anomalous pulmonary venous return:* All or part of the pulmonary venous circulation enters the right atrium rather than the left atrium, which occurs because there is direct connection of the atrium or anastomosis with systemic veins. Systemic oxygen desaturation may occur as well as right ventricular hypertrophy.
- *Transposition of the great vessels:* The aorta arises from the right ventricle and pulmonary artery is attached to the left ventricle. The body receives only deoxygenated blood from the right heart (aorta), whereas the pulmonary circulation receives fully oxygenated flood from the left heart (pulmonary artery).
- *Tricuspid atresia:* Failure of the value between the right atrium and ventricle to form, which allows oxygenated and unoxygenated blood to mix in the left side of the heart.
- *Hypoplastic left heart syndrome:* The left ventricle is poorly formed and is not functional in pumping oxygenated blood to the tissues.

CAUSE

A specific cause can sometimes be identified. Some chromosomal deficits such as Trisomy 13 or 18 may cause severe congenital cardiac anomalies, whereas others such as Trisomy 21, Turner's syndrome, and Holt-Oram syndrome may cause less severe anomalies. Material illness such as diabetes mellitus; systemic lupus erythematosus; rubella; environment exposures such as thalidomide, isotretinoin, alcohol; or a combination of these may be implicated (Beers & Berkow, 1999, p. 2198).

Incidence is about 5 to 8 per 1,000 live births (Tasso, 1999, p. 71). Ratliffe reports 8 to 10 per 1,000 (1998, p. 396).

ASSESSMENT

AREAS
- Motor development skills
- Muscle strength and endurance

INSTRUMENTS/PROCEDURES
- Denver II (Frankenburg et al, 1990)
- Pediatric Evaluation of Disability Inventory (PEDI) (Haley et al, 1992)

PROBLEMS

- Child may have congestive heart failure.
- Child may have pulmonary vascular obstructive disease.
- Child may have pulmonary hypertension.
- Child may have right ventricular hypertrophy.
- Child may have cyanosis and associated dyspnea and syncopal episodes.
- Child may have respiratory distress.
- Child may have diaphoresis (inappropriate sweating).
- Child may fatigue quickly.
- Child may have tachycardia.
- Child may have decreased blood pressure.
- Child may have cool extremities, blue lips or nail beds, or be pale in color.
- Child may breathe fast.
- Child may cough or wheeze.
- Child may be underweight.
- Child may have seizures.
- Child may require suctioning.
- Child may have damage to the nervous system or musculoskeletal system due to lack of the cardiorespiratory system's ability to meet the metabolic demands for the development of strength and gross motor skills.
- Child may have decreased muscle strength and endurance, including weakness of the cervical flexors and extensors and lack of co-contraction of the cervical muscles.
- Child may demonstrate scapular winging in weight bearing.
- Child may have difficulty with midline positions and reaching skills.
- Child may have depressed or hypoactive reflexes.
- Child may experience developmental delays as a result of poor tolerance to activity.
- Child may experience problems as a result of surgical repair including choreoathetosis, cerebral palsy, and hemiplegia.

TREATMENT/MANAGEMENT

- During infancy, the role is to teach the parents about positioning and handling.
- Increase muscle strength and endurance as cardiac condition allows.
- Promote attainment of developmental skills: sitting, standing, walking. Begin by increasing cervical flexor and extensor strength for improved antigravity head control. Progress to improving tolerance to the prone position, continue to facilitate prone on elbows with assistance. Move to improving trunk control in supported sitting, and improving upper extremity strength for reaching against gravity and for upper extremity weight bearing. Program may continue by increasing lower extremity weight bearing and strength to facilitate standing, cruising and ambulation, improving spinal extension in sitting, increasing abdominal strength to improve co-contraction of the trunk musculature in all positions, and facilitate commando crawling on the stomach and creeping in quadruped.
- Encourage participation in age-appropriate activities.
- Provide a home exercise program to promote developmental skills.
- Model to parents positioning and handling for home activities.
- As child grows older, help child learn to monitor signs of cardiac distress.
- Help child maintain a positive attitude toward exercises as well as learning specific exercise skills.

PRECAUTIONS/CONTRAINDICATIONS

- Always observe child's color, respiratory rate, level of sweating, affect, level of fatigue, and level of irritability for signs of cardiac distress. If an oxygen saturation monitor is used, observe for low saturation levels.

- Provide frequent rest periods during therapy session.
- Find alternative positions for lying prone, which children with congenital heart disease may dislike.

DESIRED OUTCOME/PROGNOSIS

- Child has age-appropriate developmental skills.
- Child has expected muscle strength for age.
- Child has expected endurance for age.
- Child performs a daily exercise program including play activities.
- Parents and child are knowledgeable about and can monitor for signs of cardiac distress.

REFERENCES

Beers MH, Berkow R, eds. *The Merck Manual of Diagnosis and Therapy.* Whitehouse Station, NJ: Merck Research Laboratories; 1999.

Carmini V, Damignani R, Brooks D, et al. Preoperative physiotherapy teaching in paediatric cardiac patients. *Physiotherapy Can.* 2000;52(4):312–314.

Ratliffe KT. Medical disorders—Heart disease in children. In: Ratliffe KT. *Clinical Pediatric Physical Therapy: A Guide for the Physical Therapy Team.* St. Louis, Mo: CV Mosby Co; 1998:396–400.

Tasso KH. Gross motor development of a child with multiple congenital heart defects. *Phys Ther Case Rep.* 2000;3(2):71–77.

Congenital Torticollis

Also known as *developmental muscular torticollis, congenital cervical torticollis,* or *muscular torticollis.*

ICD-9-CM Code: 754.1 Of sternocleidomastoid muscle (congenital sternomastoid torticollis)

APTA Guides: 4C, 4E

DESCRIPTION

An infant with congenital torticollis presents with unilateral shortening of the sternocleido-mastoid (SCM) muscle with subsequent limited cervical range of motion (ROM). The infant's head is laterally flexed toward the shortened muscle, with the chin rotated to the opposite side. Facial asymmetry and plagiocephaly (ie, flattening of the skull) may also be present. The disorder is typically noted in the first 2 to 3 weeks after birth (Stanger, 1999, p. 394). General categories (according to Cooperman in Stanger, 1999) include the following:

1. Torticollis with unilateral SCM muscle contracture and a tumor during the first 3 months of life with an otherwise normal x-ray. This is most classic presentation of congenital torticollis. The tumor usually resolves within the first year.
2. Torticollis with SCM muscle contracture without a tumor in the SCM and with a normal x-ray.
3. Head and neck asymmetry similar in appearance to classic congenital torticollis without SCM contracture and with normal x-rays. Causes include:
   - Benign paroxysmal torticollis beginning in the first few months of life which can alternate between right and left sides and is worse in the morning than at night but resolves spontaneously at about 1 year of age.

- Congenital absence of one or several cervical muscles or of the transverse ligament.
- Contracture of other neck muscles including scalenus anterior, omohyoid, or trapezius.
- Generalized neck contractures as a result of abnormal delayed neuromuscular development.
4. Congenital torticollis with abnormal spinal x-rays. Klippel-Feil syndrome, congenital scoliosis, unilateral absence of a C-1 facet, and basilar impression are examples (Cooperman, 1997, pp. 5–6).

CAUSE

The most common cause is traumatic neck injury during (but sometimes before) delivery, with hematoma, fibrosis, and contracture of the SCM muscle. Other causes include abnormalities of the bony spine, such as Klippel-Feil syndrome (fusion of the cervical vertebrae) or of the atlas to the occipital bone (atlanto-occipital fusion). CNS tumors, bulbar palsies, and ocular dysfunction are prominent neurological causes but are rarely present at birth (Beers & Berkow, 1999, p. 2219). Another possibility is an intrauterine compartment syndrome due to extreme head posturing within the birth canal. Little agreement exists on the etiology in congenital torticollis (Cooperman, 1997, p. 2). The incidence varies widely in the literature from 0.084% to 1.9% and sex ratio is reported equal in some studies while in others a higher incidence in boys than girls; about a 3:2 ratio is reported.

ASSESSMENT

AREAS
- ROM: passive and active
- Muscle tone
- Muscle strength
- Postural reactions
- Ocular eye movements
- Skeletal asymmetry
- Developmental testing

INSTRUMENTS/PROCEDURES
- goniometer
- cervical range of motion device (CROM)
- Bayley Scales of Infant Development–II (BSID–II) (Bayley, 1993)
- INFANIB: Infant Neurological International Battery (Andre-Thomas, Chesni, Dargassies, 1950)
- Movement Assessment of Infants (MAI) (Chandler, Andrews, & Swanson, 1980)
- Peabody Developmental Motor Scales, 2nd ed (PDMS–2) (Folio & Fewell, 1999)
- Test of Infant Motor Performance (TIMP) (Campbell SK, 1995)
- Torticollis Evaluation Form (Karmel-Ross K, 1997)
- photographing the face and head can document facial asymmetry and head plagiocephaly

PROBLEMS
- Child has difficulty or is unable to center the head in midline alignment.
- Child has difficulty or is unable to move into a position of active chin tuck or capital flexion.
- Child has a strong sensory and postural bias toward neck and upper body asymmetry. Child holds head in a lateral sidebend that varies in the amount of lateral neck flexion and favored side of rotation.
- Child has a unilateral SCM muscle contraction.
- Child may have facial asymmetry and plagiocephaly.

- Child rotates head to the opposite side of the contraction with lateral flexion ipsilaterally, and neck extension.
- Child is unable to turn to assume the opposite position of neck rotation and lateral flexion in supine, prone, supported sitting or supported standing.
- Child's characteristic posture includes shoulder hiking on the shortened side.
- Child may be unable to bring hands or feet together in midline position.
- Child's visual gaze is often oriented toward the side of head turning which may result in biased perceptual sensorimotor experience to one side.
- Child may have difficulty with stabilization and positioning of the head in midline or opposite position to view objects or the environment.
- In prone position, the child tends to put more weight on the arm, trunk, and pelvis on the affected side. Lateral neck flexion and shoulder hiking are pronounced.
- Child may have difficulty with trunk stability, weight shifting, and balance due to previous asymmetrical positioning and lack of symmetrical postures.
- Check for possible hip dysplagia as the two are often connected.

TREATMENT/MANAGEMENT

See: Chronological Intervention Pathway for Muscular Torticollis in Karmel-Ross and Lepp, 51; Torticollis Treatment Protocol, 52; Torticollis Exercise Sheets, 53–55; and Manual Intervention Pathway for Muscular Torticollis, 59. Generally better outcomes occur when treatment is initiated in the first year of life. Conservative treatment is recommended for the first year.

0–3 MONTHS
- Position infant so that the head turns toward the injured side (away from the contracture) and so that the child can see interesting things in the environment.
- Positioning and handling should promote midline orientation and symmetry of body.
- Stretching exercises should provide passive and active ROM to the neck. Often, it is easier to move the infant's trunk while the head is stabilized on the support surface. Parents should be taught these exercises.
- Massage can be used as a stretching technique.
- Use gravity-assisted strengthening exercises for neck and trunk.
- Encourage righting reactions supine, prone, and side-lying.
- Visual exercises can be used to promote active head rotation toward the involved side.
- Encourage normal development through age-appropriate activities.
- Instruct parents and encourage cooperation with positioning recommendations. In the infant's bedroom, the bassinet or crib should be placed so the contracture is toward the wall and the head can be turned toward the injured side. The child should be held so that he or she needs to run to the appropriate side to see or nuzzle the parent. When bottle feeding, the child should be held so that the head needs to turn to the appropriate side to see the caregiver.
- Encourage parent to socialize and play with the infant during stretching exercises.
- Therapist should learn how to console and handle a fussy infant and gain the trust of parents.

4–5 MONTHS
- In addition to the above listed steps, a cervical brace may be used if the head tilt is greater than 6 degrees. Two types are discussed and illustrated in Jacques and Karmel-Ross.
- A helmet may be used to reshape the head.

- Promote righting and equilibrium reactions in supine, prone, side-lying, sitting, and vertical suspension.
- Encourage transitional movement and symmetrical weight-shifting skills.
- Use shoulder girdle and trunk exercises.
- Promote symmetry in sacral-pelvic base.
- Specific concentric neck strengthening exercises may include:
  1. in prone: neck extension and asymmetrical neck extension
  2. in supine: neck flexion
  3. in side-lying: lateral neck flexion
- Promote active head rotation in all postures.
- Blocking visual field on the preferred side may result in improved visual engagement, fixation, and tracking.

6–8 MONTHS
- All of the above plus strengthening anti-gravity neck and trunk muscles.
- Encourage protective extension reactions.
- Promote righting and equilibrium reactions in a quadruped position.

9–12 MONTHS
- All of the above but discontinue brace wear.
- Upgrade balance and developmental exercises to include equilibrium reactions in standing.

1 YEAR PLUS
- If problems persist, surgery may be recommended.

PRECAUTIONS/CONTRAINDICATIONS
- During stretching exercises, it is important not to exercise with too much force.

DESIRED OUTCOME/PROGNOSIS

Generally, the prognosis is good using conservative treatment initiated during the first or second year of life. A full recovery may be expected. See Taylor & Norton in References.

- Child is able to bring and maintain head in midline position with no residual head tilt.
- Child is able to tuck chin and flex chin toward chest.
- Child is able to rotate head and trunk to both sides of the body to the same degree of passive and active ROM.
- Child has equal cervical muscle strength in all directions.
- Child is able to achieve a symmetrical position with head, trunk, upper and lower extremities in prone or supine.
- Child is able to bear weight evenly in sitting and standing.
- Child demonstrates equal responses on both sides of the body to righting, protective, and equilibrium reactions.
- Child's eyes are horizontal and gaze can view both right and left fields of vision.
- Residual restrictions in ROM or muscle weaknesses do not interfere with normal activities of daily living.
- Residual craniofacial asymmetry is not noticeable.
- Residual head tilt occurs only when child is fatigued.

REFERENCES

Beers MH, Berkow R, eds. *The Merck Manual of Diagnosis and Therapy.* Whitehouse Station, NJ: Merck Research Laboratories; 1999.

Cheng JC, Tang SP. Outcome of surgical treatment of congenital muscular torticollis. *Clin Orthop*. 1999;362:190–200.

Cooperman DR. Differential diagnosis of torticollis in children. *Phys Occup Ther Pediatr*. 1997;17(2):1–12.

Emery C. Conservative management of congenital muscular torticollis: a literature review. *Phys Occup Ther Pediatr*. 1997;17(2):13–20.

Hylton N. Infants with torticollis: the relationship between asymmetric head and neck positioning and postural development. *Phys Occup Ther Pediatr*. 1997;17(2):91–117.

Jacques C, Karmel-Ross K. The use of splinting in conservative and post-operative treatment of congenital muscular torticollis. *Phys Occup Ther Pediatr*. 1997;17(2):81–90.

Karmel-Ross K, Lepp M. Assessment and treatment of children with congenital muscular torticollis. *Phys Occup Ther Pediatr*. 1997;17(2):21–67.

Karmel-Ross K. Epilogue ... clinical findings in children with torticollis. *Phys Occup Ther Pediatr*. 1997;17(2):119–120.

Karmel-Ross K. Prepare ... torticollis. *Phys Occup Ther Pediatr*. 1997;17(2):xiii–xiv.

Kviberg I, Orbe A. Treatment of torticollis in infancy by manual pressure applied over the parasacro-coccygeal structures. *Physiotherapy Res Int*. 1998;3(3):228–229; discussion: 229–230.

Ho BC, Lee EH, Singh K. Epidemiology, presentation and management of congenital muscular torticollis. *Singapore Med J*. 1999;40(11):675–679.

Hylton N. Infants with torticollis: The relationship between asymmetric head and neck positioning and postural development. *Phys Occup Ther Pediatr*. 1997;17(2):91–117.

Norton ES. Developmental muscular torticollis and brachial plexus injury. In: Campbell SK, ed. *Physical Therapy for Children*. 2nd ed. Philadelphia, Pa: WB Saunders Co; 2000: 282–301.

Rajput A, Gauderer MWL. The surgical management of congenital muscular torticollis. *Phys Occup Ther Pediatr*. 1997;17(2):69–80.

Ratliffe KT. Other orthopedic disorders—Tyrone, an infant with congenital torticollis and Erb's palsy. In: Ratliffe KT. *Clinical Pediatric Physical Therapy: A Guide for the Physical Therapy Team*. St. Louis, Mo: CV Mosby Co; 1998:131–136.

Ratliffe KT. Other orthopedic disorders—The child with a congenital torticollis. In Ratliffe KT. *Clinical Pediatric Physical Therapy: A Guide for the Physical Therapy Team*. St. Louis, Mo: CV Mosby Co; 1998:139–140.

Robin NH. Congenital muscular torticollis. *Pediatr Rev*. 1996;17(10):374–375.

Saidoff DC, McDonough AL. Neonate presenting with leftward head tilt and rightward facial flattening. In: Saidoff DC, McDonough AL, eds. *Critical Pathways in Therapeutic Intervention: Extremities and Spine*. 2002;235–242.

Stanger M. Orthopedic management—congenital muscular torticollis. In: Tecklin JS, ed. *Pediatric physical therapy*. 3rd ed. Philadelphia, Pa: Lippincott Williams and Wilkins; 1999:394–396.

Taylor JL, Norton ES. Developmental muscular torticollis: outcomes in young children treated by physical therapy. *Pediatr Phys Ther*. 1997;9(4):173–178.

Cystic Fibrosis

Also known as *salty kiss disease*.

ICD-9-CM Code: 277.0 Cystic Fibrosis
APTA Guide Patterns: 6C, 6F, 6G, 6H, 6I

DESCRIPTION

Cystic fibrosis (CF) is an inherited disease of the exocrine glands, primarily affecting the gastrointestinal and respiratory systems, and usually characterized by chronic obstructive pulmonary disease, exocrine pancreatic insufficiency, and abnormally high sweat electrolytes (Beers & Berkow, 1999, p. 2366). A person with CF often has a persistent productive cough, a barrelshaped chest, and clubbed fingers and toes from hypoxia. The child tends to be small and thin for age due to disturbances in nutrient absorption (Ratliffe, 1998, p. 395). Other clinical symptoms include abnormally frequent and large stools, failure to thrive, recurrent pneumonia, rectal prolapse, and nasal polyposis (Tecklin, 2000, p. 550). Two new treatments include lung transplantation and gene therapy. Both have had limited success.

The disorder was first described in 1938 by D.H. Anderson, who published a paper about the clinical course of children who died of pulmonary and digestive problems.

CAUSE

CF is an autosomal recessive disorder. Both parents must have the recessive trait for offspring to be affected. The trait is carried by approximately 3% of the white population but is rare in Hispanic, black, and Asian children. The gene is located on chromosome 7q (the long arm). It encodes a membrane-associated protein called the cystic fibrosis transmembrane regulator (CFTR). The most common mutation leads to absence of a phenylalanine residue although many types of mutation have been identified (Beers & Berkow, 1999, p. 2366). The protein affects the exocrine (mucus-producing) glands, and the defect produces problems in multiple systems throughout the body, but most notably in the respiratory tract, gastrointestinal tract, reproductive tract, and the sweat glans of the skin. Thickened mucus results in poor ciliary action, stagnant mucus, and constant infections (Ratliffe, 1998, p. 395). The major hypothesis regarding CFTR dysfunction states that the product of the abnormal gene is responsible for a decrease in chloride and water secretion by airway epithelial cells, thereby resulting in dehydrated mucus. However, additional explanations are needed to account for the diversity of organ system involvement (Tecklin, 2000, p. 550).

CF is diagnosed in 1 in 2,000 children born to white parents. The incidence is lower in African-Americans at 1 in 17,000 and lower still in Asian society at 1 in 90,000. In the white population, the rate of heterozygote carriers is about 5% of the population (Ashwell & Agnew-Coughlin, 2001, pp. 734–735).

ASSESSMENT

AREAS
- Back pain
- Breathing pattern(s) by observation or palpation
- Breathing sounds: sonorous wheezes, harsh breath sounds, and crackles
- Chest mobility: observe for barrel appearance and fixed chest
- Cough: ability to raise secretions
- Exercise tolerance and capacity
- Posture: observe for changes caused by the hyperaeration and chronic coughing, shoulder protraction and elevation, thoracic kyphosis
- Range of motion especially of the shoulder girdle
- Quality of life
- Work capacity

INSTRUMENTS/PROCEDURES
- scale of ratings of perceived exertion (Borg, 1982)
- auscultation
- exercise tolerance testing: cycle erogmeters, treadmill test, 6- or 12-minute walk test

- expiratory reserve volume (ERV)
- forced expiratory flow (FEF)
- forced expiratory volume (FEV) or forced expiratory volume in 1 second (FEV1)
- forced vital capacity (FVC)
- function reserve capacity (FRC)
- inspiratory reserve volume (IRV)
- peak expiratory flow (PEF)
- pulmonary function testing (PFT)
- residual volume (RV)
- spirometry: vital capacity (VC), inspiratory reserve volume (IRV), and expiratory reserve volume (ERV)
- thoracic girth
- thoracic index
- total lung capacity (TLC)
- vital capacity (VC)

PROBLEMS
- Infant may have meconium ileus.
- Infant may experience failure to thrive syndrome.
- Infant may experience nutritional absorption deficiency.
- Infant may have sputum thickening.
- Infant or child may have airway and airflow obstruction related to airway inflammation, mucosal edema, mucus secretions, and increased airway tone.
- Infant or child may have difficulty clearing the airway.
- Infant or child may wheeze, indicating hyperactive airways.
- Child and adolescent may have a small stature or lower than average weight-to-height ratio due to malabsorption.
- Child may have behavior problems such as restlessness, excessive daydreaming, and inattentiveness.
- Adolescent may have arrested sexual development.
- Adolescent may have behavior problems such as rebellion against being different and a feeling of isolation, becoming withdrawn.
- Adolescent may be non-compliant or uncooperative with therapy, thus increasing risk of airway restriction.
- Adolescent may have postural changes due to CF, including increased anterior-posterior diameter of the chest, shoulder elevation, forward protraction and abdominal flexion, and thoracic kyphosis.
- Adolescent may have difficulty maintaining and gaining weight during periods of rapid growth.
- Adolescent may experience increased work of breathing and muscle fatigue, due to mechanical disadvantage caused by changes in length-tension relationships of the respiratory musculature.
- Adolescent may have back pain as a result of postural changes.
- In adult years, urinary stress incontinence may occur (White, Stiller, & Roney).

TREATMENT/MANAGEMENT

During early infancy, the major intervention is directed toward management of gastrointestinal tract symptoms because the lungs are morphologically normal at birth. Impaired respiratory function may occur within a few months often presenting at bronchiolitis with evidence of bronchoconstriction.

Infancy
- Educate the family about CF, including both the practical and psychological demands implicit in the diagnosis. Answer the family's questions.

- Encourage family not to overprotect the child but to permit the child to engage in normal activities.
- Prevent obstructive mucus plugging. Chest physical therapy may be started with chest percussion and vibration to promote postural drainage. Note that modification of the head-down position for postural drainage may be desirable to avoid gastroesophageal reflux. Also consider adjusting treatment schedule around the feeding schedule to reduce problems. Positioning may be done on the lap rather than a drainage board. Percussion can be adjusted by "tenting" the middle finger to accommodate a tiny chest wall (Ashwell & Agnew-Coughlin, 2000, p. 746).
- Instruct the family or caregivers by demonstrating treatment positions and manual techniques.
- If family members or caregivers show signs of excessive stress in coping with care of child with CF, refer such persons to social work or psychologist to assist in developing strategies to enable adjustment to the challenges.
- Order, demonstrate use, and arrange for maintenance of nebulizers used for aerosol delivery of medication.

Preschool and School-age Period
- Develop an exercise program to increase exercise tolerance, increase peak oxygen consumption, increase maximal work capacity, improve mucus expectoration, and improve expiratory flow rates. The exercise program may also improve self-concept and provide increased social interaction.
- Use techniques to mobilize and clear secretions including postural drainage, percussion, and vibration. A drainage board should be introduced when child is too large for a lap. Mechanical percussors may be used to reduce workload involved in manual percussion and permit the child to self-treat.
- Correct and maintain proper postural alignment.
- Involve child and family in goals for treatment.
- Adjust treatment to account for child's learning style, developmental stage, and family circumstances.
- Encourage child to participate in a variety of social and physical activities to promote physical and emotional health.
- Encourage family to provide an active lifestyle and interaction into the family dynamics.
- Encourage child to perform age-appropriate tasks in self-care to promote sense of self-efficacy (ie, confidence in ability to perform).

Adolescence
- Work with adolescent to develop a therapy program that the adolescent can and will follow. Creative approaches to exercise may be needed to increase adolescent's sense of "fitting in."
- Increase adolescent's sense of being "in charge" by using alternative methods: postural drainage and percussion such as active cycle of breaking technique (FET), autogenic drainage, or a positive expiratory pressure (PEP) mask.
- Encourage proper posture to provide efficient breathing mechanics. Check for postural abnormalities and determine which changes may be amenable to treatment. Addressing the benefits of good posture to a person's appearance and self-confidence may increase compliance and cooperation.
- If postural abnormalities are present, start
  1. an exercise program to improve posture
  2. a strengthening program to increase support for back and spine
  3. a stretching program for contracted musculature
  4. a training program to increase awareness of postural alignment

- Encourage good nutrition and stress the relationship of nutrition to exercise capacity and tolerance. Work with a dietitian to promote weight gain if weight is a problem.
- Instruct adolescent in energy conservation and relaxation positions to ease the work of breathing.
- Educate adolescent about possible health problems associated with CF in adulthood such as hemotysis, pneumothorax, hypertrophic pulmonary osteoarthropathy, and associated cardiopulmonary conditions. Lung transplantation may also be a consideration.
- Contribute to plans for education, employment, and independent living. Persons with CF should consider the physical demands of any work tasks and avoid jobs involving constant exposure to dust, chemical fumes, or smoke.

General
- Assist child to expel thick secretions to reduce risk of infection and improve gas exchange.
- Use postural drainage positioning and techniques to facilitate the movement of mobilized mucus from the alveolar areas toward the central bronchials to be coughed up.
- Use percussion. Percuss the child's chest firmly with tightly cupped hands. A loud popping sound should be heard as air pops out of the cupped hands. Use of a light towel or clothing can reduce bruising effects and protect the skin. For infants a small mask or percussion cap may be used instead of the hand.
- Vibration may be used if the child is unable to tolerate percussion, eg, in the neonatal intensive care unit where the infant is very fragile. Because the vibrator is less traumatic it may also be less effective.
- A combination of postural (gravity) drainage, percussion, and vibration is more effective than any of the three alone (Tecklin, 2000, 552).
- Provide training in breathing exercises—especially deep breathing. Make the exercises fun for the child. Creative approaches which are developmentally appropriate should be used.
- Alternative airway clearance techniques are being used more frequently and include:
  1. Autogenic drainage
  2. Forced expiratory technique/active cycle of breathing (see van der Schans, Williams, et al)
  3. Positive expiratory pressure (PEP) mask (McIlwaine, et al)
  4. Flutter value device or oscillating PEP (see Gondor, et al; Homnick & Marks)
  5. Mechanical vest therapy and high frequency chest compression (HFCC)
  6. Directed coughing or huffing
- Use suctioning, if necessary.
- Encourage daily exercise to improve respiratory status.
- Provide psychosocial and emotional support for patient and family.
- Provide education and instruction to family on airway clearance techniques.

PRECAUTIONS/CONTRAINDICATIONS
- Infant may experience gastroesophageal reflux if head-down position is used for postural drainage.
- The head-down position for postural drainage should not be used with a child who has increased intracranial pressure.
- Child with CF often bruises easily due to improper nutrient absorption. Reduce risk of skin injuries.
- Child may be anemic which reduces energy level and increases fatigue.

- Child is at risk for dehydration from sweating during strenuous exercise and hot temperatures. Encouraging child to drink electrolyte replacement fluids with high sodium and chloride content may help.
- All electrical equipment should be checked frequently to avoid fire danger especially when it is used in an oxygen-rich environment.
- Use of balloons to stimulate forceful deep breathing may require too much pressure and may cause a pneumothorax. Balloons also represent a choking hazard.
- Chest physical therapy is contraindicated when there is a pulmonary hemorrhage or embolism.
- Check for osteopenia, especially in adolescents, and consider risk of fractures in developing a therapy program.
- Children with minimal cardiac reserve may not be able to tolerate the energy expenditure required for chest physical therapy.
- Reduce exposure to respiratory pathogens since pulmonary infection is a major cause of death.

DESIRED OUTCOME/PROGNOSIS

Life expectancy in the United States has increased significantly from about 6 years to well into the 40s due to better understanding of the disease and medications such as antibiotics. Cause of death is typically pulmonary complications.

- Child has a clear airway.
- Child has an exercise program that is performed daily by the child or caregiver.
- Child performs functional skills that are age appropriate.
- Child participates in family, school, recreational, and community activities.
- Family and caregivers can perform suctioning as needed.
- Family and caregivers can position child to facilitate postural drainage.

REFERENCES

Ashwell JA, Agnew-Coughlin JL. Cystic fibrosis. In: Campbell SK, ed. *Physical Therapy for Children*. 2nd ed. Philadelphia, Pa: WB Saunders Co; 2000:734–763.

Beers MH, Berkow R, eds. *The Merck Manual of Diagnosis and Therapy*. Whitehouse Station, NJ: Merck Research Laboratories; 1999.

Bannigan K. Research in practice. The CF protocol. *Ther Weekly*. 1998;24(29):6.

Button BM. Postural drainage techniques and gastro-oesophageal reflux in infants with cystic fibrosis [letter]. *Eur Respir J*. 1999;14(6):1456; discussion: 1456–1457.

Button M, Heine RG, Catto-Smith AG, Phelan PD. Postural drainage in cystic fibrosis: is there a link with gastro-oesophageal reflux? *J Pediatr Child Health*. 1998;34(4):330–334.

Carr L, Smith, RE, Pryor JA, Partirdge C. Cystic fibrosis patients' views and beliefs about chest clearance and exercise—a pilot study. *Physiotherapy*. 1995;82(11):621–627.

Coates AL. Chest physiotherapy in cystic fibrosis: spare the hand and spoil the cough? [editorial; comment] *J Pediatr* 1997;131–(4):506–508.

De Jong W, van Aalderen WMC, Kraan J, Koëter GH, van der Schans CP. Skeletal muscle strength in patients with cystic fibrosis. *Physiotherapy Theory Pract*. 2001;17(1):23–28.

Fauroux B, Boule M, Lofaso F, Zerah F, Clement A, Harf A, et al. Chest physiotherapy in cystic fibrosis: improved tolerance with nasal pressure support ventilation. *Pediatr*. 1999;103(3):32.

Gondor M, Nixon PA, Mutich R, Rebovich P, Orenstein DM. Comparison of Flutter device and chest physical therapy in the treatment of cystic fibrosis pulmonary exacerbation. *Pediatr Pulmonology*. 1999;28(4):255–260.

Homnick DN, Anderson K, Marks JH. Comparison of the flutter device to standard chest physiotherapy in hospitalized patients with cystic fibrosis: a pilot study. *Chest.* 1998; 114(4):993–997.

McIlwaine PM, Wong LT, Peacock D, Davidson AG. Long-term comparative trial of conventional postural drainage and percussion versus positive expiratory pressure physiotherapy in the treatment of cystic fibrosis. *J Pediatr.* 1997;131(4):570–574.

Phillips GE, Pike SE, Rosenthal M, Bush A. Holding the baby: head downwards positioning for physiotherapy does not cause gastro-oesophageal reflux. *Eur Respir J.* 1998; 12(4):954–957.

Ratliffe KT. Medical disorders—Respiratory disorders of childhood: cystic fibrosis. In: Ratliffe KT. *Clinical Pediatric Physical Therapy: A Guide for the Physical Therapy Team.* St. Louis, Mo: CV Mosby Co; 1998:395–396.

Tecklin JS. Pulmonary disorders in infants and children and their physical therapy management—Cystic fibrosis. In: Tecklin JS, ed. *Pediatr Phys Ther.* 3rd ed. Philadelphia, Pa: Lippincott Williams and Wilkins; 1999:550–557.

van der Schans CP. Forced expiratory manoeuvres to increase transport of bronchial mucus: a mechanistic approach. *Monaldi Arch Chest Dis.* 1997:52(4):367–370.

Wallis C, Prasad A. Who needs chest physiotherapy? Moving from anecdote to evidence. *Arch Dis Child.* 1999;80(4):393–397.

White D, Stiller K, Roney F. The prevalence and severity of symptoms of incontinence in adult cystic fibrosis patients. *Physiotherapy Theory Pract.* 2000;16(1):35–42.

Williams MT, Parson DW, Martin AJ, Giles SE, Frick RA, Grant RE. Energy expenditure during physiotherapist-assisted and self-treatment in cystic fibrosis. *Physiotherapy Theory Pract.* 2000;16(2):57–67.

Developmental Coordination Disorder

ICD-9-CM Code: 781.3 Lack of coordination

APTA Guide Patterns: 4C, 5A, 5B, 5C

DESCRIPTION

The label *developmental coordination disorder* (DCD) appears in the *Diagnostic and Statistical Manual of Mental Disorders–Fourth Edition* (DSM–IV; American Psychiatric Association, 1994). The diagnosis is applied when (1) performance in daily activities that require motor coordination is substantially below the expected level for a child's chronological age and measured intelligence, and (2) significantly interferes with academic achievement or activities of daily living (ADLs), but (3) is not due to a general medical condition such as cerebral palsy or muscular dystrophy or meet the criteria for a pervasive developmental disorder, and (4) if mental retardation is present, the motor difficulties are in excess of those usually associated with it (pp. 54–55).

DCD may be involved when there are marked delays in achieving motor milestones such as walking, crawling, and sitting, when the child drops things without obvious explanation, exhibits "clumsiness," performs poorly in sports, or has poor handwriting. The condition may be recognized when the child first attempts such tasks as running, holding a knife and fork, buttoning clothes, tying shoelaces, zipping pants, or playing ball games (p. 54). In older children, the difficulties may be associated with the motor aspects of assembling puzzles and building models in addition to difficulty playing ball games, and poor printing or handwriting skills. Although delays in motor skill acquisition are required for the diagnosis, there may be delays in other nonmotor milestones and other associated disorders may be present including phonological, expressive language, and mixed

473

receptive-expressive language disorders (p. 54). In addition, a child with DCD may exhibit behavioral and psychosocial problems such as distractibility, temper tantrums, frustration, poor self-esteem, depression, and rejection from peers. Additional physical symptoms may be present without a known cause such as abdominal pain, loss of bowel and bladder control, and headaches. Parents may describe their child as "messy," "slow," and "uncoordinated." There is an overlap of emotional symptoms that may also be signs of attention deficit hyperactivity disorder (ADHD).

CAUSE

No single cause or consistent group of causes has been identified with DCD. Rather, multiple etiologies may be involved which include dysfunction of the cerebellum, of one of the two motor strips in the cerebral cortex or of the efferent motor pathways, or an imbalance in one or more of the sensory neural mechanisms which occur during the prenatal, perinatal, or neonatal period (David, 2001, p. 472). DCD is not by definition caused by muscle pathology, peripheral sensory abnormality, or central nervous system damage related to spasticity, athetosis, or ataxia. Hypotonia may be present but its relationship to DCD is unclear. The disorder has been associated with perinatal abnormalities of anoxia at birth (David, 2001, p. 473). The prevalence of DCD is estimated to be as high as 6% for children in the age range of 5–11 years (DSM–IV, 1994, p. 54).

ASSESSMENT

AREAS

- Body alignment
- Functional skills
- Gait
- Gross and fine motor skills
- Joint mobility
- Muscle strength and endurance
- Muscle tone
- Postural control and balance
- Postural transitions
- Praxis
- Righting, protective, and equilibrium responses
- Sensory integration
- Visual perceptual skills
- Rule out abnormal movements patterns and motor control problems related to neuromuscular or musculoskeletal disorders such as cerebral palsy, polyneuropathies or muscular dystrophy.
- Note different environments which facilitate or hinder performance.

INSTRUMENTS/PROCEDURES

Initial or Intake Measures
- Medical history, including pregnancy, delivery, and past and current health status; developmental history; previous musculoskeletal and neuromuscular examinations; history of the current function; and functional status from the family and school personnel
- Alberta Infant Motor Scale (AIMS) (Piper & Darrah, 1994)
- Bayley Scales of Infant Development–II (BSID–II) (Bayley, 1993)
- Brigance Diagnostic Inventory of Early Development (Brigance)
- Bruininks-Oseretsky Test of Motor Proficiency (BOTMP) (Bruininks, 1978)
- Early Learning Accomplishment Profile for Young Children (Glover et al, 1978)
- Gubbay Tests of Motor Proficiency (Gubbay, 1975). See Campbell, 2001, pp. 500–501.
- Miller Assessment for Preschoolers (MAP) (Miller, 1988)
- Movement Assessment Battery for Children (Movement ABC) (Henderson & Sugden, 1992)
- Peabody Developmental Motor Scales, 2nd ed. (PDMS–2) (Folio & Fewell, 1999)

- Sensory Integration and Praxis Test (SIPT) (Ayres, 1989)
- Clinical observation of performance in different natural environments such as a quiet or noisy area, one with an adult versus one with many children doing the same or similar tasks. Look for motor control and motor learning problems related to motor incoordination.

Outcome Measures
- Functional Independence Measure (Wee-FIM) (Granger et al, 1989)
- Gross Motor Function Measure, 2nd ed. (GMFM) (Russell et al, 1993)
- Pediatric Evaluation of Disability Inventory (PEDI) (Haley et al, 1992)
- School Function Assessment (SFA) (Coster et al, 1998)

PROBLEMS

SOFT SIGNS IMPAIRMENTS
- Abnormal muscle tone
- Decreased muscle strength and endurance
- Delayed or absent postural reactions
- Difficulty holding static balance positions
- Jerky or clumsy movements
- Joint laxity with scapular winging, elbow hyperextension, hypermobile fingers and poor trunk extension
- Immature movement patterns
- Inadequate information processing
- Inconsistent motor responses
- Motor apraxia or dyspraxia
- Poor coordination
- Poor feedback
- Poor kinesthesia
- Poor postural control
- Poor sequencing
- Poor short- and long-term memory
- Poor spatial organization
- Poor strength
- Poor visual motor, visual memory, and visual discrimination
- Reliance on feedback rather than feedforward programming

FUNCTIONAL LIMITATIONS
- Awkward gait
- Delayed and poor quality of gross motor skills such as hopping, jumping, and throwing or catching a ball, jumping rope, crossing legs in a seated position
- Delayed and poor quality of fine motor skills such as threading beads, cutting with scissors, drawing, printing, writing
- Delayed oral-motor skills
- Distractibility and poor attention-to-task
- Low self-esteem

DISABILITIES
- Delayed development of self-help skills
- Depression
- Difficulty following directions in motor tasks
- Limitations in participation in everyday physical activities
- Low academic achievement
- Poor language skills including written communication

SOCIAL LIMITATION
- Limited indoor and outdoor play with peers including sports
- Limited vocational success
- Poor social interaction skills
- Social isolation
- Strained child-parent relationships

TREATMENT/MANAGEMENT

Intervention often requires a team approach due to multiple problems. Refer to other team members when appropriate such as a physician, psychologist, classroom teacher, physical education instructor, adapted physical education teacher, speech-language pathologist, and an occupational therapist in addition to the physical therapist.

Controversy exists regarding the need for intervention and whether that intervention should be focused toward the underlying impairments, toward the functional limitations, or toward the actual disability, or even encompass a combination of all three approaches (Davis, 2001, p. 484). However, motor learning research suggests that learning specific functional tasks or motor skills requires practice in the environment in which the task or skill is expected to be performed.

- Improve functional limitations related to static balance without touching people or objects nearby. Examples: standing on one foot to put on jeans, kicking a stationary ball, or standing still in line without touching others. Provide practice situations that may be repeated with slight variation and that may include the natural environment with distractions or simultaneous activities.
- Increase muscle strength in hand muscles needed for handwriting.
- Provide motor learning training to verbally identify and remembrances for a task such as shoe-tying.
- Improve visual motor skills used for cutting, drawing, and writing.
- Improve kinesthetic performance feedback information such as watching in a mirror or listening to the sounds generated when skipping and use the information to make a different response the next time.
- Improve strength and endurance of hip and knee extensor muscles to increase speed and safety in climbing stairs in the school and at home.
- Make recommendations that may improve the child's participation in play activities such as reducing the motor demand or better match the play activity to the child's level of motor learning and skill.
- Make recommendations that can make the play environment safer to avoid accidents.
- Educate parents, teachers, and other caregivers to carry out the program in environments where the physical therapist is not present.
- Educate parents, teachers, and other caregivers to consider what expectations for motor proficiency are within the child's skill level and which exceed the skill level.
- Educate parents, teachers, and other caregivers about factors that would signal the need for additional intervention in the future.
- Assist other professionals on goals that have carryover potential, such as assisting in the improvement of word recall, retrieval, or verbal sequencing of multiple-step instructions by asking the child to name motor skills being performed or repeat instructions on how to perform a given motor skill or task.
- Coordinate goals with other professionals such as promoting oral-motor development to improve feeding and improve articulation and fluency of speech.
- Cooperate with other professionals such as with the physical education teacher to adapt motor skill requirements of a game to enable the child to participate within safe limits of motor skill demand.
- Consult with other professionals—such as a psychologist—who may be able to suggest a behavior modification program to decrease the occurrence of behaviors which interfere with achieving therapy goals.

PRECAUTIONS/CONTRAINDICATIONS
- Avoid unsafe conditions. Always be prepared to prevent falls and remove objects which may cause injury.
- Do not expect proficiency in performance beyond the child's level of motor skills; doing so may lead to frustration and unhappiness.

DESIRED OUTCOME/PROGNOSIS

Prognosis and course is variable. Lack of coordination may continue through adolescence and adulthood.

- Child demonstrates improved gross motor coordination skills on standardized tests.
- Child demonstrates improved fine motor skills.
- Child performs self-care activities at age-appropriate level.
- Child performs functional skills at age-appropriate level.
- Child performs academic skills at expected grade level.
- Child participates in recreational and leisure activities with peers.
- Parents report child can participate in home activities at age-appropriate level.
- Teachers report child can participate in school activities using age-appropriate emotional and social skills.

REFERENCES

American Psychiatric Association. *Diagnostic and Statistical Manual of Mental Disorders.* 4th ed. Washington, DC: American Psychiatric Association; 1994.

David KS. Developmental coordination disorders. In: Campbell SK, ed. *Phys Ther Child.* 2nd ed. Philadelphia, Pa: WB Saunders Co; 2000:471–501.

Leemrijse C, Meijer OG, Vermeer A. The efficacy of Le Bon Dpart and sensory integration of children with developmental coordination disorder: a randomised study of six cases. *Nederlands Tijdschrift Voor Fysiotherapie.* 2001;111(2):43–51.

Peters JM, Wright AM. Development and evaluation of a group physical activity programme for children with developmental coordination disorder: an interdisciplinary approach. *Physiotherapy Theory Pract.* 1999;15(4):203–216.

Pless M, Carlsson M, Sundelin C. Persson K. Effects of group motor skill intervention on five- to six-year-old children with developmental coordination disorder. *Pediatr Phys Ther.* 2000;12:183–189.

Ratliffe KT. Sensory, processing, and cognitive disorders of childhood—Developmental co-ordination disorder. In: Ratliffe KT. *Clinical Pediatric Physical Therapy: A Guide for the Physical Therapy Team.* St. Louis, Mo: CV Mosby Co; 1998:329–330.

Rösblad B. Visual perception in children with developmental coordination disorder. In: Cermak SA, Larkin D. *Developmental Coordination Disorder.* New York, NY: Delmar; 2002:104–116.

Developmental Dysplasia of the Hip

Also known as *congenital dislocation of the hip* or *congenital hip dysplasia.*

ICD-9-CM Code: 835 Dislocation of hip

APTA Guide Patterns: 4I, 4J

DESCRIPTION

Developmental dysplasia of the hip (DDH) occurs when the acetabulum and the femoral head are not aligned normally (Ratliffe, 1998, p. 77). The major sign of subluxation or dislocation of the hip is inability to completely abduct the thigh when the hip and knee are flexed. This is due to adductor spasm, which is often present even if the hip is not actually dislocated at the time of examination. If the hip is dislocated, abduction and external rotation of the femur may produce an audible or palpable "clunk" as the femoral head reenters the acetabulum (Ortolani's sign). The dislocation can be unilateral or bilateral. If unilateral, the involved leg is shorter and there may be asymmetric skin creases on the thigh. Partial or complete dislocation may be difficult to detect at birth. Periodic testing for limitation of hip abduction is advised during the first year of life (Beers & Berkow, 1999, pp. 2219–2220). Ultrasonography is now being used more frequently to confirm the presence or absence of dysphasia or dislocation (Leach, 2000, p. 407).

CLASSIFICATION OR GRADES OF DYSPLASIA AND DISLOCATION
(Ratliffe, 1998, p. 78; Leach, 2000, p. 407).

- *Dysphasis*: Acetabulum is shallow or small with poor lateral borders which may occur alone or with any level of femoral deformity or displacement.
- *Subluxatable:* The femoral head can be partially displaced to the rim of the acetabulum and slides laterally but does not go out of the socket.
- *Dislocatable:* The femoral head is in the socket but can be displaced completely outside the acetabulum with manual pressure.
- *Dislocated:* The femoral head lies completely outside the acetabulum but can be reduced into the acetabulum with manual pressure.
- *Teratologic:* The femoral head lies completely outside the acetabulum and cannot be reduced with manual pressure and deformity of the joint surfaces is significant, usually involving another disorder such as arthrogryposis or myelomeningocele. Surgery is needed to reconstruct the joint.

CAUSE

Congenital dislocation of the hip may be secondary to laxity of the ligaments around the joint or to in utero positioning (Beers & Berkow, 1999, p. 2219). When the term dysplasia is used, it refers to abnormal development or growth of the acetabulum or proximal femur (Ratliffe, 1998, p. 77). Congenital dislocation of the hip is more common in female than male infants and in infants with breech presentation (Beers & Berkow, 1999, p. 2219). The incidence is 1 out of every 100 births in the United States. The ratio of girls to boys is 6:1 and the left hip is affected twice as often as the right. The rationale is that in most fetal positions it is the left leg that is wedged in an adducted position against the mother's spine. Typically the dislocation or dysplasia develops in the last trimester of pregnancy (Ratliffe, 1998, p. 77).

Cultural practices may account for the diversity of occurrence in various countries. Where practices in carrying infants includes abduction of the flexion of the legs around the parent's waist or back, the incidence of dislocation is low. Where practice in carrying infants includes extension and adduction of the legs such as strapping the infant onto a cradle board, the incidence is higher (Ratliffe, 1998, p. 77).

ASSESSMENT

AREAS
- Hip range of motion (ROM)
- Joint stability
- Joint mobility and flexibility
- Muscle strength
- Positioning

INSTRUMENTS/PROCEDURES
- Barlow test involves the examiner moving the infant's hip into flexion and abduction, then slowly moving it back into adduction with pressure directed posteriorly. If a click is felt, the femur may be slipping out of the acetabulum or sliding over the posterior border of the acetabulum, indicating instability.

- Ortolani test involves first placing the hip in adduction and flexion with posterior force applied. When the hip is subsequently moved into abduction with slight traction, a click may be felt as the dislocated hip slides back into the acetabulum.

PROBLEMS
- Infant has asymmetrical hip abduction in flexion, with the affected side being tighter.
- Infant may have asymmetrical groin or buttock skin folds.
- Infant's femur may be moved in and out of the hip socket with manual traction.
- Infant's femur may appear to be shorter on the affected side.

TREATMENT/MANAGEMENT

Conservative treatment is used for the first four grades but surgery may be required if conservative treatment is not successful. The fifth type, teratologic, always requires surgery to reconstruct the joint. Treatment prior to age 18 months usually involves conservative management. After 18 months, surgery may be needed. Protocols do vary widely across the country.

GENERAL
- Maintain the hip in flexion and abduction through bracing, splinting, or diapering until the hip has remodeled so that the hip does not come out of acetabulum.
- The multiple diapering technique involves placing the child in two or three diapers holding the legs in abduction. The child is then positioned in hip flexion.
- Pavlik harness technique involves use of the harness to position the infant in moderate hip abduction and flexion but does allow for spontaneous kicking and movement of the leg. The harness is usually worn 24 hours per day for 6 to 12 weeks (Ratliffe, 1998, p. 79).
- Traction for several weeks may be used with an older child to reduce pressure on the femoral head and relax contracted muscles.
- Casting is used after closed or open reduction when the child is over 2 years of age. If open reduction involving remolding is needed, the spica cast is usually on for 6 to 12 weeks. The position in the cast is usually hip extension, moderate abduction, and knee extension. The cast may be cut back to allow for greater movement.

Pavlik Harness (use began in 1950)
- Instruct parents and family members in how to position the infant when conservative management is used.
- Instruct parents and family members in how to apply the Pavlik harness correctly to avoid too much flexion or abduction. The purpose of the harness is to restrict hip extension and adduction.
- Teach parents and family members how to handle the infant, including picking up and carrying the infant in a Pavlik harness.
- Provide information to parents on appropriate developmental intervention. The harness can decrease sensory and motor output which may lead to developmental delay. Parents may be reluctant to pick up or move the infant for fear of hurting the infant.

Spica Cast: Reclining
- Assist parents and family members to find the best way to lift and handle the child. With a spica cast on, the child may weight twice as much because of the weight of the cast itself. In addition the child's legs are extended. The combination of added weight and awkward position makes moving the child a challenge. See Ratliffe (1998) for a comprehensive set of handling strategies.
- Instruct parents and family members in care of cast.

- Discuss with parents and family members options for independent mobility while in the cast. A reclining adult wheelchair without leg rests can be used. A pillow and anti-tippers are needed to ensure safety since the center of gravity is different. Other options include a wagon with pillow and extension to support the cast, a lawn cart with extension for the cast, or a large scooter board such as the ones used in automotive repair.
- Discuss other options to increase independence such as giving the child the remote control for the TV, using a plastic basin that sits on the child's chest to facilitate face washing and brushing teeth, placing the child in the living room rather than in a secluded bedroom, and giving the child a signaling device such as a bell to call for help. Access to a computer could facilitate doing homework as well as providing recreation.
- Maintain functional ROM and strength in joints not restricted by the cast using age-appropriate games and activities which encourage active movement. Examples include scooter board races, finger (or toe) painting, playing catch, putting on a puppet show, singing, or painting at an easel.

Spica Cast: Standing
- Depending on the stability of the joint and type of surgery, passive standing can be started using a tilt table or supine stander. Usually such equipment and program will be in a hospital, clinic, or school.
- Monitor the child for pain, blood pressure, and anxiety or apprehension.
- Provide the child with an activity (toys, games, entertainment) to do while standing.
- Continue to maintain ROM and strength in joints not casted.

Walking and Gait Training
- Crutch walking can be used to maintain balance, strength, and ROM but should not be used with children under 6 years old. A walker is better for younger children. Practice in the parallel bars may make crutch walking or use of the walker easier to learn.
- Provide balance and mobility training as well as gait training after the cast is removed.

PRECAUTIONS/CONTRAINDICATIONS
- When positioning in a brace or splint do not hyperabduct or hyperflex the hip which can cause avascular necrosis as a result of excessive pressure on the femoral head. Other complications include femoral nerve palsy, inferior dislocation, and erosion of the posterior rim of the acetabulum.
- Allowing kicking and movement of the legs also reduces the pressure on the femoral head and thus reduces the possibility of avascular necrosis.
- Watch for signs of developmental delay due to a lack of interaction with the environment.

DESIRED OUTCOME/PROGNOSIS
Prognosis with the Pavlik harness is considered excellent: 90% to 95% of cases are successfully treated (Leach, 2000, p. 409).
- Child has alignment of hip joint in all functional positions.
- Child has functional ROM in the hip joint.
- Child has postural stability while kneeling or standing that is age appropriate.
- Child has mobility skills that are age appropriate with or without assistive devices.
- Child has achieved age-appropriate gross motor skills.

REFERENCES

Beers MH, Berkow R, eds. *The Merck Manual of Diagnosis and Therapy.* Whitehouse Station, NJ: Merck Research Laboratories; 1999.

Leach J. Orthopedic conditions—Developmental dysplasia of the hip. In: Campbell SK, ed. *Physical Therapy for Children.* 2nd ed. Philadelphia, Pa: WB Saunders Co; 2000:406–411.

Ratliffe KT. Disorders of the developing hip—The child with developmental dysplasia of the hip. In: Ratliffe KT. *Clinical Pediatric Physical Therapy: A Guide for the Physical Therapy Team.* St. Louis, Mo: CV Mosby Co; 1998:77–82.

Stanger M. Orthopedic management—Developmental dysplasia of the hip. In: Tecklin JS, ed. *Pediatric Physical Therapy.* 3rd ed. Philadelphia, Pa: Lippincott Williams and Wilkins; 1999:397–401.

Down Syndrome

Also known as *trisomy 21, trisomy G, mongolism.*

ICD-9-CM Code: 758 Chromosomal anomalies
APTA Guide Patterns: 5A, 5B

DESCRIPTION

A chromosomal disorder usually resulting in mental retardation, a characteristic face, and many other typical features, including microcephaly and short stature (Beers & Berkow, 1999, p. 2233). Down syndrome is named for John Langdon Down, who published a paper in 1866 on the characteristics of the syndrome. Down syndrome results in neuromotor, musculoskeletal, and cardiopulmonary pathology which require lifelong management. Neuropathology includes overall reduction in brain weight, smaller cerebellum, brain stem, microcephaly, microbrachycephaly, reduction in secondary sulci, reduction or lack of myelination, and altered synaptic morphology (Bertoti, 1999, p. 302). Some children with Down syndrome also have a seizure disorder. Common features include a flat facial profile, upward slanting eyes, a flat nasal bridge, small ears, and large tongue (Ratliffe, 1998, p. 232).

CLASSIFICATION
- *Trisomy 21:* In about 95% of cases, there is an extra whole chromosome 21 which in 95% of these cases is maternally derived.
- *Translocation:* Some persons with Down syndrome have 46 chromosomes but actually have the genetic material of 47 chromosomes; the additional chromosome 21 has been translocated or attached to another chromosome. The most common translocation is the additional chromosome 21 attached to a chromosome 14.
- *Mosaicism:* Mosaicism occurs when two different cell types are present in a person. Down syndrome mosaicism presumably results from an error in chromosomal separation during cell division in the growing embryo. Most cases have two cell lines. One normal and one with 47 chromosomes. The relative proportion of each cell line is highly variable, both between persons and within different tissues and organs in the same person (Beers & Berkow, 1999, pp. 2233–4).

CAUSE

The overall incidence among live births is about 1 in 800 but there is a marked variability depending on maternal age: for mothers under 20 years, the incidence is about 1 in 200; for mothers over age 40, it rises to about 1 in 40 overall. About 20% of infants with Down

481

syndrome are born to mothers over 35 years. Down syndrome may result from trisomy 21, translocation, or mosaicism (Beers & Berkow, 1999, p. 2233).

ASSESSMENT

- Analyze not only what the child can do but also the processes underlying the observed skills and behaviors.
- Focus on the functional aspects, using age-appropriate materials.
- Identify both the disability but also the child's abilities.
- Always assess sensory processes and attention at the same time as the item of interest.

AREAS

- Sensory systems: visual, auditory, tactile, vestibular
- Muscle strength
- Muscle tone
- Gross and fine motor skills
- Developmental testing
- Reflex/reactions and postural responses
- Autonomic reactions
- Cognitive functioning
- Functional skills
- Atlantoaxial stability
- Hip subluxation

INSTRUMENTS/PROCEDURES

No specific assessments mentioned in references.

PROBLEMS

- Child often has hypotonia in all muscle groups of extremities, neck, and trunk.
- Child often has ligamentous laxity resulting in pes planus, patellar instability, and scoliosis.
- Child often has developmental motor delay in gross and fine motor skills. Child may "W" sit, persist in using a wide base of support and toe-out.
- Child often has delays in integration of primitive reflex patterns and a slower rate of development of postural control including deficits in postural response synergies and compensatory movement strategies.
- Child often has hands and feet that tend to be small and toes are short.
- Child often has slow or poor attending skills: is slow to arouse, has difficulty staying alert, and has a short attention span to focus on task.
- Child often has difficulty with motor planning, sequential verbal processing, and auditory memory.
- Child often has difficulty with learning and memory. Generally learns fewer tasks or routines, needs a greater number of repetitions to learn, has greater difficulty with verbal-motor interactions, has greater difficulty with responses that call for auditory or vocal skills, has greater difficulty generalizing skills, has greater difficulty maintaining skills that are not practiced regularly, has slower response times, and has a more limited repertoire of responses.
- Child may have decreased grip strength, isometric strength and ankle strength.
- Child may have atlantoaxial instability due to excessive motion of C1 on C2.
- Child may have frequent respiratory and other infections due to immune deficiency.
- Child may have myopia, farsightedness, strabismus, nystagmus, astigmatism, cataracts, or other visual deficit.
- Child may have a hearing loss and difficulty with auditory processing due to narrow eustachian tubes and frequent ear infections.
- Child may have balance and gait dysfunction.
- If congenital heart defects are present, developmental motor delay may be more severe.

- Child may have decrease in velocity of growth in stature, absent palmaris longus, and supernumerary forearm flexors, lack of differentiation of distinct muscle bellies for the zygomaticus major and minor and levator labii superior, and increased deep tendon reflexes.
- Child may have oral motor delays and difficulty with feeding due to dentition delay, protruding tongue, high palate, and low muscle tone.
- Child may have delays in communication and psychosocial development.

TREATMENT/MANAGEMENT

Problems with sensory and cognitive systems often require modification of treatment and management techniques to account for variations in sensory input and cognitive processing.

- Use visual demonstration, practice and rehearsal, or multimodal sensory approaches such as visual, kinesthetic, and verbal to compensate for poor auditory processing.
- Treatment should be based on an understanding of the functional, dynamic systems perspective: control parameters most likely to cause a responsiveness shift when attempting to influence developing motor strategies.
- Use positioning and handling activities in early infancy and childhood to promote antigravity control and weight bearing.
- Facilitate antigravity extension in prone and weight shifting within and as transition from prone.
- In supine and supported sitting, encourage midline orientation, antigravity, and manual activities including eye-hand coordination and activities to promote anterior neck and trunk antigravity strength.
- Emphasize trunk extension and extremity loading, which tend to increase axial tone.
- Encourage emergence of righting and postural reactions through use of rotation within and during movement.
- Facilitate use of dynamic rather then static exploration of movement.
- Introduce developmental milestones when chronologically appropriate, including supported sitting and standing, when trunk control and alignment are established.
- Provide functional opportunities to enhance development in areas of cognition, language, and socialization.
- Use aligned compression or weight-bearing forces to stimulate longitudinal bone growth as well as thickness and density of the bone and shaft.
- Use aligned, supported weight bearing to promote joint stability and formation.
- Facilitate normal co-contraction, force production, and increased muscle tone.
- Emphasize physical fitness to increase cardiopulmonary endurance and muscle strength.
- Instruct parents and other team members about activities and position choices that will enhance the child's overall development including toys for play time.
- Provide family with suggestions for community resources.

PRECAUTIONS/CONTRAINDICATIONS

- Be aware of possible cardiopulmonary pathologies such as atrioventricular canal defects and vestibuloseptal defects which may reduce cardiopulmonary efficiency. Observe for lips or nail beds turning blue, pallid skin, lethargy, and sweating.
- If a seizure disorder is present, appropriate precautions should be applied.
- Screen for scoliosis. If present, limit asymmetrical activities.
- Avoid exaggerated neck flexion, extension, rotation, and positions of movement that may cause twisting or undue forces.

- Use caution in applying joint approximation or compression to the cervical spine in young children when a radiograph has not reliably detected whether atlantoaxial instability is present or not. In children with identified atlantoaxial instability joint compression is contraindicated.
- If atlantoaxial instability is present, participation in contact sports and physical activities that may result in cervical spine injury may be contraindicated. Examples include somersaults, diving, high jump, soccer, butterfly stroke in swimming, exercises that place pressure on the head and neck, and participation in pentathlon.

DESIRED OUTCOME/PROGNOSIS

- Child has attained gross motor milestones including rolling, sitting, standing, and walking.
- Child performs functional skills.
- Child has strength and endurance to perform activities.
- Child participates in a daily exercise program.
- Child has a role and expected tasks in the family.
- Child participates in school, community, and recreational activities.

REFERENCES

Beers MH, Berkow R, eds. *The Merck Manual of Diagnosis and Therapy*. Whitehouse Station, NJ: Merck Research Laboratories; 1999.

Dertoti, DB. Mental retardation: Focus on Down syndrome. In: Tecklin JS, ed. *Pediatr Phys Ther*. 3rd ed. Philadelphia, Pa: Lippincott Williams and Wilkins; 1999:283–313.

Lauteslager PEM, Vermeer A, Helders PJM. Disturbances in the motor behaviour of children with Down's syndrome: The need for a theoretical framework. *Physiotherapy*. 1998; 84(1):5–13.

Ratliffe KT. Genetic disorders—The child with Down syndrome. In: Ratliffe KT. *Clinical Pediatric Physical Therapy: A Guide for the Physical Therapy Team*. St. Louis, Mo: CV Mosby Co; 1998:232–236.

Stuberg WA, Sanger WG. Genetic disorders: a pediatric perspective. In: Umphred D, ed. *Neurolog Rehabil*. 4th ed. St. Louis, Mo: CV Mosby Co; 2001:287–307.

Foot Disorders

ICD-9-CM Codes:

- 755 Other congenital anomalies of limbs
- 756 Other congenital musculoskeletal anomalies

APTA Guide Patterns: 4B, 4G, 4J, 4K, 5A, 5B

DESCRIPTION

Calcaneovalgus involves dorsiflexion of the foot, eversion of valgus deformity of the hindfoot and abduction of the metatarsals. The deformity is common in cerebral palsy, spinal bifida, and arthrogryposis (Ratliffe, 1998, p. 136). Calcaneovalgus may occur as a common positional foot problem in newborns which typically corrects spontaneously or as a result of vertical talus in which the talus is vertically oriented and the navicular is displaced onto the dorsal surface of the talus. The forefoot is dorsiflexed, the hindfoot is plantar flexed, and the foot bends at the instep resulting in a "rocker-bottom" deformity of the foot (Leach, 2000, p. 403).

Flat foot occurs when the child stands and the longitudinal arch of the foot decreases or disappears (Leach, 2000, p. 405).

Metatarsus adductus (also called *metatarsus varus*) occurs when the forefoot is adducted and may be supined at rest. The forefoot is adducted in relation to the midfoot and hindfoot. The lateral border is convex with the curve beginning at the base of the fifth metatarsal. Often, the foot can be passively abducted and everted beyond the neutral position when the sole is stimulated. The appearance is one of toes curved inward and the child appears to toe-in. Resolution without treatment usually occurs in the first year of life. Fixed deformities require casting or surgery (Beers & Berkow, 1999, p. 2402; Ratliffe, 1998, p. 136; Stanger, 1999, p. 396) *Metatarsus varus* is the name given to the most severe form.

Sever's disease (apophysitis of the calcaneus) is characterized by the posterior portion of the calcaneus developing separately from the main body of the calcaneus. It is a common source of posterior heel pain in children who are active in sports during the ages of 7 to 12 years (Topham & White, 1998, p. 160).

Talipes equinovarus (also called *congenital talipes equinovarus* or *clubfoot*) is the classic form of clubfoot that involves adduction of the forefoot, varus position of the hind-foot, and equinous at the ankle. The forefoot is curved inward in relation to the heel, the heel is bent inward in relation to the leg, and the ankle is fixed in plantar flexion with the toes point down. About 50% of cases are bilateral (Ratliffe, 1998, p. 136).

Tibial torsion involves a rotation of the tibia in relation to the femur that is greater than usual. It is included under foot disorders because foot problems are associated with it.

CAUSE

Calcaneovalgus occurs in newborns and is associated with a large infant in a small space in utero (Leach, 2000, p. 403). The condition also occurs in a number of congenital disorders where the cause is unclear.

Flat foot is usually due to normal ligamentous laxity that typically can be demonstrated through the extremities as evidenced by hyperextension at the elbows and knees and ability to approximate the thumb to the forearm. In infants and toddlers the fat pad in the medial part of the foot may give the appearance of a flat foot (Leach, 2000, p. 405).

Metatarsus adductus is caused by intrauterine positioning and is usually associated with other positional deformities such as congenital muscular torticollis or hip dysplasia (Stanger, 1999, p. 396). Abnormal development of the medial cuneiform may be a pathogenic factor (Leach, 2000, p. 402).

Sever's disease (apophysitis of the calcaneus) occurs when there are predisposing factors such as abnormal stresses at the calcaneal epiphysis, microtrauma, or biomechanical abnormalities of the foot. Overuse, repetitive loading of the heel, and foot malalignments are common factors. Soccer players and runners are most often affected (Topham & White, 1998, p. 160).

Talipes equinovarus may be caused by positional deformities related to neurological disorders such as myelomeningocele or arthrogryposis, genetic predisposition or may be related to the size of infant and uterus. Often the cause is unclear. Twice as many boys as girls have clubfoot. The incidence is about 1 in every 1,000 live births (Ratliffe, 1998, p. 136; Leach, 2000, p. 402)

Tibial torsion may be related to tightness and contractures that do not stretch out normally when the child begins to walk.

ASSESSMENT

AREAS
- Alignment of foot to lower leg
- Gait
- Range of motion (ROM)
- Weight bearing

INSTRUMENTS/PROCEDURES

- Foot progression angle (FPA) or "the angle of gait": the angle between the longitudinal axis of the foot and a straight line of progression of the body in walking. In-toeing is expressed as a negative value such as −30 degrees while out-toeing is expressed as a positive value such as +20 degrees. A supported stance can be used for a child who is not yet walking independently.
- Gait analysis
- Torsional profile: Composed of 4 components: foot progression angle in standing or walking, hip rotation ROM, thigh-foot axis, and alignment of the foot
- Valgus or varus: Stand child on photocopy machine and make a photocopy of the feet

PROBLEMS

- Child may be unable to stand on the feet because of the severe angle abnormalities between the foot and tibia.
- Child may stand in abnormal positions such as severe toeing in or out.
- Child may stand totally on the lateral or medial borders of the foot.
- Child may be unable to dorsiflex the foot (ie, clubfoot).
- Child may have a foot shape that is abnormal: kidney shaped with deviates medially (metatarsus varus and clubfoot) and a banana shape with deviates laterally (calcaneovalgus).
- Child's heel position may deviate to valgus (metatarsus varus, calcaneovalgus) or varus (clubfoot).
- Child may have a "windswept" condition in which one limb toes in while the other toes out.

TREATMENT/MANAGEMENT

CALCANEOVALGUS

- If the child is expected to walk, surgical correction may be considered.
- Risks of surgery may outweigh possible benefits if the child is not expected to bear weight on the feet.

FLAT FOOT

- Corrective orthopedic shoes, Helfet heel-cuts, or custom-molded plastic inters have all been shown to be effective.
- Shoes with arch supports do not correct flat feet but can decrease wear on the medial border of the shoes, thereby decreasing expense of shoe purchases.

METATARSUS ADDUCTUS

- The decision as to when to intervene, if at all, varies. Some physicians advocate no treatment until the child is walking to see if maturation will correct the problem.
- In mild cases often no treatment is indicated. The deviance corrects itself as the child grows.
- In moderate cases, straight-last or reverse-last shoe may be used to correct the forefoot position.
- In severe cases, progressive casting or surgery may be necessary to correct foot alignment.

SEVER'S DISEASE (APOPHYSITIS OF THE CALCANEUS)

- Conservative treatment is directed toward pain relief: rest, ice, and therapeutic ultrasound.
- A half-inch heel lift may decrease the tension of the shorted Achilles tendon and plantar fascia.

- A viscoelastic heel cup may decrease the impact shock from heel strike.
- Provide a program of heel cord stretching and dorsiflexor muscle strengthening exercises.
- For more severe cases, supportive shoes and nighttime dorsiflexor splints are useful.
- If excessive pronation of the forefoot is noted, orthotics may be indicated.

TALIPES EQUINOVARUS
- Treatment involves manipulation, taping, stretching, bracing, serial casting, and surgery.
- Surgery is typically performed between 3 months and 1 year of age.
- Instruct parents in developmental activities to promote sensory experience, motor skills, and developmental experiences.

TIBIAL TORSION
- Active treatment includes braces with straps or cables that are worn at night to pull the lower leg into the opposite rotation.
- A Dennis Brown splint may be used for a young child.
- Instruct parents to provide appropriate developmental intervention.
- Instruct parents to put brace or splint onto child properly.

PRECAUTIONS/CONTRAINDICATIONS
- Correct determination as to which component(s) are causing the problem is critical. Foot disorders may be compounded by problems in other parts of the lower extremities.
- In general, surgery in infancy is not the recommended choice. Conservative measures, however, work best if started early.
- Treatment of flat foot in children should be conservative. A low arch is typically not a problem in adulthood. Rather, a high-arched (cavus) feet is often a greater problem (Leach, 2000, p. 406).
- In Sever's disease, walking barefoot should be avoided.
- In Sever's disease, surgery is not recommended because the disease is self-limiting.

DESIRED OUTCOME/PROGNOSIS

Outcomes and prognosis vary depending on the type and severity of the foot disorder and other medical conditions the infant or child may have.

- Child's foot alignment and joint tightness do not interfere with caregiving activities if there is no expectation for weight bearing or walking.
- Child's alignment of foot to tibia is within normal limits for age.
- Child has functional ROM and is free of contractures or joint tightness that restricts joint motion.
- Child is able to bear weight in standing and joint stability is good.
- Child is able to walk and gait is within accepted standards.
- Child does not experience pain while performing daily sports activities.
- Child participates in home, school, community, and recreational activities.

REFERENCES

Beers MH, Berkow R, eds. *The Merck Manual of Diagnosis and Therapy.* Whitehouse Station, NJ: Merck Research Laboratories; 1999.

Bartonek A, Saraste H, Knutson LM, Eriksson M. Orthotic treatment with Ferrari knee-ankle foot orthoses. *Pediatr Phys Ther.* 1999;11(1):33–38.

Leach J. Orthopedic conditions—Torsional conditions, angular conditions, flat foot. In: Campbell SK, ed. *Physical Therapy for Children.* 2nd ed. Philadelphia, Pa: WB Saunders Co; 2000:399–406.

Ratliffe KT. Other orthopedic disorders—The child with foot and lower leg deformities. In: Ratliffe KT. *Clinical Pediatric Physical Therapy: A Guide for the Physical Therapy Team.* St. Louis, Mo: CV Mosby Co; 1998:136–137.

Stanger M. Orthopedic management—congenital metatarsus adductus and clubfoot deformity. In Tecklin J, ed. *Pediatric physical therapy.* 3rd ed. Philadelphia, Pa: JB Lippincott Co; 1999:396–397.

Topham AE, White JA. Sever's disease. *Phys Ther Case Rep.* 1998;1(3):150–161.

Fracture of Limbs

ICD-9-CM Codes: 813, 815, 821, 823, 825, 826 Fractures
APTA Guide Patterns: 4D, 4H, 4J

DESCRIPTION

Children's bones are more flexible, more porous, and lack the density of adult bones. These factors lead to different fracture patterns in children than those seen in adults. Common fracture patterns in children are the buckle fracture, epiphyseal fracture, greenstick and bending fractures, and spiral fractures. In addition, children's periosteum is thicker and stronger than that of adults, leading to a better blood supply and therefore faster healing. Symptoms of fractures in children include swelling, redness, pain, deformity of the extremity, and muscle spasm or guarding. Very young children who cannot speak may cry or refuse to use the extremity (Ratliffe, 1998, p. 140).

CAUSE

Causes include motor vehicle accidents, falls, sports injuries, child abuse, and accidents on skateboards, rollerskates, bicycles, and trampolines. The cause of injury, direction and amount of force determine the type of fracture. Seventy-five percent of all fractures in children are in the upper extremities. Common sites are the humerus, radius, ulna, wrist, and hand. Other sites are the clavicle and femur (Ratliffe, 1998, p. 140).

ASSESSMENT

AREAS
- Gait
- Joint mobility
- Joint stability
- Muscle strength
- Range of motion (ROM)

INSTRUMENTS/PROCEDURES

None listed.

PROBLEMS
- Child may be unable to bear weight if fracture is in a lower extremity.
- Child may be reluctant to use an upper extremity.
- Child may develop contractures.
- Child may have difficulty performing functional activities such as walking or eating.

TREATMENT/MANAGEMENT

Treatment depends on the type of fracture and whether closed or open reduction is required. Typically, fractures require immobilization by splinting or casting for a specific length of time. Usually the fractures heal in 2 or 3 weeks (Ratliffe, 1998, p. 140).

If multiple fractures have occurred from a motor vehicle accident or other major trauma, additional injuries may also be present such as head injury or trauma to vital organs and soft tissue that may complicate the rehabilitation process.

- Teach crutch walking skills for lower extremity injury.
- After a sustained immobilization gentle ROM or strengthening may be necessary to help the child regain functional skills.
- Encourage child to return to normal daily activities.

PRECAUTIONS/CONTRAINDICATIONS
- Frequent sequelae to epiphyseal fractures are decreased limb length, angular deformity, joint incongruity, and premature closure. Care should be taken to minimize these problems.

DESIRED OUTCOME/PROGNOSIS

Expected outcome is complete union of the epiphyseal plate itself, the epiphyseal plate to the shaft, or parts of the shaft.

- Child has normal or functional ROM in all limbs, including the one that was fractured.
- Child has regained muscle strength and endurance expected for age or preexisting medical condition.
- Child performs functional skills that are age appropriate or where performed prior to the fracture.
- Child performs mobility and ambulation skills attained prior to fracture.
- Child's level of growth and development is age appropriate or consistent with rate attained prior to fracture.
- Child participates in home, school, community, and recreational activities.

REFERENCES

Bernhardt-Bainbridge D. Sports injuries in children—Types of injuries. In: Campbell SK, ed. *Physical Therapy for Children*. 2nd ed. Philadelphia, Pa: WB Saunders Co; 2000:445–457.

Ratliffe KT. Other orthopedic disorders—Fractures in children. In Ratliffe KT. *Clinical Pediatric Physical Therapy: A Guide for the Physical Therapy Team*. St. Louis, Mo: CV Mosby Co; 1998:140–141.

Stanger M. Orthopedic management—fractures. In: Tecklin JS, ed. *Pediatric Physical Therapy*. 3rd ed. Philadelphia, Pa: Lippincott Williams and Wilkins; 1999:406–408.

Genetic Disorders

ICD-9-CD Codes:
- 758 Chromosomal anomalies
- 759 Other and unspecified congenital anomalies

APTA Guide Patterns: 5A, 5B

DESCRIPTION

Genetic disorders include chromosomal abnormalities, single gene abnormalities, multifactorical, mitochondiral, and others in which the classification is undetermined. Chromosomal abnormalities include autosomal trisomies, sex chromosome abnormalities, and partial deletion. Single-gene abnormalities include autosomal dominant, autosomal recessive, and sex-linked abnormalities.

CAUSE

The specific cause of some genetic disorders is known while in other disorders the exact cause is unclear. For example, the cause of chromosomal and single gene disorder is clearer than disorders with multifactorical influences. The number of genetic disorders in which the cause is known has increased rapidly in the past few decades. In addition, some genetic disorders have a predictable pattern that has been and can be charted in a family tree. Other genetic disorders have not yielded such a clear picture to date.

Incidence varies widely. For example, the incidence of Down syndrome is 1 in 700, while Hurler syndrome is 1 in 100,000. Some disorders are found only in males, such as Klinefelter syndrome, while others affect only females, such as Turner syndrome. The ratio of males to females differs as well in disorders affecting both sexes. For example, fragile X syndrome is found in both sexes but males are affected more often than females. Ethnicity also plays a role. Cystic fibrosis is more common in whites than in other races.

ASSESSMENT

Note: These are general areas and instruments that are not specific to a particular disorder or individual child.

AREAS
- Developmental level
- Functional skills
- Gross and fine motor skills
- Mobility and ambulation
- Muscle strength
- Muscle tone
- Range of motion (ROM)
- Reflexes and reactions
- Sensory functions
- Soft tissue mobility

INSTRUMENTS
- Alberta Infant Motor Scale (AIMS) (Piper & Darrah, 1994)
- Bayley Scales of Infant Development–II (BSID–II) (Bayley, 1993)
- Bruninks-Oseretsky Test of Motor Proficiency (BOTMP) (Bruninks, 1978)
- Functional Independence Measure for Children (Wee FIM) (Granger, Hamilton, & Kayton, 1989)
- Gesell & Amatruda Development and Neurological Examination (Knoblock, 1987)
- Movement Assessment of Infants (MAI) (Chandler, Andrews, & Swanson, 1980)
- Peabody Developmental Motor Scales, 2nd ed. (PDMS) (Folio & Fewell, 1999)
- Pediatric Evaluation of Disability Inventory (PEDI) (Haley, et al, 1992)
- School Function Assessment (SFA) (Coster, et al, 1998)
- Tufts Assessment of Motor Performance (TAMP) (Gans, et al, 1988)

PROBLEMS
- Child may have hypertonicity including stiff or jerky movements that are limited in variety, speed, and coordination.
- Child may have total patterns of flexion or extension with limited ability for selective joint movement.
- Child may have retention of primitive reflexes that result in stereotyped movement depending on the type of sensory input.

- Child may have spasticity.
- Child may have hypotonicity and tend to lock weight-bearing joint or use a wide base of support.
- Child may have hyperextensible joints.
- Child may have contractures and deformities.
- Child may have respiratory problems.
- Child may have cognitive impairments.
- Child may have communication disorders.

TREATMENT/MANAGEMENT

Treatment and management are presented as general issues not specific to each identified genetic disorder. Usually a team approach is involved in setting goals. Team members may include family members, physicians, nursing personnel, occupational therapist, music therapist, orthotist or prosthetist, psychologist, teaching personnel, and social worker in addition to the physical therapist.

General treatment principles include focusing on functional skills, delivering services in a natural environment, incorporating therapy activities into daily routines, and using assistive technology as needed (Stuberg & Sanger, 2001, pp. 302–303).

- For hypertonicity, increase ROM and decrease effect on muscle tone through positioning.
- If primitive reflexes are present but stereotypical movements are not, facilitate functional movement that is not dominated by persistent reflexes by practicing new motor patterns to accomplish functional activity.
- If stereotypical movement is the only pattern the child uses, focus therapy activities on active movement.

   Note: Passive inhibition techniques in an attempt to "normalize" tone and movement are not cost effective and may decrease functional independence once stereotypical movement patterns are established (Stuberg, 2001, p. 296).

- Promote development of postural reactions including righting, protective extension, and tilting.
- For hypotonicity, increase joint stability, muscle strength, and energy endurance.
- For hyperextensible joint, encourage use of ROM in functional positions. Modify activities or provide external support to avoid undue stress to hyperextensible joints and surrounding ligaments, tendons, and fascia. Weight bearing should occur through neutral alignment. Vary the placement of toys, use different support surfaces, provide physical assistance, and incorporate adapted equipment (eg, a vertical stander) or orthotic devices (eg, an ankle-foot orthoses) to modify weight-bearing forces.
- Prevent contractures. Be aware of habitual positioning that may lead to restrictions in soft tissue. One example is wide abduction, external rotation, and flexion of the hips ("frog" or "reverse W" position). Soft tissue contractures can develop at the hips and knees.
- Prevent deformities. Be aware that a limited variety of postures and movements and habitual use of the same positioning pattern increases the risk of deformities. An example is the use of a constant position of hip adduction, flexion, and internal rotation that increases the risk of hip subluxation or dislocation. Abnormal muscle tone, strength, or immobility in the trunk increases the risk of excessive lumbar lordosis, thoracic kyphosis, and development of scoliosis.
- Prevent respiratory problems. Use mobilization techniques, deep breathing, chest expansion exercises, and postural drainage. For a child who is unable to tolerate one position for an extended time, find alternate positions and use adapted positioning devices.
- Increase functional skills in mobility, self-help, and communication. If possible, integrate practice into the natural environment such as the home or school at the time the activity would normally be performed. Encourage family members and teachers to

incorporate practice and application of functional skills whenever possible into the natural or normal environment in which the skill is used and within the regular daily routine.

- Recommend and provide training and practice in use of assistive technology such as mobility devices, augmentative communication devices, adapted computer keyboards, adaptive devices such as splints and bath chairs, and positioning equipment.
- Recommend and identify resources for environmental modifications to facilitate accessibility and travel.
- Support the family. Be aware that intervention can enhance or hinder the family's ability to function as a family. Recognize the multiple tasks required to care for the child with a disability including daily care, economic, recreational, social, educational, and vocational needs which must be addressed. These factors affect the whole family and not just the child. A balance of concern for the negative aspects related to the disability and for the positive elements of the child is important. Considerations include an acknowledgement of the importance of the family's priorities, respect for the family's cultural values, involvement of the family as team members, and promotion of services that build on the resources of the family and community.
- Provide information to family about the genetic disorder and help the family identify medical specialists and genetic counseling services.
- Provide information on resources available to help with management of the child's needs such as programs and services for disabilities, financial assistance, legal aid, online services, support groups, recreational activities, educational resources, and equipment and supply vendors.

PRECAUTIONS/CONTRAINDICATIONS
- Do not stretch spastic muscles.
- Avoid stress to hyperextensible joint, ligaments, tendons, and fascia. Do not allow knee or elbow joint to lock into extension during weight bearing.
- Do not focus only on the child's deficits that impact negatively on how the child is perceived in the family unit.

OUTCOME/PROGNOSIS

The outcome and prognosis varies widely in genetic disorders. Some impairments and disabilities can be treated effectively so that the individual can participate successfully in society while other disorders create severe dysfunction or multiple dysfunctions that are more difficult to treat and manage successfully. The following outcomes listed are general in nature.

- Child has independent mobility with or without mobility devices and assistance.
- Child has functional skills in self-care and communication with or without assistive devices and assistance.
- Child participates in home, school, recreational, and community activities with or without assistive technology and environmental modifications.
- Family has identified and uses legal, economic, medical, educational, online, and community resources to assist in managing the child's needs.

REFERENCES

McEwen IR. Children with cognitive impairments. In: Campbell SK, Vander Linden DW, Palisano RJ. *Physical Therapy for Children*. 2nd ed. Philadelphia, Pa: WB Saunders Co; 2001:502–532.

Ratliffe KT. Genetic disorders. In: Ratliffe, KT. *Clinical Pediatric Physical Therapy: a Guide for the Physical Therapy Team*. St. Louis, Mo: CV Mosby Co; 1998:219–274.

Stuberg WA, Sanger WG. Genetic disorders: a pediatric perspective. In: Umphred D, ed. *Neurological Rehabilitation*. 4th ed., St. Louis, Mo: CV Mosby Co; 2001:287–307.

Hemophilia

ICD-9-CM Codes:
- 286.0 Hemophilia A
- 286.1 Hemophilia B
- 286.2 Hemophilia C

APTA Guide Pattern: 4D

DESCRIPTION

Common forms of hereditary bleeding disorders caused by clotting factor deficiencies of factor VIII, IX, or XI.

LEVELS OF SEVERITY
- *Mild:* Child has 5% to 25% of normal clotting factor in the blood. The child is at risk for bleeding from moderate to severe trauma and from surgery but usually not from mild trauma resulting from falls or general sports except contact sports.
- *Moderate:* Child has between 1% and 5% of clotting factor in the blood. The child is at risk for excessive bleeding from mild to moderate trauma and will have some bleeding into joints but seldom has spontaneous bleeding. Child can participate in swimming, jogging, and golf but not contact sports.
- *Severe:* Child has less than 1% of clotting factor in the blood. The child is at risk for bleeding from very mild trauma and may have spontaneous bleeding. This is the most common type. Approximately 60% have this type.

CAUSE

Hemophilia A (factor VIII deficiency) which affects about 80% of hemophiliacs and hemophilia B (factor IX deficiency) are X-linked genetic transmission disorders and have the same clinical manifestations. About 50% of cases of severe hemophilia A result from a major inversion of a section of the tip of the long arm of the X chromosome. Because factor VIII and factor IX genes are located on the X chromosome, hemophilia affects males almost exclusively.

Daughters of hemophiliacs will be obligatory carriers but sons will be normal. Each son of a carrier has a 50% chance of being a hemophiliac, and each daughter has a 50% chance of being a carrier (Beers & Berkow, 1999, pp. 911–912).

ASSESSMENT

AREAS
- Gait
- Joint mobility
- Pain
- Muscle strength
- Range of motion (ROM)

INSTRUMENTS/PROCEDURES

None listed.

PROBLEMS

- Child can bleed into joints especially the knee, elbow, and ankle. The recurrent bleeding can lead to chronic inflammation and joint changes including damage to and loss of articular cartilage. Disability can include joint contractures, weakness of surrounding muscles, and a functional disturbance of gait.
- Child may experience pain in the joints from bleeding into joints.
- Child who receives clotting factor replacement therapy is at risk for Hepatitis B which affects 80% of children with severe hemophilia. Vaccination can help.
- Child may have attention deficit hyperactivity disorder (ADHD) and learning disabilities.
- Child with hemophilia A may develop antibodies to factor VIII. They are much more at risk for bleeding because of an ineffective response to factor therapy.
- Child with hemarthrosis usually needs to immobilize the joint and stay off the limb until the swelling and pain are reduced.
- Child may require surgery to remove hypertrophied synovial membranes in the knee and elbow.

TREATMENT/MANAGEMENT

Joint replacement surgery to the hip, joint fusion, and osteotomies may be helpful with severe joint destruction.

- Instruct parents to put helmets on toddlers with moderate and severe forms of hemophilia as they learn to walk to prevent bleeding from mild head trauma.
- Instruct child in use of crutches to allow a hemarthrosis to resolve.
- Encourage active ROM to maintain mobility and strength if child has a hemarthrosis.
- Increase muscle strength around the joint with the hemarthrosis. Exercises should be age appropriate and fun such as jumping in a swimming pool.
- Provide splinting, taping, or casting for immobilization for hemarthrosis.
- Improve functional skills such as walking.
- Encourage child to develop and follow a regular exercise program such as swimming, golf, light jogging, table tennis, or other exercise with low impact to joints.

PRECAUTIONS/CONTRAINDICATIONS

- Anyone who received clotting factor replacement therapy before 1985 is at risk for becoming HIV positive.
- Passive ROM is contraindicated for a child with hemophilia because of the risk of unintentional injury to the joint (Ratliffe, 1998, p. 412).

DESIRED OUTCOMES/PROGNOSIS

- Child has functional ROM in major joints.
- Child has muscle strength and endurance to perform daily activities.
- Child does not have pain or pain is managed to permit the performance of daily activities.
- Child performs functional skills that are age appropriate.
- Child performs self-care skills that are age appropriate.
- Child has gross motor skills that are age appropriate.
- Child participates in family, school, recreational, and community activities.
- Family, caregivers, and teachers know and can identify risks of injury.
- Family, caregivers, and teachers know procedures for managing hemophilia on a daily basis.
- Family, caregivers, and teachers know emergency procedures when bleeding occurs that is not quickly controlled.

REFERENCES

Beers MH, Berkow R, eds. *The Merck Manual of Diagnosis and Therapy.* Whitehouse Station, NJ: Merck Research Laboratories; 1999.

Beeton K, Cromwell J, Alltree J. Muscle rehabilitation in haemophilia. *Haemophilia.* 1998;4(4):532–537.

Buzzard BM. Physiotherapy for prevention and treatment of choreic hemophilic synovitis. *Clin Orthop.* 1997;343:42–46.

Buzzard BM. Proprioceptive training in haemophilia. *Haemophilia.* 1998;4(4):528–531.

Buzzard BM. Physiotherapy for the prevention of articular contraction in haemophilia. *Haemophilia.* 1999;5(suppl 1):10–15.

Gilbert MS, Radomiski TE. Management of fixed flexion contracture of the elbow in haemophilia. *Haemophilia.* 1999;5(suppl 1):39–42.

Heijnen L, & de Kleijn P. Physiotherapy for the treatment of articular contractures in haemophilia. *Haemophilia.* 1999;5(suppl 1):16–19.

McGee SM. Hemophilia. In: Campbell SK, ed. *Physical Therapy for Children.* 2nd ed. Philadelphia, Pa: WB Saunders Co; 2000:260–281.

Ratliffe KT. Medical disorders—Other medical disorders of childhood: Hemophilia. In: Ratliffe KT. *Clinical Pediatric Physical Therapy: A Guide for the Physical Therapy Team.* St. Louis, Mo: CV Mosby Co; 1998:411–413.

High-Risk/At-Risk Infant

ICD-9-CM Codes:
- 742 Other congenital anomalies of nervous system
- 756 Other congenital musculoskeletal anomalies
- 758 Chromosomal anomalies
- 759 Other and unspecified congenital anomalies
- 765 Disorders related to short gestation and unspecified low birthweight,
- 767 Birth trauma
- 768 Intrauterine hypoxia and birth asphyxia
- 771 Infections specific to the perinatal period

APTA Guide Patterns: 5A, 5B

DESCRIPTION

Risk factors include an array of medical complications: low birth weight (LBW), birth asphyxia, difficult deliveries, and brain insults. Some infants may be a "double risk" because of social or familial factors that operate to potentiate their medical problems. Examples include maternal substance use, young maternal age, and unstable family situations (Scott et al, 2000, p. 221).

High-risk infants have medical conditions that place them at risk for developmental delays, neuromotor conditions, sensory conditions, and other long-term complications (Scott et al, 2000, p. 224). In general, any infant requiring neonatal intensive care is high risk for neurodevelopmental disability such as cerebral palsy.

CAUSE

Causes include very low birth weight (eg, birth weight of 1,500 g or less); birth asphyxia; genetic conditions; meningitis or other infections that may affect the central nervous system; central nervous system malformations; certain central nervous system vascular conditions such as brain hemorrhages; and significant fetal exposures to alcohol or other drugs secondary to antenatal maternal substance use (Scott et al, 2000, p. 224). Specific high risks include premature birth, intraventricular hemorrhage (IVH), periventricular leukomalacia (PVL), perinatal asphyxia, bronchopulmonary dysplasia (BPD), respiratory distress syndrome (RDS), hyaline membranes disease (HMD), meconium aspiration, metabolic acidosis, hyperbilirubineumia, toxoplasmosis, rubella, syphilis, cytomegalovirus, herpes simplex, human immunodeficiency virus, fetal alcohol syndrome, cocaine exposure, necrotizing enterocolitis, retinopathy of prematurity, brachial plexus injury, congenital dislocation of the hip, congenital torticollis, talipes equinovarus, metatarsus varus, and tibial torsion.

ASSESSMENT

AREAS
- Body angles (popliteal angle, dorsiflexion of foot, Scarf sign, etc)
- Muscle tone
- Passive movements
- Postural control
- Reflexes and reactions
- Regulatory state
- Spontaneous or voluntary movements

INSTRUMENTS/PROCEDURES
- Alberta Infant Motor Scale (AIMS) (Piper & Darrah, 1994)
- Assessment of Premature Infant Behavior (APIB) (Als, Lester, Tronick, & Brazelton, 1982)
- Bayley Infant Neurodevelopmental Screener (BINS) (Aylward, 1995)
- Chandler Movement Assessment of Infants Screening Test (CMAI-ST) (Chandler, 1990)
- Clinical Assessment of Gestational Age (Dubowitz, Dubowitz, & Goldberg, 1970)
- Harris Infant Neuromotor Test (HINT) (Harris, 1996)
- Infant Motor Screen (IMC) (Nickel, 1987)
- Infant Neurological International Battery (INFANIB) (Andre-Thomas, Chesni, Dargassies, 1950)
- Infant Neuromotor Assessment (INA) (see Magasiner, et al, in References)
- Milani-Comparetti Motor Development Screening Test (MC) (Stuberg, 1992)
- Morgan Neonatal Neurobehavioral Examination (see Sheahan & Brockway in References, p. 88–90)
- Movement Assessment of Infants (MAI) by Chandler, Andrews, & Swanson, 1980)
- NCAST Feeding Scale (Barnard & Eyres, 1979)
- Neonatal Behavioral Assessment Scale, 3rd ed. (NBAS) (Brazelton, 1995)
- Test of Infant Motor Performance (TIMP) (Campbell, Osten, Kolobe, & Fisher, 1993)

PROBLEMS
- Infant may have poverty of spontaneous movement.
- Infant may have difficulty developing gross motor skills starting with lifting head against gravity in either prone or supine position.
- Infant may have severe asymmetry or cramped syndrony.
- Infant may have abnormal reflexes and postural tone.
- Infant may have motor coordination problems especially in maintaining midline orientation.
- Infant may have difficulty with position sense.
- Infant may have poor endurance for movement caused by severe lung disease.

- Infant may have deficits in state and behavior organization including lethargy and hyperirritability.
- Infant may have difficulty with attending behavior (focusing attention and gaze).
- Infant may have demonstrated poor visual following (tracking) of objects.
- As a child, may experience delays in attending developmental milestones.
- As a child, may have difficulty with standing balance—especially on one foot.
- As a child, may have difficulty with handwriting skills.
- As a child, may have difficulty with play activities and playing sports.

TREATMENT/MANAGEMENT
Specific treatment depends on the theoretical approach.

GENERAL GOALS
- Promote state organization and decrease stress reactions.
- Promote postural alignment and more normal patterns of movement.
- Improve postural control.
- Enhance oral-motor skills and assist with oral feedings.
- Enhance self-regulatory behavior through environmental modification.
- Use gentle range of motion (ROM) to minimize skin contractures at infiltrated intravenous site, if needed. ROM exercises may also be needed if infant is on ventilator and receiving medications to cause paralysis.
- Provide normal sensory and motor experiences to act as a basis for motor development.
- Instruct parents in handling, positioning, and feeding.

NEURODEVELOPMENTAL TREATMENT
- Use handling techniques to inhibit abnormal responses while facilitating autonomic reactions. Decrease hyperextension of the neck and trunk, reduce elevation of the shoulders, decrease retraction of the scapula, and reduce extension of the lower extremities. Activation of the primary flexor muscle groups must occur simultaneously.
- If supine, neck and trunk hyperextension can be reduced by gently flexing the hips and knees.
- If supine, elevation of shoulders can be reduced by bringing the infant's hand toward the buttocks.
- Weight bearing through the shoulder girdle can promote proximal stability. Lower extremities should be flexed and therapist's hands should be placed on the buttocks. Maintain alignment of the head and trunk.
- In side-lying, neck and trunk hyperextension can be reduced.
- In side-lying, deep proprioceptive input can be applied through the shoulders and hips to promote postural stability.
- In side-lying, scapular protraction (abduction) and upper extremity midline activities can be enhanced.
- Weight bearing through the shoulders, hips, and feet provides proprioceptive input, promotes development of more normal muscle tone, and increases proximal stability.
- Hammock handling can be used to activate flexor muscle groups, facilitate head righting, and facilitate alerting. The hammock-like sling is made with a doubled blanket whose sides have been rolled toward the infant for stability. In a supine position, the infant is placed in the hammock and very slowly elevated to a semi-sitting position and then back to supine.
- The hammock sling can also be used to active anterior neck to promote flexion, promote scapular protraction and shoulder depression while promoting upper extremity midline skills.

- In a side-lying position, begin disassociated movements between shoulder and pelvic girdles by rotating the two in opposite directions. Begin disassociation of the lower extremities by crossing one leg over the other and bending it at the knee.
- In prone position, weight bearing and weight shifting can be started. The upper extremities should be held near to the body in a flexed position while the lower extremities should be flexed and adducted at the hip so the knees can be placed in position under the abdomen. In this position, the infant's center of gravity is placed forward at a point near the cheek. The therapist's hands should be along the infant's trunk to provide tactile and proprioceptive cues.
- While holding infant in lap in hammock, use gentle downward pressure through the infant's shoulders to elongate the cervical musculature. Stroking the cervical extensor muscles promotes a head-turning reaction.
- Use supported sitting to increase alert state which provides vestibular input and encourages arousal permitting the infant to interact with the environment.
- Use therapeutic positioning to enhance flexor patterns, increase midline orientation, and promote state organization.
- Side-lying position can reduce effects of gravity and thus promote midline and flexor responses; use a blanket roll, bags of intravenous fluid, or sandbags.
- In prone position, use a small washcloth or diaper roll and place under the pelvis and below the abdomen to increase flexion of the hip and knee. This position reduces abduction and external rotation of hips.
- In supine position, place lightly rolled cloth diapers on either side of infant to support arms and legs in flexion and toward midline of body. A smaller roll can be placed below the buttocks to reinforce flexion of legs.

SENSORIMOTOR APPROACH
- Linear rocking on a small beach ball can be used to stimulate the vestibular system and promote an alert state. An alternative hammock sling may be used.
- Tightly swaddle the infant to provide deep tactile and proprioceptive input to promote calming and self-regulating behavior. Another calming technique is slow, rhythmic rocking. A pacifier may also be used.
- To increase alert state, carefully grade arrhythmic vestibular input such as bouncing, light tactile input to the face and body, and upright positioning.
- Weight bearing through the foot helps reduce tactile hypersensitivity of the foot. Cross the leg over the other and place the foot on a surface.
- Use deep rhythmic tactile and proprioceptive input rather than light touch when handling the infant. Light touch tends to disorganize.
- Deep stroke the perioral area from the temporomandibular joint toward the mouth and apply deep pressure to the upper lips to encourage oral activity even if the infant is on a ventilator.

LONG STAY INFANT
- Promote head righting. In a supported sitting position, facilitate extension of the trunk through subtle lateral shifting of weight over the ischial tuberosities. Keep head and trunk aligned. Increase anterior flexion of the neck by shifting infant's weight in a posterior direction. Increase extension of neck by anteriorly shifting infant's weight.

PRECAUTIONS/CONTRAINDICATIONS
- Avoid hyperflexion of the neck which can cause airway obstruction and pulmonary compromise.
- When promoting alert state, monitor motor and autonomic subsystems for signs of distress or instability.
- Light touch should be discouraged since it tends to disorganize.

- Do not use lotions or oils during tactile activity because they may irritate the skin.
- When positioning the infant, care must always be taken to ensure that the airway stays open.

DESIRED OUTCOME/PROGNOSIS

Outcomes vary depending on the problems that were identified during the assessment for high-risk factors. The following outcomes are general examples:

- Child has alignment of body parts that permit postural stability and functional movement.
- Child has functional ROM.
- Child has muscle strength needed to perform motor activities.
- Child has endurance to perform daily activities.
- Child has functional skills including mobility and ambulation.
- Child has attained gross motor skills that are age appropriate.
- Child performs self-care skills that are age appropriate.
- Child participates in family, school, recreational, and community activities.

REFERENCES

Burns YP, Ensbey R, O'Callaghan M. Motor abilities at eight to ten years of children born weighing less than 1,000g. *Physiotherapy*. 1999;85(7):360–369.

Campbell SK. The infant at risk for developmental disability. In: Campbell SK, ed. *Decision Making in Pediatric Neurologic Physical Therapy*. New York, NY: Churchill Livingstone; 1999:260–332.

Cott DT, Cook DS, Dinno ND, Folsom RC, Lucas BL, Swanson MW, et al. An infant at increased risk. In: Guralnick MJ. *Interdisciplinary Clinical Assessment of Young Children with Developmental Disabilities*. Baltimore, Md: Paul H. Brookes; 2000:221–250.

Darrah J, Piper M, Watt MJ. Assessment of gross motor skills of at-risk infants. Predictive validity of the Alberta Infant Motor Scale. *Dev Med Child Neurol*. 1998;40:485–491.

Magasiner VA, Molteno CD, Lachman P, et al. A neuromotor screening test for high-risk infants in a hospital or community setting. *Pediatr Phys Ther*. 1997;9:166–172. [published erratum appears in *Pediatr Phys Ther*. 1998;10(3):100].

Salokorpi T, Rajantie I, Kivikko I, Haajanen R, Rajantie J. Predicting neurological disorders in infants with extremely low birth weight using the Movement Assessment of Infants. *Pediatr Phys Ther*. 2001;13(3):106–109.

Sheahan MS, Brockway NF, Tecklin JS. The high-risk infant. In: Tecklin JS, ed. *Pediatric Physical Therapy*. 3rd ed. Philadelphia, Pa: Lippincott Williams and Wilkins; 1999:71–106.

Weindling AM, Hallam P, Gregg J, Klenka H, Rosenbloom L, Hutton JL. A randomized controlled trial of early physiotherapy for high-risk infants. *Acta Paediatrics*. 1996; 85(9):1107–1111.

Juvenile Dermatomyositis

ICD-9-CM Code: 710.3 Dermatomyositis
APTA Guide Pattern: 7E

DESCRIPTION

Systemic connective tissue disease characterized by inflammatory and degenerative changes in the muscle (polymyositis) and frequently also in the skin (dermatomyositis), leading to symmetrical weakness and some muscle atrophy, principally in the limb girdles (Beers & Berkow, 1999, p. 434). Juvenile dermatomyositis (JDM) is an inflammatory muscle disease which presents with a characteristic rash and proximal muscle weakness (Kuchta, Davidson, & Petty, 2000, p. 73).

Criteria for the diagnosis of JDM includes the following:

- Symmetric weakness of proximal musculature
- Characteristic cutaneous changes of heliotrope (violet) discoloration of the eye-lids with periorbital edema and erythematous scaly rash over the dorsal aspects of the MCP and PIP joints (Gottron's rash)
- Elevation of the serum level of one or more of the skeletal muscle enzymes: crea-tine kinase, aspartate aminotransferase, lactic dehydrogenase, and aldolase
- Electromyographic demonstration of the characteristics of myopathy and denervation
- Muscle biopsy showing histologic evidence of necrosis and inflammation (Kuchta, Davidson, & Petty, 2000, p. 74)

CAUSE

The cause is unknown. The disease may be caused by an autoimmune reaction; deposits of IgM, IgG, and the third component of complement have been found in the blood vessel walls of skeletal muscle, particularly in childhood dermatomyositis (Beers & Berkow, 1999, p. 434). The incidence is 4.3 cases per 1,000,000 in children ages 1–14 years. The disease is somewhat more common in girls than boys (Kuchta, Davidson, & Petty, 2000, p. 73).

ASSESSMENT

AREAS

- Functional abilities such as walking, eating, dressing, toileting, and social interactions
- Mobility and transfer skills
- Muscle length of two-joint muscles: flexor digitorum profundus, hamstrings, quadriceps, gastrocnemius
- Muscle strength, especially of neck flexors, abdominals, shoulder abductors, elbow flexors and extensors, hip flexors, extensors, abductions, knee flexors and extensors muscles
- Range of motion (ROM), especially of large joints: shoulders, elbows, wrists, hips, knees, ankles, trunk, and neck
- Skin: observe and palpate for pressure areas and calcinosis
- Splinting needs: wrists, ankles, elbows, and knees
- Swallowing and speech: food sticking, liquids coming out of the nose, evidence of aspiration, nasal or weak voice
- Vital capacity

INSTRUMENTS/PROCEDURES

- brief functional evaluation of muscle strength (see Kuchta, Davidson, & Petty, p. 80)
- Childhood Health Assessment Questionnaire (CHAQ) (Singh, Arthrya, Fries, & Goldsmith, 1994)
- evaluation of JDM throughout the disease course (see Kuchta, Davidson, & Petty, p. 81)
- Juvenile Arthritis Functional Status Index (JASI) (Wright, et al, 1994)
- manual muscle test or myometer

PROBLEMS

- Child often has fatigue and malaise.
- Child typically has symmetrical, progressive, and proximal muscle weakness in the shoulder and hip girdles during the early phase of the disease followed by distal musculature weakness as the disease progresses. Hip-girdle weakness is evident in the gait, difficulty climbing stairs, by the presence of a Trendelenburg sign, and by the demonstration of Gowers sign.
- Child often has neck flexor muscle weakness manifested by lead lag, inability to hold the head upright when sitting, or decreased ability to resist passive extension of the neck.
- Child often has trunk flexor weakness.
- Child often has difficulty performing motor tasks previously mastered or displays regression of motor skill milestones.
- Child often has difficulty performing gross, fine, and functional motor tasks.
- Child often has a rash: Gottrons lesions are bright pink-red, scaly, atrophic areas over the proximal interphalangeal (PIP) joints of the fingers, the metacarpophalangeal (MCP) joints, and extensor surfaces of the elbows and knees.
- Child often has heliotrope (violet or reddish-purple) discoloration of the upper eyelids and may have periorbital edema. Note that facial muscles are not usually involved.
- Child often has dilatation and distortion of the capillary loops, together with the disappearance of some loops which occurs in the periungual region (around the nail) of the fingers.
- Child often has a low-grade fever.
- Child may have joint contractures resulting from the effects of muscle inflammation.
- Child may have muscle pain or tenderness.
- Child may have weakness of the abdominal musculature making it difficulty or impossible for the child to rise from a lying position without turning onto their side.
- Child may have edema of the muscle and subcutaneous tissues.
- Child may have dyspnea and poor cough due to involvement of the respiration muscles.
- Child may have a voice that is weak, hoarse, or nasal in quality.
- Child may have dysphagia due to involvement of the swallowing muscles.
- Child may have subcutaneous, fascial, or intramuscular calcium deposits late in the disease course.
- Child may have arthritis, tenosynovitis, and tendon nodules. These problems suggest the possibility of a mixed connective tissue disease.

TREATMENT/MANAGEMENT

Treatment typically requires a multidisciplinary approach involving physicians, therapists, educators, the family, and patient.

ACUTE PHASE

- Maintain ROM. Provide or instruct parents in twice-daily passive stretching of affected muscles through tolerated ROM.
- Prevent flexion contractures of hamstrings and quadriceps muscles through stretching.
- As muscle inflammation decreases, weak muscles should be stretched with active and active-resistive exercise.
- Provide a collar for the head if neck musculature is weak.

- In severe disease, splint to maintain a normal position of joints and prevent shortening of inflamed muscles.
- Consider use of ankle foot orthosis and/or footboard in bed to maintain ankle dorsiflexion.
- Determine need for and provide protective padding over pressure areas (buttocks, scapulae, elbows, ischial tuberosities, and trochanters) to prevent pressure sores.
- Consider use of emollients to help keep the skin soft.
- Provide pain management including progressive muscle relaxation, meditative breathing, and guided imagery. Music or videotapes may also be used.
- Instruct patient and family in proper positioning.
- Provide information and support regarding the protracted, unpredictable course of the disease.

SUBACUTE PHASE
- Encourage child to normalize function within limitations.
- Minimize the development of contractures secondary to muscle weakness, atrophy, or calcinosis.
- Encourage patient to do more ADLs independently—with or without aids.
- Active ROM and stretching exercises should be initiated slowly. Consider use of pool to enhance relaxation and encourage active movement and functional patterns.

RECOVERY PHASE
- Begin muscle strengthening exercises. Focus on isometric strengthening of proximal muscle groups. Proprioceptive neuromuscular facilitation (PNF) and modified PNF trunk patterns are useful. When tolerated, balance and strengthening exercises using Swiss Balls and dynamic surfaces may be used.
- Serial casing or splinting should be continued as needed to stretch out flexion deformities of the knees, ankles, and elbows.
- Assist family in planning a home program that can be accomplished within the family members' schedule.
- Modify requirements for ADLs to encourage the child to perform as independently as possible.
- Consider use of wheelchairs, scooters, or rolling walkers for child with continued difficulty in ambulation or low endurance.
- Consider use of adapted equipment to facilitate participation in school activities and educational tasks such as a laptop computer mini keyboard. Child may also need a teacher's aide to help with bathroom tasks and transfers.

CHRONIC PHASE
- Encourage child to reach maximum potential in age-appropriate roles.
- Limit the use of aids and adaptation to those that are essential for independence.
- Recommend structural changes to home or school that are necessary to accommodate a wheelchair or scooter as needed.
- Assist in planning or re-evaluating vocational goals with team members.

PRECAUTIONS/CONTRAINDICATIONS
- Child may be subject to aspiration.
- Child may require ventilatory support due to an increased involvement of respiratory muscles.
- Child may be subject to skin breakdown and pressure sores.
- Child may resist therapy because of muscle tenderness.
- When considering splinting or stretching two-joint flexor muscles, consider the tenodesis effect.

OUTCOME/PROGNOSIS

In most children, the active disease lasts from 2 to 3 years, although there is wide variation.

- Child has functional ROM in all joints.
- Child has adequate muscle strength for activities.
- Child performs functional skills with or without assistive devices.
- Child participates in family, social, school, and community activities.

REFERENCES

Beers MH, Berkow R, eds. *The Merck Manual of Diagnosis and Therapy.* Whitehouse Station, NJ: Merck Research Laboratories; 1999.

Hall E. Arthritis in children—juvenile dermatomyositis. In: David C, Lloyd J, eds. *Rheumatological Physiotherapy.* London, England: Mosby International; 1999:210.

Hyde S. Physical therapy of muscle diseases—dermatomyositis. In Lane RJM, ed. *Handbook of Muscle Disease.* New York, NY: Marcel Dekker; 1996:668.

Kuchta G, Davidson I, Petty RE. Connective tissue diseases in children—juvenile dermatomyositis. In: Melvin JL, Wright FV, eds. *Pediatr Rheum Dis.* (Rheumatologic rehabilitation series, v. 3). Bethesda, Md: American Occupational Therapy Association; 2000: 73–83.

Wright FV. An adolescent girl with juvenile dermatomyositis. In: Melvin JL, Wright FV, eds. *Pediatr Rheum Dis.* (Rheumatologic rehabilitation series, v. 3). Bethesda, Md: American Occupational Therapy Association; 2000:284–293.

Juvenile Rheumatoid Arthritis

Also known as *juvenile chronic arthritis.*

ICD-9-CM Codes:

714.3 Juvenile chronic polyarthritis

714.30 Polyarticular juvenile rheumatoid arthritis, chronic or unspecified

714.31 Polyarticular juvenile rheumatoid arthritis, acute

714.32 Pauciarticular juvenile rheumatoid arthritis

714.33 Monoarticular juvenile rheumatoid arthritis

APTA Guide Patterns: 4C, 4D, 4F

DESCRIPTION

Juvenile rheumatoid arthritis begins at or before age 16 and is similar to adult rheumatoid arthritis. The disease tends to affect large and small joints and may interfere with growth and development. Micrognathia (receded chin) due to impaired mandible growth may occur (Beers & Berkow, 1999, p. 2401).

Systemic onset or Stills disease occurs in 10–20% of patients. High fever, rash, splenomegaly, generalized adenopathy, serositis, neurophilic leukocytosis, and thrombocytosis often occur. The number of joints involved is variable. Age of onset does not peak but occurs through childhood. Ratio of females to males is equal. Uveitis is rare.

Pauciarticular onset (Oligoarticular) occurs in approximately 40–50% of patients; typically young girls. Antinuclear antibodies are present in up to 75% of affected children. Chronic iridocyclitis (uveitis) occurs in nearly 20% of these patients; it is often asymptomatic and detected only with periodic slit-lamp examinations. Examination by an ophthalmologist is important. Chronic uveitis occurs in approximately 20% of cases. Most boys affected subsequently develop classic features of one of the seronegative spondyloarthropathies. Typically 4 joints are involved. Typical age of onset is approximately 1–2 years. Ratio of females to males is 5:1.

Polyarticular onset occurs in the remaining 40% of patients and often is similar to adult rheumatoid arthritis. Typically, 5 joints are involved but up to 20 joints have been reported. Peak age of onset is 1–3 years but can occur throughout childhood. Ratio of females to males is 3:1. Chronic uveitis occurs in approximately 5% of cases. (Beers & Berkow, 1999, p. 2402; Scull, 2000, p. 228).

Medical management involves a variety of medications used to control joint inflammation. The primary drugs of choice are NSAIDs (nonsteroidal anti-inflammatory drugs) such as naproxen, tolmetin, and ibuprofen, but several other types of drugs have been tried to control the various chemical agents produced by neutrophils in joint and lymphocytes in the synovial membrane macrophages. Surgical procedures include soft tissue releases of the hip flexors, hamstrings, hip adductors or heel cords, synovectomy, osteotomy, and arthroplasty of the hip or knee.

The following are classifications of functional limitations according to the American College of Rheumatology (Scull, 2000, p. 254). *Note:* standardized for adults but not for children.

- Class I   Completely able to perform usual ADLs (self-care, vocation, and avocation)
- Class II   Able to perform usual self-care and vocational activities but limited in avocational activities
- Class III Able to perform usual self-care activities but limited in vocational and avocational activities
- Class IV   Limited in ability to perform usual self-care, vocational, and avocational activities

CAUSE

No definitive cause is known. Multiple factors are thought to be involved. A viral or bacterial infection may trigger the autoimmune reactions. Some children may have a genetic predisposition to response. Systemic JRA usually begins with a high fever so the cause is assumed to be an infection. In all cases, the child's own immune system fights against the connective tissue, causing inflammation and resulting in pain and stiffness, especially in the joints (Ratliffe, 1998, pp. 119–120).

Incidence is estimated at 13.9 per 100,000 population. Prevalence is 113.4 cases per 100,000. There are between 160,000 to 190,000 cases in the United States (Scull, 2000, p. 228).

ASSESSMENT

AREAS
- Assessability to the environment
- General appearance
- Functional abilities
- Gait
- Joint range of motion (ROM)
- Joint stability and integrity
- Muscle strength
- Pain
- Posture
- Swelling
- Extra-articular manifestations

INSTRUMENTS/PROCEDURES
- exercise tolerance test using cycle ergonometry
- goniometer for ROM. Passive ROM provides the most accurate baseline for joint pathology. Active ROM provides the best information for functional skills.

- manual muscle test and dynamometry
- Childhood Health Assessment Questionnaire (CHAQ) (Singh et al, 1994). Scale provided in Scull, 2000, pp. 236–237.
- Health-Related Physical Fitness Test (AAHRERD, 1980)
- Juvenile Arthritis Functional Assessment Scale (JAFAS) (Lovell et al, 1989). Scale provided in Scull, 2000, p. 234.
- visual analog scale to measure pain. For sample, see Scull, 2000, p. 234.

PROBLEMS
- Child often has pain in the involved joints.
- Child typically has swelling in the involved joints.
- Child often has stiffness and loss of joint flexibility especially in the hip flexors, adductors, hamstrings, and gastrocnemius of the lower extremities and wrist and finger flexors in the upper extremities.
- Child often has loss of ROM which may be due to swelling, stiffness, pain, or loss of joint integrity.
- Child often has contractures most often in the flexor groups. If the contracture reduces ROM more than 10 degrees, functional loss predictably occurs. Long standing contractures may lead to growth abnormalities.
- Child often has loss of functional skills.
- The young child may have developmental delays in acquiring ADLs such as feeding, dressing, and toileting. The older child may have gross motor skill delays due to lack of opportunities because parents fear injury.
- Child may have laxity in the ligaments.
- Child may have joint subluxation.
- Child may have widening of joint space early in the disease which changes to narrowing after 2 or more years.
- Child may have osteoporosis.
- Child may have bony ankylosis in carpal and tarsal joints and cervical spine.
- Child may have muscle weakness secondary to disuse and pain. Strength less than 4 on a 5-point scale in the lower extremity antigravity muscles may result in gait deviations and functional limitations such as when climbing stairs.
- Child may have postural deviations: valgus or varus in the lower extremities. Coxa valga may occur due to forces across the femoral epiphysis. Avascular necrosis can occur.
- Child may have leg length discrepancy.
- Child may have gait abnormalities such as decreased velocity, cadence, and stride length. Increased anterior pelvic tilt throughout the gait cycle, decreased hip extension, and plantar flexion at toe-off may also be noted due to pain, weakness, or contractures.
- Child may have foot deformities which may include loss of subtalar motion, such as a valgus hindfoot, combined with pronation. Forefoot involvement is common. The great toe may lose extension at the metatarsophalangeal joint or may deviate into a valgus position. Toes may develop a hammertoe posture.
- Young child may have difficulty separating from the mother because of dependence by the child and overprotection by the mother.
- Child may refuse to cooperate during assessment and treatment.
- Child may lack friends and playmates because of difficulties performing normal childhood gross motor tasks.
- Adolescent may experience problems with social and work roles such as dating, driving, or career selection.
- Parents may feel frustration and/or guilt.

TREATMENT/MANAGEMENT

Treatment and management require a team approach including a pediatric rheumatologist, orthopedist, nurse, occupational therapist, and social worker. Other team members or consultants may include a psychologist, ophthalmologist, cardiologist, or physical education teacher.

- Maintain and/or improve active joint range of motion through once daily exercise regimes involving all joints. Client must be involved in planning the exercise program or he or she is likely not to participate.
- Increase muscle strength through isometric exercises if pain is present. Concentric and eccentric contractions may be taught. Resistive exercise should be restricted to weights of only a few pounds (Scull, 2000, p. 233). Elastic bands may be used. Play activities such as bicycle or tricycle riding are also useful.
- Maintain or increase cardiopulmonary endurance. Recreational activities such as swimming, cycling, or dancing may be recommended. Games such as "Simon Says" may be helpful.
- Reduce pain. Consider applying heat in the form of paraffin, ultrasound, warm water, whirlpool, and heat lamps. Behavior management techniques such as muscle relaxation, meditative breathing and guided imagery can be taught to assist in pain management.
- Reduce swelling; cold has been demonstrated to be effective.
- Reduce stiffness. A warm tub bath in the morning with exercises performed in the water may decrease morning stiffness.
- Prevent or reduce contractures. Splinting may be used to lengthen the antagonist. Night splints (typically resting type) can be used on knees, ankles, wrist, and hands. Stretching exercises to the agonist can be useful. Gentle, passive ROM exercise is indicated for contractures if joint inflammation is under medical control and contracture is believed to be muscular in nature. Flexion contractures in hips and knees can often be managed using gravity-assisted stretching in the prone position for 20 minutes per day (Kelly, 2000, p. 232). A baton held in both hands over the head can be used to perform active-assisted shoulder flexion. Dynamic splinting, which permits a slow prolonged stretch, is often more effective for elbow and knees. Serial casting or drop-out casts may be used.
- Protect joints. Instruction in joint conservation should be taught to insulate the large joints in avoiding stress on the small joints: carry objects close to the center of gravity, and use longer levers to increase torque.
- Encourage pacing. Instruct child and family in how to pace activity to reduce pain and fatigue.
- Decrease leg length discrepancy. A shoe lift may be added to correct leg length if needed to improve posture or gait.
- Decrease foot deformity and pain. Assist family in selecting comfortable yet supportive footwear. Sneakers are generally preferred because they have good arch support and are cushioned throughout the sole. A metatarsal bar may be added to provide a rocker-like surface to the sole of the forefoot, which allows a toe-off without requiring hyperextension of the toes. An AFO (ankle-foot orthosis) may be useful if there is pain in the ankles during weight bearing.
- Assist ambulation and mobility. If ambulation is a problem due to lower extremity pain, contracture, or weakness, platform crutches (Lofstrand or axillary) may be used or a wheeled walker with platform attachments to avoid weight bearing on small joints of the wrist and hand may be preferred. Additional assistance may be needed for ambulation in the community. Depending on the age of the child and distance, consider a wheelchair, stroller, wagon, or tricycle. Training in the stand-pivot-sit method may be useful. If a wheelchair is used, check that seat height is correct and

that posture is aligned and maintained to prevent hip asymmetry or spinal deformity. A brake extension may be needed if upper extremities are weak. Swing away or desk arms are useful for access to the school desk.

- Maximize normal development. Use developmentally appropriate activities, tasks, toys, and games based on the child's interests.
- Increase or maintain self-care skills. A backpack may be used to carry books or ask the school to issue two sets of textbooks: one for school and one for home; dressing aids may be used—such as a dressing stick—to assist in reaching the feet to put on pants and underwear; a zipper pull or button hook; a sock aid; a long-handled shoe-horn or elastic shoelaces can help with autonomous care. Enlarge handles on utensils and brushes to make gripping easier. Writing aids with enlarged diameters may improve writing endurance. A computer or dictating device may be preferred. Bathroom needs include a special seat in the tub and a grab bar to ensure safety. A long hose can facilitate showering and a long-handled sponge permits reaching the back. A raised toilet seat may permit independent toileting. Refitting knobs with lever type handles aids use of the sink.
- Provide support and encouragement to continue the treatment program. Behavior modification techniques may be used to encourage adaptive behaviors and discourage maladaptive behaviors.
- Instruct family about the disease process and need for cooperation in treatment.
- Provide information on accessibility to the physical environment if assistive devices are needed.

PRECAUTIONS/CONTRAINDICATIONS

- Do not use ultrasound with a child who has growth plates.
- Be aware that a young child does not always report temperature on the skin accurately. Children are at risk from agents that are too hot or cold.
- Passive stretching exercises should be avoided for acutely inflamed joints and for those that show signs of instability or mechanical derangement.
- If stretching is used, watch that the joint is protected and does not sublux. Always warm up the joint using light exercise, modalities, or passive ROM before beginning the stretching exercises.
- Recreational activities such as tumbling (especially headstands and somersaults), weight bearing on upper extremities, contact sports, and high-impact activities such as jogging are contraindicated.

DESIRED OUTCOME/PROGNOSIS

Prognosis is variable. Ten years after onset, many children still have active disease although the percentage varies with the type. Children with polyarticular disease who are rheumatoid factor positive have the worst prognosis. Children with pauciarticular disease do well functionally except for complications with vision.

- Child does not experience pain or is able to manage pain.
- Child has normal strength (5/5) in antigravity muscles.
- Child has functional ROM in all joints with no contractures greater than 10 degrees.
- Child has cardiopulmonary endurance that is expected for chronological age.
- Child has ambulation and mobility skills with or without assistive devices.
- Child is able to perform self-care activities which are age appropriate with or without assistive devices.
- Child is able to participate in school, social, and recreational activities.

REFERENCES

Beers MH, Berkow R, eds. *The Merck Manual of Diagnosis and Therapy.* Whitehouse Station, NJ: Merck Research Laboratories; 1999.

Hackett J, Johnson B, Parkin A, Southwood T. Physiotherapy and occupational therapy for juvenile chronic arthritis: custom and practice in five centres in the UK, USA and Canada. *Br J Rheumatol.* 1996;35(7):695–699.

Hall E. Arthritis in children. In: David C, Lloyd J, eds. *Rheumatological physiotherapy.* London, England: Mosby International, 1999:205–216.

Klepper SE, Scull SA. Juvenile rheumatoid arthritis. In: Tecklin JS, ed. *Pediatric Physical Therapy.* 3rd ed. Philadelphia, Pa: Lippincott Williams and Wilkins; 1999:429–467.

Matsuura K. A body with pauciarticular juvenile rheumatoid arthritis. In: Melvin JL, Wright FV, eds. *Pediatr Rheum Dis* (Rheumatologic rehabilitation series. V. 3). Bethesda, Md: American Occupational Therapy Association; 2000:267–275.

Mier RJ, Wright FV, Bouding DJ. Juvenile rheumatoid arthritis. In: Melvin JL, Wright FV, eds. *Pediatr Rheum Dis* (Rheumatologic rehabilitation series. V. 3). Bethesda, Md: American Occupational Therapy Association; 2000:1–44.

Nestor B, Figgie MP, Wright FW, Melvin JL. Surgical treatment of juvenile rheumatoid arthritis. In: Melvin JL, Wright FV, eds. *Pediatr Rheum Dis* (Rheumatologic rehabilitation series. v 3). Bethesda, Md: American Occupational Therapy Association; 2000:249–266.

Nieuwenhuis MK, van der Net J, Kuis W, et al. Assessment of wrist malalignment in juvenile rheumatoid arthritis. *Adv Physiotherapy.* 1999;1(2):99–109.

Ratliffe KT. Developmental orthopedic disorders—Camilla, a young girl with juvenile rheumatoid arthritis. In Ratliffe KT. *Clinical Pediatric Physical Therapy: A Guide for the Physical Therapy Team.* St. Louis, Mo: CV Mosby Co; 1998:99–105.

Ratliffe KT. Developmental orthopedic disorders—The child with juvenile rheumatoid arthritis. In Ratliffe KT. *Clinical Pediatric Physical Therapy: A Guide for the Physical Therapy Team.* St. Louis, Mo: CV Mosby Co; 1998:119–124.

Scull SA. Juvenile rheumatoid arthritis. In: Campbell SK, ed. *Physical Therapy for Children.* 2nd ed. Philadelphia, Pa: WB Saunders Co; 2000:227–246.

Scull SA. Physical therapy for the child and adolescent with juvenile rheumatoid arthritis. In: Melvin JL, Wright FV, eds. *Pediatr Rheum Dis* (Rheumatologic rehabilitation series. V. 3). Bethesda, Md: American Occupational Therapy Association; 2000:199–222.

Wright EV. Measurement of outcome in juvenile rheumatoid arthritis. In: Melvin JL, Wright FV, eds. *Pediatr Rheum Dis* (Rheumatologic rehabilitation series. V. 3). Bethesda, Md: American Occupational Therapy Association; 2000:231–248.

Kyphosis

Also known as *hunchback.*

ICD-9-CM Codes:
- 756.19 Anomalies of spine, Other
- 737.30 Kyphoscoliosis

APTA Guide Patterns: 4A, 4B, 6F

DESCRIPTION

Kyphosis is an abnormal posterior convexity of a segment of the spine (Patrick, 2000, p. 272). The most common site is the thoracic spine which leads to a thoracolumbar or lumbar kyphosis. Kyphosis should not be confused with roundback. In roundback the posture is not fixed and there are no end-plate irregularities on x-ray.

- *Congenital kyphosis* results when the anterior part of the vertebra is aplastic or hypoplastic and posterior elements form normally. An anterior unsegmented failure of formation or unsegmented bar leads to progressive kyphosis (Patrick, 2000, p. 273). The condition is progressive and deformity increases as the child grows (Ratliffe, 1998, p. 146).
- *Scheuermann's disease* develops during childhood and adolescence and is usually attributed to poor posture but may be transmitted by an autosomal dominant trait. Posture is characterized by an excessive lumbar lordosis and a forward head, with an excessive cervical lordosis (Ratliffe, 1998, p. 146). Criteria include irregular vertebral end-plates, narrowing of the intervertebral disk space, anterior wedging of 5 degrees or greater of one or more vertebrae, and kyphosis greater than 40 degrees that is uncorrected on active hyperextension (Patrick, 2000, p. 273). The child is unable to extend the spine to a neutral position.
- *Neuromuscular kyphosis* results from asymmetrical muscle pull on the spine caused by weakness, lack of innervation, or lack of control of certain muscle groups (Ratliffe, 2000, p. 146).

CAUSE

Primary causes include congenital kyphosis or Scheuermanns disease. A secondary cause may be the previous treatment of spinal tumors with laminectomy. Kyphosis may also be found in children with osteochrondrodystrophies, rickets, osteogenic imperfecta, idiopathic juvenile osteoporosis, neurofibromatosis, myelomeningocele, spondyloepiphyseal dysplasia, or trauma to the spine (Patrick, 2000, p. 272). Incidence is reported as 4% of children (Ratliffe, 1998, p. 146).

ASSESSMENT

AREAS
- Pain
- Range of motion (ROM)

INSTRUMENTS/PROCEDURES

No specific instruments mentioned.

PROBLEMS
- Child often has back pain.
- Child often has a cosmetic deformity.
- Child may have spinal cord compression which results in paresis or paraplegia.
- Child may have hip contracture.
- Child may have scoliosis.

TREATMENT/MANAGEMENT

For congenital kyphosis, surgery is usually the preferred option. Physical therapy may be ordered after surgery. For Scheuermanns disease, both orthotic management and surgery are often used. Orthotic management is used when the kyphosis is greater than 50-60 degrees. A modified Milwaukee-type brace or custom-molded body jack (ie, a thoracic lumbar sacral orthosis [TLSO]) have been used successfully. Two-stage surgical management involves anterior discectomy and intravertebral grafting coupled with a posterior compression arthrodesis. For neurological conditions with kyphosis, see the individual disorder. Treatment suggestions apply primarily to Scheuermann's disease.

- Use exercise to strengthen active trunk extension using prone lifts with arms straight ahead. Lower abdominals are important to maintain an upright posture and decrease lumbar lordosis. Bent knee lifts in supine are one exercise. Muscles include gluteals, abdominals, and spinal extensor muscle group.
- Use stretching to increase trunk extension and improve overall alignment. Muscles include hamstrings, pectoral, and abdominal muscles.
- Use exercise to improve posture, especially for the abdominals and gluteals. Use gravity to assist the posture rather than fighting gravity to maintain an upright position. An example is tilting or reclining the back surface of any adapted seating or wheelchair. Be sure to maintain pelvic alignment. A wedge behind the head or other positioning device should keep the neck in slight flexion, allowing the child to see forward rather than upward.
- Instruct child to extend at the kyphotic section of the spine, usually thoracic, while maintaining a neutral or slightly flexed cervical and lumbar spine.
- Reduce hip contractures, if present, resulting from increased lumbar lordosis and increased anterior pelvic tilt along with limited hamstring length as measured by straight leg raising.

PRECAUTIONS/CONTRAINDICATIONS

- In positioning the child, watch for strong flexor tone or righting reactions that pull the child into flexion when placed in a semi-reclined position. Other positioning options will be needed.

DESIRED OUTCOME/PROGNOSIS

- Child has more normal alignment of body segments.
- Child has more normal posture in sitting, standing, and ambulation.
- Child has increased strength in anterior muscles of the trunk.

REFERENCES

Patrick C. Spinal conditions—Kyphosis. In: Campbell SK, ed. *Physical Therapy for Children.* 2nd ed. Philadelphia, Pa: WB Saunders Co; 2000:272–275.

Ratliffe KT. Other orthopedic disorders—Kyphosis. In Ratliffe KT. *Clinical Pediatric Physical Therapy: A Guide for the Physical Therapy Team.* St. Louis, Mo: CV Mosby Co; 1998: 146–7.

Legg-Calvé-Perthes Disease

Also known as *Legg Perthes disease* or *Perthes disease.*

ICD-9-CM Code: 732.1 Juvenile osteochondrosis of hip and pelvis
APTA Guide Patterns: 4F, 4H, 4J

DESCRIPTION

Idiopathic aseptic necrosis of the femoral capital epiphysis. Legg-Calvé-Perthes disease (LCPD) is the most common of the osteochondroses, has a maximum incidence between the ages of 5 and 10 years with a predilection for males, and is usually unilateral (Beers &

Berkow, 1999, pp. 2413–2414). There are 4 stages to the disease: initial, fragmentation, re-ossification, and healed. During the *initial* stage, the femoral head stops growing because there is a lack of blood supply. There is a high risk of deformity if not treated. During the *fragmentation* stage, the epiphysis appears fragmented. New bone begins to form on the old bone as revascularization of the femoral head occurs. During the *reossification* stage, the bone density returns to normal but the femoral head and neck may show changes in shape and structure even after remodeling has occurred. During the *healed* stage, the femoral head will continue to retain any residual deformity from the repair process. The process takes 2–4 years to complete (Ratliffe, 1998).

Because the disease is self-limiting, treatment options vary. Conservative treatment consists of observation and monitoring, limiting involvement in contact sports, and the rec-ommendation to participate in swimming for range of motion (ROM) and strengthening. Aggressive treatment includes splinting and bedrest but more modern approaches use ac-tive splinting which allows the child to participate in daily living. The child may be allowed partial weight bearing or be non-weight bearing, depending on the severity of the disease. Surgery is the most aggressive treatment and is performed when there is inadequate con-tainment of the femoral head in the acetabulum. Proximal femoral varus osteotomy, in-nominate pelvic osteotomy, or Pemberton pelvic osteotomy are used.

CAUSE

Etiology is unknown but it is thought that certain children may be susceptible to develop-ing the disease as a result of genetic predisposition. The assumption is that variations in the anatomy cause the blood supply to the femoral head to be interrupted. Other possibil-ities are recurrent synovitis of the hip, or multiple infarctions of arteries supplying the femoral head (Ratliffe, 1998).

The disease occurs in boys 4–5 times more frequently than girls and is found more frequently in children of Northern European or Asian ancestry than those of Native Ameri-can, Polynesian, or African-American ethnicity. It is also more common in urban rather than rural settings. Disease usually occurs between ages 3 and 12 with most boys between 5 and 7. Twenty percent of cases are bilateral.

ASSESSMENT

AREAS
- Functional skills
- Gait
- Muscle strength
- Pain
- ROM
- Reflexes and reactions

INSTRUMENTS/PROCEDURES
- Positive Trendelenburg: the pelvis drops lower on one side during gait because of muscle weakness
- Gait analysis

PROBLEMS
- Child begins to limp.
- Child has mild pain in the groin, medial thigh, or medial knee (referred pain).
- Child has decreased ROM especially in hip abduction and internal rotation.
- Child may have atrophy from disuse in the thigh, calf, or buttocks.
- Child may have limb length inequality from collapse of the femoral head on the affected side.

TREATMENT/MANAGEMENT

If splints are used, the leg or legs will be splinted in the abducted position. Common types of splinting include broomstick, Petrie, and Toronto orthoses. A Petrie cast has two long leg casts with a bar positioned between holding the hips abducted and internally rotated.

- Depending on the treatment options used, daily stretching for hip extension, abduction, and hip internal rotation or strengthening exercises must be done by the therapist or by a member of family whom the therapist has taught.
- If crutches are used, teach proper crutch-walking; teaching the child to keep one crutch in front and one in the back of the abducted legs.
- If the child is in school, the teacher may need advice on managing a child on crutches in the classroom. Seating and access to work surface may be issues to address as well as mobility around the school especially if the classroom is not on the main floor or there are stairs to the school entrance.
- If the child has a spica cast after surgery, the family will to be taught how to turn the child over, lift the child, assist in strengthening and ROM activities, and how to help the child be as independent as possible in daily tasks such as self-help, school work, and recreation. A mechanical lift may be useful.
- Once the child is out of the spica cast, the goals will be to regain lost ROM and strength and relearn ambulation skills.
- Provide gait retraining if gait will be altered as a result of the disease.
- Once the healing stage has started recommend a strengthening program such as swimming, driving, water polo, and walking for 30 minutes. Other exercises may include side-lying, supine, and seated straight-leg raises and squats.

PRECAUTIONS/CONTRAINDICATIONS
- A child in a walking cast may need extra time to move about in the school hallway and need to avoid crowds of other children.
- Child may develop scoliosis from asymmetrical weight bearing when crutches are used.

DESIRED OUTCOME/PROGNOSIS

A child with middle or moderate involvement (Catterall grades 1 or 2) usually has good results. A child in grades 3 or 4 may have greater deformity of the femur and thus have more limitation in ROM, residual pain, and decreased function. Long-term studies suggest that degenerative arthritis of the hip is common in adults who had LCPD in childhood.

- Child has functional ROM.
- Child has regained muscle strength.
- Child has regained ambulation skills.
- Child has a normal gait pattern.
- Child does not have pain or pain does not interfere with daily activities.
- Child participates in a daily exercise program.
- Child participates in school, community, and recreational activities.

REFERENCES

Beers MH, Berkow R, eds. *The Merck Manual of Diagnosis and Therapy*. Whitehouse Station, NJ: Merck Research Laboratories; 1999.

Leach J. Orthopedic conditions—Perthes disease. Patrick C. Spinal conditions—scoliosis. In: Campbell SK, ed. *Physical Therapy for Children*. 2nd ed. Philadelphia, Pa: WB Saunders Co; 2000:414–415.

Ratliffe KT. Disorders of the developing hip—The child with Legg-Calve-Perthes disease. In: Ratliffe KT. *Clinical Pediatric Physical Therapy: A Guide for the Physical Therapy Team*. St. Louis, MO: CV Mosby Co; 1998:82–85.

Ratliffe KT. Disorders of the developing hip—Shelly, a girl with Legg-Calve-Perthes disease. In: Ratliffe KT. *Clinical Pediatric Physical Therapy: A Guide for the Physical Therapy Team*. St. Louis, MO: CV Mosby Co; 1998:71–77.

Stanger M. Legg-Calves-Perthes disease. In: Tecklin JS, ed. *Pediatric Physical Therapy*, 3rd ed. Philadelphia, Pa: Lippincott Williams and Wilkins; 1999:410–415.

Limb (Leg) Length Discrepancy

Also known as *leg length inequality* (LLI).

ICD-9-CM Codes:
- 736.81 Unequal leg length (acquired)
- 755 Other congenital anomalies of limbs

APTA Guide Patterns: 4H, 4J, 4K

DESCRIPTION

Leg length discrepancy (LLD) is defined as a 2.5-centimeter or greater difference in length of the two limbs (Leach, 2000, p. 420). Intervention is generally not indicated for leg length differences of less than 2 centimeters; a lift inside the shoe may be used for these differences. Leg length discrepancies are a cosmetic and functionality problem (Stanger, 1999, p. 419).

Treatment depends on the age of the child and growth remaining, severity of the leg length differences, and preferences of the family and child. Surgical options involve either shortening the longer limb or lengthening the shorter limb. To shorten the leg of a young child, the physes or epiphyses are surgically destroyed to arrest growth in the longer leg. Epiphysiodesis is used for discrepancies of 2 to 5 centimeters. In adolescents, an osteotomy can be performed where 5 to 6 centimeters of the femur and/or 2 to 4 centimeters are removed. For greater discrepancies, the choice is usually to lengthen the shorter limb.

Limb lengthening techniques involve either metaphyseal or disphyseal distraction. They are based on the principles of fixation of the fragments that allow vascular ingrowth. The best known techniques for children are the Wagner and Ilizarov methods. The Wagner technique uses the diaphyseal approach and the Ilizarov method uses the metaphyseal lengthening.

CAUSE

A limb length discrepancy may be caused by the shortening or overgrowth of one or more bones in the leg. Inequality may result from congenital conditions such as limb deficiencies or hemihypertrophy, infections or fractures that injure the physes, neuromuscular disorders, tumors, or trauma that results in overgrowth and disease process. Leg length differences may range from 1 to 10 centimeters or greater (Stanger, 1999, p. 419).

Specific congenital causes include hemihypertrophy in which one side of the body is larger than the other, hemiatrophy in which one side is smaller than the other, proximal focal femoral deficiency, congenital coxa vera, fibular and tibial hemimelia, and other focal dysplasias. Examples of muscle weakness or paralysis include myelodysplasia, poliomyelitis, and hemiplegia caused by cerebral palsy. Acquired conditions include Legg-Calvé-Perthes disease and Slipped Capital Femoral Epiphysis. Other causes include fibrous dysplasia and tumors.

ASSESSMENT

AREAS
- Functional activities: rising from a chair, getting down on the floor and back up
- Gait
- Leg length

- Muscle strength
- Posture and postural alignment: observe for substitution patterns
- Range of motion (ROM)

INSTRUMENTS/PROCEDURES
- Body measurements: sitting and standing height; weight; arm span
- Gait analysis: with and without assistive devices and shoe lift
- Leg length:
  1. *block measurement:* blocks of known height are placed under the shorter leg
  2. *tape measurement:* measure from the medial malleolus to the anterior superior iliac spine when the pelvis has been set level prior to recording the measurement
  3. *radiographic measurement:* none by the physician

PROBLEMS
- Child walks with a limp that is noticeable.
- Child has an inefficient and awkward gait.
- Child may have postural compensations of the pelvis and spine.
- Child may experience developmental delays.
- Child may have difficulty performing functional skills.

TREATMENT/MANAGEMENT
- After surgery, provide gait training activities.
- Promote early weight bearing for the child that has undergone the Ilizarov procedure.
- Provide instruction in pin care.
- Minimize joint ROM limitations, especially ankle dorsiflexion.
- Consider an ankle splint to maintain the ankle in a plantigrade position and to stretch the soft tissue.
- Provide muscle strengthening exercises throughout the lengthening procedure.

PRECAUTIONS/CONTRAINDICATIONS
- During the lengthening procedure, the family must be able to make multiple appointments over a period of time, perform daily pin care, and carry out an exercise program.
- Infection can occur at the pin sites, joint stiffness can occur, and there may be subluxation or dislocation of the proximal tibia, nonunion, and fractures.

DESIRED OUTCOME/PROGNOSIS
- Child walks independently with or without bracing or assistive devices.
- Child has a smoother, more normal gait with decreased energy expenditure.
- Child has increased agility in sports participation.
- Child has improved cosmetic and physical appearance.
- Future disability resulting from the disparity in leg length is prevented.

REFERENCES

Leach J. Orthopedic conditions—Leg length inequality. In: Campbell SK, ed. *Physical Therapy for Children.* 2nd ed. Philadelphia, Pa: WB Saunders Co; 2000:420–425.

Stanger M. Orthopedic management—Limb length discrepancy. In: Tecklin JS, ed. *Pediatric Physical Therapy.* 3rd ed. Philadelphia, Pa: Lippincott Williams and Wilkins; 1999:419–21.

Muscular Dystrophy in Children

ICD-9-CM Codes:
- 359   Muscular dystrophies and other myopathies
- 359.1 Hereditary progressive muscular dystrophy

APTA Guide Patterns: 4C, 6B, 6F, 6G

DESCRIPTION

A group of inherited, progressive muscle disorders, distinguished clinically by the selective distribution of weakness (Beers & Berkow, 1999; p. 1499). There are 4 primary elements: (1) muscular dystrophy is primarily a disease of muscle tissue, (2) the course is progressive, (3) the disease process involves degeneration and death of muscle fibers, and (4) there is a genetic basis for the disorder (Ratliffe, 1998; p. 241).

Duchenne muscular dystrophy (pseudohypertrophic) is an X-linked recessive disorder characterized by progressive proximal muscle weakness with destruction and regeneration of muscle fibers and replacement by connective tissue (Beers & Berkow, 1999; p. 1499).

Becker muscular dystrophy is a less severe variant of Duchenne muscular dystrophy.

Facioscapulohumeral (Landouzy-Dejerine) *muscular dystrophy* is an autosomal dominant disorder characterized by weakness of the facial muscle and shoulder girdle, usually beginning between the ages of 7 and 20 years (Beers & Berkow, 1999; p. 1499).

Limb-Girdle muscular dystrophy results in weakness developing in a limb girdle and with proximal limb distribution (Beers & Berkow, 1999; p. 1499).

Congenital muscular dystrophy (CMD) is not a single clinical entity, and 4 different forms have been reported: 1) CMD with central nervous system disease (Fukuyama type), 2) CMD without CNS damage, 3) atonic sclerotic type, and 4) stick man type (Stuber, 2000; p. 353)

Myotonic dystrophy, in its typical form, is first noticed during adolescence and is characterized by myotonia, a delay in muscle relaxation time, and muscle weakness. *Congenital myotonic dystrophy* is a more severe form with mental retardation, speech disturbances, delayed motor milestones, distal weakness, and spinal deformities commonplace (Florence, 1999; p. 241).

CAUSE

Duchenne dystrophy is caused by a mutation at the Xp21 locus, which results in the absence of dystrophin, a protein found inside the muscle cell membrane. It affects 1 in 3,500 live male births. Most patients are confined to a wheelchair by age 10 or 12, and die of respiratory complications by 20 years of age (Beers & Berkow, 1999; p. 1499). Most children affected are boys, but girls can be affected either by monosomy of their sex chromosome pairs or due to an inactivate X chromosome from their father. The absence of the dystrophin protein causes increased permeability of the muscle cell membranes and a resultant build-up of calcium level. The calcium activates enzymes that cause a breakdown of muscle cells. Muscle cells are replaced with fat and connective tissue. The breakdown of muscle cells causes weakness, which increases over time (Ratliffe, 1998; p. 242).

Becker muscular dystrophy is a less severe variant, but also due to a mutation at the Xp21 locus. Dystrophin is reduced in quantity or in molecular weight. Patients usually remain ambulatory, and most survive into their 30s and 40s (Beers & Berkow, 1999; p. 1499). Incidence is about 1 in 20,000 births with a prevalence of 2 to 3 cases per 100,000 population (Stuberg, 2000; p. 352).

Facioscapulohumeral muscular dystrophy is caused by a gene located on chromosome 4q35 in most facilities, but the genetic defect has not been identified and pathogenesis is unknown (Beers & Berkow, 1999; p. 1499).

Limb-girdle muscular dystrophy is the result of structural (dystrophin-associated glycoproteins) or nonstructural (protenses) proteins being affected. Several chromosomal loci have been identified for autosomal dominant (5q [no known gene product]) and recessive (2q, 4q [beta-sarcoglycan], 13q [gamma-sarcoglycan], 15q [calpain, a calcium-activated protease], and 17q [alpha-sarcogycan, or adhalin]) forms (Beers & Berkow, 1999; p. 1499).

Myotonic dystrophy is an autosomal dominant disorder whose location is on chromosome 19. *Congenital myotonic dystrophy* is characterized by maternal transmission only (Florence, 1999; p. 241).

Congenital muscular dystrophy is an autosomal recessive disorder but the range of severity and disability varies significantly among the four types (Stuberg, 2000; p. 353).

ASSESSMENT

AREAS
- Gait
- Muscle strength
- Range of motion (ROM)
- Activities of daily living (ADLs)
- Adapted equipment and orthotic devices

INSTRUMENTS/PROCEDURES
- Functional Rating Scale for Boys with Duchenne Muscular Dystrophy

PROBLEMS
- In early childhood, parents may notice that the child trips or falls frequently or is considered clumsy.
- Child may toe walk.
- Child may walk later than the expected norm.
- Child may complain of fatigue while walking or climbing stairs.
- Child may be reluctant to run, climb, hop, or jump.
- Child may show hypertrophy in calves and deltoids, weakness of neck flexor, abdominals, shoulder, and hip extensor muscles.
- Child may demonstrate Gower sign: walking up their legs with their hands to stand up from the floor indicating weak quadriceps and hip extensor musculature.
- At school age, parents and others may notice the lack of reciprocal arm swing while walking and defined lordosis. Child often toe walks with abducted legs and weight on lateral borders of the feet.
- Child has gait deviation beginning with increased lateral trunk lean and arm swing to compensate for gluteus medius weakness, then leaning his trunk backward to compensate for weak hip extensor muscles. Child will begin to take smaller steps, increase lordosis, and move his arms backward to compensate for more forward center of gravity.
- Child may be unable to climb stairs without support.
- Child may walk with a wide-based gait.
- Child may be unable to rise from the floor without help.
- Child may be unable to ambulate distances.
- Child may tire easily.
- Child may demonstrate Trendelenburg sign.
- Child may demonstrate intellectual impairment.
- Child may have cardiac myopathy.
- In preadolescence, child may need braces to walk.
- Child may develop scoliosis.
- Child may have respiratory insufficiency.
- Child may lose ambulation skills.

- In adolescence, child may become obese.
- Child may develop contractures at the hips, knees, ankles, and elbows.
- Child may develop osteoporosis.
- Child may become dependent in transfers.
- Child may have an increasing need for assistance in ADLs.
- Child may require assisted ventilation.

TREATMENT/MANAGEMENT

Most services will be provided by an outpatient facility, in a home-based program, or school-based program. Usually a team approach will be used including physician, nurse, teacher, other therapists, and family members. Other persons who may need to be consulted are the school bus driver, dance teacher, or baseball coach.

GENERAL GOALS
- Maintain or improve muscle strength.
- Prevent or retard the secondary complications of contractures and deformity.
- Promote and prolong ambulation.
- Promote and maintain function.
- Facilitate psychosocial development and interaction.

Birth to 2 Years
- Unless there is a family history, there may not be a recognized need for treatment during this age range.
- Monitor developmental milestones and acquisition of functional skills.
- Monitor muscle strength, signs of hypotonia, and ROM.
- Watch for Gower sign; may be noticed as early as 15 months.

Ages 3–5
- Instruct family on daily ROM and stretching exercises for gastrosoleus (especially ankle dorsiflexion) and tensor fascia latae groups. Time and place in daily schedule should be discussed. Ratliffe (1998) suggests twice daily doing at least 10 repetitions, and holding each for 20 seconds. Each should be done slowly and should never be forced or cause pain.
- Instruct family in positioning to encourage functional skills.
- Instruct family in a general exercise program, such as swimming, rather than a specific prescribed program. Encourage participation in normal play activities and settings.
- Continue monitoring muscle strength and ROM—especially ankle dorsiflexion.
- Continue monitoring development milestones and acquisition of functional skills.
- Encourage developmentally appropriate activities such as jumping on 2 feet, standing and balancing on 1 foot, walking on heels, squatting to play, or walking up an angled balance beam or ramp. Incorporate activities into normal routines and play games such as "Simon Says" for balancing, jumping, and squatting or using a balance beam as a gangplank to a pirate ship to overcome child's reluctance to engage in motor activities.
- Suggest specific activities which promote and improve ankle and hip range of motion as well as balance and motor planning skills.
- Examples of goals: child will maintain ankle ROM of at least 90 degrees or child will play on playground equipment safely.

Ages 6–8
- Continue above goals plus consult with family and school about modifying school activities to avoid fatigue and conserve energy for tasks identified as high priority. Physical education instructor may be able to assist with ROM exercises.

- Develop a standing/walking program. A total of 3–5 hours is needed per day while the child is walking and 1 hour per day when walking is no longer possible (Tecklin).
- Teach breathing exercises.
- Consider night splints for ankles to decrease contractures.
- Monitor spinal alignment for signs of scoliosis.
- Continue a regular exercise program such as swimming or riding a bicycle.
- Consider alternate strategies, appropriate equipment, and appropriate exercises to maintain or increase the child's ability to perform ADLs.
- Splints may need to be made before surgery for lengthening the Achilles tendon, iliotibial band, or hamstrings, permitting therapy to begin as soon as possible afterwards to begin standing and walking.
- A behavioral management program may be useful to encourage the child to perform exercises and activities; provide a reward or incentive for good performance.
- Example goal: Child will breathe efficiently in the pool or child will swim 25 yards in the pool.

Ages 9–11
- Consider use of KAFOs (knee-ankle-foot orthoses) and TLSO (thoracic-lumbar-sacral orthosis) to provide better leg and trunk stability.
- Teach use of a Relater walker, parapodium, or reciprocating gait orthosis.
- Develop a program to integrate walking into school activities.
- Provide gait training and strengthening if surgery is performed.
- Teach breathing exercises.
- Suggest using a manual wheelchair for longer distances with appropriate seating positioning supports; the wheelchair should be as lightweight as possible.
- Consider a motorized scooter for independent seated mobility.
- Consider ROM exercises, positioning for function, monitoring scoliosis, and limb contractures.

Ages 12–14
- Continue a standing program as long as possible.
- Work with family and other professionals to manage obesity.
- Consider use of a power wheelchair for independent mobility. The wheelchair should have a proportional joystick control with the ability to change controls, speed, and power as the child's function changes. It should also have a manual or power tilt-in-space option to provide for pressure relief, postural relief, and repositioning. The back-to-seat angle should be greater than 90 degrees to allow for a slight extension of the spine and resultant locking of spinal facets in a neutral position. A biangled back is ideal. Safety features should include chest straps for stability when riding. The chair should accommodate a mechanical ventilator and oxygen canister when needed. The child should be involved in selecting the colors, features, and customization.
- Instruct family in the use of mechanical lifting devices such as a Hoyer lift.
- Consider recommending the use of a commode chair, shower chair, or other adapted equipment to facilitate performance of daily activities.
- Consult with teacher and other team members to develop positioning in the classroom and access to computer to facilitate academic work.
- Example goal: Child will tolerate an upright seated position for 3 hours.

Ages 15–17
- Consider the use of ball-beaning feeder and other adapted equipment to assist with ADLs.
- Develop a regular schedule and method for pressure relief and monitoring skin condition.

- Consider adapting power or manual chair for mechanical ventilation.
- Instruct family in assisted coughing, breathing exercises, and postural drainage.
- Consider recommending a power-controlled bed with air flow or an alternating pressure pad.
- Assist family and team members to plan for vocational goals.
- Example goal: Child will dance at the prom.

Age 18 Plus
- Consider adapting the controls of power chair to sip and puff or other control method for weak trunk and extremity muscles.
- Continue programs of skin care, management of contractures, and positioning.
- Consult with family regarding higher education or vocational activities, including accessible transportation.

PRECAUTIONS/CONTRAINDICATIONS
- A consistent program of exercise and stretching is necessary to avoid contractures—especially in the ankle and hip joints.
- Force in ROM and stretching should be monitored closely to avoid damaging muscle fibers and causing more destruction. Have parent exert level of force on you to assess how strong it should be.
- Because of balance problems in upright position, safety considerations should always be implemented to prevent injuries during standing and walking.

DESIRED OUTCOME/PROGNOSIS

There is no cure for MD. Death typically occurs from respiratory failure or pulmonary infection.
- Child is able to ambulate with or without assistive equipment.
- Child is able to perform ADLs with or without assistive devices.
- Child is able to maintain ankle dorsiflexion and hip extension to avoid contractures.

REFERENCES

Beers MH, Berkow R, eds. *The Merck Manual of Diagnosis and Therapy.* Whitehouse Station, NJ: Merck Research Laboratories; 1999.

Closs C, Gibbs F. Contractures of the hand in a boy with Duchenne muscular dystrophy associated with use of a computer game console. *Physiotherapy.* 1999;85(11):595–596.

Florence JM. Neuromuscular disorders in childhood and physical therapy intervention. In: Tecklin JS, ed. *Pediatric Physical Therapy.* 3rd ed. Philadelphia, Pa: Lippincott Williams and Wilkins; 1999:223–246.

Hallum A. Neuromuscular diseases—muscular dystrophy. In: Umphred DA, ed. *Neurological Rehabilitation.* 4th ed. St Louis, Mo: CV Mosby Co; 2001:397–415.

Heap R, Bond J, Hander M, Bushby K. Management of Duchenne muscular dystrophy in the community: Views of physiotherapists, GPs and school teachers. *Physiotherapy.* 1996; 82(4):258–263.

Hyde S. Physical therapy of muscle diseases. In: Lane, RJM, ed. *Handbook of Muscle Disease.* New York, NY: Marcel Dekker; 1996:663–669.

Kakulas BA. Problems and solutions in the rehabilitation of patients with progressive muscular dystrophy. *Scand J Rehabil Med Supplement.* 1999;39:23–37.

Kroksmark AK. Physiotherapy in muscular dystrophy. *Scand J Rehabil Med Supplement.* 1999;39:65–68.

Ratliffe KT. Genetic disorders—The child with Duchenne muscular dystrophy. In: Ratliffe KT. *Clinical Pediatric Physical Therapy: A Guide for the Physical Therapy Team.* St. Louis, Mo: CV Mosby Co; 1998:241–249.

Stuberg WA. Muscular dystrophy and spinal muscular atrophy. In: Campbell SK, ed. *Physical Therapy for Children.* 2nd ed. Philadelphia, Pa: WB Saunders Co; 2000:339–369.

Myelodysplasia

Also known as *spina bifida* or *neural tube disorder.*

ICD-9-CM Codes:
- 741 Spina bifida
- 756.17 Spina bifida occulta

APTA Guide Patterns: 5A, 5B

DESCRIPTION

The term *myelodysplasia* encompasses a group of central nervous system disorders in which there is defective development of the spinal cord and which have different functional outcomes. *Note:* Useful terms are defined as follows:

- *Arnold-Chiari (Chiari II) malformation:* deformity of the cerebellum, medulla, and cervical spinal cord in which the posterior cerebellum herniates downward through the foramen magnum, and brain stem structures are also displaced in a caudal direction (Tappit-Emas, 1999, p. 166).
- *Canalization:* the spinal cord distal to the S2 vertebra develops by canalization, a process of cells clumping together into masses and developing cystic structures that join to form many canals. Failure of proper canalization explains the occurrence of skin-covered meningoceles, lipomas of the spinal cord, and myelocystroceles, all of which develop caudal to the L3 vertebra (Hinderer et al, 2000, p. 624).
- *Diastematomyelia:* a fibrous, cartilaginous, or bony band or spicule separating the spinal cord into hemicords, each surrounded by a dural sac (Hinderer et al, 2000, p. 622).
- *Hydrocephalus:* abnormal accumulation of cerebral spinal fluid in the cranial vault (Tappit-Emas, 1999, p. 166).
- *Lipoma:* large or small subcutaneous masses of fat that are frequently associated with abnormal pigmentation of skin, hirsutism, skin appendages, and dimples above the gluteal cleft. A lipomatous or fibrous tract descends ventrally from the subcutaneous lipoma into the subdural space adjacent to the spinal cord (Hinderer et al, 2000, p. 622).
- *Lipomeningocele:* a superficial fatty mass in the low lumbar or sacral level. Neurological deficits and hydrocephalus are not usually associated with lipomeningoceles. Bowel and bladder dysfunction resulting from a tethered spinal cord may occur (Tappit-Emas, 1999, p. 165).
- *Meningocele:* a sac of skin usually located on the dorsal side of the spinal column which contains meninges (membranes) and spinal fluid but no functional neural elements (Gram, 1999, p. 1999; Hinderer, 2000, p. 622).
- *Myelocele:* a protruding sac confining meninges and cerebrospinal fluid but not nerve roots (Tappit-Emas, 1999, p. 165).
- *Myelocystoceles:* separated or septated cysts that separate from the central canal of the spinal cord and from the subarachnoid space. If associated with the primitive gut and an open abdomen it is called an exstrophy of the cloaca. If bony elements of the sacrum are missing or abnormal it is called a sacral agenesis (Hinderer, 2000, p. 622).

- *Myelolipomas:* lipomas within the dural sheath usually associated with paralysis (Hinderer et al, 2000, p. 622).
- *Myelomeningocele:* a sac of skin usually on the dorsal side of the spinal column which contains meninges, spinal fluid, and neural elements resulting in loss of neural innervation of the structures below the level of the sac (Gram, 1999, p. 199; Hinderer, 2000, p. 622).
- *Neurulation:* the folding of ectoderm (primitive skin and associated structures) on each side of the notochord (primitive spinal cord) to form a tube that extends from the hindbrain to the second sacral vertebra. Myelomeningoceles can occur from C1 to S2 vertebrae and are the result of a failure to complete entubuation with associated abnormal mesodermal (primitive connective tissue, muscle, and nervous tissue) development. Abnormal mesodermal development produces epidermal sinus tracts, lipomas, and diastematomyelia (Hinderer, 2000, pp. 622–623).
- *Spina bifida:* means split spine and is classified into two types: aperta (visible or open) lesion or occulta (hidden or not visible) lesion. The result may be no sensory or motor loss or there may be severe involvement (Hinderer, 2000, p. 622).
- *Spina bifida aperta:* a visible or open lesion in the spinal column. Usually the severe involvement occurs in spina bifida aperta and will result in myelomeningocele (Hinderer, 2000, p. 622).
- *Spina bifida occulta:* no visible lesion or the lesion is hidden in the spinal column. The condition occurs when there is nonfusion of the halves of the vertebral arch usually in the lumbar or sacral spine, eg but with no disturbance to the underlying neural tissue (Hinderer 2000, p. 622).
- *Spinal cord tethering or tethered cord:* occurs when adhesions anchor the spinal cord at the site of the back lesion. The child continues to grow but the cord is not free to slide upward as normally occurs but instead remains bound at the level of the back defect. Excessive stretch to the spinal cord causes metabolic changes and ischemia of the neural tissues with associated degeneration to muscle function (Tappit-Emas, 1999, p. 209).

CAUSE

The cause of canalization is unknown. The cause of neurulation is unclear but probably involves a combination of genetic and environmental factors. The neural tube defect probably occurs between 22 and 28 days of gestation and is the result of the failure of the process of neurulation in which the ectoderm folds over the primitive spinal cord to form a tube. The failure may occur from spinal levels C1 to S2. Incidence is highest for persons of Celtic background (Irish-Scottish-Welsh) and lowest for African blacks. In the United States, the incidence is from 0.4 to 0.9 per 1000 births. Environmental factors such as alcohol and drug abuse have been studied but results are not conclusive. Folic acid supplements may decrease the incidence 50% to 70% (Gram, 1999, pp. 198–199; Hinderer, 2000, pp. 624–625)

ASSESSMENT

AREAS
- Muscle strength
- Range of motion (ROM)
- Sensation
- Motor development and function
- Reflex and balance reactions

INSTRUMENTS/PROCEDURES
- manual muscle testing; in infants observe play activities
- ROM testing: passive and active

- sensory testing for touch, pain, or temperature; child needs to be 5 or older for accurate testing
- Alberta Infant Motor Scale (AIMS) (Piper & Darrah, 1994)
- Functional Reach Test (Duncan et al, 1990)
- Gross Motor Function Measure, 2nd ed. (GMFM) (Russell et al, 1993) See Gram, 1999, pp. 219–221 for sample.
- Peabody Developmental Motor Scales–2nd ed. (PDMS–2) (Folio & Fewell, 1999)
- Pediatric Evaluation of Disability Inventory (PEDI) (Haley et al, 1992)
- Seated Postural Control Measure (Story & Fife, 1992)

PROBLEMS

IMPAIRMENTS

- Disruption of nerve conduction below the level of the lesions resulting in loss of muscle function and paralysis of lower extremity muscles; specific loss depends on the level of involvement.
- Joint contractures due to muscle imbalance or the result of chronic positions of paralyzed limbs and the trunk in response to the pull of gravity. Common contractures include hip flexion, abduction, and external rotation contractures, knee flexion contractures, and ankle plantar flexion contractures. The neonate may have extreme tightness of the hip flexors.
- Decreased bone density related to decreased standing leading to osteoporosis.
- Loss of sensation with reduced ability to respond to touch, pain, and temperature.
- Loss of bowel and bladder sphincter control, flaccid bladder, urinary reflux, and kidney damage.
- Postural problems include forward head, rounded shoulders, kyphosis, scoliosis, excess lordosis, anterior pelvic tilt, rotational deformities of the hip or tibia (in-toeing, out-toeing, or windswept positions), flexed hips and knees, and pronated feet.
- Crouch standing is a typical postural deviation characterized by persistent hip and knee flexion and increased lumbar lordosis due to muscle weakness in the soleus and orthopedic deformities including calcaneal valgus.
- Spinal deformities include scoliosis, kyphosis, and lordosis.
- Hip deformities include subluxation or dislocations.
- CNS malformation: Arnold-Chiari malformation, hydrocephalus which may require a shunt.
- Motor paralysis: paraplegia resulting from the spinal cord malformation. Upper limb weakness can also occur.
- Hydromyelia (enlargement of the spinal canal): increases scoliosis, necrosis of peripheral nerves, upper extremity weakness, and hypertonus.
- Spinal cord tethering (tethered cord): increases spasticity and muscle tone, scoliosis, lumbar lordosis, pain, changes in urologic function and gait pattern, and weakening leg musculature.
- Sensory deficits: loss of sensation including light touch, pinprick, vibration, thermal, proprioception, and kinesthetic sensation.
- Hydrocephalus: excessive accumulation of cerebral spinal fluid in the ventricles of the brain occurring in approximately 85% of cases.
- Cognitive dysfunction: problems have been documented in knowledge, integration of right-left hemisphere functions, speed of motor response, and memory.
- Language dysfunction: higher frequency of irrelevant utterances and poorer performance with abstract language.
- Upper limb dyscoordination: difficulty with timed fine motor skill tasks. Movement is halting and deliberate. Mixed hand dominance may exist.
- Visuoperceptual deficits: results are mixed. Poor performance may be related to poor coordination.

- Cranial nerve palsies: most frequent is cranial nerve VI (oculomotor), IX (glossopharyngeal), and X (vagus). Optical problems may result in amblyopia, squint, palsy, nystagmus, papilledema, and atrophy. Pharyngeal and laryngeal dysfunction can include a croupy, hoarse cry and swallowing difficulty. Apneic episodes and bradycardia may occur.
- Spasticity: upper motor neuron signs are present in approximately two-thirds of affected children. The other third have lower motoneuron presentation with scattered upper motoneuron signs.
- Progressive neurologic dysfunction: changes include loss of sensation, loss of strength, pain at the site of the sac repair, pain radiating along a dermatome, initial onset or worsening of spasticity, development or rapid progression of scoliosis, development of a lower limb deformity, and changes in bowel or bladder sphincter control.
- Seizures: 10% to 30% of children and adolescents have seizures which are associated with brain malformation, cerebral spinal fluid shunt malfunction or infection, and residual rain damage from shunt infection or malfunction.
- Neurogenic bowel and bladder: 95% or more of children with myelodysplasia have bowel and bladder dysfunction.
- Skin breakdown: decubitus ulcers and other types of skin breakdown occur in 85% to 95% of all children with myelodysplasia by the time they reach young adulthood.

FUNCTIONAL LIMITATIONS
- Child may have reduced mobility due to loss of muscle function.
- Child may have delay in attaining motor milestones.
- Child may have decreased muscle function or increased spasticity with loss of previously learned motor skills.
- Child may have a tendency to become obese because fewer calories are used.
- Child may develop pressure sores due to bracing or long periods of sitting.
- Recovery from pressure sores requires prone positioning and/or hospitalization.
- Child may have fractures, kyphosis, or scoliosis requiring immobility.
- Child may have reduced ability to sense changes in temperature of hot or cold.
- Child may have reduced proprioception for balance in standing.
- Child may have incontinence and the need for diapers or self-catheterization.
- Child may have urinary tract infections.
- Child may have shunt malfunctions and periods of illness.
- Child may have visual perceptual and visual motor problems.
- Child may have "cocktail party" speech (child "chatters" for social interaction without engaging in meaningful communication).

DISABILITY
- Child may have reduced ability to keep up physically with peers.
- Child may have social isolation or ineffective social interaction.
- Child may have reduced ability to walk and possible limited access if destination areas are not wheelchair accessible.
- Child may have loss of time from school or work while recovering from surgery or injury.
- Child may have limitation of participation in outdoor activities and sports.
- Child may have difficulty with learning school work or job skills, especially if a shunt is present.

LEVEL OF LESION
- Thoracic (T6-T12): no lower extremity muscles, and may have the loss of some thoracic muscles as well depending on level of lesion; may have muscle imbalance because involvement is different on the two sides, external rotation of the

legs, kyphoscoliosis, contractures of the hip abductors and hip external rotation, and clubfeet.

- Upper lumbar (L1-L3): has hip flexors, hip adductors, and limited knee extensors. May have hip flexor contractures, hip dislocation, "wind drift," and scoliosis.
- Lower lumbar (L4): has knee extensors, ankle invertors, and dorsiflexors. May have flexor contractures and hip dislocation.
- Lower lumbar (L5): has hip abductors, knee extensors, and minimal knee flexors. May have lumbar lordosis and calcaneovarus.
- Sacral (S1-S2): has knee flexor, hip extensors, ankle evertors, plantar flexor, and toe flexor. May have calcaneovarus, toe clawing, and heel ulcers.

TREATMENT/MANAGEMENT

Treatment is usually a team management effort including a neurosurgeon, orthopedist, pediatrist, urologist, nurse, teacher, occupational therapist, and physical therapist. Before treatment, the physical therapist should interview the parents and the client to identify the family's information needs, support structure, and goals.

Therapy is divided into 4 groups according to the level of lesion: thoracic, high lump (Li-L3), low lumbar (L4-L5), and sacral.

THORACIC
- Prevent contractures in the hip abductors and external rotators through daily passive ROM, stretching exercises, splinting, orthoses, or all of these for 15 minutes a day. The tensor fasciae latae are the primary source of contractures. Contractures can limit use of bracing or other mobility aids and make dressing and transfers difficult.
- Night splint (leg wraps) may be useful in limiting external rotation. Wrap the baby's legs together from hip to knee with a cloth diaper and pin it securely for overnight and naptimes. Another method is placing both legs into one pajama-bottom leg.
- Clubfoot or other foot deformities may be corrected with serial casting or passive ROM exercises. An ankle-foot orthoses (AFO) may be needed to prevent recurrence of the contractures. Surgery may be needed if conservative measures do not work.
- A TLSO may be useful to prevent the progression of a spinal curve such as kyphoscoliosis which can compromise sitting stability and function of internal organs. Spinal fusion may be needed.
- Prevent pressure sores due to loss of sensation to the lower body—especially over the ischium from long periods of sitting—at the toes or knees. If the child is allowed to crawl, apply shoes for the toes or protective covering for the knees or any other part of the body that experiences excess pressure from orthoses such as a poorly fitting TLSO or AFO.
- Facilitate motor skills of rolling, prone (commando) crawling, and moving to a sitting position. Sitting is usually attained by pushing backward from a prone-on-hands posture until the child has pushed "through" the legs and into a sitting posture because the hip flexors and adductors are not functional. The child usually props both elbows on the thighs to maintain the sitting position which limits the use of the hands. A corner chair may be needed to provide trunk support or a caster cart to provide mobility while maintaining trunk support to free the upper extremities for exploration and play activities.
- Facilitate standing with a parapodium Toronto or Rochester and ambulation with a reciprocating gait orthoses (RGO). A hip-knee-ankle-foot orthoses (HKAFO) or a reverse Rollator walker or parallel pusher (very elongated walker) may be used. Weight-bearing and movement promote bone growth and reduce loss of bone density and potential for fractures. Standing posture also frees the hands.
- Provide a stroller and/or wheelchair (manual or powered) when distance and outdoor travel is involved. Factors may include age, size, and weight of child, ability and

maturity for propelling a chair without danger to self and others, and what type of vehicle the family has available to transport. Wheelchair must have a seatback which provides trunk support, include a pressure-relief cushion, be lightweight if child is to self-propel, be expandable for growth, and reduce or eliminate the need for bracing.

- Instruct and encourage parents in techniques for picking up, handling, and positioning infant or child—especially after surgery for a shunt.
- Instruct parents in daily exercise program.
- Instruct parents to provide sensory stimulation through handling, positioning, singing, and talking while the child is unable to provide for self due to limitations in movement.
- Instruct parents on the value of "floor time." Infant should not always be placed in an infant seat, swing, backpack, frontpack, and so on. Floor time is critical for the infant to develop postural patterns and the control needed for rolling and prone crawling and for development of perceptual skills such as calibrating distances and depth perception.
- Discuss with parents techniques for play development and skills. Suggest toys and social interaction activities the child can learn and enjoy.
- Encourage parents to develop a daily routine in which everyone participates.
- Encourage parents to allow the child to try to do things independently and not to do everything for the child. The child should be challenged within an appropriate ability level.
- Provide information to teachers as needed regarding the child's abilities, precautions to be observed, and modifications that may be needed in the classroom to facilitate participation in normal school activities.

HIGH LUMBAR LESION

- Prevent hip flexor contractures by passive positioning for 30 or more minutes per day and using manual ROM exercises. If hip flexion contracture develops, the child will stand with hyperextended trunk posture which reduces stability and can cause back pain.
- Prevent femoral valgus and hip dislocation by using an abduction splint to promote development of acetabulum. Surgery may be necessary.
- Prevent "wind drift" effect in which one leg becomes adducted while the other is abducted by use of positioning, splinting, and manual ROM exercises. The imbalance produced by "wind drift" reduces standing balance and ambulation, and may cause dislocation.
- Facilitate motor skills including rolling, crawling, and sitting. Child may be able to move from a prone to four-point position which can then be used to drop into a sitting position. Child may be able to pull to knees using a support such as a couch which increases opportunity for exploration of the environment and improves visual perceptual abilities. Sitting may limit exploration and play activities because the lack of hip extensors decreases stability. Child needs trunk support to maximize interaction with the environment.
- Facilitate standing and ambulation using a parapodium, RGO, or HKAFO. Three-point pressure is needed (anterior chest, posteriorly at the hip, and anteriorly at the knee) to achieve an upright trunk for standing and walking. A walker may provide additional support. A standing table may permit better use of the hands. A wheelchair may be useful for long distances and travel in the community.
- Instruct child and family in transfer skills: in and out of a chair, and from the floor to standing.
- Determine if the home is accessible for ambulation. If a wheelchair is used, child and family should be able to access the home and community.
- Instruct parents and child in transfer skills.
- Discuss appropriate toys and activities, the value of play skills, and a daily routine.

LOW LUMBAR LESION

- Prevent hip flexion contractures through prone positioning and manual stretching exercises.
- Prevent hip dislocation through use of a hip abduction splint.
- Prevent lumbar lordosis by the use of a chest pad during standing.
- Reduce back pain through correct positioning.
- Encourage motor skills development. Child should crawl for exploration, pull to stand, and walk holding on to furniture. All motor and transition skills should be practiced but the schedule for attainment will be delayed when compared to a normal sequence.
- Encourage ambulation. A chest strap may be needed to counteract the lack of hip extension and a pelvic band is needed because of weak or absent hip rotators. Child should be able to walk about the house and do some community walking. A wheelchair may be needed for long distances, especially in the community. The chair should be lightweight, have seating that relieves pressure over the ischium, be durable, and be adjustable for growth.
- Discuss with parents whether a brace is needed, how long it should be worn, and what kind of walker is needed.
- Discuss appropriate toys, development of play skills, and the use of a daily routine.

SACRAL-LEVEL LESIONS

- Prevent contractures due to imbalance of strength between everts and inverters and between dorsiflexors and plantar flexors of the foot.
- Prevent pressure sores on the feet, especially the heel. An AFO, supramalleolar orthoses, or shoe insert may be helpful. Child and parents should be taught to inspect the feet daily.
- Encourage development of all motor skills. Rate and sequence of development should be slower than normal but can be attained. Gait pattern will be of a Trendelenburg type in which the child's trunk sways from side to side to compensate for lack of hip stability. Assistive devices such as a walker or wheelchair should be considered if long distances are involved. Condition of the feet, general strength, lifestyle, and personality are considerations in the decision.
- Positioning should be observed and abnormal positions, especially of the feet, should be corrected.
- Encourage parents to facilitate the development of play skills.

PRECAUTIONS/CONTRAINDICATIONS

- Watch for signs of shunt failure or blockage. Examples include vomiting, irritability, headaches, lethargy, seizures, edema, or redness along the shunt tract, new nystagmus, squint or "sunset" sign of eyes, high-pitched cry, decreased school performance, and personality changes.
- Observe for signs of tethered spinal cord including increased tone on passive ROM, asymmetric changes in manual muscle testing, areas of decreased strength, and discomfort in the back or buttocks.
- Watch for signs of hip dislocation.
- Do not force legs through passive ROM. May tear soft tissues or cause fracturing.
- If pain occurs, evaluate source and evaluate the need for corrective posture or positioning.
- When child is on the floor, feet and knees should have protective padding to reduce abrasions and pressure since there is no sensation. Child should not sit for long periods of time on the floor without a cushion for the buttocks.
- Home and yard should be evaluated for safety considerations including sources of heat (floor vents, radiators) and other dangers to which a normal child would respond by crying due to pain sensation or avoid by moving.
- Watch for signs of latex allergy or use latex-free products.

DESIRED OUTCOME/PROGNOSIS

Prognosis was poor prior to 1970 because of complications such as hydrocephalus or kidney damage. Since 1970, prognosis has improved into adulthood although actual life span is unknown at this time due to the limited number of surviving individuals into their middle years.

- Child has attained expected motor skills with or without assistive devices.
- Child has mobility and ambulation with or without assistive devices.
- Child has expected ROM and does not have contractures.
- Child has attained independence in ADLs with or without assistive devices.
- Child is able to participate in school, leisure, and community activities.

REFERENCES

Gram MC. Myelodysplasia (Spina Bifida). In: Campbell SK. *Decision Making in Pediatric Neurologic Physical Therapy*. New York, NY: Churchill Livingstone; 1999:198–234.

Hinderer KA, Hinderer SR, Shurtleff DB. Myelodysplasia. In: Campbell SK, ed. *Physical Therapy for Children*. 2nd ed. Philadelphia, Pa: WB Saunders Co; 2000:621–670.

Ratliffe KT. Developmental orthopedic disorders—The child with spina bifida. In: Ratliffe KT. *Clinical Pediatric Physical Therapy: A Guide for the Physical Therapy Team*. St. Louis, Mo: CV Mosby Co; 1998:109–115.

Schneider JW, Krosschell KJ. Congenital spinal cord injury. In: Umphred DA, ed. *Neurological Rehabilitation*. 4th ed. St. Louis, Mo: CV Mosby Co; 2001:449–476.

Tappit-Emas E. Spina Bifida. In: Tecklin JS, ed. *Pediatric Physical Therapy*. 3rd ed. Philadelphia, Pa: Lippincott Williams and Wilkins; 1999:163–222.

Myotonic Dystrophy

ICD-9-CM Code: 359.2 Myotonic disorders

APTA Guide Patterns: 6B, 6F, 6G

DESCRIPTION

A form of progressive muscle dystrophy which is inherited as a autosomal dominant genetic disorder and results in a delayed or slowed muscle relaxation. Myotonic dystrophy is rarer than Duchenne.

CAUSE

Congenital myotonic muscular dystrophy is almost exclusively inherited from the mother. Childhood or adult onset may be inherited from either parent. Both are due to a genetic abnormality on the 29 chromosome at the 19q13.3 locus. The cause is an expanded number of trinucleotide repeats of cytosine, thymine, and guanine (CTG). The abnormality has been designated as myotonin protein kinase. The genetic abnormality demonstrates somatic mosaicism. This means different tissues have different numbers of CTG repeats that account for the variability of symptoms seen in subjects with similar size abnormalities of DNA analysis of peripheral blood leucocytes (Nitz, 1999, p. 597).

The incidence is reported to be 3 to 5 cases per 100,000 population and affects males and females equally (Stuberg, 2000, p. 355).

ASSESSMENT

AREAS
- Muscle testing
- Developmental progress

INSTRUMENTS/PROCEDURES

No specific instruments mentioned.

- Manual muscle testing
- Developmental testing

PROBLEMS
- Child often has myotonia which results in slowed muscle relaxation (eg, difficulty in grip release). However the myotonia may not be evident until age 3–5 and is not the major cause of functional limitations when compared to muscle weakness. Symptoms may increase with fatigue, cold, or stress.
- Child often has progressive weakness which progresses from distal to proximal that may cause poor head control, decreased hand function, gait problems, and delays in achieving developmental milestones.
- Child often has talipes equinovarus contractures.
- Child typically has a short median part of the upper lip giving it an inverted-V shape; facial movements, including sucking, are limited due to cranial nerve involvement.
- Child may have central and peripheral nervous system dysfunction including cerebral atrophy and multifocal white matter loss.
- Child may have slow conduction in both sensory and motor nerves.
- Child may have decreased or absent tendon reflexes.
- Child may have cardiovascular disorders including conduction defects, arrhythmias, ventricular hypertrophy, and mitral value prolapse.
- Child may have hypotension.
- Child may have respiratory problems due to muscle weakness and myotonia leading to reduced lung volumes and respiratory excursion that may result in retained secretions, atelectasis, decreased PAO2, and increased PACO2.
- Child may have sleep apnea.
- Child may have endocrine problems such as diabetes mellitus, gonadal atrophy, adrenal androgenic dysfunction. Some have thyroid impairment or altered hypophyseal pituitary-adrenal function.
- Child may have gastro-intestinal dysfunction due to smooth muscle involvement including myotonia and failure to function, mainly affecting the pharynx, esophagus, gall bladder, and less commonly the small and large intestines.
- Child may have dysphagia, vomiting, or aspiration.
- Child may have abdominal pain, constipation or diarrhea, volvulus, or gall stones.
- Child may have intellectual problems including attention and concentration deficits and special orientation and visual sequencing disability.
- Child may require surgery for gall stones.

TREATMENT/MANAGEMENT

Respiratory management may require consultation with a respiratory therapist, especially if a ventilator is needed. Other team members may include a family physician, orthopedic surgeon, occupational therapist, teacher, and family members. Most intervention will be consultation and the family's education, except for specific surgical interventions.

- Facilitate sucking through positioning and helping with jaw and lip closure.
- Instruct parents in positioning and the stimulation of postural responses to facilitate postural stability and promote achievement of developmental milestones.

Note: If mother has myotonic muscular dystrophy, other family members may need to be instructed on carrying out the infant program.

- Instruct family in a home instruction program for ROM activities to manage contractures.
- Instruct family in a general program of activities to promote gross motor skills development.
- Talipes equinovarus contractures should be managed with casting, taping, and exercises. Orthopedic intervention may be required.
- Positioning for seating may be needed to facilitate use of upper extremities when writing.

Note: The use of exercise to increase muscle strength is controversial. Literature reports state there is no successful treatment for muscle weakness and wasting but also suggest that the child should be encouraged to be involved in activities to decrease the problem of obesity.

- Consider recommending the use of ankle-foot orthoses to increase standing balance and reduce bilateral foot drop. Night splints may be helpful.
- Consider recommending the use of a wheelchair for distances when manual muscle test grades for muscles such as quadriceps and tibialis anterior is less than 3, since functional gait over distances is no longer practical.
- Child may require management of fractures after falls.
- Child may require chest physical therapy after surgery for atelectasis due to poor air entry and retained secretions as a result of low respiratory volumes and weak muscles. Facilitate coughing and improve air entry.
- Child will require assistance with mobilization after surgery, including assistance in raising head from the pillow.

PRECAUTIONS/CONTRAINDICATIONS
- Watch for signs of contractures: hip abduction, external rotation, and talipes equinovarus.
- If knee surgery is performed, child may be unable to participate in a standard exercise program due to muscle weakness which may delay recovery.
- If endocrine dysfunction is present, care with exercising, electrotherapeutic, and thermal modality application should be observed.
- Raynauds type circulatory problems may be present requiring consideration when exercising or using electrotherapeutic and thermal modalities.

DESIRED OUTCOME/PROGNOSIS

Disorder will demonstrate progression similar to adult forms. Weakness in distal upper and lower extremities will progress, limiting activities unless adapted equipment or techniques are used.

- Child usually improves in motor function over the first decade and most walk independently but may require a wheelchair for distances.
- Child attains normal developmental milestones although the sequence may be delayed.
- Child does not have contractures.
- Child is able to attend school and participate in regular school activities although sports activities will necessarily be limited.

REFERENCES

Florence JM. Neuromuscular disorders in childhood and physical therapy intervention—Myotonic dystrophy. In: Tecklin JS, ed. *Pediatric Physical Therapy*. 3rd ed. Philadelphia, Pa: Lippincott Williams and Wilkins; 1999:241.

Nitz JC. Physiotherapy for myotonic dystrophy. *Physiotherapy*. 1999:85(11):597–602.

Stuberg WA. Muscular dystrophy and spinal muscular atrophy—congenital myotonic muscular dystrophy. In: Campbell SK, ed. *Physical Therapy for Children*. 2nd ed. Philadelphia, Pa: WB Saunders Co; 2000:355–356.

Near Drowning

ICD-9-CM Code: 994.1 Drowning and nonfatal submersion
APTA Guide Patterns: 5A, 5B, 5G

DESCRIPTION

Near-drowning is defined as survival for a minimum of 24 hours after submersion in a fluid medium (Ratliffe, 1998, p. 285). Near-downing is an episode in which someone survives a period of underwater submersion; also called a submersion injury (Kerkering & Phillips, 2000, p. 600).

CAUSE

Ventilatory insufficiency is the most critical problem for near-drowning victims. Severe hypoxia is due to aspiration of fluid or to acute reflex laryngospasm, which may result in asphyxia without aspiration of fluid. Aspiration of fluid and particulate matter may cause chemical pneumonitis, damaging cells lining the alveoli, and may impair alveolar secretion of surfactant, resulting in patchy atelectasis (Beers & Berkow, 1999, p. 2459).

The most common causes are swimming pools; bathtubs; large bodies of water such as ponds, lakes, or oceans; or very small bodies of water such as toilets or buckets. The incidence is estimated at 2.8 per 1,000,000. Children under 5 and adolescents 15–18 are at the highest risk (Ratliffe, 1998, pp. 285–286).

ASSESSMENT

AREAS

- Cardiovascular status
- Cognitive state: arousal, attention, cognition
- Cranial nerve integrity
- Functional skills
- Motor coordination and balance
- Muscle tone
- Muscle strength
- Range of motion (ROM)
- Sensory systems

INSTRUMENTS/PROCEDURES

- Bayley Scales of Infant Development–II (BSID–II) (Bayley, 1993)
- Bruininks-Oseretsky Test of Motor Proficiency (BOTMP) (Bruininks, 1978)
- Function Independence Measure for Children (WeeFIM) (Granger et al, 1989)
- Peabody Developmental Motor Scales–2nd ed. (PDMS–2) (Folio & Fewell, 1999)
- Pediatric Evaluation of Disability Inventory (PEDI) (Haley et al, 1992)

PROBLEMS

- Child is often hypoxic—too little oxygen to the brain and other organs. Child usually experiences hypoxemia due to inactivate of pulmonary surfactant which leads to a decrease in lung compliance.
- Child often experiences apnea due to fluid being introduced into the airways.
- Child may have damage to the brain or cardiac system as a result of the lack of oxygen.
- Child often has irreversible damage after 4 to 6 minutes of anoxia unless the diving reflex occurs in very cold water.
- Child may have aspiration of fluid into the lungs causing pulmonary edema, inflammation, or a further decrease in oxygen supply.
- Child may have hypothermia—depending on the temperature and length of time submerged—if submerged in water with a temperature lower than the body's.
- Child may have infections from the aspirated fluid, especially from toilets and hot tubs.
- Child may experience cardiac arrest.
- Child may have rigidity, spasticity, and abnormal posturing.
- Child may be comatose.
- Child may have cerebral edema caused by increased intercranial pressure.
- Child may have cognitive impairments if the motor system is damaged.

TREATMENT/MANAGEMENT

Note: Details of treatment for near-drowning are not provided in the textbooks. Generally the therapist should follow the guidelines provided for traumatic brain injury.

- Prevent contractures by providing ROM exercise.
- Prevent pressure sores.
- Provide splinting.
- Provide positioning.
- Work toward improving postural control.
- Work toward promoting equilibrium responses.
- Work toward functional use of extremities.
- Encourage weight bearing through arms and legs.
- Encourage weight shifting in prone, supine, and sitting positions using play activities such as reaching for toys.
- Encourage sitting, standing and mobility; these activities will also increase the level of alertness.
- Consider use of assistive devices for child that does not regain ambulation skills. Focus on positioning while seated and facilitate mobility.
- Focus on functional goals that facilitate the child attending school and participating in an educational environment.
- Instruct parents on home program.
- Prevent recurrence of drowning through family education to childproof the environment and a community awareness of regulations.

PRECAUTIONS/CONTRAINDICATIONS

- None specifically stated. Follow guidelines for traumatic brain injury.

DESIRED OUTCOME/PROGNOSIS

Outcome depends on the length of time submerged: 5 minutes or less—a good chance of recovery; after 10 minutes—severe neurological impairment or death is likely. In addition, such children may be comatose, have seizures, dysthymias of the heart, and abnormal posturing.

- Child has functional ROM.
- Child has muscle strength and endurance within expected limits.

- Child performs functional skills.
- Child is mobile with or without assistive devices.
- Child participates in family, school, recreation, and community activities.
- Parents and child know and practice methods to prevent submersion accidents.

REFERENCES

Beers MH, Berkow R, eds. *The Merck Manual of Diagnosis and Therapy.* Whitehouse Station, NJ: Merck Research Laboratories; 1999.

Kerkering GA, Phillips WE. Brain injuries: Traumatic brain injuries, near-drowning, and brain tumors. In: Campbell SK, ed. *Physical Therapy for Children.* 2nd ed. Philadelphia, Pa: WB Saunders Co; 2000:597–620.

Ratliffe KT. Traumatic disorders—The child with a near-drowning injury. In: Ratliffe KT. *Clinical Pediatric Physical Therapy: A Guide for the Physical Therapy Team.* St. Louis, Mo: CV Mosby Co; 1998:285–286.

Osteogenesis Imperfecta

Also known as *fragilitas ossium, osteogenesis imperfecta tarda, osteogenesis imperfecta congenita,* and *brittle bone disease.*

ICD-9-CM Code: 756.51 Osteogenesis imperfecta

APTA Guide Patterns: 4A, 4B, 4C, 4D, 4G, 4H, 4I, 4J, 5F

DESCRIPTION

Osteogenesis imperfecta—an abnormal fragility of bone—is a serious disease that diffusely affects bone and connective tissue. Several forms have been described, but the neonatal type (congenital) is the most severe. Infants are born with multiple fractures, which lead to shortening of the extremities (Beers & Berkow, 1999, p. 2220). Major clinical characteristics include fragility of bone, osteopenia, variable degrees of short stature, and progressive skeletal deformities. Other clinical manifestations are blue sclerae, dentinogenesis (teeth) imperfecta, joint laxity and maturity-onset deafness (Engelbert et al, 2001). Intelligence is usually normal to above normal.

CLASSIFICATION

There are 4 types of osteogenesis imperfecta based on clinical, radiographic, and genetic characteristics according to Sillence, et al (1994):

- Type I   Most common type, which is characterized by osteopenia leading to fractures, distinctly blue sclerae, and a high incidence of adult-onset conductive hearing loss. Type IA has normal teeth and type IB has dentinogenesis imperfecta.
- Type II   Usually lethal in the perinatal period. Also known as osteogenesis imperfecta congenita (OIC).
- Type III Characterized by severe osteopenia leading to multiple fractures, progressive deformity of bones and spine, and severely decreased height.
- Type IV   Rarest type characterized by osteopenia leading to fractures but sclerae are normal. Short stature and deforming of long bones and spine tend to be more marked than in Type I. May have either normal teeth or have dentinogenesis imperfecta.

CAUSE

Genetic cause is generally autosomal dominant but Types II and III may also be caused by autosomal recessive inheritance. It is not a single genetic disorder but is heterogeneous. There is a defect in the collagen synthesis that affects the formation of both enchondral and intramembranous bone. Prevalence is 1 in 5,000 to 10,000 individuals without racial or ethnic preference according to Engelbert et al (2001, p. 943).

ASSESSMENT

AREAS

- Handling of infant during routine care
- Joint integrity
- Joint range of motion (ROM): active or functional
- Mobility and ambulation
- Muscle strength
- Positioning during routine care and rest and sleep periods
- Self-care

INSTRUMENTS/PROCEDURES

- ambulation—see Bleck EE. Nonoperative treatment of osteogenesis imperfecta: orthotic and mobility management. *Clin Orthop.* 1981;159:111-122. (Classified as nonwalking, therapy walking, household walking, neighborhood walking, and community walking with or without use of crutches)
- Bayley Scales of Infant Development–II (BSID–II) (Bayley, 1993)
- goniometer for active ROM
- joint alignment and motion scale
- manual muscle test
- Peabody Developmental Motor Scales–2nd ed. (PDMS–2) (Folio & Fewell, 1999)
- Pediatric Evaluation of Disability Inventory (PEDI) (Haley et al, 1992)
- Perceived Competence Scale for Children (also known as the Harter Self-Perception Profile for Children) (Harter, 1982)

PROBLEMS

- Generally, involvement is greater in Types III and IV than in Type I.
- Child often has joint laxity.
- Child often has osteoporosis which can result in multiple recurrent fractures.
- Child typically has delayed growth (short stature for age) and development (gross motor skills).
- Child often has a relatively large head, a soft and membranous skull, and short deformed limbs.
- Often, bones in the infant are short and wide with thin cortices, and the diaphyses are as wide as the metaphyses. Crepitation can be palpated at fracture sites.
- Child may have a triangular face with a broad forehead and faciocranial disproportions.
- Child may have decreased range of motion, which may be severe—especially in LEs.
- Child may have deformities in joints, teeth, and bones—especially long bones.
- Child may have decreased mobility and ambulation.
- Child may have decreased muscle strength—especially in LEs.
- Child may have bowing occurring in the anterolateral direction in the femur and anteriorly in the tibia.
- In sitting, child may show joint laxity and bony deformities including femoral anterolateral bowing and tibial anterior bowing.
- Child may have decreased ability in self-care skills.

- Child may have negative perceived competence in athletic performance and romance.
- Hearing loss may occur—especially as adults.
- Child may bruise easily.
- Child may have excessive sweating.
- Child may have hernias.
- Child may be overprotected by family because of fractures.
- Child may be socially isolated as a result of family overprotection.

TREATMENT/MANAGEMENT

Treatment management is typically through a team of professionals. Pharmacologic management for recurrent fractures is of dubious efficacy.

INFANT
- Provide a home program to facilitate developmentally age-appropriate gross motor skills such as head and trunk control, rolling, reaching for toys, and sitting without support. Prone over a roll placed under the chest can increase head control; gently place one arm along head to encourage rolling. Supported sitting can be accomplished with seat inserts or corner chair. Use of a small pool may be helpful.
- Instruct caregivers in handling and carrying the child especially during bathing, diapering, dressing, and carrying since these are at-risk activities for fractures. Bathing should be done in a padded, plastic basin. Diapering should be done by rolling the infant off the diaper and supporting the buttocks with one hand with the infant's legs supported on the caregiver's forearm while the other hand positions the diaper. Clothing should be loose fitting with front or side Velcro closures. Overdressing should be avoided to reduce excessive sweating. Using a pillow or custom-molded foam cushion is recommended for carrying. Head, shoulders, trunk, and legs should be well supported to reduce the risk of fractures, development of further muscle weakness, and joint laxity. A variety of positions, however, should be explored to allow for visual input, vestibular input, and opportunity for movement against gravity.
- Instruct caregivers in positioning and alignment of child's body to minimize risk of fractures and maximize social interaction. Crib should be well padded. Infant seat should provide full support and be well padded. Side-lying position should be supported with towel rolls along the spine and the extremities aligned. A prone position over a towel roll or soft wedge under the chest is an alterative. In supine, the hips should be in neutral rotation with knees over a roll. Positions should be changed frequently and not restrict active spontaneous movement.
- Provide modeled plastic splints to the lower leg to keep legs in neutral alignment.
- In cooperation with an occupational therapist, recommend safe toys and comfortable play positions that will increase sensorimotor and cognitive skills but minimize fractures, injury, and bruising. For example, the child can lie prone on a soft roll or over a parent's leg which allows for weight-bearing use of the arms, co-contraction of shoulder musculature, and promotes active neck and back extensor muscle control while maintaining good body alignment. This position also promotes the development of protective and equilibrium responses.
- Provide support and act as a resource to caregivers regarding strategies to meet the challenges of safe handling, mobility, and developmental facilitation.

TODDLER AND PRESCHOOLER
- Continue proper positioning, handling, and transferring.
- Continue active exercise through developmental and age-appropriate play. Straddling a bolster or towel roll can facilitate sit-to-stand activity for extremity strengthening and weight bearing. Begin with a high roll and gradually decrease the height of the roll. Light weights can be added if they are attached close to the large joints.

- Swimming and other aquatic exercises can be helpful in maintaining or improving cardiovascular fitness and respiratory function while providing a relatively safe environment.
- Encourage independent mobility: creeping, cruising, scooting on buttocks, walking, and moving through space.
- Encourage normal growth and development in gross motor skills within the limits of the disorder.
- Encourage weight bearing and other joint compression through the arms and legs to promote active bone strengthening even if walking is not feasible to reduce the impact of osteoporosis. Contour-molded orthoses may be used to provide compression and support.
- Consider a scooter, a wheelchair, or other powered mobility such as a caster cart when speed or distance is needed.
- Consider bracing to support extremities and minimize fractures or bowing which can facilitate mobility. Air splints may be an effective alternative.
- Consider assistive devices such as rolling walkers or crutches to increase balance and support. Standing frames are also useful.
- Instruct child in safety if a powered chair is used.
- Air splints such as pneumatic trouser splints or "vacuum pants" may be used to prevent fractures and for fracture management However, there is limited availability in the United States and they can be hot as well as bulky.

SCHOOL AGE
- Begin or continue gait training with long leg braces or other assistive devices such as prone, supine stander, or splints. Consider using a pool as a place to begin gait training activities.
- Develop and provide a daily exercise program to maintain independent mobility, gait training, bone density, muscle strength and endurance. Walking and standing activities are useful. Involve the child in decisions about the exercise program to increase cooperation. Sports and other avocational interests should be considered, provided the risk of fracture or other injury can be prevented or minimized. Swimming and wheelchair court sports such as tennis, badminton, or ping pong are possibilities.
- Facilitate child's participation in school and social activities such as joining in physical education activities, walking to the lunch room, and going on field trips.
- Recommend adapted equipment such as adapted chair for floor activities, a reacher to get materials without assistance, and modification of a computer to accommodate limited ROM.
- Provide bracing with thermoplastic materials as an adjunct to surgically implanted intramedullary rods to provide external stability.
- Recommend a wheelchair for distances and instruct the child in the safe use of a wheelchair.
- Instruct child and caregivers in how to remove and put on braces.
- Instruct caregivers and other team members in signs on slippage of intramedullary rode slippage (see Precautions/Contraindications following).
- Encourage the family to include the child in home responsibilities the same as other children. The child should have chores to do as well as expectations for behavior and participation in family life.

ADOLESCENCE
- Provide strengthening exercises before surgery for internal fixation of scoliosis, and rehabilitation after surgery to minimize loss of bone demineralization and osteoporosis.
- As a team member, explore with the child and caregivers all options for work, further education, social opportunities, and recreation after high school. Volunteer work

and social opportunities such as Boy Scouts or Girl Scouts encourage emotional growth and develop leadership skills.
- Provide information on adaptive equipment, community transportation, community programs, local colleges with programs for students with disabilities, and strategies for adapting work sites for accessibility.

ADULT
- Facilitate educational interests and career placement considering intellectual capacity and physical constraints. Note that hearing loss may become a factor.
- Continue to promote independent mobility and ambulation. Note that some adults may no longer need wheelchairs because of improved functional mobility.

PRECAUTIONS/CONTRAINDICATIONS
- Do not measure passive ROM: only active or functional ROM due to potential for fractures.
- Never lift the infant by the ankles because fractures may occur. Roll the child to one side or the other.
- Do not allow legs to dangle over the edge of a carrier. Legs should be fully supported to minimize injury and fracture.
- Pull-to-sit maneuver is contraindicated. Maneuver should be modified and facilitated by supporting the child around the shoulders while the child attempts to sit up.
- Caution parents against using baby walkers and jumping seats because they do not provide proper positioning and weight bearing.
- Fractures: once a fracture has occurred, the bone is more susceptible to refracture. Observe for crying, vacant stare, hypersensitivity to touch, and decreased interaction with parents or caregivers. Classic signs of fracture include redness, swelling, heat, and discoloration at the sight of the fracture.
- If intramedullary rods have been surgically inserted, monitor the rod sites for rod slippage, ie, a change in the orientation of the limb, length of the limb, or a bruise or bump at the end of the long bone. The physician should be notified immediately if one or more signs of slippage have occurred.
- Because the heat of a pool may increase metabolism which is already high in most children with OI, pool therapy sessions are usually limited to 20–30 minutes.
- Contact sports such as football, soccer, or baseball must be avoided.

DESIRED OUTCOME/PROGNOSIS
- Child has independent mobility with or without assistive devices.
- Child is progressing in the achievement of developmental and age-appropriate skills.
- Child has a daily exercise program which maintains strength and endurance while providing enjoyable recreational activity with or without assistive devices.
- Child is able to participate in family life as a contributing member with or without assistive devices.
- Child is able to engage in school, social, and community activities with or without assistive devices and adapted equipment.

REFERENCES

Beers MH, Berkow R, eds. *The Merck Manual of Diagnosis and Therapy*. Whitehouse Station, NJ: Merck Research Laboratories; 1999.

Bleakney DA, Donohoe M. Osteogenesis imperfecta. In: Campbell SK, ed. *Physical Therapy for Children*. 2nd ed. Philadelphia, Pa: WB Saunders Co; 2000:320–338.

Engelbert RH, Custers JWH, van der Net J, Van der Graff Y, Beemer FA, Helders PJM. Functional outcome in osteogenesis imperfecta: disability profiles using the PEDI. *Pediatr Phys Ther*. 1997:9(1):18–22.

Englebert RH, Gulmans VA, Uiterwaal CS, Helders PJ. Osteogenesis imperfecta in childhood: perceived competence in relation to impairment and disability. *Arch Phys Med Rehabil*. 2001;82(7):943–948.

Ratliffe KT. Genetic disorders—The child with osteogenesis imperfecta. In: Ratliffe KT. *Clinical Pediatric Physical Therapy: A Guide for the Physical Therapy Team*. St. Louis, Mo: CV Mosby Co; 1998:254–259.

Stanger M. Orthopedic management: Osteogenesis imperfecta. In: Tecklin JS, ed. *Pediatric Physical Therapy*. 3rd ed. Philadelphia, Pa: Lippincott Williams and Wilkins; 1999: 404–406.

Prader-Willi Syndrome

ICD-9-CM Code: 759.8 Other and unspecified congenital anomalies, Other specified anomalies

APTA Guide Patterns: 5A, 5B

DESCRIPTION

Prader-Willi syndrome is characterized by diminished fetal activity, obesity, muscular hypotonia, mental retardation, and hypogonadotropic hypogonadism. Abnormalities of growth in infancy include "failure to thrive" due to hypotonia and feeding difficulties, which generally improve after 6 to 12 months of age. From 12 to 18 months onward, uncontrollable hyperphagia causes worsening weight gain as well as psychological problems; insatiable hunger with plethoric obesity becomes the most striking feature (Beers & Berkow, 1999, p. 2384). Typically, the hair is light in color and eyes are blue with almond-shaped eyelids, a thin upper lip, mouth turned downward, narrow forehead, and fair skin. *Note*: The syndrome was first named in 1956 by Prader, Labhart, and Willi.

CAUSE

The syndrome is caused by deletion or disruption of a gene or genes on the proximal long arm of the paternal chromosome 15 or by maternal uniparental disomy of chromosome 15 (Beers & Berkow, 1999, p. 2384). Prevalence is 1 in 10,000 live births.

ASSESSMENT

AREAS
- Gait
- Gross and fine motor skills
- Muscle and grip strength
- Muscle tone
- Range of motion (ROM)
- Reflex/reactions: righting, protective, equilibrium
- Self-care skills

INSTRUMENTS
- dynamometer
- Peabody Developmental Motor Scales, 2nd ed. (PDMS–2) (Folio & Fewell, 1999)
- School Function Assessment (SFA) (Coster et al, 1998)

PROBLEMS

INFANCY
- Child often is hypotonic at birth.
- Child often has difficulty with sucking and feeding at birth.
- Child may require tube or gavage feedings in infancy.
- Child may show signs of "failure to thrive."
- Child may have abnormal or absent cry.
- Child may have hypoplasia or small genitals—undescended testicles in boys.
- Child may have delayed motor milestones.
- Child may have delayed speech development.
- Child may have sticky saliva which contributes to dental caries.

TODDLER
- At approximately age 2 to 3 years, the child develops an insatiable appetite.
- Child tends to become morbidly obese.
- Gross motor milestones continue to be delayed due to hypotonia but fine motor skills are often age appropriate.
- Child may be difficult to understand due to poor articulation and weak voice quality which is high pitched with a nasal quality.

CHILDHOOD
- Child often has delays in gross and fine motor skills.
- Child often has short stature.
- Child typically has small hands and feet.
- Child often bruises easily.
- Child often has impaired intelligence. Even those with normal intelligence do not perform to their intelligence potential. Math is typically more difficult than reading.
- Child often has learning disabilities.
- Child often is sleepy during the day.
- Child may develop scoliosis.
- Child may have an ulnar boarder in the hands.
- Child may have strabismus (eyes do not work together).
- Child may be myopic (near-sighted) and squint to see.
- Child may have difficulty learning and performing self-care skills.
- Child may have behavioral problems such as temper tantrums, stubbornness, manipulative personality, negativism, and depression.

ADOLESCENT
- Child often demonstrates creativity and perseverance when it comes to finding food including stealing, ordering from catalogs over the telephone, forging checks, and eating from garbage cans.
- Child typically has a lower metabolic rate and engages in less physical activity, resulting in weight gain.
- Child may have a poor self-image due to obesity, poor performance in school, poor athletic performance, poor communicative skills, and difficulty with self-help skills.
- Child may have poor peer relationships.
- Child may become easily frustrated.
- Child may have difficulty dealing with changes in routine.
- Child may ask the same question repeatedly.
- Puberty is delayed or incomplete.
- 60% to 80% of girls do not menstruate and boys have small genitals.

ADULT
- Often, adults are infertile.
- Adult may have osteoporosis due to decreased hormonal levels.

TREATMENT/MANAGEMENT

INFANT
- Instruct caregivers in positioning for feeding: head should be midline and chin should be slightly tucked for easy swallowing. Head should be higher than stomach. May feed in the parent's lap or in an infant seat. Encourage face-to-face interaction to promote social skills. Talk to, smile, and touch the infant often.
- Improve oral-motor tone. Activities may include stroking the lips, gums, and tongue; provide light pressure around the mouth and facial massage. Observe amount of time the infant sucks before taking a break and encourage caregiver to recognize the infant's patterns and rhythm.
- Instruct caregivers on techniques for static positioning and carrying. Head should be midline, legs in flexion, and arms close to the sides of the body to approximate position of a child with normal tone.
- Facilitate gross motor milestones such as rolling, sitting without support, and standing. Activities might include wheelbarrow walks, push/pull a wagon, throwing, lifting objects, scooter board, and playground.
- Encourage aerobic conditioning. Activities might include bunny-hopping; long jumping; running up and down steps, inclines or hills; riding a tricycle; and sitting on a scooter board while propelling with the feet.

CHILD
- Facilitate the gross and fine motor skills needed for educational activities. Activities might include dance, swimming, trampoline activities, dynabands, therabands, or hand weights.
- Behavioral control has been most effective in controlling weight gain.
- Increase independence in self-care skills such as dressing and tying shoes. May need larger buttons or Velcro for shoes.

ADOLESCENT
- Continue strength training. Activities might include the use of weight machines, hand weights, exercises for upper and lower limbs and trunk including biceps and hamstring curls, triceps and quad extensions, latissimus pulls, abdominal crunches, squats, and toe rises.
- Increase activity level to counter hypoactivity. Encourage a routine of daily physical activity such as aerobic conditioning including bike riding, brisk walking, water aerobics, roller skating, roller blading, ice skating, cross country skiing, or downhill skiing.

PRECAUTIONS/CONTRAINDICATION
- During weight-training exercises, monitor blood pressure in those who are obese due to the risk of developing hypertension.

DESIRED OUTCOME/PROGNOSIS

AEROBIC CONDITIONING
- Child is able to improve time or timed performance tests.
- Child is able to increase distance or number of laps.
- Child's heart range decreases during work or activity and returns to baseline quickly after activity.

STRENGTH TRAINING
- Child's grip strength increases as measured by the dynamometer.
- Child is able to increase the number of repetitions performed.
- Child is able to increase the distance for long jumps, swimming, or running.

REFERENCES

Beers MH, Berkow R, eds. *The Merck Manual of Diagnosis and Therapy.* Whitehouse Station, NJ: Merck Research Laboratories; 1999.

Belt AB, Hertel TA, Mante JR, Marks T, Rockett VL, Wade C, et al. Movement characteristics of persons with Prader-Willi syndrome rising from supine. *Pediatr Phys Ther.* 2001; 13(3):110–121.

Holm VA, Douglass T, Lucas BL, Washington KA, Hay A, Coggins TE. A child with Prader-Willi syndrome. In Guralnick MJ, ed. *Interdisciplinary Clinical Assessment of Young Children with Developmental Disabilities.* Baltimore, Md: Paul H Brookes; 2000:327–349.

Lewis CL. Prader-Willi syndrome: a review for pediatric physical therapists. *Pediatr Phys Ther.* 2000;12(2):87–95.

Ratliffe KT. Genetic disorders—the child with Prader-Willi syndrome. In: Ratliffe KT. *Clinical Pediatric Physical Therapy: A Guide for the Physical Therapy Team.* St. Louis, Mo: CV Mosby Co; 1998:249–254.

Premature Infant

Also known as *prematurity.*

ICD-9-CM Code: 765 Disorders relating to short gestation and unspecified low birthweight

APTA Guide Patterns: 5A, 5B

DESCRIPTION

Any infant born before 37 weeks gestation. Note that the weight criteria of <2.5 kg (5.5 lbs) has been discontinued. The premature infant is small, usually weighs <2.5 kg, and tends to have thin, shiny, pink skin through which the underlying veins are easily seen. Little subcutaneous fat, hair, or external ear cartilage exists. Spontaneous activity and tone are reduced, and extremities are not held in a flexed position (Beers & Berkow, 1999, pp. 2127–2128).

CLASSIFICATION OF INFANTS BASED ON SIZE

- AGA: Appropriate for gestational age infants who are between the 10th and 90th percentiles of infants the same age
- ELBW: Extremely low birth weight. Infants below 1000 g (2 lbs, 3.5 oz)
- IUGR: Intrauterine growth retardation. May be used interchangeably with SGA
- LBW: Low birth weight. Infants below 2500 g (5 lbs, 8 oz)
- LGA: Large for gestational age. Infants who are above the 90th percentile for infants the same age
- SGA: Small for gestational age. Infants who are below the 10th percentile for infants the same age
- VLBW: Very low birth weight. Infants below 1500 g (3 lbs, 5 oz)
- VVLBW: Same as ELBW

COMMON COMPLICATIONS OF PREMATURITY

(Scott et al, 2000, pp. 226–228; Ratliffe, 1999, p. 361).

- *Intraventricular hemorrhage* (IVH), *Germinal matrix-Intraventricular hemorrhage* (GM-IVH): bleeding into the germinal matrix region of the brain, with possible rupture of blood into the ventricles.

- *Periventricular hemorrhage:* lesion is a hemorrhagic venous infarction with the major cause being obstruction of blood flow in the trigerminal vein caused by GM-IVH (Kahn-D'Angelo & Unanue, 2000, p. 847).
- *Necrotizing enterocolitis* (NEC): an intestinal condition with symptoms of abdominal distention, blood in the stool, vomiting, diarrhea, and retention of feedings in the stomach.
- *Respiratory Distress Syndrome* (RDS) or *Hyaline Membrane Disease:* results from the immaturity of the lungs.
- *Patent Ductus Arteriosus* (PDA): failure of the patent ductus arteriosus to close so that blood is still shunted to the descending aorta instead of to the pulmonary artery.
- *Bronchopulmonary dysplasia* (BPD) or *Chronic Lung Disease:* an advanced lung disease in infants caused by damage to lung tissues from mechanical ventilation.
- *Hyperbilirubinemia:* an excessive level of bilirubin in the infant's blood serum.
- *Periventricular leukomalacia:* a lesion caused by a reduction in cerebral blood flow in the periventricular region of the brain (Kahn-D'Angelo & Unanue, 2000, p. 846).
- *Hypoxic-Ischemic encephalopathy* (HIE): perinatal asphyxia and ischemia form of oxygen deprivation (Kahn-D'Angelo & Unanue, 2000, p. 848).
- *Status Marmoratus:* neuronal loss, gliosis, and hypermyelinization of the basal ganglia and thalamus (Kahn-D'Angelo & Unanue, 2000, p. 850).
- *Parasagittal Cerebral Injury:* a lesion of the cerebral cortex and subcortical white matter.
- *Focal Ischemic Brain Necrosis and Cavitation:* large, localized areas of neuronal death in the distribution of single or multiple major blood vessels in the cerebral cortex and subcortical white matter (Kahn-D'Angelo & Unanue, 2000, p. 851).

CAUSE

The cause of premature labor, whether or not preceded by premature rupture of the membranes, is typically unknown. However, maternal histories commonly show low socioeconomic status, inadequate prenatal care, poor nutrition, poor education, unwed state, and intercurrent, untreated illness or infection. Other risk factors include untreated maternal bacterial vaginosis and a previous preterm birth (Beers & Berkow, 1999, p. 2128).

ASSESSMENT

AREAS
- Behavioral state assessment
- Gross motor skills
- Manual muscle testing
- Pain
- Range of motion (ROM)
- Reflexes/reactions
- Sensory Testing

INSTRUMENTS/PROCEDURES
- Apgar score at 1 and 5 minutes
- Assessment of Preterm Infant Behavior (APIB) (Als et al, 1982)
- Bayley Scales of Infant Development–II (BSID–II) (Bayley, 1993)
- Milani-Comparetti Motor Development Screening Test, 3rd ed. rev. (MCMDST) (Stuberg, 1993)
- Morgan Neonatal Neurobehavioral Examination (MNNE) (Morgan et al, 1988) Scale printed in Sheahan & Brockway, 1999, pp. 88–91.
- Movement Assessment of Infants (MAI) (Campbell et al, 1980)
- Naturalistic Observation of Newborn Activity (Als, 1984)
- Neonatal Behavioral Assessment Scale, 3rd ed. (NBAS) (Brazelton, 1995)
- Neonatal Oral–Motor Assessment Scale (NOMAS) (Braum & Palmer, 1985)
- Neurobehavioral Assessment for Preterm Infants (NAPI) (Korner et al, 1992)

- Neurologic Assessment of the Preterm and Full-Term Newborn Infant (Dubowitz & Dubowitz, 1981)
- Nursing Child Assessment Feeding Scale (NCAFS) (Barnard & Eyres, 1979)
- Test of the Infant Motor Performance (TIMP) (Campbell et al, 1993)

PROBLEMS

- Infant is often hypotonic. The degree depends on the amount of prematurity.
- Infant often has an increased ROM. The degree depends on the amount of prematurity. Increased ROM and flexibility is evident in the shoulders, elbows, hips, and knees.
- Infant's posture in supine or prone is often in extension with abduction.
- Infant often has difficulty with flexor patterns and midline orientation.
- Infant often has hypotonic or floppy muscle tone and does not achieve the full degree of flexor muscle tone seen in the full-term infant (Sheahan & Brockway, 1999, p. 73).
- Infant often lacks the counterbalance of flexor tone to offset the normal progression of extensor muscle tone; there is an imbalance between extensor and flexor muscle groups.
- Infant often has minimal spontaneous movement. What movement occurs is typically jerky and unorganized.
- Infant may have absent, reduced, or inconsistent primitive reflexes.
- Infant may have difficulty with midrange control of head, sitting balance, reaching skills, and bilateral coordination.
- Infant may have respiratory distress syndrome (RDS)—also known as hyaline membrane disease—due to lack of surfactant.
- Infant may have cardiac problems due to fetal heart circulation patterns which have not changed, eg, patent ductus arteriosus (PDA).
- Infant may have an intracranial hemorrhage (ICH), eg, an intraventricular hemorrhage (IVH), which may cause brain damage resulting in neurological deficits including cerebral palsy.
- Infant may have retinopathy of prematurity due to the prolonged use of oxygen which results in visual impairment or blindness.
- Infant may have a hearing loss or be profoundly deaf.
- Infant may have apnea or episodes of "forgetting" to breathe due to immature respiratory regulation which may result in bradycardia, slowing the heart rate. Sometimes known as "A's and B's"
- Infant may have poor state control and is easily overwhelmed by sensory stimuli.
- Infant on mechanical ventilation may show increased hypertension of the neck, scapular elevation, retraction of the shoulders and upper extremities, arching of the trunk and immobility of the pelvis.

TREATMENT/MANAGEMENT

Treatment is often conducted with a transdisciplinary approach including a physician, nurse, nutritionist, occupational therapist, and physical therapist. Occupational and physical therapists frequently work together. Cross training is common between nurses and therapists in tasks related to feeding, positioning, gross and fine motor skills.

- Promote and instruct parents in proper positioning including emphasis on physiological flexion to increase and improve flexion of joints against gravity using towel or diaper rolls to position limbs and body in flexion positions.
- Promote and instruct parents in handling techniques for parent-child interaction including holding, touching, and communicating with the infant, eg, watching the infant for an open, alert expression, pursed lips, and a steady gaze which can facilitate the bonding process and encourage positive relations between parent and child.

- Promote postural alignment and more normal patterns of movement through therapeutic handling and positioning.
- Instruct parents to recognize signs of distress and loss of state control including crying, arching the back, turning away from the person or object, hiccups, sneezing, holding an arm straight out as if to say "stop," change in skin color, excessive increase in heart rate, gagging, choking, and gasping. Help parents learn techniques to calm the child and help the child regain state control by tuning out stressful stimuli, eg, a water bed, audiotapes of sounds heard in utero, wrapping or bundling the child in blankets, and skin-to-skin contact.
- Promote and instruct parents in techniques to enhance self-regulatory behavior through environment modification.
- Promote and instruct parents in methods of facilitating the development of gross motor skills: head and trunk control, push up on arms, and supported sitting.
- Promote and instruct parents in methods of facilitating fine motor skills development: reaching, grasping, and releasing objects, and bringing hands to midline to examine toys.
- Instruct parents in techniques to increase infant awareness of the environment by providing sensations including weight bearing on feet and hands similar to kicking in utero, vestibular input through rocking, holding the arms and legs in flexion, gentle massage, and talking to the infant.
- Modify the environment and instruct parents in how to modify the environment to facilitate the child's development.
- Modulate sensory input such as oral-motor stimulation, hydrotherapy, and the use of water mattresses.
- Instruct parents in feeding-related activities since the infant is usually tube fed due to the lack of strength, endurance, and sensorimotor organization. Activities include providing face-to-face interaction, helping the baby suck on something during the feeding, and providing touch or stroking.

PRECAUTIONS/CONTRAINDICATIONS
- Infant should be monitored closely for signs of stress and loss of state control such as oxygen saturation, heart rate, respiration rate, and to identify behavioral signs of stress during treatment. Treatment and active intervention should be terminated and efforts to regain state control instituted.

DESIRED OUTCOME/PROGNOSIS
- Child has reduced or no impairments.
- Child has normal or functional ROM, postural adaptation, and control of extremities.
- Child has improved regulation and organization of motor behavior, interactions with caregivers and the environment, and family.
- Parents and caregivers are involved in the development of goals and outcomes.

REFERENCES
Beeby PJ, Henderson-Smart DJ, Lacey JL, Rieger I. Short- and long-term neurological outcomes following neonatal chest physiotherapy. *J Pediatr Child Health.* 1998;34(1): 60–62.

Beers MH, Berkow R, eds. *The Merck Manual of Diagnosis and Therapy.* Whitehouse Station, NJ: Merck Research Laboratories; 1999.

Boivin J. Preemies need PT, too. *Nurs Spectrum.* 1997;7(15):18.

Carmichael KM, Burns YR, Gray PH, O'Callaghan MJ. Neuromotor behavioural assessment of preterm infants at risk for impaired development. *Aust J Physiotherapy*. 1997;43(2): 101–107.

Gray PH, Flenady VJ, Blackwell L. Potential risks of chest physiotherapy in preterm infants [letter; comment]. *J Pediatr*. 1999;135(1):131; discussion 132.

Harding JE, Miles FK, Becroft DM, Allen BC, Knight DB. Chest physiotherapy may be associated with brain damage in extremely premature infants. *J Pediatr*. 1998;132:(3 pt 1): 440–444.

Kahn-D'Angelo L, Unanue RA. The special care nursery. In: Campbell SK, ed. *Physical Therapy for Children*. 2nd ed. Philadelphia, Pa: WB Saunders Co; 2000:840–880.

Kaisor-Szerszen I. Home-based physical therapy intervention for a premature infant born at very low birthweight. *Phys Ther Case Rep*. 2000;3(6):280–282.

Lekskulchai R, Cole J. Scarf ratio: a method of measuring the Scarf sign in preterm born infants. *Aust J Physiotherapy*. 2000;46(2):85–90.

Lekskulchai R, Cole J. Effect of a developmental program on motor performance in infants born preterm. *Aust J Physiotherapy*. 2001;47(3):169–176.

Maynard V, Bignall S, Kitchen S. Effect of positioning on respiratory synchrony in non-ventilated pre-term infants. *Physiotherapy Res Int*. 2000;5(2):96–110.

Oberwaldner B. Physiotherapy for airway clearance in paediatrics. *Eur Respir J*. 2000;15(1): 196–204.

Ratliffe KT. Neonatal disorders—Matthew, a boy born prematurely. In: Ratliffe KT. *Clinical Pediatric Physical Therapy: A Guide for the Physical Therapy Team*. St. Louis, Mo: CV Mosby Co; 1998:351–358.

Ratliffe KT. Neonatal disorders—Prematurity. In: Ratliffe KT. *Clinical Pediatric Physical Therapy: A Guide for the Physical Therapy Team*. St. Louis, Mo: CV Mosby Co; 1998:359–367.

Scott DT, Cook DS, Dinno ND, Folsom RC, Lucus BL, Swanson MW, et al. An infant at increased risk. In: Guralnick MJ, ed. *Interdisciplinary Clinical Assessment of Young Children with Developmental Disabilities*. Baltimore, Md: Paul H Brookes; 2000:221–250.

Sheahan MS, Brockway NF. The high-risk infant. In: Tecklin JS, ed. *Pediatr Phys Ther*. Philadelphia, Pa: JB Lippincott Co; 1999:71–106.

Sweeney JK, Swanson MW. Low birthweight infants: Neonatal care and follow-up. In: Umphre DA, ed. *Neurological Rehabilitation*. 4th ed. St Louis, Mo: CV Mosby Co; 2001: 203–258.

Sweeney JKI, Heriza CB, Reilly MA, Smith C, VanSant AF. Practice guidelines for the physical therapist in the neonatal intensive care unit (NICU). *Pediatr Phys Ther*. 1999;11(3): 119–132.

Vincon C. Potential risks of chest physiotherapy in preterm infants [letter, comment]. *J Pediatr*. 1999;135(1):131–132.

Respiratory Failure

ICD-9-CM Codes:
- 508 Respiratory condition due to unspecified and external agents
- 514 Pulmonary congestion and hypostasis
- 516 Other alveolar and parietoalveolar pneumonopathly
- 518 Other disease of lung

- 553 Other hernia of abdominal cavity without mention of obstruction of gangrene
- 769 Respiratory distress syndrome
- 770 Other respiratory conditions of fetus and newborn
- 786 Symptoms involving respiratory system and other chest symptoms

APTA Guide Pattern: 6J

DESCRIPTION

Respiratory failure is the impairment of gas exchange between ambient air and circulating blood occurring in intrapulmonary gas exchange or in the movement of gases in and out of the lungs (Beers & Berkow, 1999, p. 544). Respiratory failure occurs when the infant or child's pulmonary system is unable to exchange carbon dioxide and oxygen between the body and its environment.

CAUSE

Causes include acute respiratory conditions, abnormal control mechanisms, traumatic injuries, and progressive degenerative neurological and muscular disorders. Diffuse pathology of the CNS such as viral encephalitis, acute polyneuritis (Guillain-Barré syndrome) or barbiturate intoxication may lead to respiratory failure by paralyzing the voluntary and involuntary positions of the respiratory muscles. Abnormal neural control mechanisms and reflexes may also reduce the physiologic response to chemical and mechanical stimuli. Examples of childhood disorders that result in a reduced response include familial dysautonomia, sleep apnea, and obesity-hypoventilation syndrome. Spinal cord lesions above the C-4 level may result in total ventilatory paralysis. Progressive degenerative disorders may lead to respiratory failure such as Werdnig-Hoffmann and Duchenne muscular dystrophy (Tecklin, 1999, pp. 540–541).

ASSESSMENT

AREAS
- Airway clearance
- Breathing patterns: resting, exertion
- Chest and shoulder mobility and range of motion (ROM)
- Coughing: inspiration, glottic closure, expiratory force
- Respiratory muscle strength: inspiratory, expiratory
- Sensorimotor development: overall strength, mobility, and coordination and developmental level
- Oral motor skills including swallowing of solids and semisolids

INSTRUMENTS/PROCEDURES
- *Minute ventilation:* the product of the respiratory rate and the tidal volume; determines the arterial PaCO2.
- *Respiratory rate:* count respirations for 30 seconds or 1 minute.
     Note: Normal respiratory rate at rest varies with age. A younger child will have a higher rate.
- *Tidal volume:* measure with a spirometer or a Wright respirometer.
     Note: Tidal volume varies with height. Compare pattern and symmetry of each hemithorax.
- *Respiratory muscle strength:* measure lung volumes, maximal static inspiratory and expiratory pressures, or use electromyography.

- *Chest mobility:* measure chest during inspiration and expiration.
- *Shoulder girdle and shoulder ROM:* functional ROM or goniometry.
- *Auscultation of the lungs:* listen for decreased breath sounds, areas with absent sounds, rhonchi, or wheezes.
- *Cough:* evidence of integral components of a cough: sufficient active inspiration effort and coordinated closure of the glottis, followed by sudden contraction of the abdominal muscles to increase intrathoracic pressure.

PROBLEMS
- Airway obstruction
- Airway resistance
- Poor or inadequate gas exchange
- Increased work of breathing
- Loss of lung capacity

TREATMENT/MANAGEMENT
- Increase respiratory muscle strength: provide instruction in the use of two incentive spirometers, one calibrated for diaphragmatic breathing and lateral costal breathing and the second, a blow bottle for use in expiratory exercise.
- Decrease spasticity.
- Increase chest wall movement.
- Facilitate accessory muscle breathing while in an upright posture.
- Increase diaphragmatic breathing. Provide instruction in diaphragmatic breathing and lateral costal expansion.
- Facilitate assisted coughing.
- Increase or maintain ROM of respiratory muscles.

PRECAUTIONS/CONTRAINDICATIONS
- Intervention which increases bronchospasm or pulmonary hypertension should be stopped and re-evaluated.
- Avoid repositioning a foreign body unless directed by a physician.
- Avoid destabilizing a sick infant.

DESIRED OUTCOME/PROGNOSIS
- Child has a clear, unobstructed airway.
- Child has minimal airway resistance.
- Child has enhanced gas exchange.
- Child expends minimal effort in breathing.

REFERENCES

Beers MH, Berkow R, eds. *The Merck Manual of Diagnosis and Therapy.* Whitehouse Station, NJ: Merck Research Laboratories; 1999.

Ratliffe CE. Chest physical therapy. In: Ratliffe KT. *Clinical Pediatric Physical Therapy: A Guide for the Physical Therapy Team.* St. Louis, Mo: CV Mosby Co; 1998:376–383.

Tecklin JS. Pulmonary disorders in infants and children and their physical therapy management—Respiratory muscle weakness. In: Tecklin JS, ed. *Pediatric Physical Therapy.* 3rd ed. Philadelphia, Pa: Lippincott Williams and Wilkins; 1999:540–545.

Wallis C, Prasad A. Who needs chest physiotherapy: Moving from anecdote to evidence. *Arch Dis Child.* 1999;50:393–397.

Scoliosis

ICD-9-CM Code:

- 737.30 Scoliosis, idiopathic
- 754.2 Certain congenital musculoskeletal deformities, Of spine

APTA Guide Patterns: 4A, 4B, 6F

DESCRIPTION

A structural, lateral curvature of the spine. Scoliosis may be first suspected when one shoulder seems higher than the other or when clothes do not hang straight, but is often detected during routine physical examination.

The spinal curve is more pronounced when the child or adolescent bends forward. Most curves are convex to the right in the thoracic area and to the left in the lumbar area, so that the right shoulder is higher than the left (Beers & Berkow, 1999, p. 2419).

Curves that progress beyond 10 degrees should be treated (Ratliffe, 1999, p. 143). Common surgical procedures for spinal stabilization use either anterior or posterior methods. The Dwyer and Zielke instrumentation procedures use anterior fusion. The Cotrel-Bubousset, Harrington Rod, and Luque instrumentation systems are posterior fusion procedures. Common braces include the Boston brace which is an underarm TLSO (thoracolumbosacral orthosis), and the Milwaukee brace which is a CTLSO (cervical-thoracic-lumbar-sacral orthosis). Other TLSO types are the Wilmington, Lyon, and Charleston models.

CAUSE

The cause is unknown. Sixty to eighty percent of cases occur in girls. Two to three percent of children aged 10 to 16 years have detectable idiopathic scoliosis. Incidence of scoliosis that requires medical treatment is approximately 2 per 1,000 (Ratliffe, 1999, p. 141).

Classification systems include age of onset; magnitude of curve; direction, location, size and number of curves; and type and etiology of the curve (Ratliffe, 1999, p. 142). See Table 12.3.

ASSESSMENT

AREAS

- Gait
- General activity level
- General alignment
- Leg length
- Muscle strength: especially leg and trunk
- Muscle tone
- Posture: standing and bending at the waist
- Range of motion (ROM), especially lower extremity
- Reflex/reactions
- Shoulder, trunk, and pelvic symmetry
- Spinal alignment during forward bend
- Spinal rotation
- Trunk compensation
- Trunk flexibility

INSTRUMENTS/PROCEDURES

- *Cobb method:* Used to measure curve on a radiograph. Lines are drawn at the beginning and end of the curve. Next, lines are drawn parallel to both the beginning and end lines. The angle formed by the intersection of the perpendicular lines is measured to determine the degree of curvature.
- *Plumb line:* Measure for trunk compensation.

TABLE 12.3
Scoliosis Diagnostic Markers

	Value	**Qualification**
Age of Onset	Birth to 5 years	Congenital
	3 years to puberty	Juvenile
	During or after puberty	Adolescence
Magnitude of Curve	0 to 20 degrees	Mild
	20 to 40 degrees	Moderate
	> 40 degrees	Severe
Direction, Location, Size, and Number of Curves	Directions	Right or left apex
	Location	Cervical, cervicothoracic, thoracic, throacolumbar, lumbar curves
	Size	Minor or major curve
	Number	Single or double curve
Type and Etiology of Curve	Functional, postural, nonstructural	No structural changes, may be related to poor posture or musculoskeletal anomalies, correctable with bending or postural correction
	Structural	Changes in vertebrae and supporting tissue
		Decreased flexibility
		Rotation of vertebrae is often present
		Related changes to rib cage, pelvis, hips
Etiology of Structural Types	Congenital	Malformation of vertebrae at 3 to 5 weeks of gestation
	Neuromuscular (paralytic)	Associated with neuromuscular diseases such as cerebral palsy, muscular dystrophy, or myelomeningocele. Diseases with orthopedic manifestations such as arthrogryposis, and osteogenesis imperfecta may also be included here
	Traumatic onset	Associated with spinal fractures, irradiation, tumors, or metabolic disorders (rickets)
	Idiopathic	Causes include unknown etiologies and familial tendency for scoliosis

- *Risser sign:* Measured by a radiograph of the iliac crest; indicates the amount of ossification as it correlates to the level of skeletal maturity. Grades 0 to 5 indicate skeletal maturity levels starting with the absence of any ossification of grade 0 and ending with complete maturation and cessation of skeletal growth at grade 5.
- *Scoliometer:* Measure for rotation.

- *Screening* (Ratliffe, 1999, p. 143)
    - *Standing:* Child is standing and facing away from therapist.
        - Assess symmetry of the shoulders (look for elevation on the convex side of the curve).
        - Assess symmetry of scapulae and posterior rib cage (scapula may be higher and rib cage may be prominent on the convex side).
        - Assess symmetry of the waist and gluteal folds (waist may appear fuller on the convex side; gluteal folds may be asymmetrical).
        - Assess symmetry of the hips (one hip may protrude).
        - Drop plumb line from occiput to assess trunk alignment (plumb line may fall lateral to gluteal crease; if it falls over gluteal crease, check for a compensatory curve).
        - Assess symmetry of spinous processes.
    - *Bending forward:* Child bends forward from the waist as if to touch the ground. The arms should swing freely.
        - As the child bends forward, assess symmetry of the ribcage (rib hump may appear posteriorly on the convex side).
- Measuring the angle of trunk rotation.
- Rib hump height.
- Moire photography.

PROBLEMS
- Child may have decreased trunk flexibility in all planes.
- Child may have limited hamstring length.
- Child may have reduced cardiopulmonary fitness and endurance.
- Child may have reduced sitting tolerance or ischial skin breakdown due to pelvic obliqueness.
- Child may use upper extremities to maintain sitting balance due to collapsing curves.
- Child may experience pain due to rib impingement against the iliac crest.
- Child may have difficulty performing daily activities due to the curves and rotation of the spine; parents may have more difficulty caring for the child.
- Child has a misshaped body due to wedge-shaped vertebrae which are higher and rotated on the convex side and compressed on the concave side.
- Child may have unequal muscle strength and tone on the two sides of the body due to shortened muscles on the concave side and lengthened muscles on the convex side.
- Child may have reduced vital capacity or difficulty breathing due to ribs that are rotated from their normal position.
- Child may develop contractures, especially hip flexion contractures.
- Child may have difficulty with transitional movements such as from sitting to standing.

TREATMENT/MANAGEMENT

BEFORE AND AFTER SURGICAL INTERVENTION
- Instruct family and child how to put on and remove the brace/orthosis.
- Instruct family and child in good body mechanics, posture, and positioning techniques while brace/orthosis is being worn in prone, supine, sitting, and standing positions.
- Instruct family and child in techniques for getting in and out of bed with the brace/orthosis in place.
- Instruct family and child in transfer techniques such as sit-to-stand and getting in and out of car.

- Instruct family and child in how to pick up objects from the floor while brace/orthosis is worn.
- Instruct family and child in dressing techniques while brace/orthosis is worn.
- Instruct family and child in the need for ROM and strengthening exercises permitted while brace/orthosis is on the child's body. Provide examples of good choices such as swimming.

Note: Use of a chart showing progress may encourage cooperation and compliance.

- Prevent contractures and encourage child to participate in appropriate activities to maintain flexibility.
- Instruct child in techniques to improve balance and muscle tone during sitting and standing.
- Instruct family and child in exercises that can be done with the family, peers, or in group situations that are meaningful to the child; encourage compliance. Use of video tapes and/or music may be helpful as well as individualizing the exercise program for the child. Adapting any physical education program the child already has is a useful idea to allow and encourage the child to continue to participate with peers. Examples of exercises include knees to chest, pelvic tilts, 4-point trunk extensor strengthening, curl-ups, oblique curl-ups, lateral flexion, and trunk shift to address trunk flexion, extension, rotation, and abdominal strength.
- Encourage early ambulation by explaining its importance and demonstrating techniques such as how to go up and down stairs.
- Discuss with family and child what clothing is appropriate to wear and how to minimize the impact of the brace in social situations.

TREATMENT FOR NEUROMUSCULAR CAUSES
- Instruct family or caregiver on 3-point method of trunk positioning. Pressure is applied over the apex of the curve and ribs at the cephalic and caudal end of the curve. Optimal alignment may be facilitated with custom-molded seating systems, gravity-assisted positioning, or trunk orthoses.
- Maintain optimal alignment when positioning in bed or lying down. Alternative positions may be needed such as side-lying.
- Adaptive devices such as the Vac-Pac (Olympic Medical), Versa Form Plus Positioning Pillows (Tumbleforms), or similar devices can provide custom positioning in side-lying, supine, prone, or sitting positions.

PRECAUTIONS/CONTRAINDICATIONS
- Check and monitor the fit of the brace/orthosis for areas of pressure or abrasions on the skin and report to orthotist or physician.
- Participation in contact sports is contraindicated.
- Monitor child for abnormal neurological signs and report to physician.
- Monitor brace/orthosis for stability; note any changes or shifts in position and report to physician.
- Child with neuromuscular disease may have low or high muscle tone, weakness, persistence of primitive reflexes, soft tissue contractures, and behavioral, cognitive, or developmental issues which must be considered in the treatment of the scoliosis.

DESIRED OUTCOME/PROGNOSIS

Note: The younger the child is at diagnosis, the greater the risk of progression. Double-curve patterns have a greater risk for progression than single-curve patterns. The lower the Risser sign, the greater the risk of progression. Curves with greater magnitude are at a greater risk of progress. Risk of progression in females is approximately 10 times that of males with curves of comparable magnitude. Greater risk of progression is present when curves develop before menarche (Patrick, 2000, p. 264).

- Child has normal or expected muscle strength for age which is equal on both sides of the body.
- Child has good sitting and standing postural alignment and symmetry considering the amount of surgical fusion, if surgery was performed.
- Child has equal leg length or discrepancy is correctable by shoe insert.
- Child has good ROM in all joints except those vertebrae which were fused, if surgery was performed.
- Child participates in a daily exercise program to maintain fitness and endurance.
- Child is able to perform daily activities without pain.
- Child is able to participate in school, recreational, social, and community activities within restrictions based on surgical fusion, if surgery was performed.

REFERENCES

Beers MH, Berkow R, eds. *The Merck Manual of Diagnosis and Therapy.* Whitehouse Station, NJ: Merck Research Laboratories; 1999.

Patrick C. Spinal conditions—scoliosis. In: Campbell SK, ed. *Physical Therapy for Children.* 2nd ed. Philadelphia, Pa: WB Saunders Co; 2000:261–272.

Ratliffe KT. Other orthopedic disorders—Scoliosis. In: Ratliffe KT. *Clinical Pediatric Physical Therapy: A Guide for the Physical Therapy Team.* St. Louis, Mo: CV Mosby Co; 1998: 141–146.

Stanger M. Orthopedic management—scoliosis (idiopathic). In: Tecklin JS, ed. *Pediatric Physical Therapy.* 3rd ed. Philadelphia, Pa: Lippincott Williams and Wilkins; 1999: 421–425.

Weiss HR, Lohschmidt K, El-Obeidi N, Verres C. Preliminary results and worst-case analysis of inpatient scoliosis rehabilitation. *Pediatr Rehabil.* 1997;1(1):35–40.

Wright A. The conservative management of adolescent idiopathic scoliosis. *Phys Ther Rev.* 1997;2(3):153–163.

Sensory Disorders: Visual and Visual-Perceptual Disorders

ICD-9-CM Code: 360–379 Disorders of the eye and adnexa
APTA Guide Patterns: 5A, 5B

DESCRIPTION

Visual disorders can be related to the structure of the eye or visual centers of the brain and the central nervous system (CNS) itself. Structures include the eye muscles, cornea, retina, optic nerve, and optic chiasma. Visual centers include the pathways and the optic cortex. The result of visual disorders is some degree of deficient visual skills.

CAUSE

Causes include structural problems, malformations of the brain, in utero infections, and events occurring after birth. Malformation includes cerebral palsy. In utero infections include toxoplasmosis and rubella. Events include head trauma, eye infections, tumors, vitamin A deficiency, meningitis, encephalitis, or anoxia.

Structural problems include refraction errors causing hyperopia (farsightedness), myopia (nearsightedness), and astigmatism (blurry vision), cataracts, and glaucoma. A common structural problem in cerebral palsy and other developmental disorders is strabismus—a disorder of the muscles of the eye causing abnormal alignment. Both eyes may turn in, out, or only one eye may deviate. The problem may occur intermittently or continuously. The result may be a blurring of vision or double image and an attempt to suppress the visual input from one eye to avoid this blur or double vision.

Retinopathy of prematurity is another example of a structural program in which the development of normal blood vessels in the retina is disrupted. There may be too many blood vessels extending from the retina and the detachment of a portion of the retina occurs causing partial or complete blindness in one or both eyes.

CNS problems can include cortical blindness due to brain infection, visual field deficits such as hemianopsia (unable to see one half of each eye's visual field), tunnel vision (lack of peripheral vision), or lack of central vision (seeing only with peripheral vision).

ASSESSMENT

AREAS
- Development milestones
- Gross motor skills
- Mobility skills
- Muscle strength
- Muscle tone
- Visual perception

INSTRUMENTS/PROCEDURES
- Developmental Test of Visual Perception, 2nd ed. (DTVP–II) (Hammill et al, 1993)
- Motor-Free Visual Perception Test–Revised (MVPT–R) (Colarusso & Hammill, 1996)

PROBLEMS
- Child may tilt the head to see or see more clearly.
- Child may turn the head so that peripheral vision may be used when central vision is not available.
- Child may have an eye that turns in toward the nose (esotropia); turns out toward the temple (exotropia); turns upward (hypertropia), or downward (hypotropia).
- Child may respond intermittently to visual stimuli, depending on the location of the stimulus.
- Child who is blind often has low muscle tone, and gross motor milestones are reached later than in sighted children: examples include reaching for objects and development of language and social skills.
- Child may develop self-stimulatory behaviors such as pressing the eyes, flicking fingers in front of the eyes, or rolling the head.
- Child may have a figure-ground deficit (difficulty distinguishing a given form from the background) which impairs transition in different types of terrain depth.
- Child may have visiospatial deficit which can interfere with activities of daily living such as putting on an orthotic device.
- Child may have difficulty developing a mental map (topographical map) of the environment and thus may experience difficulty moving independently from place to place without getting lost.

TREATMENT/MANAGEMENT

Note: Work with trainers who are skilled in teaching mobility skills to the blind, if available.
- Promote development of gross motor skills.
- Promote development of muscle strength.
- Support confidence in ability to move about the environment.
- Encourage movement transitions: pulling to stand, cruising, and independent walking.

- Assist family members in identifying motivators for the child, such as assistive technology, voice cueing, and structuring the environment.
- Consider different levels of cognitive ability when promoting mobility skills.
- Recommend that obstacles in the environment be reduced, such as throw rugs, rocking chairs with long rockers, or other protrusions into open space that might trip or impede progress.
- Facilitate a young child's use of trailing (use of a hand on the wall to assess position in the environment).
- Facilitate an older child's use of assistive devices such as canes, guide dogs, or laser devices to identify obstacles.

PRECAUTIONS/CONTRAINDICATIONS
- Child with visual disorders may be at risk for safety concerns in the environment.
- Child with visual disorders is at risk for delays and poor performance in motor skills.

DESIRED OUTCOME/PROGNOSIS
- Child is able to move about the environment with visual devices, such as glasses or with use of compensatory skills such as trailing.
- Child has acquired normal developmental milestones.
- Child is able to perform age-equivalent gross motor skills.
- Child has assistive devices needed to perform daily tasks.

REFERENCES

Ratliffe KT. Sensory, processing, and cognitive disorders of childhood—Sensory disorders of childhood. In: Ratliffe KT. *Clinical Pediatric Physical Therapy: A Guide for the Physical Therapy Team.* St. Louis, Mo: CV Mosby Co; 1998:335–337.

Sensory Disorders: Hearing Impairment

Also known as *hearing loss, hard of hearing, deaf, deafness.*

ICD-9-CD Code: 380–389 Disorders of the ear and mastoid process
APTA Guide Patterns: 5A, 5B

DESCRIPTION

Hearing impairment occurs when a child is unable to hear sounds that others can hear. Of those with hearing impairment, about 40% have mild, 20% have moderate, 20% have severe, and 20% have profound hearing loss. The timing of the loss is important. Those who lose hearing prior to their third birthday are considered to be in a "prelinginal" phase for the development of language and speech and are likely to have problems in the development of effective language and speech. The earlier the hearing loss occurs, the poorer the prognosis. Children with developmental disabilities and cognitive impairments are often in this group (Redcliffe, 1999, p. 337).

Note: Classification is based on type and amount of hearing loss in decibels.

TYPE
- *Conductive hearing loss:* occurs when the structures of the external or middle ear are involved due to repeated ear infections, buildup of fluid in the middle ear, or

damage to the tympanic membrane, all of which reduce the conduction of sound from the external environment to the inner ear.

- *Sensorineural learning loss:* occurs when there is a disorder in the cochlea or the auditory nerve, such as from brain hemorrhage, asphyxia in premature infants, cerebral malformation, trauma, infections, and ototoxic antibiotics.
- *Mixed:* any combination of conductive and sensorineural loss.

AMOUNT OF HEARING OF LOSS

- *Slight:* 16–25 decibels. Miss about 10% of speech sounds.
- *Mild:* 26–40 decibels. Miss 25–40% of speech sounds, distant sounds, unvoiced consonants (p, t, f), plurals, and tenses.
- *Moderate:* 41–55 decibels. Miss 50–80% of speech sounds.
- *Moderate-severe:* 56–70 decibels. Miss most speech sounds and all speech information.
- *Severe:* 71–90 decibels. Miss all speech sounds. Can hear loud environmental noises.
- *Profound:* >90 decibels. Miss all speech and environment sounds. Can feel vibration.

CAUSE

Causes include environmental, genetic, and unknown factors. Environmental factors include maternal infections, such as rubella, toxoplasmosis, or CMV; postnatal infection, such as meningitis or encephalitis; trauma; exposure to ototoxic antibiotics; and prematurity. Genetic elements include primary and secondary factors. An example of a primary factor is an autosomal recessive inherited hearing loss. Secondary factors often involve chromosomal disorders in which hearing impairment is one of a cluster of symptoms. For example, 60% to 80% of children with Down syndrome have a conductive hearing loss because of narrow ear canals and a high incidence of middle ear infections. Finally, about one-third of cases with hearing loss are unknown (Redcliffe, 1999, p. 337).

ASSESSMENT

AREAS

- Language skills: listening, follow sounds
- Communication skills
- Pre-speech sounds
- Speech

INSTRUMENTS/PROCEDURES

Note: Physical therapists are not the primary evaluators of speech and language but may notice signs or symptoms of hearing loss during testing for balance reactions, developmental levels, or interactions with a child while determining motor skill acquisition.

PROBLEMS

- Child may not turn toward or follow sounds.
- Child may have a temper tantrum caused by the frustration of being unable to communicate.
- Child may become sad and withdrawn or noncompliant because he or she cannot hear or cannot make self understood.

TREATMENT/MANAGEMENT

- Therapist can learn basic sign language useful for communicating with children (see example in Redcliffe, 1999, p. 340). Use the signs as the child learns them.

- Therapist should make sure the child is looking at the therapist before the therapist speaks.
- Encourage the child to wear the hearing aid(s) if prescribed for the child. Therapist should learn to adjust the hearing aid(s) to avoid feedback and ensure the aid or aids are in good working order.
- Encourage early language activities when possible such as signing, use of computers, naming toys, looking at books and pictures, and so on.
- Encourage use of residual hearing through talking, singing, playing music, and use of rhythm and vibration during therapy activities.
- Encourage movement in space such as rocking, bouncing, swinging, or jumping.
- Use other sensory input, especially proprioception and vision. Proprioceptive activities include jumping, marching, stamping, wheelbarrow walking, and pushing activities. Vision activities can include the use of toys with bright visual appeal and visual references to external objects to facilitate orientation.

PRECAUTIONS/CONTRAINDICATIONS

- Child with a hearing impairment is at risk for safety considerations in the environment.
- Child with a hearing impairment is at risk for the decreased effective communication of needs and understanding of social demands.

DESIRED OUTCOME/PROGNOSIS

- Child is able to understand communication necessary to participate in therapy program.
- Child is able to communicate individual needs during therapy program.

REFERENCES

Rine RM, Lindeblad S, Donovan P, Vergara K, Gostin J, Mattson K. Balance and motor skills in young children with sensorineural hearing impairment: a preliminary study. *Pediatr Phys Ther.* 1996;8(1):55–61.

Ratliffe KT. Sensory, processing, and cognitive disorders of childhood—sensory disorders of childhood. In: Ratliffe KT. *Clinical Pediatric Physical Therapy: A Guide for the Physical Therapy Team.* St. Louis, Mo: CV Mosby Co; 1998:337–345.

Ratliffe, KT. Matthew, a boy born prematurely. In: Ratliffe KT. *Clinical Pediatric Physical Therapy: A Guide for the Physical Therapy Team.* St. Louis, Mo: CV Mosby Co; 1998:351–357.

Slipped Capital Femoral Epiphysis

Also known as *coxa vara* or *epiphyseal hip fracture.*

ICD-9-CM Code: 732.2 Nontraumatic slipped upper femoral epiphysis
APTA Guide Patterns: 4D, 4H, 4J

DESCRIPTION

Movement of the femoral neck upward and forward on the femoral epiphysis. Onset is typically insidious, and symptoms are associated with the stage of slippage. Initially, there may be hip stiffness that improves with rest, followed by a limp, and then hip pain that radiates down the antemedial thigh to the knee (Beers & Berkow, 1999, p. 2430). Management often includes stabilization of the growth plate to prevent further displacement. Complications can include avascular necrosis, chondrolysis, and early osteoarthritis (Stanger, 1999, p. 417).

CLASSIFICATION
- Grade I: 1%–33% slippage of the epiphysis from the femoral head
- Grade II: 33%–50% slippage
- Grade III: >50% slippage

CAUSE

This disorder often occurs in overweight adolescents—usually boys. The cause is unknown but may be related to the effects of growth hormone and estrogen on the thickness of the epiphyseal plate (Beers & Berkow, 1999, p. 2430). Occurrence is 0.71 to 3.41 per 100,000 children and in boys is 2 to 3 times more common than in girls.

ASSESSMENT

AREAS
- Gait
- Muscle strength
- Range of motion (ROM)

INSTRUMENTS/PROCEDURES

No specific instruments mentioned or listed.

PROBLEMS
- Child often has pain in groin, medial thigh, or knee.
- Child may limp and/or be unable to bear weight on the leg.
- Child may have external rotation of the leg (hip joint).
- Child may have limited ROM especially in hip flexion, abduction, and internal rotation.

TREATMENT/MANAGEMENT
- Instruct child in crutch walking or wheelchair mobility skills (whichever is to be used) before child is discharged to home.
- Instruct parents or caregivers in transfer training in a spica cast if used.
- Instruct parents or caregivers in upper extremity exercises to help child maintain strength and mobility.
- A home evaluation is useful to asses the home accessibility and help the family determine care for the child at home; a hospital bed and mechanical lift may be needed.
- After spica cast is removed, progressive gait training is typically needed to facilitate independent mobility.
- Muscle strength may need to be increased in lower extremities after spica cast is removed.
- Increased passive and active ROM may be needed to regain lost range.

PRECAUTIONS/CONTRAINDICATIONS
- During acute recovery period, child is usually not allowed to bear weight.

DESIRED OUTCOME/PROGNOSIS

Outcome and prognosis depend in part on the degree of slippage and the success in surgical stabilization of the growth plate.

- Child is able to bear weight evenly on both legs.
- Child has a normal gait pattern.
- Child does not report pain in the groin.

REFERENCES

Beers MH, Berkow R, eds. *The Merck Manual of Diagnosis and Therapy.* Whitehouse Station, NJ: Merck Research Laboratories; 1999.

Leach J. Orthopedic conditions—slipped capital femoral epiphysis. In: Campbell SK, ed. *Physical Therapy for Children.* 2nd ed. Philadelphia, Pa: WB Saunders Co; 2000:415–417.

Ratliffe KT. Disorders of the developing hip—the child with slipped capital femoral epiphysis. In: Ratliffe KT. *Clinical Pediatric Physical Therapy: A Guide for the Physical Therapy Team.* St. Louis, Mo: CV Mosby Co; 1998:85–88.

Stanger M. Orthopedic management—slipped capital femoral epiphysis. In: Tecklin JS, ed. *Pediatric Physical Therapy.* 3rd ed. Philadelphia, Pa: Lippincott Williams and Wilkins; 1999:415–417.

Spinal Cord Injuries

ICD-9-CM Codes:
- 952 No evidence of spinal bone injury
- 952.0 Cervical
- 952.1 Dorsal [thoracic]
- 952.2 Lumbar

APTA Guide Pattern: 5F

DESCRIPTION

Spinal cord injury is the result of a partial or complete injury to the spinal cord. The mechanism of injury, the effects of development on functional skills, and the effects of the spinal cord injury on development are very different in a child than an adult (Redcliffe, 1998, p. 287).

Children younger than 16 years of age account for less than 5% of spinal cord injuries. Ages 10–15 are the most common age (Shakhazizian et al, 2000, p. 571). See Table 12.4 for classifications.

STAGES OF RECOVERY

- Immediately after injury, child experiences edema and trauma to the spinal cord, leading to the appearance of a complete transection of the cord which is called *spinal shock syndrome*: an absence of reflexes below the level of the injury, flaccidity of deinnervated muscles, loss of sensation and autonomic dysfunction including hypertension, abnormal body temperature, loss of bladder and bowel function, and autonomic dysreflexia.
- The second stage occurs when the flaccidity of affected muscles ends and spasticity begins along with neurological return.
- The third stage involves stabilization of loss and the recovery of spinal functions.

CAUSE

Most injuries occurring to children after birth are the result of trauma. The most common mechanism for spinal cord injury in a child is incurred during a motor vehicle accident.

TABLE 12.4
Spinal Cord Injury Classifications

Level A	complete injury—no sensory or motor function is present below sacral levels 4 and 5
Level B	incomplete injury—sensory but no motor function present below sacral levels 4 and 5
Level C	incomplete injury with motor and sensory preservation below the level of injury—motor strength is less than grade 3
Level D	motor and sensory preservation with strength greater than grade 3 below the level of injury
Level E	complete recovery—child has complete recovery of sensory and motor tracts
Brown-Séquard	injury to half the spinal cord causing hemiplegia
Anterior cord injury	impairment of motor functions as well as sensation of pain and temperature but sparing of proprioception, kinesthesia, and vibration
Central cord syndrome	disability in sensory functions, especially pain and temperature as well as motor dysfunction which is more severe in the upper extremities than the lower
Cauda equina injury	flaccid paralysis of muscles in the lower extremities

Young children can sustain cervical cord injuries when involved in an accident even when restrained in a car seat, if facing forward. Older children who are restrained by lap and shoulder belts may sustain a cervical cord injury as a result of the poor placement of an adult-sized shoulder belt or because of securely restrained torso, weak neck muscles, and a large head resulting in hyperflexion.

Other causes include falls, diving into shallow water, sports injuries such as football or surfing, young infant trauma from shaking, birth trauma, gunshots, and stabbing with a knife. Mechanisms that are not traumatic including tumors of the spinal cord and transverse myelitis (Redcliffe, 1998, p. 287).

ASSESSMENT

AREAS
- Cardiorespiratory endurance
- Mobility skills
- Motor skills
- Muscle strength
- Range of motion (ROM), passive

INSTRUMENTS/PROCEDURES
- Functional Independence Measure (FIM) (Hamilton et al, 1987)
- Functional Independence Measure for Children (WeeFIM) (Granger et al, 1989)
- goniometer
- manual muscle testing (over age 5)
- Pediatric Evaluation of Disability Inventory (PEDI) (Haley et al, 1992)

PROBLEMS

GENERAL
- Child may be fearful of movement.
- Child may have pain in certain muscles or during certain movements.

C1–C3
- No voluntary musculoskeletal control below chin level
- No respiratory control: Dependent on ventilator for breathing
- May have cardiac problems including bradycardia and tachycardia
- May be nauseated and may vomit
- No mobility or functional skills; total dependence

C4
- No voluntary control of upper extremities, trunk, or lower extremities
- Dependent on ventilator support for breathing
- No mobility or functional skills; dependent on others for total care

C5
- Must use abdominal respiration due to lack of accessory respiratory muscles; result is poor respiratory reserve
- Cannot roll over or get into a sitting position independently
- Incomplete shoulder motion (no rotation) and limited or poor elbow and wrist flexion
- No elbow extension, forearm, finger motion, trunk control, or lower limb motion
- No functional use of hands for grasp and release

C6
- Must use abdominal breathing: no accessory respiratory muscles; poor respiratory reserve
- Limited or weak elbow extensors and hand functions

C7
- Has weak hand grasp, release, and coordination
- Needs assistance with transfers and lower extremity dressing

T1-T10
- Has poor trunk balance
- Needs braces for standing

T10-L2
- Poor control of lower limbs
- Limited endurance for walking with long leg braces

L3 OR BELOW
- Has poor control of ankles
- May have lumbar lordosis
- May have difficulty getting up from a sitting position

TREATMENT/MANAGEMENT

Intervention requires a team of medical and rehabilitation professionals including nurses, physicians, therapists, social service personnel, teachers, and family members.

BY RECOVERY STAGES

Initial Stage of Recovery
- Provide or recommend ankle splints to prevent contractures in the calf muscles during initial period of flaccidity.
- Provide or instruct others to do ROM at least once or twice per day to avoid contractures from immobility.

- Position child to maintain good alignment while reducing pain and stiffness. Examples include positioning shoulder to permit scapular freedom, positioning upper extremity in abduction and external rotation, and positioning lower arm on a pillow during ROM exercises. Poor spinal stability may limit use of some positions.
- Provide chest physical therapy in all children with injuries above T12 to encourage deep breathing and mobilization of secretions to reduce pulmonary infections. Assisted coughing, quick stretches to assist expiration and inspiration, intercostal mobilization to maintain rib mobility, and incentive spirometry can assist in maintaining pulmonary hygiene (Ratliffe, p. 291). Use games to encourage breathing, such as blowing a ping pong ball across a table, singing loudly, and spitting contests.
- Assist child in getting into an upright position using a tilt table. Process must be gradual to avoid orthostatic hypotension (low blood pressure). Note if child reports being nauseous or lightheaded, is disoriented, or starts breathing faster.
- Involve the family in the rehabilitation process. Initially, family may prefer to observe but should be encouraged to participate as they feel more comfortable being with medical and rehabilitation personnel.

Second Stage of Recovery

- Monitor child for signs of sensory function, muscle tone, muscle strength, and ROM.
- Prevent contractures through positioning, ROM exercise, orthotic devices, and changing position throughout the day. Watch for contractures in ankle-plantarflexion and flexion in the hip, knee, elbow, and fingers.
- Increase strength and balance with weight-training group or individual mat training using pulleys with weights, Theraband (an elastic material with variable resistance), or other specific activities. For shoulder abduction and flexion—writing or drawing on a chalk board, and for wrist extension—fingerpainting in shaving or whipped cream sprayed on a vertical board or wall, or painting on an easel.
- Monitor skin with decreased or absent sensation for potential pressure sores (decubitus ulcers). Instruct child to relieve pressure on ischium by pushing down with his or her hands to lift hips off the support surface every 2 hours, if possible. A child with a high thoracic or cervical injury may be able to lean forward by hooking an arm through a strap for a few seconds every hour or two. A child with a higher injury needs a mechanical means to relieve pressure such as a tilt-in-space or power recliner.
- Increase ROM through use of play activities, such as asking a child to reach for a toy that is held in the air.
- Observe child for changes in muscle tone as flaccidity changes to spasticity which may increase potential for contractures, and create difficulty in maintaining or changing positions.
- Improve mobility skills in bed, on the mat, or the floor including rolling, sitting up with or without assistance, and scooting.
- Instruct child in independent transfers or with minimum assistance if lesion is at C7 or below. A transfer, sliding board, or a board with a "lazy Susan" device to permit pivoting may be useful. Include standing pivot with assistance or a mechanical lift for children unable to stand. If a lift is to be used at home, help team consult with family to find one which best fits the needs and space available in the home. Transfers to and from a car should also be explored. Modifications to the car or different vehicle may be desirable, such as van with ramp or electric lift to accommodate a wheelchair.
- Instruct child in wheelchair mobility using a manual or power wheelchair. Consider cognitive status, child's age, level of injury, and location of use when selecting a wheelchair. Teach safety in using a wheelchair, especially a powered chair. Child with a high-level injury will require a powered chair but also a child with a midthoracic injury may need a powered chair for distance because of low strength and endurance.

A manual chair or stroller may be needed as backup when the powered chair breaks down. Check for proper positioning frequently to maintain good alignment.

- If lesion is low, work on ambulation with use of assistive devices.
- Instruct child and family/caregivers in techniques for inhibiting clonus by pressing down firmly through the joint so the muscle has no excursion when it contracts, taking the foot off the supporting surface so gravity cannot provide a stretch when the muscle relaxes, and stretching the muscle to its full range (Ratliffe, p. 292).
- Instruct child and family/caregivers in techniques to reduce the effect of hypertonicity by placing limbs in reflex-inhibiting postures such as flexion and abduction to avoid spasms into extension. Other techniques include warm baths, relaxation techniques, ROM exercise, and massage.
- For high lesions, continue chest physical therapy with percussion, drainage, and assistance with coughing.
- Perform a home evaluation to ensure access in a wheelchair, help family plan where the child will sleep, determine access to the bathroom for bathing, and assist in planning for other activities in the home.

Third Stage of Recovery

- Continue with ROM and strengthening to maximize function.
- Promote independence in mobility and other functional skill such as the use of an ecological control device to turn on and off equipment, and facilitate computer access including adapted switches, keyboards, or other input devices.
- If ambulation is an option, assist team in selecting equipment such as crutches, a parapodium, platform walker, knee-ankle-foot orthosis (KAFO), and surface or implanted electrodes. Considerations include balance, strength, age, level of injury, energy required, and cost.
- Assist child and family in coping with new challenges, such as accessibility at a summer camp, selection of new equipment, and adapting devices as the child grows.
- In adolescence, the issues may include driving, sexuality, intimacy, having children, higher education, and vocational choice. Physical therapists can provide information, work with other team members, and suggest resources.

BY LEVEL OF INJURY

C1–3

- Position child in midline seating position with ventilator tray.
- Provide a pressure relief mechanism in seating.

C4

- Consider use of Sip 'n Puff control mechanism for power mobility and a chin control.
- Provide an environmental control system (environmental ADL device).
- Facilitate performance of functional skills with a mouthstick.
- Provide or instruct parents and caregivers in respiratory hygiene.
- Provide alternative positioning and cushions to prevent pressure sores.
- Provide or instruct parents and caregivers in ROM exercises to prevent contractures.

C5

- Consider adapted joystick on power wheelchair and environmental control device.
- Instruct child and parents/caregivers in use of standing pivot transfers with assistance.
- Recommend use of adapted devices such as universal cuff, mouthstick, switch interface for grooming, self-feeding, and accessing a computer.
- Provide or instruct parents/caregivers in respiratory hygiene.

- Provide or recommend use of pressure relief cushions.
- Instruct older child in how to do independent pressure relief by hooking arm and leaning if biceps are strong enough.

C6

- Instruct child to propel wheelchair independently using hand rim extensions.
- Instruct child in independent pressure relief.
- Instruct child and parents/caregivers in use of a sliding board for transfers with assistance.
- Instruct child and parents/caregivers in use of standing pivot transfers.
- Recommend use of adapted devices such as universal cuff, mouthstick, switch interface for grooming, self-feeding, and accessing a computer.
- Provide or instruct parents/caregivers in respiratory hygiene.
- Provide or recommend use of pressure relief cushions.

C7

- Instruct child to independently propel manual wheelchair.
- Instruct child and parents/caregivers in transfers using minimal assistance.
- Instruct child in mobility skills such as how to scoot on mat or floor, roll over, and sit up independently.
- Encourage child to participate in lower extremity dressing.

T1-T10

- Instruct child to propel wheelchair independently.
- Instruct child in mobility skills such as scooting, rolling, and coming to sitting position.
- Provide practice in trunk balance.
- Increase upper extremity muscle strength.
- For adolescent, instruct or recommend instruction in use of hand controls to drive a car or van.

T10-L2

- Instruct child in ambulation with bilateral long leg braces and crutches within level of endurance.
- Instruct child in mobility skills including scooting, rolling, and coming to sitting position.
- Increase trunk strength and balance skills for standing and walking.
- Recommend that a wheelchair be used for distances.

L3 OR BELOW

- Instruct in ambulation using walker, crutches, or cane.
- Recommend use of short leg braces or ankle foot orthoses for walking to provide ankle stability.
- Encourage mobility skills including creeping on all fours, rolling, coming to sitting position, and pushing up to stand.

PRECAUTIONS/CONTRAINDICATIONS

- Manual muscle testing is considered unreliable in children younger than 5 years of age.
- Determine degree of spinal stability before beginning mobilization.
- When performing ROM, do not stress the spine.
- If a hip flexion contracture is present, a pillow may be needed when lying prone to avoid causing an increased lumbar lordosis.
- Limit shear force in recliners to reduce skin friction and rubbing.
- Always provide information on skin inspection, use of positioning to reduce skin breakdown, and safety to reduce possibility of sores and cuts.

- Know causes, signs, and symptoms of autonomic dysreflexia and instruct child and parents/caregivers.
- Check wheelchair or stroller positioning: pelvis should be level in the seat and trunk supported laterally to avoid slumping. Foam blocks, plywood, vinyl, or cloth covering can be used to provide inserts as needed.

DESIRED OUTCOME/PROGNOSIS

- Child has ROM in all joints above level of injury.
- Child has maximum muscle strength in all muscle groups above level of injury.
- Child does not have contractures.
- Child has balance and equilibrium responses consistent with level of injury.
- Child has mobility skills with or without assistive devices.
- Child has functional skills consistent with level of injury.
- Child is able to use mobility devices correctly and safely.
- Parents and child know how to repair assistive devices or know resources to complete required repairs.
- Child participates in family, school, community, and recreational activities.

REFERENCES

Creitz L, Nelson VS, Haubenstricker L, Backer G. Orthotic prescriptions. In: Betz RR, Mulcahey MJ, eds. *The Child with a Spinal Cord Injury*. Rosemont, Ill: American Academy of Orthopaedic Surgeons; 1996:537–554.

Kelly MA, Stokes KS. Standing and ambulation for the child with paraplegia or tetraplegia. In: Betz RR, Mulcahey MJ, eds. *The Child with a Spinal Cord Injury*. Rosemont, Ill: American Academy of Orthopaedic Surgeons; 1996:519–532.

Moynahan M, Hunt M, Halden E. Evaluation of standing and ambulation: Needs and outcomes. In: Betz RR, Mulcahey MJ, eds. *The Child with a Spinal Cord Injury*. Rosemont, Ill: American Academy of Orthopaedic Surgeons; 1996:503–518.

Nelson VS, Driver LE, Backer G, Hilker DF, Howell B, Walfe BB. High tetraplegia. In: Betz RR, Mulcahey MJ, eds. *The Child with a Spinal Cord Injury*. Rosemont, Ill: American Academy of Orthopaedic Surgeons; 1996:791–802.

Perrin JCS, Johnstone KS. Prevention of spinal cord injury in children. In: Betz RR, Mulcahey MJ, eds. *The Child with a Spinal Cord Injury*. Rosemont, Ill: American Academy of Orthopaedic Surgeons; 1996:13–22.

Ratliffe KT. Traumatic disorders—The child with a spinal cord injury. In: Ratliffe KT. *Clinical Pediatric Physical Therapy: A Guide for the Physical Therapy Team*. St. Louis, Mo: CV Mosby Co; 1998:286–295.

Rheault S, Dagenais. Standing and ambulation: An overview. In: Betz RR, Mulcahey MJ, eds. *The Child with a Spinal Cord Injury*. Rosemont, Ill: American Academy of Orthopaedic Surgeons; 1996:501–502.

Shakhazizian KA, Massagli ML, Southard TL. Spinal cord injuries. In: Campbell SK, ed. *Physical Therapy for Children*. 2nd ed. Philadelphia, Pa: WB Saunders Co; 2000:571–596.

Triolo RJ. Clinical perspective. Neuromuscular stimulation in children with incomplete spinal cord injuries. *Pediatr Phys Ther*. 1997;9(3):139–143.

Spinal Muscular Atrophy

ICD-9-CM Code: 335.1 Spinal muscular atrophy
APTA Guide Patterns: 4a, 4B, 4C, 4D, 4G, 4H

DESCRIPTION

Spinal muscular atrophy (SMA) is a disorder that may begin in infancy or childhood, characterized by skeletal muscular wasting due to progressive degeneration of anterior horn cells in the spinal cord and motor nuclei in the brain stem (Beers & Berkow, 1999; p.1488).

CLASSIFICATION

- *Type I spinal muscular atrophy.* Also known as *Werdnig-Hoffman disease, infantile SMA,* or *acute SMA.* Disorder is present in utero or becomes symptomatic by 2 to 4 months of age. Most affected infants are hypotonic at birth and all have delayed motor milestones by 6 months of age. Death occurs in 95% by age 18 months and in all by age 4 years, usually from respiratory failure (Beers & Berkow, 1999, p. 1488). Infants with SMA type ROM 1 have decreased movements, especially against gravity, lie in a typical "frogged" posture of externally rotated hips and flexed knees and have a weak cry and cough. Their breathing is usually diaphragmatic because the intercostal and accessory muscles are weak. Deep tendon reflexes are absent or decreased. Intelligence and alertness are normal (Redcliffe, 1998; p. 236).

- *Type II (intermediate) spinal muscular atrophy.* Most infants and children are symptomatic by about age 5 to 12 months and all by 2 years, <25% learn to sit, and none walk or crawl. *Note:* Not all authors agree that none can walk. Children are hypotonic with flaccid muscle weakness, absent deep tendon reflexes, and fasciculations, which may be hard to see in young children. Dysphagia may be present. The disorder is often fatal in early life, frequently from respiratory complications. However, progression can stop spontaneously, leaving the child with permanent, nonprogressive weakness (Beers & Berkow, 1999; p. 1488). Symptoms include weakness and delayed or regressed gross motor milestones. A pervasive problem for children with SMA type II is scoliosis because of weak trunk muscles. Those who walk will need braces (Redcliffe, 1998; p. 237).

- *Type III spinal muscular atrophy.* Also known as *Wohlfart-Kugelberg-Welander disease.* Disorder begins between 2 and 30 years of age. Pathologic finds and mode of inheritance are similar to the acute form, but disease evolution is slower and life expectancy longer. Weakness and wasting are most evident in the legs, beginning in the quadriceps and hip flexors. Later, the arms are affected. Weakness often progresses from proximal to distal parts. Some familial cases are secondary to specific enzyme defects (eg, hexosaminidase deficiency) (Beers & Berkow, 1999; p. 1488). Children with SMA type III usually walk with braces for a time but will eventually need a wheelchair for mobility as they get weaker. They exhibit many signs of low muscle tone and weakness during gait, including lumbar lordosis, genu recurvatum or hyperextended knees, and a waddling gait. Some, but not all, will have scoliosis and the severity of the scoliosis is often milder (Redcliffe, 1998; p. 237).

- *Type IV spinal muscular atrophy.* Disorder has a variable inheritance pattern (recessive, dominant, X-linked), with adult onset (age 30–60 years) and slow progression. *Note:* Differentiating it from the lower motor neuron form of amyotrophic lateral sclerosis may be impossible (Beers & Berkow, 1999; p. 1488).

CAUSE

Most cases are autosomal recessive and appear to be allelic mutations of a single gene locus on chromosome 5 (Beers & Berkow, 1999; p. 1488). SMA has an incidence of 1 in 10,000.

ASSESSMENT

AREAS

- Joint range of motion (ROM)
- Muscle strength
- Muscle tone
- Reflexes and reactions
- Mobility skills
- Transfer skills
- Activities of daily living (ADLs)
- Recreation and leisure
- Adaptive equipment

INSTRUMENTS/PROCEDURES

None stated.

PROBLEMS

- Muscle weakness, especially in antigravity muscles in the pelvic or shoulder anti-gravity musculature and typical posturing in a gravity-dependent position; proximal musculature of the neck, trunk, and pelvic and shoulder girdles demonstrate the greatest weakness.
- Delays in attaining developmental milestones including head control and rolling over.
- Some developmental milestones such as prone on elbows are not attained.
- Mobility may be limited, ambulation may be delayed or not attained.
- Respiratory distress and difficulty with coughing.
- Lack of flexibility and limitations in ROM.
- Contractures may occur in the chronic forms.
- Scoliosis is common in the chronic forms.
- Fasciculations of the tongue.
- Difficulty performing ADLs including feeding, dressing, and hygiene.
- Tremor may be present.
- Difficulty in breast feeding.

TREATMENT/MANAGEMENT

Note: Treatment/management is usually in the home or on an outpatient basis.

INFANT

- Therapy should be tailored to the individual child based on his or her strengths and interests.
- Positioning and handling to prevent deformity and discomfort are essential due to weakness and to permit infant access to environment. Traditional infant seats, rolled towels, cutout foam pads, or a commercially purchased car seat with infant head supports may be used. Special adaptive equipment from durable medical equipment vendors may be necessary or useful, if available.
- Encourage small periods of active movement to maintain strength and support normal intellectual development. Watch for signs of fatigue.
- Use ROM and stretching exercises to promote movement and prevent contractures. Aquatic therapy may be useful for both ROM and active movement.
- Use normal developmental activities such as reaching for toys, reaching for and playing with feet, rolling, and sitting with or without support.
- Chest physiotherapy and suctioning to mobilize secretions may be needed in SMA type 1.
- Goals should be functional such as holding a bottle, bringing a toy to the mouth, sitting up with or without support to be fed with a spoon.
- Instruct family on positioning and handling techniques that work best for that infant. Positioning for sleeping, for watching others, for meals, in the car, and while outside should be discussed.

- Provide family support. If child has SMA type I, family will be dealing with losing the child likely within a year and needs to recount day-to-day emotions as well as talking about impending death.
- Provide family with information about community resources including support groups and literature about SMA.
- Therapist should be aware of his or her own feelings about the child and the prognosis and may need to take advantage of counseling services at the workplace or in the community.
- Examples of short-term objectives might be child will sit with support for 10 minutes, child will hold head up without support for 5 minutes, or child will be able to grasp finger foods and bring to the mouth.

TODDLER AND PRECHOOLER

- Functional ability in this age group will vary widely depending in part on the type of SMA and in part on the individual child: one may be too weak to eat independently while another is walking well.
- Promote motor development and movement within child's limitations, especially functional mobility skills including walking, walking with assistive devices, or mobility using a wheechair. Aquatic therapy has been shown to encourage active movement and balance.
- Encourage upright mobility, including the use of knee-ankle-foot orthoses (KAFOs), reciprocating gait orthoses, parapodiums, crutches, and walkers. When upright mobility is not feasible, consider seated mobility including manual and powered wheelchairs to facilitate independent mobility.
- Provide progressive strengthening for SMA types II and III. Aquatic therapy may be useful since the water provides buoyancy to decreased joint loading or weight bearing.
- Increase or maintain vital capacity. Breathing exercises in the pool can provide resistance.
- Promote normal cognitive and socialization skills by using or facilitating the use of activities that are developmentally appropriate, including blocks, pictures, crayons, singing recitation, and aquatic activities.
- Consider adaptive equipment including standers, wheelchairs, braces, and orthotic devices to improve positioning and accessibility.
- Goals may focus on the child's ability to access the environment through toys, switches, and manipulative tools.
- Facilitate and promote attendance at a preschool or kindergarten program whether for special children with disabilities or a regular preschool or kindergarten. In a regular school, setting recommendations for assistive devices, adapted equipment and materials, or additional personnel may be needed if therapy services are not provided within the educational setting. Rearrangement of existing materials or school layout for accessibility may also be needed.
- Examples of short-term objectives are: child will learn to operate joy-stick; child will maintain full, functional ROM in upper and lower extremities; child will paint independently; and child will accompany class on field trips.

SCHOOL-AGED AND ADOLESCENCE

- Positioning should be designed to prevent scoliosis or limited progression of spinal deformity.
- Positioning should also consider respiratory function and comfort.
- Chest physical therapy may be needed for respiratory hygiene due to poor cough and lack of movement. Alternate positioning may be necessary during the day by standing in a standing frame or tilt table, or lying supine on a wedge or cot. Lying prone over a wedge is frequently not tolerated well by children with SMA.

- Proximal weakness in the trunk and extremities requires adjustments in the positioning relative to environmental interactions. Adjustments may be needed for the height of the arm rests, lap tray, or table to permit writing, keyboarding on a computer, or using a trackball.
- Continue support for academic tasks. Adaptive devices may become more important to facilitate performance in the classroom.
- Examples of short-term objectives: the child will drive up and down curb cuts in power wheelchair; child will drive power wheelchair at a safe speed and not hit other children; child will drive power wheelchair on uneven ground; child will negotiate small doorways in power chair; child will be able to tell someone how to change wheelchair and perform basic maintenance activities; child will tolerate alternative positions during the school day; child and family will develop opportunities to provide positioning and percussion for postural drainage each day.

PRECAUTIONS/CONTRAINDICATIONS
- Stabilization of head and trunk must be considered in all activities since child is usually unable to actively regain postural control independently.
- Because of respiratory limitations, activities should be monitored closely for signs of respiratory distress. In the pool, child should be slowly immersed in the water.
- Because children with SMA are prone to serious respiratory infection, they should be protected from water- and air-borne pathogens in all therapy activities.

DESIRED OUTCOME/PROGNOSIS
- Child increases or maintains active ROM and movement without contractures.
- Child increases or maintains muscle strength.
- Child increases or maintains vital capacity.
- Child increases or maintains mobility whether performed independently or with assistive equipment.
- Child is able to attend school and participate in educational activities.
- Child is able to engage in play and recreational activities using normal or adapted techniques.

REFERENCES

Beers MH, Berkow R, eds. *The Merck Manual of Diagnosis and Therapy.* Whitehouse Station, NJ: Merck Research Laboratories; 1999.

Cunha MC, Oliveira AS, Labronici RH, Gabbai AA. Spinal muscular atrophy type II (intermediary) and III (Kugelberg-Welander). Evolution of 50 patients with physiotherapy and hydrotherapy in a swimming pool. *Arguivos de Neuro-psiquiatry.* 1996;54(3):402–406.

Figuers CC. Aquatic therapy intervention for a child diagnosed with spinal muscular atrophy. *Phys Ther Case Rep.* 1999;2(1):109–112.

Florence JM. Neuromuscular disorders in childhood and physical therapy intervention. In: Tecklin JS, ed. *Pediatric Physical Therapy.* 3rd ed. Philadelphia, Pa: JB Lippincott Co; 1999:223–246.

Ratliffe KT. Genetic disorders—Rik, a boy with spinal muscular atrophy. In: Ratliffe KT. *Clinical Pediatric Physical Therapy: A Guide for the Physical Therapy Team.* St. Louis, Mo: CV Mosby Co; 1998:219–227.

Ratliffe KT. Genetic disorders—The child with spinal muscular atrophy. In: Ratliffe KT. *Clinical Pediatric Physical Therapy: A Guide for the Physical Therapy Team*. St. Louis, Mo: CV Mosby Co; 1998:236–241.

Stuberg WA. Muscular dystrophy and spinal muscular atrophy. In: Campbell SK, ed. *Physical Therapy for Children*. 2nd ed. Philadelphia, Pa: WB Saunders Co; 2000:339–369.

Sports or Recreational Athletic Injuries in Children

ICD-9-CM Codes:

- 524   Dentofacial anomalies, including maloclusion
- 717   Internal derangement of knee
- 719.7   Difficulty in walking
- 726.1   Rotator cuff syndrome of shoulder and allied disorders
- 726.10   Disorders of bursae and tendons in shoulder region, unspecified
- 7270   Synovitis and tenosynovitis
- 727.61   Complete rupture of rotator cuff
- 727.31   Contracture of tendon (sheath)
- 728.2   Muscle wasting and disuse atrophy, not elsewhere classified
- 728.85   Spasm of muscle
- 729.2   Myalgia and myositis, unspecified
- 729.81   Swelling of limb
- 781.2   Abnormality of gait
- 781.3   Lack of coordination
- 811–816   Fractures of upper extremities
- 820–825   Fractures of lower extremities
- 830–839   Dislocations of limb joints
- 840–848   Sprains and strains

APTA Guide Patterns: 4C, 4D, 4E, 4H, 4I, 4J

DESCRIPTION

Children differ from adults in terms of the injuries that may occur in sports and athletics. Children have different physiological capacities than adults which must be considered in training and recovery. Children are growing, which results in musculosketetal, normal, and physiological changes that take place at a much faster pace than in adults. Because a child's musculoskeletal system is different from that of an adult, some orthopedic injuries are different from those of adults (Ratliffe, p. 147). Children with disabilities who participate in sports have special needs such as extra physical examinations to rule out congenital defects, adapted or specialized equipment, or changes in the rules (Ratliffe, p. 149). Common sports in which injuries occur are baseball, basketball, gymnastics, football, ice hockey, soccer, skateboarding, skiing, swimming and diving, tennis, track, and wrestling. Recreational activities include dancing, dirt biking, and tag football.

Sports can be classified as contact or noncontact. Contact includes contact collision type sports such as boxing, field and ice hockey, football, lacrosse, martial arts, rodeo, soccer, and wrestling; and limited contact impact such as baseball, basketball, bicycling, diving, pole vaulting, gymnastic, horseback riding, ice skating, roller skating, skiing, softball, squash or handball, and volleyball. Noncontact sports include three categories: strenuous, moderately strenuous, and nonstrenuous. Strenuous includes aerobic dancing; crew or rowing; fencing; field sports such as discus, javelin, and shot put; running; swimming; track; and weight lifting. Moderately strenuous includes badminton, curling, and table tennis. Nonstrenuous sports include archery, golf, and riflery (Bernhardt-Bainbridge, p. 436).

CAUSE

The two primary types of orthopedic injuries occurring in children while playing sports are high-impact injury and the overuse or repetitive trauma injury. A third category is lacerations and abrasions which can be treated by medical means. A fourth category is traumatic injuries to the brain and spinal cord which are discussed in other sections (see preceding sections on spinal cord injuries and traumatic brain injuries).

High-impact injuries occur as a result of contact between players or between the player and a solid surface such as the ground, wall, fence, or post. Sprains, strains, contusions (bruises) and fractures constitute the bulk of high-impact injuries. Overuse injuries most commonly damage the epiphyseal growth centers and sites of tendon insertion (aprophyses). Diseases associated with overuse in sports include *Osgood-Schlatter disease*, apophysitis or epiphysis of the tendon insertion of the tibial tubercle—thought to be caused by rapid growth of the long bones combined with stress or traction on the patellar tendon during sports activities; *Sever's disease*, apophysitis or epiphysitis of the calcaneous; and *osteochondritis dissecans*—microdegeneration of the articular cartilage and ischemic neurosis thought to be caused by repetitive shear forces especially to the distal femur although other sites can occur. Other overuse syndromes in children include "Little League shoulder," a fracture of the proximal humeral growth plate due to repetitive rotational stresses on the shoulder during pitching or catching, and "Little League elbow," a stress fracture due to hypertrophy of the medial condyle of the elbow.

Risk factors for overuse injuries include training errors; musculotendinous imbalances of strength, flexibility, or bulk; anatomic malalignment of the lower extremity; improper footwear; faulty playing surface; and associated disease states of the lower extremity such as old injury or arthritis and growth factors (Bernhardt-Bainbridge, p. 445).

ASSESSMENT

AREAS

- Agility and flexibility
- Balance
- Body composition
- Cardiovascular performance
- Edema
- Endurance
- Muscle power
- Muscle strength
- Pain
- Posture
- Range of Motion (ROM)
- Speed
- Tenderness
- Vision

INSTRUMENTS/PROCEDURES

- active knee extension test
- athletic fitness scorecard for boys and girls (see Bernhardt-Bainbridge, p. 439)
- cycle ergometer
- girth measurement
- Lachman's test
- palpation
- postural alignment
- preparticipation physical examination: individual or multistation (for recommendations, see Bernhardt-Bainbridge, pp. 437–438)
- sit and reach test
- treadmill
- upper-body ergometer
- Osgood-Schlatter disease: child may limp, complain of acute, severe pain in the knee
- osteochondritis dissecans: child often has pain, swelling around the knee, and an antalgic gait

- Sever's disease: posterior heel pain is elicited with a medial/lateral calcaneal squeeze test. A tight heel cord is apparent with active and passive dorsiflexion of the ankle with the knee extended.

PROBLEMS

- Child complains of pain or discomfort in the affected joint.
- Child may have swelling at the site of the injury or disease.
- Child may have tenderness at the site of the injury.
- Child may limp or have an antalgic gait.
- Child may be unable to bear weight on a leg.
- Child may have limitation(s) in mobility.
- Child may have decreased flexibility.
- Child may have decreased muscle strength.
- Child may have decreased muscle endurance and cardiovascular fitness.
- Child may have difficulty performing purposeful, controlled movements.
- Child may have decreased speed and agility.

TREATMENT/MANAGEMENT

Note: General program: weekly increase should not be greater than 10% of the previous level.

- Maintain cardiovascular skills.
- Increase mobility and flexibility to normal limits.
- Increase endurance to normal limits both in the injured area and the entire extremity.
- Increase muscle strength to normal limits with exercises, such as the use of Theraband.
- Direct attention to resumption of purposeful, controlled movement at the appropriate speed.

CONTUSIONS

- Treat with ice and elevation.
- For deep hematoma, ultrasound may be used after 48 hours but not over an epiphysis.

SPRAINS

- Treated symptomatically with rest, ice, compression, and elevation (RICE).
- Consider use of sling for upper extremity.
- Increase mobility and strength with exercises.

STRAINS

- Initially treat with rest, immobilization, ice, and elevation (RICE) to reduce swelling.
- Gentle active mobilization may be applied after healing to maintain ROM.
- Restrict play during acute phase of injury to avoid long-term injury.

OVERUSE INJURIES

- Decrease irritation: rest, ice, compression or elevation (RICE) may be needed.
- Reduce adhesions using stretching.
- Increase strength using exercises against resistance.
- Recommend alteration of technique and equipment.

PRECAUTIONS/CONTRAINDICATIONS

- Ultrasound should not be used over any epiphysis, including the ends of long bones (Ratliffe, p. 150).
- Thermoregulatory capability: a child's ability to exercise in conditions of high humidity or heat is less than an adult because a child has decreased cardiac output compared with an adult, a proportionately greater surface area, and does not sweat like an adult (Ratliffe, p. 150).
- In cold conditions and particularly in water, a child should be monitored closely because a child cannot maintain body heat as well as an adult.
- Cardiovascular training: A child's response to training to improve cardiorespiratory fitness is limited compared to adults. For example, a prepubescent child does not increase maximum oxygen uptake significantly with training and may not benefit significantly from short intensive aerobic training or workouts. Low-intensity, long-duration training improves performance to a greater degree (Ratliffe, p. 151; Bernhardt-Bainbridge, p. 436).
- Strength training using weights continues to be controversial. Recommendations are that training should occur 2 to 3 times a week for 20–30 minutes and that weights should be increased in small increments of 1–3 pounds after a child demonstrates ability to do 15 repetitions at the previous weight. Also, proper lifting techniques should be stressed (Ratliffe, p. 151; Bernhardt-Bainbridge, p. 438).
- In Osgood-Schlatter disease, the child should avoid deep knee bending.

DESIRED OUTCOME/PROGNOSIS

- Child has attained the component skills needed to participate in the sport of choice.
- Child is able to return to play the sport in a safe manner.
- Child does not have edema.
- Child has full, pain-free and biomechanically normal mobility.
- Child has normal strength as measured by objective testing.
- Child completes appropriate function tests such as vertical leap, hopping, running, or cutting activities.
- Child uses supportive or protective devices designed to provide stability and anatomic alignment.

REFERENCES

Bernhardt-Bainbridge D. Sports injuries in children. In: Campbell SK, ed. *Physical Therapy for Children*. 2nd ed. Philadelphia, Pa: WB Saunders Co; 2000:429–464.

Lear LJ, Gross MT. An electromyographical analysis of the scapular stabilizing synergists during a push-up progression. *J Orthop Sports Phys Ther*. 1998;28(3):146–157.

Ratliffe KT. Other orthopedic disorders—The child athlete. In: Ratliffe KT. *Clinical Pediatric Physical Therapy: A Guide for the Physical Therapy Team*. St. Louis, Mo: CV Mosby Co; 1998:147–151.

Saidoff DC, McDonough AL. Obese, early adolescent with insidious onset of mechanical obstruction in knee extension that is accompanied by knee swelling, and pain that varies in location, in the absence of acute trauma or giving-way. In: Saidoff DC, McDonough AL, eds. *Critical Pathways in Therapeutic Intervention: Extremities and Spine*. St. Louis, Mo: CV Mosby Co; 2002:709–720.

Topham AF, White JA. Severs disease. *Phys Ther Case Rep*. 1998;1(3):160–161.

Wightman AB. A ballet dancer with chronic hip pain due to a lesser trochanter bony avulsion: the challenge of a differential diagnosis. *J Orthop Sports Phys Ther*. 1998;28(3):168–173.

Substance Exposure in Utero

ICD-9-CM Code: 760.7 Noxious influences affecting fetus via placenta or breast milk
APTA Guide Patterns: 5A, 6C

DESCRIPTION

In utero exposure to teratogens, such as alcohol, tobacco use, prescription drugs, street drugs, and certain viruses can affect fetal development.

CAUSE

Cause is the ingestion by the mother of the substance into the gastrointestinal or pulmonary system.

ASSESSMENT

AREAS

- Gross motor skills
- Interaction skills: eye contact and bonding skills
- Muscle tone
- Neurobehavior
- Reflexes and reactions
- Regulatory behavior

INSTRUMENTS

- Alberta Infant Motor Scale (AIMS) (Piper & Darrah, 1994)
- Bayley Scales of Infant Development–II (BSID–II) (Bayley, 1993)
- Miller Assessment for Preschoolers (MAP) (Miller, 1998)
- Movement Assessment of Infants (MAI) (Chandler et al, 1980)
- Neonatal Behavioral Assessment Scale–3rd ed. (NBAS) (Brazelton, 1995)
- Peabody Developmental Motor Scales, 2nd ed. (PDMS–2) (Folio & Fewell, 1999)
- Performance Qualifying Scale (PQS) for use with the Bayley. See Rose-Jacobs, Frank, & Brown, 1996, p. 79.

PROBLEMS

- Child may be born prematurely.
- Child may be born with low to very low birth weight.
- Child may have congenital malformations.
- Child may have respiratory distress.
- Child may have poor state regulation, especially difficulty in regulating the arousal state in novel or stimulating situations (ie, environmental stimulation).
- Child may have seizures.
- Child may experience developmental delays, especially in antigravity skills.
- Child may have decreased perceptual-cognitive abilities.

TREATMENT/MANAGEMENT

The need for treatment and management of infants exposed in utero is controversial. Cocaine exposure has been studied extensively with mixed results. The results tend to reflect the instrument used to measure the infants' responses and the theory or rationale on which the instrument was developed. The MAI has demonstrated delays but other assessments (eg, AIMS, BSID, PDMS, and NBAS) have not.

- Instruct parents and caregivers in techniques to calm an oversensitive infant including swaddling, holding arms and legs in flexion against the body, minimizing

sensory input such as eye contact and talking, and putting the infant in a darkened room with external sounds muted.
- Facilitate prone motor activities.
- Use multisystem (multisensory) approaches.
- Enhance gross and motor skills through exercise, including play activities and opportunity for exploration.

DESIRED OUTCOME/PROGNOSIS
- Child has attained normal motor performance for age.
- Child has attained visual-motor, fine motor, and sensory orientation and processing within normal limits.
- Child is able to function in school environment.
- Child is able to participate in play activities that are age appropriate.

REFERENCES

Blanchard Y, Suess PE, Beeghly M. Effects of prenatal drug exposure on neurobehavioral functioning in young infants. *Phys Occup Ther Pediatr.* 1998;18(3/4):19–37.

Blanchard Y. Neurobehavioral and neuromotor long-term sequelae of prenatal exposure to cocaine and other drugs: an unresolved issue. *Pediatr Phys Ther.* 1999;11(3):140–146.

Fetters L, Tronick EZ. Neuromotor development of cocaine-exposed and control infants from birth though 15 months: poor and poorer performance. *Pediatrics.* 1996;98:938–943.

Fetters L, Tronick EZ. Trajectories of motor development: polydrug exposed infants in the first fifteen months. *Phys Occup Ther Pediatr.* 1998;18(3/4):1–18.

Fetters L, Tronick EZ. Discriminative power of the Alberta Infant Motor Scale and the Movement Assessment of Infants for prediction of Peabody Gross Motor Scale scores of infants exposed in utero to cocaine. *Pediatr Phys Ther.* 2000;12(1):16–23.

Grattan MP, Hans SL. Motor behavior in children exposed prenatally to drugs. *Phys Occup Ther Pediatr.* 1996;16(1/2):89–109.

Ratliffe KT. Sensory, processing, and cognitive disorders of childhood—Exposure to environmental threats. In: Ratliffe KT. *Clinical Pediatric Physical Therapy: A Guide for the Physical Therapy Team.* St. Louis, Mo: CV Mosby Co; 1998:330–334.

Riegger-Krugh C, Blaire A, Sparling JW. Assessment of fetal knee angular velocity as a possible method to determine the effect of prenatal exposure to cocaine. *Phys Occup Ther Pediatr.* 1996;16(1/2):173–186.

Rose-Jacobs R, Frank DA, Brown ER. Issues of developmental measurement in clinical research and practice settings with children who were prenatally expose to drugs. *Phys Occup Ther Pediatr.* 1996;16(1/2):73–87.

Solomon M, Orlin M, Morrissey K, Cockerill M. Motor performance of infants born prematurely: a comparison at age six months of those exposed and not exposed to cocaine. *Pediatr Phys Ther.* 1996;8(2):80–86.

Swanson MW. Neuromotor outcome of infants exposed to cocaine: issues of assessment and intervention. *Phys Occup Ther Pediatr.* 1996;16(1/2):35–60.

Traumatic Brain Injuries

ICD-9-CM Codes:
- 853 Other and unspecified intracranial hemorrhage following injury
- 854 Intracranial injury of other and unspecified nature

APTA Guide Patterns: 5A, 5B, 5C, 5G, 6G, 6I

DESCRIPTION

Note: Traumatic brain injuries (TBIs) are a major cause of death in children.

CLASSIFICATION ACCORDING TO HOW INJURY WAS INTRODUCED
- Acceleration-deceleration (closed head injuries): occurs when the head hits an immobile object or a mobile object hits an immobile head
- Crush injuries
- Penetration injuries

CLASSIFICATION ACCORDING TO TYPE OF DAMAGE
- *Primary injury:* diffuse and focal injuries
- *Secondary injury:* hypoxic-ischemic injury
- *Diffuse axonal injury (DAI or diffuse):* often due to shearing forces most often involving the brainstem and corpus callosum.
- *Focal:* often involves frontal and/or temporal lobes resulting in contusion or hematoma
- *Contusion:* transient loss of awareness without gross lesions to the brain or neurologic damage
- *Hematoma:* may be subdural or extradural
- *Hypoxic-ischemic:* usually due to intracranial factors such as mass lesions or cerebral edema, or extracranial factors such as hypoxemia or hypotension

CLASSIFICATION OF TYPES OF RECOVERY
- *Restitution:* involves resolution of cellular toxicity, metabolic dysfunction, diaschisis, edema, and absorption of blood products which allow the neural network to recover and function to return. Therapy has little impact here but pharmacologic agents may help.
- *Substitution:* involves adaptation at the neuronal level or within the neural network to access spared portions of the brain. Neuronal changes may include synaptic sprouting, axonal and dendritic regeneration, remyelination, changes in the number of receptors, ion channel changes, changes in actions of neurotransmitters and neuromodulators, changes in the uptake and release of neurotransmitter, and increased neuronal responsiveness resulting from denervation hypersensitivity. Therapy has primary impact here.

CLASSIFICATION SYSTEM FOR ADULTS
- Rancho Los Amigos: original scale is 8 levels; revised is 10 levels.

CLASSIFICATION SYSTEM FOR CHILDREN
- Rancho Pediatric Levels. *Note:* lower number corresponds to better performance on the children scale whereas in the adult scale lower number corresponds to poorer performance.
  - I *Infant (6 months to 2 years):* interacts with environment
       Preschool (2 to 5 years): oriented to self and surrounds
       School-age (5 years and older): oriented to time and place; records ongoing

    II   *Infant:* demonstrates awareness of environment
        Preschool and school-age: is responsive to environment
    III *All ages:* gives localized response to sensory stimuli
    IV *All ages:* gives generalized response to sensory stimuli
    V   *All ages:* no response to stimuli
- Ommaca Scale

CAUSE

Most common cause is blunt trauma due to a motor vehicle accident (MVA) followed by falls and assaults.

ASSESSMENT

AREAS
- Functional skills and impairments
- Cognition
- Motor control
- Postural control
- Somatosensory: light touch, proprioception, sharp-dull, two-point discrimination
- Musculoskeletal
- Physiologic control: heart rate, blood pressure, respiratory rate, rhythm and pattern, pain
- Dysphagia
- Child's goals and motivation
- Family or caregiver's expected involvement in recovery process
- Family or caregiver's understanding of the injury and expected outcome
- Family and community resources
- Discharge destination

INSTRUMENTS/PROCEDURES

Cognitive Skills
- Glasgow Coma Scale
- Rancho Pediatric Level (infant to about 12 years)
- Rancho Adult Level (12 and older)

Functional Skills
- Alberta Infant Motor Scale (AIMS)
- Bruininks-Oseretsky Test of Motor Proficiency (BOTMP)
- Functional Independence Measure (FIM)
- Functional Independence Measure for Children (WeeFIM)
- Functional Reach Test
- Gross Motor Function Measure (GMFM)
- Movement Assessment of Infants (MAI)
- Peabody Developmental Motor Scales–2nd ed. (PDMS–2)
- Pediatric Evaluation of Disability Inventory (PEDI)
- Timed Up and Go (TUG)
- Upright Motor Control Test

Musculoskeletal
- dynamometry
- goniometer
- manual muscle testing
- modified Ashworth test

Other
- Glasgow Outcome Scale
- coma/near-coma
- Western Neuro Sensory Stimulation Profile

PROBLEMS
- Impaired level of consciousness: level of arousal, orientation
- Changes in cognitive function:
  1. *Attention:* alertness, sound mental processing, selective attention, and sustained attention such as shortened attention span, distractibility
  2. *Memory and learning:* memory (immediate, delayed, cued) and visual and verbal learning
  3. *Executive function:* planning, initiation, maintenance, and monitoring of goal orientation; problem solving; abstract reasoning, such as poor judgment, difficulties with problem solving
  4. *Motor control impairments:* velocity-dependence muscle stiffness (spasticity), ataxia, contractures, paralysis; hypotonicity, fatigability
  5. *Postural control and somatosensory impairments:* static and dynamic balance, hemianopsia, diplopia, impaired proprioception, impaired tactile sensation
  6. *Musculoskeletal complications and limitations:* may also have brachial plexus injury, spinal cord injury, fractures or dislocation. May develop contractures in plantar flexion, hip adduction, and knee flexion resulting in range of motion limitations; pressures sores; heterotrophic ossification; scoliosis; limb-length discrepancies; muscle atrophy; and muscles weakness
  7. *Swallowing dysfunction or dysphagia:* difficulty with chewing and swallowing
  8. *Behavioral changes:* irritability, hyperactivity, low tolerance of frustration, poor social judgment, lack of impulse control, aggression
  9. *Impaired sensory and perception:* decreased vision and hearing, poor visual perception, visual spatial relations
  10. *Difficulty with functional tasks:* ADLs, schoolwork, participation in the community
  11. *Impaired speech and communication skills:* difficulty with receptive and expressive language
  12. *Abnormal physiological responses:* hypertension, impaired ventilatory efficiency such as reduced vital capacity, inspiratory capacity, total lung capacity, and forced expiratory volumes at 1 second.

See Table 12.5 for additional relevant information.

TREATMENT/MANAGEMENT
- Treatment generally involves a team approach which may include physician, nurse, psychologist, speech pathologist, social worker, and an occupational therapist.
- Treatment is usually focused on activity-dependent "unmasking" of previously ineffective synapses, and activity-dependent changes in synaptic strength tied to memory and learning.

RANCHO PEDIATRIC LEVEL II OR RANCHO ADULT LEVEL IV OR V
- Use simple one-step commands with structure and cuing.
- Use of automatic activities (eg, catch a ball) is more successful during initial treatment than asking client to follow a verbal instruction such as "lift your arms."
- Several short treatment sessions when client is alert and attentive will produce better results than one long session.

TABLE 12.5
Rancho Pediatric Levels of Consciousness (Infants, Preschool, and School-Age)

Rancho Pediatric Levels	Infants: 6 Mo to 2 Yr	Preschool: 2–5 Yr	School-age: 5 Yr and Older
I	Interacts with environment a. Shows active interest in toys; manipulates or examines before mouthing or discarding b. Watches other children at play; may move toward them purposefully c. Initiates social contact with adults; enjoys socializing d. Shows active interest in bottle e. Reaches or moves toward person or object	Oriented to self and surroundings a. Provides accurate information about self b. Knows he or she is away from home c. Knows where toys, clothes, etc., are kept d. Actively participates in treatment program e. Recognizes own room, knows way to bathroom, nursing station, etc. f. Is potty trained g. Initiates social contact with adult; enjoys socializing	Oriented to time and place; records ongoing events a. Provides accurate, detailed information about self and present situation b. Knows way to and from daily activities c. Knows sequence of daily routine d. Knows way around unit; recognizes own room e. Finds own bed; knows where personal belongings are kept f. Is bowel and bladder trained
II	Demonstrates awareness of environment a. Responds to name b. Recognizes mother or other family members c. Enjoys imitative vocal play d. Giggles or smiles when talked to or played with e. Fussing is quieted by soft voice or touch	Is responsive to environment a. Follows simple commands b. Refuses to follow commands by shaking head or saying "no" c. Imitates examiner's gestures or facial expressions d. Responds to name e. Recognizes mother or other family members f. Enjoys imitative vocal play	Is responsive to environment a. Follows simple verbal or gestured requests b. Initiates purposeful activity c. Actively participates in therapy program d. Refuses to follow request by shaking head or saying "no" e. Imitates examiner's gestures or facial expressions

(continued)

- To reduce confusion and agitation, use a calm environment with structured stimuli.

RANCHO PEDIATRIC I OR RANCHO ADULT LEVEL VII OR VIII
- Initially, use a quiet environment with minimal distractions to enhance accuracy and reproducibility of motor control; however, treatment will need to progress to dealing with distractions.
- Longer treatment sessions up to 30 minutes may be possible.

TABLE 12.5 *Continued.*

Rancho Pediatric Levels	Infants: 6 Mo to 2 Yr	Preschool: 2–5 Yr	School-age: 5 Yr and Older
III	Gives localized response to sensory stimuli a. Blinks when strong light crosses field of vision b. Follows moving object passed within visual field c. Turns toward or away from loud sound d. Gives localized response to painful stimuli	Gives localized response to sensory stimuli a. Blinks when strong light crosses field of vision b. Follows moving object passed within visual field c. Turns toward or away from loud sound d. Gives localized response to painful stimuli	Gives localized response to sensory stimuli a. Blinks when strong light crosses field of vision b. Follows moving object passed within visual field c. Turns toward or away from loud sound d. Gives localized response to painful stimuli
IV	Gives generalized response to sensory stimuli a. Gives generalized startle to loud sound b. Responds to repeated auditory stimulation with increased or decreased activity c. Gives generalized reflex response to painful stimuli	Gives generalized response to sensory stimuli a. Gives generalized startle to loud sound b. Responds to repeated auditory stimulation with increased or decreased activity c. Gives generalized reflex response to painful stimuli	Gives generalized response to sensory stimuli a. Gives generalized startle to loud sound b. Responds to repeated auditory stimulation with increased or decreased activity c. Gives generalized reflex response to painful stimuli
V	No response to stimuli a. Complete absence of observable change in behavior to visual, auditory, or painful stimuli	No response to stimuli a. Complete absence of observable change in behavior to visual, auditory, or painful stimuli	No response to stimuli a. Complete absence of observable change in behavior to visual, auditory, or painful stimuli

Source: Campbell SK. Decision making in pediatric neurologic physical therapy. New York: Churchill Livingstone, 1999:92.

FAMILY
- Educate family to increase understanding of disabilities, expected future needs, and methods to access available community resources.
- Ensure that family demonstrates competence in the provision of appropriate supervision and daily care.

FUNCTIONAL MOBILITY
- Maximize age-appropriate independence with self-care, mobility, and cognition.
- Independence with bed mobility activities: rolling, scooting, and coming to sitting position.
- Facilitate learning transfers (eg, to and from bed, toilet, tub, and floor).
- Facilitate ambulation.

PRECAUTIONS/CONTRAINDICATIONS

- Cognitive deficits limit client's awareness and actions necessary for physical safety.
- Therapist must always screen the environment for safety considerations and be prepared to take actions to protect the client.
- Distractibility, limited attention span, and memory impairments will reduce quality of performance in both assessment and treatment.

DESIRED OUTCOME/PROGNOSIS

- Recovery of function depends on the extent of primary and secondary injury and on neuroplasticity of the residual areas.
- Glasgow Outcome Scale uses 5 categories: death, persistent vegetative state, severe disability, moderate disability, and good recovery.
- Duration of coma is a major predictor of recovery: shorter lengths of coma historically result in improved outcomes.
- Child with Rancho Pediatric Levels V to III or Rancho Adult Levels I to III are generally dependent in all functional mobility, self-care, and social interactions (Blaskey & Jennings, 1999, pp. 97–98).
- Child with Rancho Pediatric Level II or Rancho Adult Level IV or V with only minimal physical limitation is often able to perform previously well-learned activities such as rolling, sitting up, crawling, or walking but executive functions necessary for judgment and problem solving necessitate constant supervision and assistance to prevent injury. If physical limitations are moderate to severe, cognitive deficits in memory and learning limit implementation of compensatory strategies to perform functional mobility activities. Procedural memory is generally better than declarative, allowing learning to occur through observation but sequencing ability may limit performance and generalization to other tasks in the environment may not occur.
- A child functioning at Rancho Pediatric Level I or Rancho Adult Levels VI to VIII with only minimal physical limitations may be independent in self-care activities and functional mobility. Supervision may still be needed in the community because of deficits in executive functioning such as low frustration tolerance, poor problem-solving abilities, poor judgment, and poor impulse control.

REFERENCES

Blaskey J, Jennings MC. Traumatic brain injury. In: Campbell SK. *Decision Making in Pediatric Neurologic Physical Therapy*. New York, NY: Churchill Livingstone; 1999:84–140.

Both A. Traumatic brain injury in childhood. In: Tecklin JS, ed. *Pediatric Physical Therapy*. 3rd ed. Philadelphia, Pa: Lippincott Williams and Wilkins; 1999:247–282.

Brewer K, Geisler T, Moddy K, Wright V. A community mobility assessment for adolescents with an acquired brain injury. *Physiotherapy Can.* 1998;50(2):118–122.

Halley SM, Duman HM, Ludlow LH. Variation by diagnostic and practice pattern groups in the mobility outcomes of inpatient rehabilitation programs for children and youth. *Phys Ther.* 2001;81(8):1425–1436.

Harris SR. The effectiveness of early intervention for children with cerebral palsy and related motor disabilities. In: Guralnick MJ. *The Effectiveness of Early Intervention*. Baltimore, Md: Paul H. Brookes; 1997:327–347.

Kerkering GA, Phillips WE. Brain injuries: Traumatic brain injuries, near-drowning, and brain tumors. In: Campbell SK, ed. *Physical Therapy for Children*. 2nd ed. Philadelphia, Pa: WB Saunders Co; 2000:597–620.

Ratliffe KT. Traumatic disorders—The child with a traumatic brain injury. In: Ratliffe KT. *Clinical Pediatric Physical Therapy: A Guide for the Physical Therapy Team*. St. Louis, Mo: CV Mosby Co; 1998:279–285.

Sandstedt JA. Contracture management for a pediatric patient with a severe traumatic brain injury. *Phys Ther Case Rep*. 2000;3(6):283–287.

Ventilator Dependence

ICD-9-CM Codes:
- 770.7 Chronic respiratory disease arising in the perinatal period
- 770.8 Other respiratory problems after birth

APTA Guide Patterns: 6C, 6E, 6J

DESCRIPTION

A ventilator-dependent child is one who needs mechanical breathing assistance to compensate for loss of respiratory function and respiratory failure. Clinical signs of failure of the respiratory system include altered depth and pattern of respiration, chest wall retractions, cyanosis, decreased or absent breath sounds, expiratory grunting, nasal flaring, tachypnea and wheezing, or prolonged expiration. Signs of cardiac involvement include bradycardia, cardiac arrest, hypertension, hypotension, and tachycardia. Cerebral signs include coma, headache, irritability, mental confusion, papilledema, restlessness, and seizures. Chronic respiratory failure is defined as treatment with mechanical ventilation for more than 28 days (Kelly, p. 712).

Mechanical ventilation and the artificial airway used to facilitate ventilation are designed in 2 ways. The ventilators either assist or substitute for a person's respiratory effects by moving air into and out of the lungs. Ventilators can be classified into those that provide positive-pressure ventilation (PPV) or negative-pressure ventilation (NPV). With PPV, pressurized gas is delivered into the vent circuit and airways during inspiration. With NPV, a pressure gradient is created to form a negative pressure around the person's entire body from the neck down during inspiration, causing air to enter the lungs. PPV is more commonly used with children. It can be delivered with either a nasal mask or a tracheostomy. The mask is not secure which limits its use to children who are not moving about such as in an intensive care setting (Kelly, p. 716).

PPV has 4 types of cycling ventilation mechanisms: flow-cycled, pressure-cycled, time-cycled, and volume-cycled. In flow-cycled, the mechanical ventilation is terminated when the inspiratory flow rate delivered by the ventilator decreases to a critical value. With pressure-cycled ventilation, the mechanical ventilation terminates when a preselected peak inspiratory pressure achieved with the breathing circuit tubing. With time-cycled ventilation, the mechanical ventilation terminates after a preselected inspiratory time has elapsed. With volume-cycle ventilation, the mechanical inhalation terminates after a preselected volume has been ejected from the ventilator (Kelly, p. 717).

CAUSE

There are 4 major pathophysiologic mechanisms leading to chronic respiratory failure and potential ventilator dependence: central nervous system conditions, intrinsic muscle disease, intrinsic pulmonary disease, and congenital airway abnormalities. Central nervous system conditions include anterior horn cell disease, apnea of prematurity, Arnold-Chiari malformation, brain tumors, congenital central hypoventilation syndrome (CCHS; also known as Ondine's curse), hypoxic encephalopathy, intracranial hemorrhage, traumatic spinal cord injuries, and viral encephalitis. Intrinsic muscle diseases include botulism, congenital abnormalities of the thoracic rib cage, congenital myopathies, diaphragmatic dysfunction, Duchenne muscular dystrophy, myasthenia gravis, and phrenic nerve trauma. Intrinsic pulmonary diseases include aspiration syndromes, congenital heart disease, pneumothorax, respiratory distress syndrome or bronchopulmonary dysplasia, and tumors. Congenital airway abnormalities include choanal atresia, laryngomalacia, subglottic stenosis, tracheoesophageal fistula, and various syndromes (Kelly, p. 713).

ASSESSMENT

AREAS
- Adaptive behavior
- Aerobic capacity and endurance
- Arousal, attention, and cognition
- Basic and instrumental activities of daily living (ADLs)
- Breathing pattern: diaphragmatic and intercostal
- Chest wall mobility
- Coughing ability: inspiration, glottic closure, expiratory force
- Environment: home, school, play
- Functional skills: general mobility, communication
- Integumentary integrity
- Motor function/neuromotor development
- Muscle performance
- Neuromotor development and motor control
- Oral motor functions: swallowing of solids and semisolids
- Posture
- Range of motion/joint integrity and mobility
- Reflex integrity
- Respiratory muscle strength: inspiratory and expiratory
- Role of child in family structure and integration into family
- Sensory integrity
- Soft tissue and muscle flexibility
- Ventilation and circulation

INSTRUMENTS/PROCEDURES
- Maximum expiratory pressure
- Vital capacity
- Gross Motor Function Measure, 2nd ed. (GMFM) (Russell et al, 1993)
- Peabody Developmental Motor Scales–2nd ed. (PDMS–2) (Folio & Fewell, 1999)

Note: Developmental tests, although useful, are inadequate because they fail to consider the effects of medical and physiological instability; long-term hospitalization; decreased mobility; and separation from "normal" social, emotional, and physical life experiences (Kelly, p. 722).

PROBLEMS
- Child often has impaired gas exchange.
- Child often has decreased endurance.
- Child often has delayed acquisitions of motor skills.
- Child often has experienced a lack of opportunity for "normal" learning due to restrictions imposed by the ventilator and airway attachments.
- Child may have primary lung failure usually associated with acute respiratory disease.
- Child may have failure of the respiratory pump system due to impaired neural control of respiratory or inadequate force generation.
- Child may have developmental delays.
- Child may have generalized weakness.

- Child may have sensory defensiveness or hypersensitivity especially in the oral motor area.
- Child may have soft tissue and muscle tightness.
- Child may have neurologic damage such as an intraventricular hemorrhage.

TREATMENT/MANAGEMENT

Management requires a team approach including a physician such as a neonatologist, nurse, pharmacist, nutritionist, family members, physical therapist, occupational therapist, speech language pathologist, teachers, and others. The specific needs of the child will vary due to the nature of the condition which lead to use of a ventilator. The goals listed below are general. One child is unlikely to need all. The team will determine the mode, intensity, and frequency of activity.

- Increase tolerance to physical interaction without desaturation.
- Increase aerobic capacity and endurance to motor activity and feeding.
- Decrease spasticity, if present.
- Increase chest wall movement.
- Improve accessory muscle breathing while upright.
- Increase diaphragmatic breathing.
- Facilitate assisted cough.
- Provide opportunity to practice motor skills in a variety of environments.
- Encourage child to explore environment.
- Increase general activity level to counter the inactivity cycle of reluctance to move and explore, leading to decreased endurance and "fitness" with more inactivity.
- Prevent deprivation of sensory and motor experiences by providing movement challenges and exercise.
- Provide assistive devices, if needed, for positioning and ambulation.
- Support development of cognitive and communication skills.
- If ventilator is used at home, provide family with instructions on use, potential complications, and emergency procedures.
- If therapy is done in the home, it should be integrated into the family's daily routine.
- Instruct the family on idea of lifelong fitness and the benefits of regular exercise that is individualized and graded to the child's level of tolerance.
- Encourage the family to focus on the child's abilities, not disabilities.
- Provide information to school personnel about the child's abilities as well as disabilities.

PRECAUTIONS/CONTRAINDICATIONS

- Monitor child for all signs of distress since child may not have communication skills. Areas to monitor include respiratory distress, skin color changes, changes in respiratory rate, breathing patterns, symmetry of chest expansion, posture, and general comfort.
- During use of the ventilator, efforts should be made to preserve physiological function, especially the diaphragm which is subject to atrophy. Always work within safe physiologic parameters. Monitor heart rate, respiratory rate, and oxygen saturation.
- Therapist should be familiar with equipment and purpose including cardiorespiratory monitors, oxygen analyzers, pulse oximeters, sphygmomanometers, transcutaneous Po_2 and Pco_2, ventilators, and ventilator alarms.
- Therapist should be alert to possible respiratory complication associated with mechanical ventilation including accidental endotracheal tube displacement, actual extubation, air leaks (eg, pneumothorax, pneumomediastrium, interstitial emphysema), excess secretions or atelectasis, infection (eg, tracheitis, pneumonities) oxygen hazards (eg, bronchopulmonary dysplasia, depression of ventilation), pulmonary

hemorrhage, and tracheal lesions (eg, edema, erosion, granuloma, obstruction, perforation, stenosis).

- Therapist should be alert for possible circulatory complications including hyperventilation (ie, decreased cerebral blood flow), impairment of venous return (ie, decreased cardiac output and systemic hypotension), intracranial hemorrhage, oxygen hazard (eg, cerebral vasoconstriction, retrolental fibroplasia), and septicemia.
- Therapist should be alert to possible metabolic complications including alkalosis, excessive bicarbonate therapy, potassium depletion, and increased work of breathing ("fighting the ventilator").
- Therapist should be alert to possible signs of renal and fluid balance problems including antidiuresis and excess water in inspired gas.
- Therapist should be alert to equipment malfunctions including improper humidification (eg, inspiratory line condensation, overheating of inspired gas), improper tubing connections (eg, disconnection, kinked line), power source failure, and ventilation malfunction (eg, leaks, value dysfunction).
- Therapist should monitor the amount of physical exertion that can be tolerated for safety and avoid muscular and respiratory fatigue (Kelly, p. 718).

DESIRED OUTCOME/PROGNOSIS

Note: If no neurologic damage has occurred, child has a good chance for normal growth and development.

- Child has adequate gas exchange.
- Child is medically stable with adequate growth and healing of lung.
- Child can be withdrawn from assisted ventilation.
- Family or child knows how to operate the ventilator and recognize signs of dysfunction.
- Child has age-appropriate gross motor skills.
- Child has age-appropriate oral motor skills.
- Child has age-appropriate endurance level.
- Child can participate in play groups and structured social groups.
- Child can participate in school and community activities.

REFERENCES

Kelly MK. Children with ventilator dependence. In: Campbell SK, ed. *Physical Therapy for Children*. 2nd ed. Philadelphia, Pa: WB Saunders Co; 2000:711–733.

Tecklin JS. Pulmonary disorders in infants and children and their physical therapy management—Asthma. In: Tecklin JS, ed. *Pediatric Physical Therapy*. 3rd ed. Philadelphia, Pa: Lippincott Williams and Wilkins; 1999:540–541.

Disorders with Limited Information

REFERENCES

Attention Deficit Hyperactivity Disorder

Ratliffe KT. Sensory, processing, and cognitive disorders of childhood—Attention-deficit hyperactivity disorder. In: Ratliffe KT. *Clinical Pediatric Physical Therapy: A Guide for the Physical Therapy Team.* St. Louis, Mo: CV Mosby Co; 1998:329.

Child Abuse

Ratliffe KT. Traumatic disorders—Child abuse. In: Ratliffe KT. *Clinical Pediatric Physical Therapy: A Guide for the Physical Therapy Team.* St. Louis, Mo: CV Mosby Co; 1998:278–279.

Dermatomyositis

Wright FB. An adolescent girl with juvenile dermatomyositis. In: Melvin JL, Wright FV, eds. *Pediatr Rheum Dis.* (Rheumatologic rehabilitation series. V. 3). Bethesda, Md: American Occupational Therapy Association; 2000:284–293.

Dyspraxia

Lee MG, Smith GN. The effectiveness of physiotherapy for dyspraxia. *Physiotherapy.* 1998; 84(6):276–284.

Epilepsy

Beckung E. Development and validation of a measure of motor and sensory function in children with epilepsy. *Pediatr Phys Ther.* 2000;12(1):24–35.

Fetal Alcohol Syndrome

Ratliffe KT. Sensory, processing, and cognitive disorders of childhood—Fetal alcohol syndrome and fetal alcohol effects. In: Ratliffe KT. *Clinical Pediatric Physical Therapy: A Guide for the Physical Therapy Team.* St. Louis, Mo: CV Mosby Co; 1998:330–331.

HIV

Lowenthal B. HIV infection: Transmission, effects on early development, and intervention. *Infant-Toddler Intervention: The Transdisciplinary Journal.* 1997;7(3):191–200.

Potterton JL. Prevalence of developmental delay in infants who are HIV positive. *S Afr J Physiotherapy.* 2001;57(3):11–15.

Inflammation/Infection of the Brain

Porter RE. Inflammatory and infection disorders of the brain—Pediatric HIV infection. In: Umphred DA, ed. *Neurolog Rehabil.* 4th ed. St Louis, Mo: CV Mosby Co; 2001:564–565.

Learning Disorders

Ratliffe KT. Sensory, processing, and cognitive disorders of childhood—learning disabilities. In: Ratliffe KT. *Clinical Pediatric Physical Therapy: A Guide for the Physical Therapy Team*. St. Louis, Mo: CV Mosby Co; 1998:328–329.

Meckel-Gruber Syndrome

Kamunker MK. School-based physical therapy for a child with Meckel-Gruber syndrome. *Phys Ther Case Rep*. 1999;2(5):188–194.

Medical Disorders

Ratliffe KT. Medical disorders—acquired/infectious neurological disorders of childhood: meningitis and encephalitis, Guillain-Barré Syndrome, Infantile Botulism. In: Ratliffe KT. *Clinical Pediatric Physical Therapy: A Guide for the Physical Therapy Team*. St. Louis, Mo: CV Mosby Co; 1998:400–404.

Minimal Cerebral Dysfunction

Williams J, Unwin J. Physiotherapy management of minimal cerebral dysfunction in Australia: current practice and future challenges. *Aust J Physiotherapy*. 1997;43(1): 135–143.

Myositis Ossificans

Hartigan BJ, Benson LS. Myositis ossificans after a supracondylar fracture of the humerus in a child. *Amer J Orthop*. 2001;30(2):152–154.

Rett Syndrome

Budden SS. Rett syndrome. *Eur Child Adolesc Psychiatry*. 1997;6 (suppl 1):103–107.

Rubinstein-Taybi Syndrome

Young JR, Hunter D, Baylor D. Rubinstein-Taybi Syndrome and physical therapy. *Phys Ther Case Rep*. 1998;1(4):181–190.

Sickle Cell Anemia

Ratliffe KT. Medical disorders—other medical conditions of childhood: Sickle cell anemia. In: Ratliffe KT. *Clinical Pediatric Physical Therapy: A Guide for the Physical Therapy Team*. St. Louis, Mo: CV Mosby Co; 1998:413–415.

Spondylarthropathies

Davidson I, Kuchta G, Petty RE. Spondylarhropathies in children. In: Melvin JL, Wright FV, eds. *Pediatr Rheum Dis*. (Rheumatologic rehabilitation series. V. 3), Bethesda, Md: American Occupational Therapy Association; 2000:45–66.

Spondylolisthesis

Patrick C. Spinal conditions—spondylolisthesis. In: Campbell SK, ed. *Physical Therapy for Children*. 2nd ed. Philadelphia, Pa: WB Saunders Co; 2000:275–277.

Sudden Infant Death Syndrome

Knight AK. Positioning to reduce the risk of Sudden Infant Death Syndrome (SIDS): current trends and research. *Phys Occup Ther Pediatr.* 1998;18(3/4):137–148.

Thoracic Surgery

Howell BA. Thoracic surgery. In: Campbell SK, ed. *Physical Therapy for Children.* 2nd ed. Philadelphia, Pa: WB Saunders Co; 2000:786–810.

Chapter 13

Pulmonary Disorders

Asthma

DESCRIPTION

Asthma is a disease of excessive airway responsiveness to stimuli that are otherwise harmless. This hyperreactivity leads to recurrent inflammation and narrowing of the airways that can be reversed with medication or spontaneously. Asthma is one of a number of disorders considered obstructive, including bronchiectasis, chronic bronchitis, cystic fibrosis, and emphysema.

CAUSE

Obstructive diseases are caused either by reversible factors, such as inflammation, or irreversible factors, such as damaged alveoli. A localized lesion, such as a foreign body, can also cause airway obstruction. Causes can be considered extrinsic or intrinsic. Extrinsic asthma is caused by hypersensitivity to a triggering substance and usually develops early in life. Intrinsic asthma begins in adulthood and is considered more intense and harder to control with treatment. Factors that can trigger or exacerbate asthma include anxiety, history of stress at birth or early hospitalization, respiratory irritants like smoke, exercise-induced temperature change in airways, premenstrual changes, hyperventilation, changes in weather temperature, and certain foods such as dairy foods, caffeine drinks, or products with the additives of salt or aspirin. Genetic predisposition may also be a factor.

ASSESSMENT

Note: See APTA's Guide to Physical Therapist Practice. 2nd ed. *Physical Therapy.* 2001;81.

Cardiovascular/Pulmonary Preferred Practice Patterns: C, F

Cardiovascular/Pulmonary Preferred Practice Patterns: B, C, F, G, H, I

AREAS
- History
- General appearance
- Equipment, including use of oxygen, humidification, drips, and any chest tubes
- Vital signs, including temperature, resting heart rate, resting BP, resting respiratory rate and rhythm
- Cardiovascular, including results of exercise testing
- Musculoskeletal, including posture, head and neck musculature, and chest shape
- Skin and soft tissue, including edema and condition of hands, especially nails

Pulmonary Tests and Measures
- aerobic capacity and endurance, including vital signs and palpation of pulses
- auscultation of heart, lungs and major vessels
- breathing patterns, including thoracoabdominal movements and chest wall mobility
- claudication time tests
- cough/sputum production and airway clearance
- edema assessment
- functional level (see following)
- quality of life measures (see following)
- rating of perceived exertion (RPE) scales
- response to positional changes
- skin coloration including cyanosis

- size and body fat composition
- ventilatory muscle ability

INSTRUMENTS/PROCEDURES

Functional Level
- Chronic Respiratory Disease Questionnaire
- Classes of Respiratory Impairment
- Klein Bell Activities Scale
- Living with Asthma Questionnaire
- Pulmonary Functional Status Scale
- Pulmonary Functional Status and Dyspnea Questionnaire
- St. George's Respiratory Questonnaire
- visual analog scale for dyspnea and/or pain

Special Tests to Which the Physical Therapist May or May Not Have Access
- arterial blood gas analysis (ABG)
- bacterial and cytological tests of sputum
- chest x-ray (CXR)
- exercise tests (walk test, cycle test, treadmill test)
- flexible bronchoscopy
- oximetry
- Ventilation/Perfusion Scan
- pulmonary function tests (PFTs):
  airways resistance (Raw)
  alveolar ventilation (AV)
  body plethysmography
  diffusion capacity of lungs for carbon monoxide (DL co)
  graded exercise tests (GXT)
  expiratory reserve volume (ERV)
  flow-volume loop (F-V loop)
  forced expiratory volume in 1 second (FEV1)
  forced vital capacity (FVC)
  functional residual capacity (FRC)
  helium dilution method
  inspiratory reserve volume (IRV)
  maximum voluntary ventilation (MVV)
  maximum minute expired volume (VE)
  methacholine provocation test
  nitrogen washout test
  peak expiratory flow rate (PEFR)
  residual volume (RV)
  spirogram
  spirometry
  tidal volume (TV)
  total lung capacity (TLC)
  vital capacity (VC)
  Ventilation/Perfusion Scan

Clinical Measures of Risk Assessment for Exercise
- ECG monitoring (continuous or intermittent)
- rate of perceived exertion and effort tolerance
- signs/symptoms
- telemetry (continuous or intermittent)
- vital signs

PROBLEMS

ACUTE ASTHMA

- The client often has decreased breath sounds and wheezing.
- The client typically feels breathless, and breathing is labored with prolonged expiration.
- The client may have overexpansion of the chest.
- The client may feel anxious.

SEVERE ACUTE ASTHMA

- The wheeze often lessens.
- The client often has difficulty in talking.
- The skin can feel clammy.
- The client can look blue and have a rapid heart rate.
- The client may feel confused.
- The client often has tachypnea.
- The client often has increased use of accessory muscle tone.
- The client may have cough and increased secretions.
- There may be pulsus paradoxus.

CHRONIC ASTHMA

- The client often has a dry cough at night or morning wheezing.
- The client can have an exaggerated bronchial response to a cold room at night, leading to a morning dip in peak flow.

TREATMENT/MANAGEMENT

ACUTE ASTHMA

Aim to control the disease. Attacks may be avoided by offering the following suggested instructions to the client:

- Assess peak expiratory flow rate (PEFR) upon waking (within 1/2 hour) daily, if chronic; may need to seek medical help if PEFR is below 80 and does not rise to above 200 following medication.
- Keep a log of symptoms to gain better understanding of when to seek medical help.
- If in a high-risk group, be prepared for an attack with equipment ready needed for self-treatment.

Provide the following instructions to the client on how to deal with an attack:

- Lean forward with arms supported in an upright position. An alternative position is to straddle a chair facing backwards.
- Fresh air, but not too cold, may help.
- Try to breathe slowly through the nose, controlling the rate and rhythm of breath.
- Place emphasis on exhalation, perhaps using pursed-lip breathing.
- Use relaxation techniques.
- Use secretion removal techniques as indicated.

CHRONIC ASTHMA

- Provide the client with education about the disease.
- Help the client identify avoidable precipitating factors.
- Encourage regular exercise.
- Teach relaxation and stress reduction techniques.
- Encourage the client to try different sleeping postures and temperatures if he or she has nocturnal asthma.
- Inform the client about support groups.

Activity and exercise are generally prescribed in more frequent, shorter sessions monitored by rating perceived exertion and O_2 saturation. Supplemental O_2 may be indicated as needed.

PRECAUTIONS
- Deep breathing can exacerbate bronchospasm in those with acute asthma.
- Improperly used nebulizers can trigger bronchospasm.

DESIRED OUTCOME/PROGNOSIS
- The client will experience a reduction in the number and intensity of asthma attacks.
- The client will have an increased capacity for ADLs.
- The client will have an increased sense of control over symptoms.

REFERENCES

Assessment

American Physical Therapy Association. Guide to physical therapist practice. 2nd ed. *Phys Ther.* 2001;81.

Bourgeois MC. Diagnosing pulmonary impairment: a lung volume reduction surgery case that uses the patient management model. *CardioPulmonary Phys Ther J.* 1999;10:98–100.

Brooks D, Wilson L, Kelsey C, et al. Accuracy and reliability of specialized physical therapists in auscultating tape recorded lung sounds. *Physiotherapy Can.* 1993;45:21–24.

Frownfelter D, Dean E. *Principles and Practice of Cardiopulmonary Physical Therapy.* 3rd ed. New York, NY: CV Mosby Co; 1996.

Goodman C, Snyder TE. *Differential Diagnosis in Physical Therapy.* Philadelphia, Pa: WB Saunders Co; 2000.

Hill J, Johansen J, Pedersen S, LaPier TK. Site of measurement and subject position affect chest excursion measurements. *CardioPulmonary Phys Ther J.* 1997;8:12–17.

Hillegass EA, Sadowsky HS. *Essentials of Cardiopulmonary Physical Therapy.* 2nd ed. Philadelphia, Pa: WB Saunders Co; 2001.

Pasterkamp H, Montgomery M, Wiebicke W, et al. Nomenclature used by health care professionals to describe breath sounds in asthma. *Chest.* 1993;92:346–352.

Rothstein JM, Roy SH, Wolf SL. *The Rehabilitation Specialist's Handbook.* 2nd ed. Philadelphia, Pa: FA Davis Co; 1998.

Singh S. The use of field walking tests for assessment of functional capacity in patients with chronic airway obstruction. *Physiotherapy.* 1992;78:102–104.

Treatment

Emtner M. Physiotherapy and intensive physical training in rehabilitation of adults with asthma. *Phys Ther Rev.* 1999;4:229–240.

Emtner M, Hedin A, Stalenheim G. Asthmatic patients' views of a comprehensive asthma rehabilitation programme: a three-year follow-up. *Physiotherapy Res Int.* 1998;3:175–193.

Emtner M, Herala M, Stalenheim G. High-intensity physical training in adults with asthma. A 10-week rehabilitation program. *Chest.* 1996;109:323–330.

Goodman C, Snyder TE. *Differential Diagnosis in Physical Therapy*. Philadelphia, Pa: WB Saunders Co; 2000.

Hondras MA, Linde K, Jones AP. Manual therapy for asthma. *The Cochrane Collaboration*. 2000;1.

Jenkins S. Pulmonary rehabilitation. *Physiotherapy Singapore*. 2000;3:106–112.

Nielsen KE, Neilsen DH, Lin S, Fieseler KCR, et al. Changes in exercise responses and tolerance following an eight week pulmonary rehabilitation program. 1997;8:3–11.

Parsons M. Spotlight on asthma. *Physiotherapy Moves*. 1999;11:17.

Webber BA, Pryor JA. *Physiotherapy for Respiratory and Cardiac Problems*. New York, NY: Churchill Livingstone; 1993.

Zadai CC. *Pulmonary Management in Physical Therapy*. New York, NY: Churchill Livingstone; 1992.

Bronchiectasis

DESCRIPTION

Bronchiectasis is an obstruction of airways that have become damaged and chronically dilated. Airway obstruction is characterized by an increased resistance to airflow occurring during forced expiration. Other disorders considered obstructive include asthma, chronic bronchitis, cystic fibrosis, and emphysema.

CAUSE

Obstructive diseases are caused either by reversible factors—such as inflammation, or irreversible factors—such as damaged alveoli. A localized lesion, such as a foreign body, may cause airway obstruction. Bronchiectasis can be caused by accidental inhalation of a foreign object or by a viral infection such as severe pneumonia.

ASSESSMENT

Note: See APTA's Guide to Physical Therapist Practice. 2nd ed. *Physical Therapy*. 2001;81.

Cardiovascular/Pulmonary Preferred Practice Patterns: B, C, F, H

AREAS
- History
- General Appearance
- Equipment, including use of oxygen, humidification, drips, and any chest tubes
- Vital signs including temperature, resting heart rate, resting BP, resting respiratory rate and rhythm
- Cardiovascular, including results of exercise testing
- Musculoskeletal, including posture, head and neck musculature, and chest shape
- Skin and soft tissue, including edema and condition of hands, especially nails
- Selected pulmonary tests and measures

Pulmonary Tests and Measures

- aerobic capacity and endurance including vital signs and palpation of pulses
- auscultation of heart and lungs and major vessels
- breathing patterns including thoracoabdominal movements and chest wall mobility

- claudication time tests
- cough/sputum production and airway clearance
- edema assessment
- functional level (see following)
- quality of life measures (see following)
- rating of perceived exertion (RPE) scales
- response to positional changes
- skin coloration including cyanosis
- size and body fat composition
- ventilatory muscle ability

INSTRUMENTS/PROCEDURES

Functional Level
- Chronic Respiratory Disease Questionnaire
- Classes of Respiratory Impairment
- Klein Bell Activities Scale
- Pulmonary Functional Status Scale
- Pulmonary Functional Status and Dyspnea Questionnaire
- St. George's Respiratory Questonnaire
- visual analog scale for dyspnea and/or pain

Special Tests to Which the Physical Therapist May or May Not Have Access
- arterial blood gas analysis (ABG)
- bacterial and cytological tests of sputum
- chest x-ray (CXR)
- exercise tests (walk test, cycle test, treadmill test)
- flexible bronchoscopy
- oximetry
- Ventilation/Perfusion Scan
- pulmonary function tests (PFTs):
  airways resistance (Raw)
  alveolar ventilation (VA)
  body plethysmography
  diffusion capacity of lungs for carbon monoxide (DL co)
  graded exercise tests (GXT)
  expiratory reserve volume (ERV)
  flow-volume loop (F-V loop)
  forced expiratory volume in 1 second (FEV1)
  forced vital capacity (FVC)
  functional residual capacity (FRC)
  helium dilution method
  inspiratory reserve volume (IRV)
  maximum voluntary ventilation (MVV)
  maximum minute expired volume (VE)
  methacholine provocation test
  nitrogen washout test
  peak expiratory flow rate (PEFR)
  residual volume (RV)
  spirogram
  spirometry
  tidal volume (TV)
  total lung capacity (TLC)
  vital capacity (VC)
  Ventilation/Perfusion Scan

Clinical Measures of Risk Assessment for Exercise
- ECG monitoring (continuous or intermittent)
- rate of perceived exertion and effort tolerance
- signs/symptoms
- telemetry (continuous or intermittent)
- vital signs

PROBLEMS
- The client often has hoarse wheezes and altered breath sounds.
- There may be clubbing at the fingers.
- The client may be short of breath and fatigued.
- There can be a large quantity of pus-filled sputum that may also contain blood.
- The client may have sinusitis.
- The client may experience anemia, weight loss, malaise, and fatigue.
- There may be fever.

TREATMENT/MANAGEMENT
- Educate the client in sputum clearance.
- Encourage daily exercise if the disease is in the moderate stage.
- The client will probably need daily postural drainage to improve impaired sputum clearance.

CHEST PT IN GENERAL
- Provide education on disease control and pain management.
- Provide clearance of secretions via hydration, humidification, nebulization, mobilization, breathing exercises, postural drainage, manual techniques, mechanical aids, cough and forced expiratory techniques, and nasopharyngeal suction.
- Consider mechanical devices to aid ventilation, such as continuous positive airways pressure (CPAP) and intermittent positive-pressure breathing (IPPB). In general, additional oxygen therapy is needed only for hypoxemia. It can be delivered through low-flow or high-flow masks, large-capacity masks, reservoir bags, nasal cannulas, transtracheal oxygen catheters, tents, head boxes, or clear plastic hoods. Medication delivery devices include inhalers and nebulizers.
- Provide advice on appropriate activity level.
- Implement the following chest physical therapy techniques: positioning, controlled mobilization, and breathing exercises, as indicated.

POSITIONING
- Modify functional residual capacity using the following posture sequence, which gradually increases volume: supine, slumped sitting, half-lying, side-lying, toward prone, sitting upright, standing.
- Regular position changes should be part of the client's management plan.

CONTROLLED MOBILIZATION WITH EXERCISE
- Use controlled mobilization with exercise while the client is in an upright posture.
- Control activity level to increase depth of respiration slightly, and follow by relaxed standing to regain breath.
- Modify activity with transfers or walking depending on the client's abilities.
- Progress to regular graded exercise.

BREATHING EXERCISES
- Techniques can include deep breathing, end-inspiratory hold, sniff technique, single percussion, and abdominal breathing.

PRECAUTIONS/CONTRAINDICATIONS

- Oxygen is a drug that has both side effects and risks. It should be carefully administered, precisely prescribed, and routinely monitored. Substernal pain, dyspnea, and cough may signal oxygen toxicity. In neonates, high concentrations of oxygen may cause eye damage.
- Some degree of atelectasis can develop in clients who cannot take deep breaths due to low lung volumes but are required to perform forced expiratory maneuvers.

CONTRAINDICATIONS TO CPAP AND IPPB

- These devices are not intended to be used with subcutaneous emphysema, facial trauma, bronchopleural fistula, bullae, undrained pneumothorax, and recent esophageal or bronchial surgery.
- For IPPB, other cautions include pneumothorax, large emphysematous bullae in the lung, hemoptysis, active tuberculosis, or a bronchial tumor in the proximal airway.
- Clients with cystic fibrosis or emphysema can be susceptible to air trapping or pneumothorax, gastric distention, or infection.
- Improperly used nebulizers can trigger bronchospasm.

CONTRAINDICATIONS TO HEAD-DOWN POSITION IN POSTURAL DRAINAGE

- abdominal distention
- acute spinal cord lesion
- arrhythmias
- breathlessness
- cardiovascular instability
- cerebral edema
- headache
- hemoptysis (recent)
- hiatal hernia
- hypertension
- obesity
- pregnancy
- pneumothorax, undrained
- pulmonary edema
- subcutaneous emphysema
- seizures

CONTRAINDICATIONS TO POSTURAL DRAINAGE IN ANY POSITION

- head injuries
- post esophagectomy
- aortic aneurysm
- during the filling cycle of peritoneal dialysis
- facial edema from burns, post eye surgery

Note: Discuss with medical staff if contraindicated technique should be risked for potential benefit.

CONTRAINDICATIONS TO PERCUSSION AND VIBRATION

- arrhythmias or angina (unstable)
- hemoptysis (recent)
- skin not intact due to trauma
- osteoporosis
- rib fracture or an increased risk of fracture

CONTRAINDICATIONS TO COUGHING THERAPY

- aneurysm
- increased intracranial pressure
- eye surgery (recent)
- subcutaneous emphysema
- pneumonectomy (recent)

Note: Spasm of multiple coughs can lead to fatigue, bronchospasm, and airway closure.

CONTRAINDICATIONS AND
PRECAUTIONS TO NASOPHARYNGEAL SUCTIONING
- Avoid with a client with a cerebrospinal fluid leak, clotting disorders, stridor, or pulmonary edema.
- Use caution with clients with recent esophagectomy or pneumonectomy.
- Suctioning may aggravate bronchospasm.
- Hypoxia and cardiac arrhythmias can occur during nasopharyngeal suctioning.
- Atelectasis or obstruction of the airway can be caused by suction that is too strong or too prolonged.

DESIRED OUTCOME/PROGNOSIS
- The client will have an increase in lung volume.
- The client will experience a relief of symptoms.
- The client will increase capacity for ADLs.
- The client will experience a decrease in episodes of attacks, leading to a sense of control over symptoms.

Note: Bronchiectasis may be reduced by childhood vaccination for whooping cough and measles.

REFERENCES

Assessment

American Physical Therapy Association. Guide to physical therapist practice. 2nd ed. *Phys Ther.* 2001;81.

Brooks D, Wilson L, Kelsey C, et al. Accuracy and reliability of specialized physical therapists in auscultating tape recorded lung sounds. *Physiotherapy Can.* 1993;45:21–24.

Frownfelter D, Dean E. *Principles and Practice of Cardiopulmonary Physical Therapy.* 3rd. New York, NY: CV Mosby Co; 1996.

Goodman C, Snyder TE. *Differential Diagnosis in Physical Therapy.* Philadelphia, Pa: WB Saunders Co; 2000.

Hill J, Johansen J, Pedersen S, LaPier TK. Site of measurement and subject position affect chest excursion measurements. *CardioPulmonary Phys Ther J.* 1997;8:12–17.

Hillegass EA, Sadowsky HS. *Essentials of Cardiopulmonary Physical Therapy.* 2nd ed. Philadelphia, Pa: WB Saunders Co; 2001.

Pasterkamp H, Montgomery M, Wiebicke W, et al. Nomenclature used by health care professionals to describe breath sounds in asthma. *Chest.* 1993;92:346–352.

Rothstein JM, Roy SH, Wolf SL. *The Rehabilitation Specialist's Handbook.* 2nd ed. Philadelphia, Pa: FA Davis Co; 1998.

Singh S. The use of field walking tests for assessment of functional capacity in patients with chronic airways obstruction. *Physiotherapy.* 1992;78:102–104.

Treatment

Chen HC, et al. Chest physiotherapy does not exacerbate gastroesophageal reflux in patients with chronic bronchitis and bronchiectasis. *Chang Keng I Hsueh Tsa Chih.* 1998; 21:409–414.

Conway JH. The effects of humidification for patients with chronic airways disease. *Physiotherapy.* 1992;78:97–101.

Gallon A. The use of percussion. *Physiotherapy.* 1992;78:85–89.

Goodman C, Snyder TE. *Differential Diagnosis in Physical Therapy*. Philadelphia, Pa: WB Saunders Co; 2000:145–180.

Harding J, Kemper M, Weissman C. Alfentanil attenuates the cardiopulmonary response of critically ill patients to an acute increase in oxygen demand induced by chest physiotherapy. *Anesth Analg*. 1993;77:1122–1129.

Hardy KA, Anderson BD. Noninvasive clearance of airway secretions. *Respir Care Clin North Am*. 1996;2:323–345.

Hough A. *Physiotherapy in Respiratory Care*. London, England: Chapman & Hall; 1991.

Irwin S, Tecklin JS. *Cardiopulmonary Physical Therapy*. 3rd ed. St Louis, Mo: CV Mosby Co; 1995.

Jenkins S. Pulmonary rehabilitation. *Physiotherapy Singapore*. 2000;3:106–112.

Jones A, Rowe BH. Issues in pulmonary nursing. Bronchopulmonary hygiene physical therapy in bronchiectasis and chronic obstructive pulmonary disease: a systematic review. *Heart Lung J Acute Crit Care*. 2000;29:125–135.

Zadai CC. *Pulmonary Management in Physical Therapy*. New York, NY: Churchill Livingstone; 1992.

Chronic Bronchitis

DESCRIPTION

Chronic bronchitis is chronic inflammation of the tracheobronchial tree. This disorder is characterized by mucus hypersecretion leading to a chronic productive cough and structural changes of the bronchi. To be considered a chronic condition, the symptoms must have been present for at least 3 months for 2 consecutive years.

Chronic bronchitis is considered an obstructive disorder and is generally progressive. Airway obstruction is characterized by an increased resistance to airflow occurring during forced expiration. Other disorders considered obstructive include asthma, bronchiectasis, cystic fibrosis, and emphysema. The disease combination of chronic bronchitis and emphysema is called various names, including *chronic obstructive pulmonary disease* (COPD) and *chronic airways obstruction*.

CAUSE

Obstructive diseases are caused either by reversible factors—such as inflammation, or irreversible factors—such as damaged alveoli. A localized lesion, such as a foreign body, may also cause airway obstruction. Chronic bronchitis can be caused by repeated exposure to pollutants that irritate the airway's sensitive lining. It is most commonly associated with cigarette smoking.

ASSESSMENT

Note: See APTA's Guide to Physical Therapist Practice. 2nd ed. *Physical Therapy*. 2001;81.

Cardiovascular/Pulmonary Preferred Practice Patterns: B, C, F, H, I

AREAS
- History
- General Appearance
- Equipment, including use of oxygen, humidification, drips, and any chest tubes
- Vital signs, including temperature, resting heart rate, resting BP, resting respiratory rate, and rhythm

- Cardiovascular, including results of exercise testing
- Musculoskeletal, including posture, head and neck musculature, and chest shape
- Skin and soft tissue, including edema and condition of hands, especially nails
- Selected pulmonary tests and measures

Pulmonary Tests and Measures may include:

- aerobic capacity and endurance including vital signs and palpation of pulses
- auscultation of heart and lungs and major vessels
- breathing patterns including thoracoabdominal movements and chest wall mobility
- claudication time tests
- cough/sputum production and airway clearance
- edema assessment
- functional level (see following)
- quality of life measures (see following)
- rating of perceived exertion (RPE) scales
- response to positional changes
- skin coloration including cyanosis
- size and body fat composition
- ventilatory muscle ability

INSTRUMENTS/PROCEDURES

Functional Level
- Chronic Respiratory Disease Questionnaire
- Classes of Respiratory Impairment
- Klein Bell Activities Scale
- Pulmonary Functional Status Scale
- Pulmonary Functional Status and Dyspnea Questionnaire
- St. George's Respiratory Questonnaire
- visual analog scale for dyspnea and/or pain

Special Tests to Which the Physical Therapist May or May Not Have Access
- arterial blood gas analysis (ABG)
- bacterial and cytological tests of sputum
- chest x-ray (CXR)
- exercise tests (walk test, cycle test, treadmill test)
- flexible bronchoscopy
- oximetry
- Ventilation/Perfusion Scan
- pulmonary function tests (PFTs):
  airways resistance (Raw)
  alveolar ventilation (VA)
  body plethysmography
  diffusion capacity of lungs for carbon monoxide (DL co)
  graded exercise tests (GXT)
  expiratory reserve volume (ERV)
  flow-volume loop (F-V loop)
  forced expiratory volume in 1 second (FEV1)
  forced vital capacity (FVC)
  functional residual capacity (FRC)
  helium dilution method
  inspiratory reserve volume (IRV)
  maximum voluntary ventilation (MVV)
  maximum minute expired volume (VE)
  methacholine provocation test

nitrogen washout test
peak expiratory flow rate (PEFR)
residual volume (RV)
spirogram
spirometry
tidal volume (TV)
total lung capacity (TLC)
vital capacity (VC)
Ventilation/Perfusion Scan

Clinical Measures of Risk Assessment for Exercise
- ECG monitoring (continuous or intermittent)
- rate of perceived exertion and effort tolerance
- signs/symptoms
- telemetry (continuous or intermittent)
- vital signs

PROBLEMS
- The client often has a productive cough, which is usually a morning cough.
- The client may have breathlessness and fatigue.
- The breath sounds are often decreased with crackles and wheezes.
- The disorder may lead to sleep disturbance.
- There is often poor tolerance to exercise and labored breathing, with a decreased functional capacity and expiratory flow rates.
- The client often has frequent respiratory infections and may have a fever.
- There may be cor pulmonale.

TREATMENT/MANAGEMENT

CHEST PT IN GENERAL
- Provide education on disease control and pain management.
- Provide clearance of secretions via hydration, humidification, nebulization, mobilization, breathing exercises, postural drainage, manual techniques, mechanical aids, cough and forced expiratory techniques, and nasopharyngeal suction.
- Consider mechanical devices to aid ventilation, such as continuous positive airways pressure (CPAP) and intermittent positive-pressure breathing (IPPB). In general, additional oxygen therapy is needed only for hypoxemia. It can be delivered through low-flow or high-flow masks, large-capacity masks, reservoir bags, nasal cannulas, transtracheal oxygen catheters, tents, or clear plastic hoods. Medication delivery devices include inhalers and nebulizers.
- Provide advice on appropriate activity level.
- Implement the following chest physical therapy techniques: positioning, controlled mobilization, and breathing exercises, as indicated.

POSITIONING
- Modify functional residual capacity using the following posture sequence, which gradually increases volume: supine, slumped sitting, half-lying, side-lying, toward prone, sitting upright, and standing.
- Regular position changes should be part of the client's management plan.

CONTROLLED MOBILIZATION WITH EXERCISE
- Use controlled mobilization with exercise while in upright posture.
- Control activity level to slightly increase depth of respiration, and follow by relaxed standing to regain breath.
- Modify activity with transfers or walking depending on the client's abilities.
- Progress to regular graded exercise.

BREATHING EXERCISES
- Techniques may include deep breathing, end-inspiratory hold, sniff technique, single percussion, and abdominal breathing.

PRECAUTIONS/CONTRAINDICATIONS
- Oxygen is a drug that has both side effects and risks. It should be carefully administered, precisely prescribed, and routinely monitored. Substernal pain, dyspnea, and cough may signal oxygen toxicity. In neonates, high concentrations of oxygen may cause eye damage.
- Some degree of atelectasis can develop in clients who cannot take deep breaths due to low lung volumes but are required to perform forced expiratory maneuvers.

CONTRAINDICATIONS TO CPAP AND IPPB
- These devices are not intended to be used with subcutaneous emphysema, facial trauma, bronchopleural fistula, bullae, undrained pneumothorax, and recent esophageal or bronchial surgery.
- For IPPB, other cautions include pneumothorax, large emphysematous bullae in the lung, hemoptysis, active tuberculosis, or a bronchial tumor in the proximal airway.
- Clients with cystic fibrosis or emphysema can be susceptible to air trapping or pneumothorax, gastric distention, or infection.

Note: Improperly used nebulizers can trigger bronchospasm.

CONTRAINDICATIONS TO HEAD-DOWN POSITION IN POSTURAL DRAINAGE
- abdominal distention
- acute spinal cord lesion
- arrhythmias
- breathlessness
- cardiovascular instability
- cerebral edema
- headache
- hemoptysis (recent)
- hiatal hernia
- hypertension
- obesity
- pregnancy
- pneumothorax, undrained
- pulmonary edema
- subcutaneous emphysema
- seizures

CONTRAINDICATIONS TO POSTURAL DRAINAGE IN ANY POSITION
- head injuries
- post esophagectomy
- aortic aneurysm
- during the filling cycle of peritoneal dialysis
- facial edema from burns, post eye surgery

Note: Discuss with medical staff if contraindications should be risked for potential benefit.

CONTRAINDICATIONS TO PERCUSSION AND VIBRATION
- arrhythmias or angina (unstable)
- hemoptysis (recent)
- skin not intact due to trauma
- osteoporosis
- rib fracture or an increased risk of fracture

CONTRAINDICATIONS TO COUGHING THERAPY
- aneurysm
- increased intracranial pressure
- eye surgery (recent)

- subcutaneous emphysema
- pneumonectomy (recent)

Note: Spasm of multiple coughs can lead to fatigue, bronchospasm, and airway closure.

CONTRAINDICATIONS AND PRECAUTIONS TO NASOPHARYNGEAL SUCTIONING

- Avoid in a client with a cerebrospinal fluid leak, clotting disorders, stridor, or pulmonary edema.
- Use caution with clients with recent esophagectomy or pneumonectomy.
- Suctioning may aggravate bronchospasm.
- Hypoxia can occur during nasopharyngeal suction as well as cardiac arrhythmias.
- Atelectasis or obstruction of the airway can be caused by suction that is too strong or too prolonged.

DESIRED OUTCOME/PROGNOSIS

- The client will have an increase in lung volume.
- The client will experience a relief of symptoms.
- The client will increase capacity for ADLs.
- The client will experience a decrease in episodes of attacks, leading to a sense of control over symptoms.

Note: The advent of peripheral edema with chronic bronchitis is an initial sign of cor pulmonale, which carries a grim prognosis.

REFERENCES

Assessment

American Physical Therapy Association. Guide to physical therapist practice. 2nd ed. *Phys Ther.* 2001;81.

Brooks D, Wilson L, Kelsey C, et al. Accuracy and reliability of specialized physical therapists in auscultating tape recorded lung sounds. *Physiotherapy Can.* 1993;45:21–24.

Frownfelter D, Dean E. *Principles and Practice of Cardiopulmonary Physical Therapy.* 3rd ed. New York, NY: CV Mosby Co; 1996.

Goodman C, Snyder TE. *Differential Diagnosis in Physical Therapy.* Philadelphia, Pa: WB Saunders Co; 2000.

Hill J, Johansen J, Pedersen S, LaPier TK. Site of measurement and subject position affect chest excursion measurements. *CardioPulmonary Phys Ther J.* 1997;8:12–17.

Hillegass EA, Sadowsky HS. *Essentials of Cardiopulmonary Physical Therapy.* 2nd ed. Philadelphia, Pa: WB Saunders Co; 2001.

Pasterkamp H, Montgomery M, Wiebicke W, et al. Nomenclature used by health care professionals to describe breath sounds in asthma. *Chest.* 1993;92:346–352.

Rothstein JM, Roy SH, Wolf SL. *The Rehabilitation Specialist's Handbook.* 2nd ed. Philadelphia, Pa: FA Davis Co; 1998.

Singh S. The use of field walking tests for assessment of functional capacity in patients with chronic airways obstruction. *Physiotherapy.* 1992;78:102–104.

Treatment

Bellone A, et al. Chest physical therapy in patients with acute exacerbation of chronic bronchitis: effectiveness of three methods. *Arch Phys Med Rehabil.* 2000;81:558–560.

Chen HC, et al. Chest physiotherapy does not exacerbate gastroesophageal reflux in patients with chronic bronchitis and bronchiectasis. *Chang Keng I Hsueh Tsa Chih.* 1998;21:409–414.

Conway JH. The effects of humidification for patients with chronic airways disease. *Physiotherapy.* 1992;78:97–101.

Gallon A. The use of percussion. *Physiotherapy.* 1992;78:85–89.

Goodman C, Snyder TE. *Differential Diagnosis in Physical Therapy.* Philadelphia, Pa: WB Saunders Co; 2000.

Harding J, Kemper M, Weissman C. Alfentanil attenuates the cardiopulmonary response of critically ill patients to an acute increase in oxygen demand induced by chest physiotherapy. *Anesth Analg.* 1993;77:1122–1129.

Irwin S, Tecklin JS. *Cardiopulmonary Physical Therapy.* 3rd ed. St Louis, Mo: CV Mosby Co; 1995.

Jenkins S. Pulmonary rehabilitation. *Physiotherapy Singapore.* 2000;3:106–112.

Zadai CC. *Pulmonary Management in Physical Therapy.* New York, NY: Churchill Livingstone; 1992.

Emphysema

DESCRIPTION

Emphysema is a disease of the alveoli with accompanying permanent damage to the airways, particularly to the air spaces distal to the terminal bronchioles. Emphysema is considered an obstructive disorder. Airway obstruction is characterized by an increased resistance to airflow occurring during forced expiration. Other disorders considered obstructive include asthma, bronchiectasis, cystic fibrosis, and chronic bronchitis. The disease combination of chronic bronchitis and emphysema is known by various names, including *chronic obstructive pulmonary disease* (COPD) and *chronic airways obstruction.*

CAUSE

Obstructive diseases are caused either by reversible factors—such as inflammation—or irreversible factors—such as damaged alveoli. A localized lesion, such as a foreign body, may also cause airway obstruction. Emphysema is caused by smoking or occasionally by a congenital destruction of alveoli. The development of emphysema may also be affected by genetics, gender, and ethnicity.

ASSESSMENT

Note: See APTA's Guide to Physical Therapist Practice. 2nd ed. *Physical Therapy.* 2001;81.

Cardiopulmonary Preferred Practice Patterns: B, C, F, G, H

Musculoskeletal Preferred Practice Pattern: C

AREAS
- History
- General Appearance
- Equipment, including use of oxygen, humidification, drips, and any chest tubes
- Vital signs, including temperature, resting heart rate, resting BP, resting respiratory rate and rhythm
- Cardiovascular, including results of exercise testing
- Musculoskeletal, including posture, head and neck musculature, and chest shape

- Skin and soft tissue, including edema and condition of hands, especially nails
- Selected pulmonary tests and measures

Pulmonary Tests and Measures

- aerobic capacity and endurance including vital signs and palpation of pulses
- auscultation of heart and lungs and major vessels
- breathing patterns including thoracoabdominal movements and chest wall mobility
- claudication time tests
- cough/sputum production and airway clearance
- edema assessment
- functional level (see below)
- quality of life measures (see below)
- rating of perceived exertion (RPE) scales
- response to positional changes
- skin coloration including cyanosis
- size and body fat composition
- ventilatory muscle ability

INSTRUMENTS/PROCEDURES

Functional Level

- Chronic Respiratory Disease Questionnaire
- Classes of Respiratory Impairment
- Klein Bell Activities Scale
- Pulmonary Functional Status Scale
- Pulmonary Functional Status and Dyspnea Questionnaire
- St. George's Respiratory Questionnaire
- visual analog scale for dyspnea and/or pain

Special Tests to Which the Physical Therapist May or May Not Have Access

- arterial blood gas analysis (ABG)
- bacterial and cytological tests of sputum
- chest x-ray (CXR)
- exercise tests (walk test, cycle test, treadmill tests)
- flexible bronchoscopy
- oximetry
- Ventilation/Perfusion Scan

Pulmonary Function Tests (PFTs)

- airways resistance (Raw)
- alveolar ventilation (VA)
- body plethysmography
- diffusion capacity of lungs for carbon monoxide (DL co)
- graded exercise tests (GXT)
- expiratory reserve volume (ERV)
- flow-volume loop (F-V loop)
- forced expiratory volume in 1 second(FEV1)
- forced vital capacity (FVC)
- functional residual capacity (FRC)
- helium dilution method
- inspiratory reserve volume (IRV)
- maximum voluntary ventilation (MVV)
- maximum minute expired volume (VE)
- methacholine provocation test
- nitrogen washout test
- peak expiratory flow rate (PEFR)

- residual volume (RV)
- spirogram
- spirometry
- tidal volume (TV)
- total lung capacity (TLC)
- vital capacity (VC)
- Ventilation/Perfusion Scan

Clinical Measures of Risk Assessment for Exercise
- ECG monitoring (continuous or intermittent)
- rate of perceived exertion and effort tolerance
- signs/symptoms
- telemetry (continuous or intermittent)
- vital signs

PROBLEMS

- The client is often breathless, with labored breathing and prolonged expiration.
- There may be weight loss.
- The client often has a barrel-like chest shape.
- There may be altered breath sounds, usually decreased and/or wheezing.
- There is often strong use of accessory muscles.
- There may be clubbing of nails and cyanosis.
- There may be cor pulmonale.
- There may be an accompanying cough.
- There may be hypoxemia and hypercapnea.

TREATMENT/MANAGEMENT

CHEST PT IN GENERAL

- Provide education on disease control and pain management.
- Provide clearance of secretions via hydration, humidification, nebulization, mobilization, breathing exercises, postural drainage, manual techniques, mechanical aids, cough and forced expiratory techniques, and nasopharyngeal suction.
- Consider mechanical devices to aid ventilation, such as continuous positive airways pressure (CPAP) and intermittent positive-pressure breathing (IPPB). In general, additional oxygen therapy is needed only for hypoxemia. It can be delivered through low-flow or high-flow masks, large-capacity masks, reservoir bags, nasal cannulas, transtracheal oxygen catheters, tents, head boxes, or clear plastic hoods. Medication delivery devices include inhalers and nebulizers.
- Provide advice on appropriate activity level.
- Implement the following chest physical therapy techniques: positioning, controlled mobilization, and breathing exercises as indicated.

POSITIONING

- Modify functional residual capacity using the following posture sequence, which gradually increases volume: supine, slumped sitting, half-lying, side-lying, toward prone, sitting upright, and finally standing.

Note: Regular position changes should be part of the client's management plan.

CONTROLLED MOBILIZATION WITH EXERCISE

- Use controlled mobilization with exercise while in upright posture.
- Control activity level to slightly increase depth of respiration, and follow by relaxed standing to regain breath.
- Modify activity with transfers or walking depending on client's abilities.
- Progress to regular graded exercise.

BREATHING EXERCISES
- Techniques may include deep breathing, end-inspiratory hold, sniff technique, single percussion, and abdominal breathing.
- Pulmonary rehabilitation program may be initiated in clients who are medically stable, have minimal complications and have moderate to moderately severe pulmonary disease. In addition, begin the administration of an exercise program; a complete program involves weight control, nutrition smoking cessation and psychological support. The exercise component of the program may include warm-up session, cardiovascular exercise for 20 to 60 minutes followed by cool-down period. Resistance training my also be included if client has no contraindications and has previous aerobic conditioning for at least 4 to 6 weeks.

PRECAUTIONS/CONTRAINDICATIONS
- Oxygen is a drug that has both side effects and risks. It should be carefully administered, precisely prescribed, and routinely monitored. Substernal pain, dyspnea, and cough may signal oxygen toxicity. In neonates, high concentrations of oxygen may cause eye damage.
- Some degree of atelectasis can develop in clients who cannot take deep breaths due to low lung volumes but are required to perform forced expiratory maneuvers.

CONTRAINDICATIONS TO CPAP AND IPPB
- These devices are not intended to be used with subcutaneous emphysema, facial trauma, bronchopleural fistula, bullae, undrained pneumothorax, or recent esophageal or bronchial surgery.
- For IPPB, other cautions include pneumothorax, large emphysematous bullae in lung, hemoptysis, active tuberculosis, and a bronchial tumor in the proximal airway.
- Clients with cystic fibrosis or emphysema can be susceptible to air trapping or pneumothorax, and gastric distention or infection can occur.

Note: Improperly used nebulizers can trigger bronchospasm.

CONTRAINDICATIONS TO HEAD-DOWN POSITION IN POSTURAL DRAINAGE
- abdominal distention
- acute spinal cord lesion
- arrhythmias
- breathlessness
- cardiovascular instability
- cerebral edema
- headache
- hemoptysis (recent)
- hiatal hernia
- hypertension
- obesity
- pregnancy
- pneumothorax, undrained
- pulmonary edema
- subcutaneous emphysema
- seizures

CONTRAINDICATIONS TO POSTURAL DRAINAGE IN ANY POSITION
- head injuries
- post esophagectomy
- aortic aneurysm
- during the filling cycle of peritoneal dialysis
- facial edema from burns, post eye surgery

Note: Discuss with medical staff if contraindications should be risked for potential benefit.

CONTRAINDICATIONS TO PERCUSSION AND VIBRATION
- arrhythmias or angina (unstable)
- hemoptysis (recent)

- skin not intact due to trauma
- osteoporosis
- rib fracture or an increased risk of fracture

PRECAUTIONS FOR COUGHING THERAPY

- aneurysm
- increased intracranial pressure
- eye surgery (recent)
- subcutaneous emphysema
- pneumonectomy (recent)

Note: Spasm of multiple coughs can lead to fatigue, bronchospasm, and airway closure.

CONTRAINDICATIONS AND PRECAUTIONS TO NASOPHARYNGEAL SUCTIONING

- Avoid in a client with a cerebrospinal fluid leak, clotting disorders, stridor, or pulmonary edema.
- Use caution with recent esophagectomy or pneumonectomy.
- Suctioning may aggravate bronchospasm.
- Hypoxia can occur during nasopharyngeal suction as well as cardiac arrhythmias.
- Atelectasis or obstruction of the airway can be caused by suction that is too strong or too prolonged.

DESIRED OUTCOME/PROGNOSIS

- The client will have an increase in lung volume.
- The client will experience a relief of symptoms.
- The client will increase capacity for ADLs.
- The client will have a decrease in episodes of attacks, leading to a sense of control over symptoms.

REFERENCES

Assessment

American Physical Therapy Association. Guide to physical therapist practice. 2nd ed. *Phys Ther.* 2001;81.

Blaney F, English CS, Sawyer T. Sonographic measurement of diaphragmatic displacement during tidal breathing manoeuvres—a reliability study. *Aust J Physiotherapy.* 1999; 45:41–43.

Brooks D, Wilson L, Kelsey C, et al. Accuracy and reliability of specialized physical therapists in auscultating tape recorded lung sounds. *Physiotherapy Can.* 1993;45:21–24.

Frownfelter D, Dean E. *Principles and Practice of Cardiopulmonary Physical Therapy.* 3rd ed. New York, NY: CV Mosby Co; 1996.

Goodman C, Snyder TE. *Differential Diagnosis in Physical Therapy.* Philadelphia, Pa: WB Saunders Co; 2000.

Hill J, Johansen J, Pedersen S, LaPier TK. Site of measurement and subject position affect chest excursion measurements. *Cardiopulmonary Phys Ther J.* 1997;8:12–17.

Hillegass EA, Sadowsky HS. *Essentials of Cardiopulmonary Physical Therapy.* 2nd ed. Philadelphia, Pa: WB Saunders Co; 2001.

Pasterkamp H, Montgomery M, Wiebicke W, et al. Nomenclature used by health care professionals to describe breath sounds in asthma. *Chest.* 1993;92:346–352.

Rothstein JM, Roy SH, Wolf SL. *The Rehabilitation Specialist's Handbook*. 2nd ed. Philadelphia, Pa: FA Davis Co; 1998.

Singh S. The use of field walking tests for assessment of functional capacity in patients with chronic airways obstruction. *Physiotherapy*. 1992;78:102–104.

Treatment

Bellet N, Tucker B, Jenkins S. Breathing exercises. *Aust J Physiotherapy*. 1997;43:61–65.

Blazey S, Jenkins S, Smith R. Rate and force of application of manual chest percussion by physiotherapists. *Aust J Physiotherapy*. 1998;44:257–264.

Cahalin LP, LaPier TK, Salley E. Physiologic response to upright and forward leaning leg cycle ergometry in subjects with chronic obstructive pulmonary disease: a preliminary study. *CardioPulmonary Phys Ther J*. 1998;9:13–15.

Calhoun K, Burlis T, Piquard S. Lung volume reduction surgery: a review. *Cardiopulmonary Phys Ther J*. 1996;7:12–14.

Conway JH. The effects of humidification for patients with chronic airways disease. *Physiotherapy*. 1992;78:97–101.

Criner GJ, Cordova FC, Furukawa S, Kuzma AM, et al. Prospective randomized trial comparing bilateral lung volume reduction surgery to pulmonary rehabilitation in severe chronic obstructive pulmonary disease. *Am J Crit Care Med*. 1999;160:2018–2027.

Dallimare K, Jenkis S, Tucher B. Respiratory and cardiovascular responses to manual chest percussion in normal subjects. *Aust J Physiotherapy*. 1998;44:267–274.

Downs AM. Physical therapy in lung transplantation. *Phys Ther*. 1996;76:626–642.

Fuchs-Climent D, Le Gallais D, Varray A, Desplan J, et al. Quality of life and exercise tolerance in chronic obstructive pulmonary disease: effects of a short and intensive inpatient rehabilitation program. *Am J Phys Med Rehabil*. 1999;78:330–335.

Fujimoto H, Kubo K, Miyahara T, Matsuzawa Y, et al. Effects of muscle relaxation therapy using specially designed plates in patients with pulmonary emphysema. *Intern Med*. 1996;35:756–763.

Gallon A. The use of percussion. *Physiotherapy*. 1992;78:85–89.

Goodman C, Snyder TE. *Differential Diagnosis in Physical Therapy*. Philadelphia, Pa: WB Saunders Co; 2000.

Grabois M, Garrison SJ, Hart KA, Lehmkuhl LD. *Physical Medicine and Rehabilitation: The Complete Approach*. Malden, Mass: Blackwell Science; 2000.

Harding J, Kemper M, Weissman C. Alfentanil attenuates the cardiopulmonary response of critically ill patients to an acute increase in oxygen demand induced by chest physiotherapy. *Anesth Analg*. 1993;77:1122–1129.

Hardy KA, Anderson BD. Noninvasive clearance of airway secretions. *Respir Care Clin North Am*. 1996;2:323–345.

Hodgson C, Carroll S, Denehy L. A survey of manual hyperinflation in Australian hospitals. *Aust J Physiotherapy*. 1999;45:185–193.

Irion GL, Finch VP. Effect of supplemental oxygen and muscle contraction on tissue oxygen tension and delivery of oxygen by the microcirculation-clinical implications from a rodent model. *CardioPulmonary Phys Ther J*. 1997;8:13–19.

Irwin S, Tecklin JS. *Cardiopulmonary Physical Therapy*. 3rd ed. St Louis, Mo: CV Mosby Co; 1995.

Jenkins S. Pulmonary rehabilitation. *Physiotherapy Singapore*. 2000;3:106–112.

Jones A, Rowe BH. Issues in pulmonary nursing. Bronchopulmonary hygiene physical therapy in bronchiectasis and chronic obstructive pulmonary disease: a systematic review. *Heart Lung J Acute Crit Care*. 2000;29:125–135.

Jones A, Tse E, Cheung L, To C, et al. Restoration of lung volume using the flutter VRP1 or breathing exercise. *Aust J Physiotherapy*. 1997;43:183–189.

Kurabayashi H, Kubota K, Machida I, Tamura K, et al. Effective physical therapy for chronic obstructive pulmonary disease: pilot study of exercise in hot spring water. *Am J Phys Med Rehabil*. 1997;76:204–207.

LaPier TK, Donovan C. Sitting and standing position affect pulmonary function in patients with COPD: a preliminary study. *CardioPulmonary Phys Ther J*. 1999;10.

Lindsay KLB. Management of the medically complex patient: chronic obstructive pulmonary disease. *CardioPulmonary Phys Ther J*. 1999;10:48–49.

McCarren B, Chow CM. Manual hyperinflation: a description of the technique. *Aust J Physiotherapy*. 1996;42:203–208.

Pasterkamp H, et al. Nomenclature used by health care professionals to describe breath sounds in asthma. *Chest*. 1993;92:346–352.

Petta A, Jenkins S, Allison F. Ventilatory and cardiovascular responses to unsupported low-intensity upper limb exercise in normal subjects. *Aust J Physiotherapy*. 1998;44:123–129.

Resnikoff PM, Ries AL. Maximizing functional capacity. Pulmonary rehabiliation and adjunctive measures. *Respir Care Clin North Am*. 1998;4:475–492.

Ries AL, Kaplan RM, Limberg TM, Prewitt LM. Effects of pulmonary rehabilitation on physiologic and psychosocial outcomes in patients with chronic obstructive pulmonary disease. *Annals Intern Med*. 1995;122:823–832.

Rusterhoz B, Ellis E. The effect of lung compliance and experience on manual hyperinflation. *Aust J Physiotherapy*. 1998;44:23–28.

Sally ER, Bailery M, Streubel D, LaPier TK. Physiologic response to upright and forward leaning leg cycle ergometry in subjects with chronic obstructive pulmonary disease: a preliminary study. *CardioPulmonary Phys Ther J*. 1997;8:3–7.

Savie S, Ince DI, Arikan H. A comparison of autogenic drainage and the active cycle of breathing techniques in patients with chronic obstructive pulmonary diseases. *J Cardiopulmonary Rehabil*. 2000;20:37–43.

Strijbos JH, Postma DS, van Altena R, Gimeno F, et al. A comparison between an outpatient hospital-based pulmonary rehabilitation program and a home-care pulmonary rehabilitation program in patients with COPD. *Chest*. 1996;109:299–300.

Thomas HM III. Pulmonary rehabilitation. Does the site matter? *Chest*. 1996;109:299–300.

Tucker B, Jenkins S. The effect of breathing exercises with body positioning on regional lung ventilation. *Aust J Physiotherapy*. 1996;42:219–227.

Wijkstra PJ, Strijbos JH. Home-based rehabiliation for patients with chronic obstructive pulmonary disease. *Monaldi Arch Chest Dis*. 1998;53:450–453.

Zadai CC. *Pulmonary Management in Physical Therapy*. New York, NY: Churchill Livingstone; 1992.

Pneumonia

DESCRIPTION

Pneumonia is an acute infection of the lung that involves the alveolar spaces and interstitial tissue. The infection may involve only a segment of a lobe or the entire lobe. Alveolar involvement in conjunction with the bronchi is called bronchopneumonia and in conjunction with interstitial tissue is known as interstitial pneumonia.

CAUSE

Pneumonia is usually caused by bacteria. In infants and children, the main pulmonary pathogens are usually viral. A client may be predisposed to pneumonia if his or her history includes any of the following factors: alcoholism, chronic obstructive airways disease, compromised consciousness, debility, dysphagia, exposure to transmissible agents, extreme age, or immunosuppressive disorder and therapy.

ASSESSMENT

Note: See APTA's Guide to Physical Therapist Practice. 2nd ed. *Physical Therapy.* 2001;81.

Cardiovascular/Pulmonary Preferred Practice Patterns: C, F

Cardiovascular/Pulmonary Preferred Practice Patterns: B, C, F, H, I

Musculoskeletal Preferred Practice Pattern: B

AREAS

- History
- General Appearance
- Equipment, including use of oxygen, humidification, drips, and any chest tubes
- Vital signs including temperature, resting heart rate, resting BP, resting respiratory rate and rhythm
- Cardiovascular, including results of exercise testing
- Musculoskeletal including posture, head and neck musculature, and chest shape
- Skin and soft tissue, including edema and condition of hands, especially nails
- Selected pulmonary tests and measures

Pulmonary Tests and Measures

- aerobic capacity and endurance including vital signs and palpation of pulses
- auscultation of heart and lungs and major vessels
- breathing patterns including thoracoabdominal movements and chest wall mobility
- claudication time tests
- cough/sputum production and airway clearance
- edema assessment
- functional level (see following)
- quality of life measures (see following)
- rating of perceived exertion (RPE) scales
- response to positional changes
- skin coloration including cyanosis
- size and body fat composition
- ventilatory muscle ability

INSTRUMENTS/PROCEDURES

Functional Level

- Chronic Respiratory Disease Questionnaire
- Classes of Respiratory Impairment
- Klein Bell Activities Scale
- Pulmonary Functional Status Scale
- Pulmonary Functional Status and Dyspnea Questionnaire
- St. George's Respiratory Questonnaire
- visual analog scale for dyspnea and/or pain

Special Tests to Which the Physical Therapist May or May Not Have Access
- arterial blood gas analysis (ABG)
- bacterial and cytological tests of sputum
- chest x-ray (CXR)
- exercise tests (walk test, cycle test, treadmill tests)
- flexible bronchoscopy
- oximetry
- Ventilation/Perfusion Scan
- pulmonary function tests (PFTs):
 airways resistance (Raw)
 alveolar ventilation (VA)
 body plethysmography
 diffusion capacity of lungs for carbon monoxide (DL co)
 graded exercise tests (GXT)
 expiratory reserve volume (ERV)
 flow-volume loop (F-V loop)
 forced expiratory volume in 1 second (FEV1)
 forced vital capacity (FVC)
 functional residual capacity (FRC)
 helium dilution method
 inspiratory reserve volume (IRV)
 maximum voluntary ventilation (MVV)
 maximum minute expired volume (VE)
 methacholine provocation test
 nitrogen washout test
 peak expiratory flow rate (PEFR)
 residual volume (RV)
 spirogram
 spirometry
 tidal volume (TV)
 total lung capacity (TLC)
 vital capacity (VC)
 Ventilation/Perfusion Scan

Clinical Measures of Risk Assessment for Exercise
- ECG monitoring (continuous or intermittent)
- rate of perceived exertion and effort tolerance
- signs/symptoms
- telemetry (continuous or intermittent)
- vital signs

PROBLEMS

BACTERIAL
- The client often has a cough, fever, and shaking chills.
- The client may have chest pain and dyspnea.
- The client may have tachypnea.
- The client often has excess sputum production that is purulent and rusty colored or blood streaked.
- The client often has hypoxemia and hypocapnea initially leading to hypercapnea.
- The client may have shoulder or knee pain.

VIRAL
- The client often has a fever and chills.
- The client often has a dry cough.

- The breath sounds are often decreased.
- The client often has hypoxemia and hypocapnea.
- The client may have shoulder or knee pain.

Note: Older clients may have an atypical presentation of symptoms such as angina, mental confusion, decline in function.

TREATMENT/MANAGEMENT

GENERAL
- Teach positioning techniques and forward-leaning postures. Teach client how to splint during cough if it is painful.
- Use relaxation exercises and work adjustment strategies.
- Instruct in breathing exercises: abdominal (diaphragmatic) breathing, pursed-lips breathing, segmental breathing, low-frequency breathing, and sustained maximal breathing.
- Provide secretion clearance via traditional or modified postural drainage.
- Enhance cough by using forced expiration, manual ventilation, mechanical stimulation with suctioning, neuromuscular facilitation with ice along the paraspinal region on the thoracic spine, positioning, or pressure.
- Consider use of transcutaneous electrical nerve stimulation (TENS) for pain relief.
- Consider supplemental oxygen or mechanical ventilation as indicated.

EFFECT OF SPECIFIC TECHNIQUES
- Abdominal (diaphragmatic) breathing exercises eliminate accessory muscle activity, decrease respiratory rate, increase tidal ventilation, increase distribution of ventilation, and decrease postoperative treatment.
- Pursed-lips breathing exercises eliminate use of accessory muscles, decrease respiratory rate, increase arterial oxygen tension, decrease carbon dioxide tension, and increase tolerance to exercise.
- Segmental breathing exercises prevent excessive pleural fluid and secretions, diminish panic, decrease paradoxical breathing, and enhance chest mobility.
- Low-frequency and sustained maximal inspiration breathing slow down the respiratory rate.
- Reduced oxygen consumption increases the dyspnea threshold for a specific activity, improves tolerance to functional activity, and increases quality of life.
- Postural drainage, percussion, and vibration increase the volume of sputum expectorated, increase the clearance of secretions, decrease airway resistance, increase lung compliance, decrease work used for breathing, increase oxygenation and ventilation, and decrease hospitalization and the number of postoperative pulmonary complications.
- Cough techniques evoke a reflex cough, decrease the risk of cough complications, and diminish retained secretions.
- Exercise conditioning increases endurance and duration of activity.
- TENS decreases pain medication and increases forced vital capacity.

PRECAUTIONS/CONTRAINDICATIONS
- Stop exercise if the following phenomena occur: premature ventricular contraction (coupled, several, or in increased frequency), atrial dysrhythmias, heart block (second- or third-degree), changes in ST-segment (greater than 2 mm), decline in heart rate or blood pressure or heart rate greater than target, increase in diastolic pressure greater than 20 mm Hg, dyspnea, nausea, fatigue, dizziness, headache, blurred vision, palor, or diaphoresis.
- TENS may possibly lead to electrocardiogram (ECG) or pacemaker interference.

DESIRED OUTCOME/PROGNOSIS

- The client will improve ventilation.
- The client will increase oxygenation and decrease oxygen consumption.
- The client will increase secretion clearance.
- The client will increase exercise tolerance.
- The client will experience a decrease in pain.

REFERENCES

Assessment

American Physical Therapy Association. Guide to physical therapist practice. 2nd ed. *Phys Ther*. 2001;81.

Brooks D, Wilson L, Kelsey C, et al. Accuracy and reliability of specialized physical therapists in auscultating tape recorded lung sounds. *Physiotherapy Can*. 1993;45:21–24.

Frownfelter D, Dean E. *Principles and Practice of Cardiopulmonary Physical Therapy*. 3rd ed. New York, NY: CV Mosby Co; 1996.

Goodman C, Snyder TE. *Differential Diagnosis in Physical Therapy*. Philadelphia, Pa: WB Saunders Co; 2000.

Hill J, Johansen J, Pedersen S, LaPier TK. Site of measurement and subject position affect chest excursion measurements. *Cardiopulmonary Phys Ther J*. 1997;8:12–17.

Hillegass EA, Sadwsky HS. *Essentials of Cardiopulmonary Physical Therapy*. 2nd ed. Philadelphia, Pa: WB Saunders Co; 2001.

Pasterkamp H, Montgomery M, Wiebicke W, et al. Nomenclature used by health care professionals to describe breath sounds in asthma. *Chest*. 1993;92:346–352.

Rothstein JM, Roy SH, Wolf SL. *The Rehabilitation Specialist's Handbook*. 2nd ed. Philadelphia, Pa: FA Davis Co; 1998.

Singh S. The use of field walking tests for assessment of functional capacity in patients with chronic airways obstruction. *Physiotherapy*. 1992;78:102–104.

Treatment

Boissonnault WG. Prevalence of comorbid conditions, surgeries, and medication use in a physical therapy outpatient population: a multicentered study. *J Orthop Sports Phys Ther*. 1999;29:509–525.

Gallon A. The use of percussion. *Physiotherapy*. 1992;78:2:85–89.

Goodman C, Snyder TE. *Differential Diagnosis in Physical Therapy*. Philadelphia, Pa: WB Saunders Co; 2000.

Irwin S, Tecklin JS. *Cardiopulmonary Physical Therapy*. 3rd ed. St Louis, Mo: CV Mosby Co; 1995.

Jenkins S. Pulmonary rehabilitation. *Physiotherapy Singapore*. 2000;3:106–112.

Krause MW, van Aswegen H, de Wet E H. Postural drainage in intubated patients with acute lobar atelectasis: A pilot study. *S Afr J Physiotherapy*. 2000;56:29–32.

Piper A, Willson G. Nocturnal nasal ventilatory support in the management of daytime hypercapic respiratory failure. *Aust J Physiotherapy*. 1996;42:17–29.

Smith MCL, Ellis ER. Is retained mucus a risk factor for the development of postoperative atelectasis and pneumonia? Implications for the physiotherapist. 2000;16:69–80.

Zadai CC. *Pulmonary Management in Physical Therapy*. New York, NY: Churchill Livingstone; 1992.

Chapter 14

Skin Disorders

Burns

DESCRIPTION

Burns cause localized injury to tissues through wound edema, protein denaturation, and diminished intravascular fluid volume. Burns lead to erythema, increased capillary permeability, and cell death. They also lead to systemic, life-threatening problems such as hypovolemic shock, infection, and inhalation injury. After a burn injury, the client has usually suffered many losses, but the most critical to the client is often the loss of former appearance.

Burns are described most precisely by the depth of skin tissue destroyed, although they are also classified by the degree system (see Table 14.1).

CAUSE

Burns are caused by a chemical, electrical, or thermal mechanism of injury. Children aged 1 to 5 are most often burned by scalds from liquids. Home fires account for less than 5% of hospitalizations for burns.

ASSESSMENT

Note: See APTA's Guide to Physical Therapist Practice. 2nd ed. *Physical Therapy.* 2001;81.

Cardiovascular/pulmonary Preferred Practice Patterns: C, E

Integumentary Preferred Practice Patterns: B, C, D, E

AREAS
- History
- Psychological state
- Pain
- Posture
- Extent of burns: degree, percentage of body surface burned
- Mobility, including active and passive range of motion (ROM), including any contractures
- Strength

TABLE 14.1
Classification of Burns

Degree	Description
Superficial (first-degree)	epidermis layer is involved
Partial-thickness (second-degree)	
Superficial	outer level of the dermis is involved
Deep	much of the dermis is involved, and there may be alteration in hair follicles and sweat glands
Full-thickness (third-degree)	all of the dermis has been burned
Subdermal (fourth-degree)	all of the tissue from the epidermis to and through the subcutaneous tissue is destroyed. This may include muscle and bone.

- Pulmonary, including any inhalation injury
- Neurological, including sensation
- Functional level, including activities of daily living (ADLs), transfers
- Gait, if indicated

INSTRUMENTS/PROCEDURES

Extent of Burns
- Lund-Browder charts for estimating areas
- Rule of nines
- Vancouver Burn Scar Assessment Scale

Functional Level
- Barthel index
- PULSES profile

Strength
- manual muscle testing (only appropriate to areas not burned)
- voluntary motion

PROBLEMS
- The client has often suffered many losses, but the most critical to the client is often the loss of former appearance.
- The client will have pain.
- The client may show signs of shock.
- There may be infection.
- The client may have pulmonary injury.
- The client often has metabolic complications.
- The client may suffer kidney damage.
- The client may have circulatory problems due to the physiological changes post burn.

TREATMENT/MANAGEMENT

EMERGENT PHASE (FIRST 72 HOURS AFTER INJURY)
- Physical therapy is primarily concerned with positioning to maintain proper length as the burn heals and to assist with control of edema through elevation.
- Begin active ROM exercises as soon as the client is able to tolerate them; these can be combined with hydrotherapy sessions. It is usually beneficial to have clients medicated for pain in preparation for the session.
- Clients with extensive burns will need breathing exercises.

ACUTE PHASE
- Assess for the need for splints or positioning devices.
- Monitor skin for areas of increased pressure. Use of special beds/mattresses can assist in prevention of pressure points.
- Elevate any burned extremities.
- Provide wound care with whirlpool (containing a chemical agent) and mechanical debridement if indicated, typically for 20 minutes. Sussman reports burns and wounds have a similar management and that the key components of management relate to depth of tissue injury, and the presence of necrosis, edema, and infection (see pressure ulcers for more details on wound care).
- Debridement is followed by wound dressing with topical agents, if indicated.
- Continue active and functional exercise, but switch to passive exercise if the client is unable to perform active exercise.
- The skin should blanch if a stretch is applied to the area.

- Use adaptive equipment as indicated. Consult with the occupational therapist as needed.
- Exercise is usually contraindicated after skin grafting for 3 to 7 days, or 7 to 10 days after a cultured epithelial autograft. Assess for postoperative splinting.
- Ambulate as soon as possible. Consult with surgeon before ambulating post skin grafting in lower extremities. See Precautions for contraindications. Proper dressing and elastic support are needed if the client has burns on the lower extremities. Use protective and assistive devices as indicated.
- Consider use of a tilt table if the client has postural hypotension.

LONG-TERM REHABILITATION PHASE

Select exercise and stretching appropriate to the client's needs, ranging from passive to resistive. Consider use of continuous passive machines, isokinetic exercise, aquatics, proprioceptive neuromuscular facilitation patterns, open- or closed-chain exercise, and functional activities. Prescribe a conditioning program and advice on use of equipment such as a stationary bicycle, a treadmill, and free-standing weights.

- Assess for use of serial splinting, casting, or dynamic splinting to avoid contractures.
- Educate the client about scar management through use of pressure therapy via appliances or garments. An ideal pressure of 25 mm Hg is recommended. Garments are usually worn 23 hours a day for over a year. Scar management equipment should be fitted by experienced personnel and can include light dressings, elastic pressure devices, gloves, stockings, and clothing with a high-pressure component such as bicycle shorts and custom garments.
- Scar massage, especially deep friction massage, may be used to mobilize scar tissue.
- Referral to a support group, such as the Phoenix Society, is recommended.
- Referral to a cosmetologist who specializes in corrective makeup can be helpful for some clients, especially women with facial burns.
- Establish a discharge plan, including a home exercise program of exercise, skin care, and use of pressure garments and splints. Use of written materials and/or videotapes may be helpful.

Physical therapy may be continued on an outpatient basis:

1. Continue exercise: ROM, strengthening, and conditioning.
2. Monitor the use of pressure garments and splints.
3. Provide modalities such as paraffin for scar tissue softening and ROM.
4. Educate the client about edema prevention and skin care.
5. Provide gait training as indicated.
6. Treat associated injuries.
7. Assist in preparation to return to work, such as work tolerance screening, job analysis, and work hardening.

PRECAUTIONS/CONTRAINDICATIONS

Note: Clients with diabetes prior to the burn are at higher risk for metabolic complications.

- Mechanical debridement should not cause bleeding.
- Avoid side effects of improper positioning:
  1. Prolonged use of a lower extremity position with hips abducted and externally rotated, knees in flexion, and ankles inverted with plantar flexion can result in peroneal nerve stretch with weakness of dorsiflexors.
  2. Avoid prolonged use of shoulder abduction of more than 90 degrees to prevent brachial plexus stretch.

3. Avoid pressure on the ulnar nerve at the cubital space in the elbow.
4. Avoid prolonged stretch to exposed tendon until the wound is sufficiently healed.

- Splints should not leave any pressure points.
- Monitor vital signs during initial endurance activities.
- Minimize hand contact with burned area due to pain.
- For clients with recent skin grafting, exercise is usually contraindicated after grafting for 3 to 7 days.
- Do not use direct heat. Caution client to use proper skin care protection when in the sun.

Contraindications to ambulation post burn include the following:

- cellulitis or thrombophlebitis
- fractures
- lower extremity tendon damage
- burned weight-bearing surface on soles of feet
- medically unstable condition, such as very low hemoglobin or severe burn wounds

DESIRED OUTCOME/PROGNOSIS

ACUTE PHASE
- The client will avoid infection.
- The client will have a decrease in scarring and contracture.
- Therapy will facilitate healing and protect tissue.
- The client will maintain strength and endurance.
- Therapy will prevent pulmonary complications.
- The client will remain active.

LONG-TERM PHASE OF REHABILITATION
- The client will be independent in self-care and transfers and ambulation.
- The client will have normal strength.
- The client will be independent in a home exercise program.
- Pressure therapy will provide control of hypertrophic scarring.
- The client will be competent in skin care.
- The client will resume functioning in life.

Notes: Scars continue to mature for 1 to 2 years after initial wound healing. At maturation, the scar should no longer appear inflamed but should have a faded appearance. It is advisable for the client to use pressure garments until the scar matures.

Long-term recovery depends heavily on a client's compliance with the home program. Adjustment to alterations in appearance due to the burn usually takes much time and support.

In all phases of treatment, 2 key components for success are team approach and education.

REFERENCES

Assessment

American Physical Therapy Association. Guide to physical therapist practice. 2nd ed. *Phys Ther.* 2001;81.

Brandsma JW. Development of a uniform record for patients with burns of the hand. *J Hand Ther.* 1999;12:333–336.

Grabois M, Garrison SJ, Hart KA, Lehmkuhl LD. *Physical Medicine and Rehabilitation: The Complete Approach.* Malden, Mass: Blackwell Science; 2000.

Keck TL, Jones JL, Yowler CJ, Yurko L, et al. Physical therapy acute burn evaluation tool. *J Burn Care Rehabil.* 1999;20:321–324.

Rothstein JM, Roy SH, Wolf SL. *The Rehabilitation Specialist's Handbook.* Philadelphia, Pa: FA Davis Co; 1998.

Silverberg R, Lombardo G, Gorga D, et al. Gait variables of patients after lower extremity burn injuries. *J Burn Care Rehabil.* 2000;21:259–267.

Treatment

Ang ES, Tan KC. Full-thickness of the palm caused by hot wax. *Burns.* 1997;23:458–459.

Bahnof R. Intra-oral burns: rehabilitation of severe restriction of mouth opening: case report. *Physiotherapy.* 2000;86:263–266.

Biggs KS. Determining the current roles of physical and occupational therapists in burn care. *J Burn Care Rehabil.* 1998;19:442–449.

Byl N, Zellerbach LR, Pfalzer LA. Systemic issues and skin conditions: wound healing, oxygen percutaneous drug delivery, burns, and desensitized skin. In: Myers RS, ed. *Saunders Manual of Physical Therapy Practice.* Philadelphia, Pa: WB Saunders Co; 1995:610.

Chang JK. Assistive devices in the rehabilitation of patients with electrical burns—three case reports. *J Burn Care Rehabil.* 2001;22:90–96.

Demling RH, DeSanti L. Increased protein intake during the recovery phase after severe burns increases body weight gain and muscle function. *J Burn Care Rehabil.* 1998;19: 161–168.

Dobbs ER. Burn therapy of years ago. *J Burn Care Rehabil.* 1999;20:62–66.

Keilty SEJ. Inhalation burn injured patients and physiotherapy management. *Physiotherapy.* 1993;79:87–90.

Luce EA. The acute and subacute management of the burned hand. *Clin Plast Surg.* 2000; 27:49–63.

Marquez RR. Acute care of the adult burn patient. *Phys Ther Pract.* 1994;3:37–61.

Nussbaum E. The influence of ultrasound on healing tissues. *J Hand Ther.* 1998;11:140–147.

Patina O, Novick C, Merlo A, Benaim F. Massage in hypertrophic scars. *J Burn Care Rehabil.* 1999;268–271.

Phillips BJ, Kassir A, Anderson B, et al. Recreational-outdoor burns: the impact and severity—a retrospective review of 107 patients. *Burns.* 1998;6:559–561.

Richard RL, Staley MJ. *Burn Care and Rehabilitation: Principles and Practice.* Philadelphia, Pa: FA Davis Co; 1994.

Richards AM, Klaassen MF. Heterotopic ossification after severe burns: a report of three cases and review of the literature. *Burns.* 1997;23:64–68.

Serghiou M, Staley M. Proceedings of the physical and occupational therapy special interest group meeting. *J Burn Care Rehabil.* 1998;19:147–150.

Silverberg R, Johnson J, Moffat M. The effects of soft tissue mobilization on the immature burn scar; results of a pilot study. *J Burn Care Rehabil.* 1996;17:252–259.

Staley M. Casting guidelines, tips, and techniques: proceedings from the 1997 American Burn Association PT/OT casting workshop. *J Burn Care Rehabil.* 1997;254–260.

Staley M, Richard R. The elderly patient with burns: treatment considerations. *J Burn Care Rehabil.* 1993;14:559–565.

Staley M, Richard R, et al. Functional outcomes for the patient with burn injuries. *J Burn Care Rehabil.* 1996;17:362–367.

Staley M, Richard RL, Falkel JE. Burns. In: O'Sullivan SB, Schmitz TJ, eds. *Physical Rehabilitation.* 3rd ed. Philadelphia, Pa: FA Davis Co; 1994;509–532.

Sussman C, Bates-Jensen BM. *Wound Care. A Collaborative Practice Manual for Physical Therapists and Nurses.* Gaithersburg, Md: Aspen Publishers; 1998.

Tilley W, McMahon S, Shukalak B. Rehabilitation of the burned upper extremity. *Hand Clin.* 2000:16:303–318.

Van Zuijlen PP, Kreis RW, Vloemans AF, et al. The prognostic factors regarding long-term functional outcome of full-thickness hand burns. *Burns.* 1999;25:709–714.

Ward RS. Reasons for the selection of burn-scar support suppliers by burn centers in the United States: a survey. *J Burn Care Rehabil.* 1993;14:360–367.

Ward RS, Hayes-Lundy C, Reddy R, et al. Influence of pressure supports on joint range of motion. *Burns.* 1992;18:60–62.

Ward RS, Hayes-Lundy C, Reddy R, et al. Evaluation of topical therapeutic ultrasound to improve response to physical therapy and lessen scar contracture after burn injury. *J Burn Care Rehabil.* 1994;15:74–79.

Wetzel JL, Giuffrida C, Petrazzi A, et al. Comparison of measures of physiologic stress during treadmill exercise in a patient with 205 lower extremity burn injuries and healthy matched and non-matched individuals. *J Burn Care Rehabil.* 2000;21:359–366.

Woo SH. Optimizing the correction of severe postburn hand deformities by using aggressive contracture releases and fascioucutaneous free-tissue transfers. *Plast Reconstr Surg.* 2001;107:1–8.

Pressure Ulcers

Also known as *decubitus ulcers, pressure sores,* or *bedsores.*

DESCRIPTION

A pressure ulcer is an area of ulcerated tissue with exudate and ischemic necrosis. Sores typically occur in tissue that covers a bony prominence that has been exposed to prolonged pressure from lying in bed or pressure from a cast, splint, bed, or wheelchair. Clients who are paralyzed or debilitated or who have desensitized skin are especially vulnerable to injury. Pressure sores can increase the length of hospitalization, interfere with rehabilitation, and lead to amputation. In extremes cases, a pressure sore can be life threatening. Pressure ulcers are commonly located in the area of bony prominences such as the occiput, scapulae, olecranon, sacrum, trochanter, malleolus, heel, and metatarsals.

CAUSE

Pressure sores may be triggered by intrinsic or extrinsic factors. Intrinsic factors include diminished sense of pain and pressure, loss of tissue, disuse atrophy, malnutrition, infection, fever, spasticity, and loss of vasomotor control. Of extrinsic factors, pressure is the primary risk factor due to interruption of local circulation, lack of changing position due to immobility, friction, wrinkles in clothing or bedding, or moisture leading to maceration of the skin.

ASSESSMENT

Note: See APTA's Guide to Physical Therapist Practice. 2nd ed. *Physical Therapy.* 2001;81.

Integumentary Preferred Practice Patterns: A, C, E

Musculoskeletal Preferred Practice Patterns: D, K

AREAS
- History
- Skin surrounding wound, including cleanliness, color, dryness, edema, elasticity, moisture and temperature changes, hair growth patterns, nail beds, sensation
- Abnormal skin response, including blanching, pressure marks or areas, presence of pressure sores
- Grade/status of wound (see Table 14.2), including wound location, color, size and dimensions, and presence of any drainage, foul odor, tunneling, or wound contraction.
- Functional level

INSTRUMENTS/PROCEDURES
Edema
- girth measurements and volumetric edema measurement
- palpation grading system

Infection
- culture

Pain
- questionnaires
- visual analog scale
- pain diary

Sensation
- Semmes-Weinstein monofilaments for protective sensation (lower than 5.07 level)

Size and depth measurements
- clock technique
- wound stick tunnels
- wound stick wand
- wound tracings
- overall undermined estimated size
- wound assessment graphs
- wound photography

TABLE 14.2
Grades of Pressure Sores

Grade	Description
1	Limited to superficial epidermis and dermal layers
2	Involves the epidermal and dermal layers and extends into the adipose tissue
3	Extends through the superficial structures and adipose tissue down to and including muscle
4	Destroys all soft tissue structures down to bone, with communication with bone or joint structures or both

Source: Reprinted courtesy of the National Spinal Cord Injury Association. Thorofare, NJ.

Temperature
- thermistor
- liquid crystal thermography
- infrared scanner
- skin fever thermometer

Vascular condition
- laser doppler
- transcutaneous partial pressure of oxygen level (tcpO2)
- ankle-brachial index
- pulse exam (0 to 4+)
- digital plethysmography

Risk Assessment Scales
- Norton Scale
- The Braden Scale
- Pressure Sore Status Tool (PSST)

Scales
- The Sussman Wound Healing Tool (SWHT)
- Sessing scale
- Pressure Ulcer Scale for Healing (PUSH)
- Wound Healing Scale (WHS)
- The National Pressure Ulcer Advisory Panel (NPUAP)
- Wagner Ulcer Grade Classification system
- partial thickness/full-thickness skin loss criteria
- Marion Laboratories system of classification by color
- edema severity scale (0 to 3+)

PROBLEMS
- The client has an area of skin ulceration with exudate and necrosis.
- Pressure sores can eventually affect muscle and bone.

Characteristics of arterial disease include the following symptoms: Pain (walking and/or at rest), foot cool or cold, weak or absent pulses, absence of leg hair, shin shiny, dry, pale, thickened toenails, ulcer location usually below ankle (pressure areas, toes), ulcer necrotic with minimal drainage, Ankle-brachial index less than 0.5 (if diabetic, can be greater than 1.0), elevation pallor/dependent rubor, history of diabetes, hypertension, smoking, claudication, history of foot trauma.

Characteristics of venous disease include the following symptoms: Foot warm, edema, brawny skin pigment changes, varicose veins, ulcer location usually above ankle (medial malleolus), venous ulcers generally not painful, ulcer granulating, drainage, ABI greater than 1.0, history of trauma, deep vein thrombosis, varicose veins, malignancy.

TREATMENT/MANAGEMENT
- Prevention is critical. Instruct client and caregivers in abnormal skin responses to identify early changes.
- Perform daily skin inspection regularly, such as when bathing, dressing, and undressing, after using toilet, and after transfers.
- Check main pressure points, including areas where cast, brace, or clothing may rub. Use dorsum of hand or mirror to assist in areas hard to see.
- Use positioning, turning, and pressure-relieving devices and wound care if a sore develops. Avoid smoking and promote optimal nutrition.

TREATMENT OF PRESSURE SORES

- Debridement interventions include autolytic, enzymatic, mechanical, and sharp and will depend the type and amount of necrotic tissue involved.
- For edema control, consider the use of gentle exercise, elevation of limb, compressions therapy, bandaging (tubular/paste, multi-layer), graduated compression stockings, compression pump therapy.
- Dressings for wound care may include film dressing, foam dressings, hydrogel products, dyrocolloids, alginates, hydroactive dressings depending on the color, depth, and exudate.
- Use topical therapy debridement and dressing technique for pressure sores, grade III or grade IV, a minimum of twice daily.
- Consider use of whirlpool, hyperbaric oxygen, electrical stimulation, and laser therapy.

AHCPR RECOMMENDED GUIDELINES FOR PRESSURE ULCER CLEANSING*

- Cleanse wound initially and at each dressing change.
- Use minimal mechanical force when cleansing ulcer with gauze, cloth, or sponges.
- Do not clean wounds with skin cleansers or antiseptic agents (providone-iodine, sodium hypochlorite solution, hydrogen peroxide, and acetic acid).
- Use normal saline for cleansing most ulcers.
- Use enough irrigation pressure to enhance wound cleansing without causing trauma to the wound bed. Safe and effective ulcer irrigation pressures range from 40 to 15 psi.
- Consider whirlpool treatment for cleansing ulcers that contain thick exudate, slough, or necrotic tissue. Discontinue whirlpool when ulcer is clean.
- Immobility can be countered with pressure relieving devices, frequent repositioning either actively or passively by caregiver. Key areas to cushion include under the legs to raise the heels, between the ankles and knees, behind back, and under the head.
- Consider the use of the following physical agents for tissue repair: diathermy, electrical stimulation, pulsed radio frequency stimulation, pulsed short wave diathermy, ultrasound. Ideally, the first 72 hours post injury is the optimal time to begin intervention.

PRECAUTIONS/CONTRAINDICATIONS

The client should be referred to a vascular surgeon or lab if there is:

- ABI > 1.0 or <0.5
- TcpO2> 30 mm Hg
- Gangrene
- Exposed bony or tendinous structures
- Cellulitis
- Nonhealing wound

Debridement is contraindicated in arterial/ischemic ulcer unless there is sufficient circulation.

Donut type ring cushions are contraindicated because they can actually lead to increased pressure and edema via venous congestion.

---

* Source: AHCPR Guidelines. Bergstrom N, Bennett MA, Carlson CE, et al. *Treatment of Pressure Ulcers.* Clinical Practice Guideline No. 15, December 1994, U.S. Department of Health and Human Services, Public Health Service Agency for Health Care Policy and Research, AHCPR Publication No. 95-0652.

DESIRED OUTCOME/PROGNOSIS

Healing progresses through the phases of wound healing which include inflammation, proliferation and epitheliazation. Sussman lists 12 possible wound healing phase diagnoses to label impairments in wound healing: chronic inflammation, inflammation, absence of inflammation, chronic proliferation, proliferation, absence of proliferation, chronic epithelialization, epithelialization, absence of epithelialization, chronic remodeling, remodeling, and absence of remodeling. Prognosis generally includes progression from an impaired phase of repair to a more advanced phase of repair. This progression results in a wound that is minimally, acceptable, or ideally healed. The client will experience healing of pressure sore. Normal wound healing takes 3–4 weeks. However, a pressure sore may take up to a year to heal.

REFERENCES

Assessment

American Physical Therapy Association. Guide to physical therapist practice. 2nd ed. *Phys Ther*. 2001;81.

AHCPR Guidelines. Bergstrom N, Bennett MA, Carlson CE, et al. *Treatment of Pressure Ulcers*. Clinical Practice Guideline No. 15, December 1994, U.S. Department of Health and Human Services, Public Health Service Agency for Health Care Policy and Research, AHCPR Publication No. 95–0652.

Bates-Jensen BM. Indices to include in wound healing assessment. *Adv Wound Care*. 1995; 8:25–33.

Bergstrom N, Braden B. A prospective study of pressure sore risk among institutionalized elderly. *J Am Geriatr Soc*. 1992;40:747–758.

Ferrell BA, Artinian BM, Sessing D. The Sessing scale for assessment of pressure ulcer healing. *J Am Geriatr Soc*. 1995;43:37–40.

Grabois M, Garrison SJ, Hart KA, Lehmkuhl LD. *Physical Medicine and Rehabilitation: The Complete Approach*. Malden, Mass: Blackwell Science; 2000.

Maklebust J. Pressure ulcer staging systems: NPUAP proceedings. *Adv Wound Care*. 1995; 8:1–14.

Myers RS, ed. *Saunders Manual of Physical Therapy Practice*. Philadelphia, Pa: WB Saunders Co; 1995.

Sussman C, Bates-Jensen BM. *Wound Care: A Collaborative Practice Manual for Physical Therapists and Nurses*. Gaithersburg, Md: Aspen Publishers; 1998.

Sussman C, Swanson G. The utility of Sussman wound Healing Tool in predicting wound healing outcomes in physical therapy. *Adv Wound Care*. 1997;10:74–77.

Wagner FW. The dysvascular foot: a system for diagnosis and treatment. *Foot and Ankle*. 1981;64:122.

Treatment

Albeln S. Reporting risk check-up. *PT Magazine*. October 1997;5:38.

Bergstrom N, Bennett MA, Carlson CE, et al. *Treatment of Pressure Ulcers*. Clinical Practice Guideline No. 15, December, 1994, U.S. Department of Health and Human Services, Public Health Service, Agency for Health Care Policy and Research, AHCPR Publication No. 95–0652.

Burke DT, Ho CH, Saucier MA, Stewart G. Effects of hydrotherapy on pressure ulcer healing. *Am J Phys Med Rehabil.* 1998;77:394–398.

Burks RI. Providone-iodine solution in wound treatment. *Phys Ther.* 1998;78:212–218.

Byl N, McKenzie A, Stern R, et al. Amniotic fluid modulates wound healing. *Eur J Rehabil Med.* 1993;2184–190.

Byl N, McKenzie A, et al. Pulsed micro amperage stimulation: a controlled study of healing of surgically induced wounds in Yucatan pigs. *Phys Ther.* 1994;74:201–218.

Byl N, Zellerbach LR, Pfalzer LA. Systemic issues and skin conditions: wound healing, oxygen percutaneous drug delivery, burns, and desensitized skin. In: Myers RS, ed. *Saunders Manual of Physical Therapy Practice.* Philadelphia, Pa: WB Saunders Co; 1995: 619.

Dean E. Oxygen transport deficits in systemic disease and implications for physical therapy. *Phys Ther.* 1997;77:187–202.

Feedar JA. Pressure sores. *Top Geriatr Rehabil.* 1994;9:4:1–16;35–82.

Feedar JA. Wound evaluation and treatment planning. *Top Geriatr Rehabil.* 1994;9:4:35–42.

Fitzgerald GK, Newsome D. Treatment of a large infected thoracic spine wound using high voltage pulsed monophasic current. *Phys Ther.* 1993;73:355–360.

Gogia PP. *Clinical Wound Management.* Thorofare, NJ: Slack Inc; 1995.

Gogia PP. Physical therapy modalities for wound management. *Ostomy Wound Manage.* 1996;42:46–48.

Grabois M, Garrison SJ, Hart KA, Lehmkuhl LD. *Physical Medicine and Rehabilitation: The Complete Approach.* Malden, Mass: Blackwell Science; 2000.

Hudson KD, Long L. Management of chronic venous ulcers. *Phys Ther Case Rep.* 2000;3: 45–56.

Kalinowski DP, Brogan MS, Sleeper MD. A practical technique for disinfecting electrical stimulation apparatuses used in wound treatment. *Phys Ther.* 1996;12:1340–1347.

Kierney PC, Engrav LH, Isik FF, Esselman PC, et al. Results of 268 pressure sores in 158 patients managed jointly by plastic surgery and rehabilitation medicine. *Plast Reconstr Surg.* 1998;102:765–772.

Klyscz T, Ritter-Schempp C, Junger M, Rassner B. Biomechanical stimulation therapy as physical treatment of arthrogenic venous insufficiency. *Hautarzt.* 1997;48:318–322.

Manser S, Boeker C. Seating considerations: spinal cord injury. *PT Magazine.* December 1993;47–51.

McCulloch J. Health and wound care in The Netherlands. *Ostomy Wound Manage.* 2000; 46:25–27.

McCulloch J, Kloth L. Wound care management. *Rehabil Manage.* 1997;10:46–58.

McCulloch JM. The role of physiotherapy in managing patients with wounds. *J Wound Care.* 1998;7:241–244.

McCulloch JM, Kloth L, Feedar JA. *Wound Healing: Alternatives in Management.* 2nd ed. Philadelphia, Pa: FA Davis Co; 1995.

Mosher BA, Cuddigan J, Thomas DR, et al. Outcomes of four methods of debridement using a decision analysis methodology. *Adv Wound Care.* 1999;12:81–88.

Myer AH. Exploring a new path toward global understanding of wound care. *Ostomy Wound Manage.* 1999;45:22–26.

National Report of Subacure Care. Court enjoins HCFA from enforcing non-coverage decision on electrical stimulation for wound care. *National Report of Subacure Care.* 1997;10:1–3.

Rappl L. A conservative treatment for pressure ulcers. *Ostomy Wound Manage.* 1993;39: 722–725.

Sparks B. Collaboration in wound care: a nursing and physical therapy team approach. *Ostomy Wound Manage.* 1996;42:94.

Sussman C. *Ultrasound for Wound Healing: A Monograph.* Chattanooga, Tenn: Chattanooga Corp; 1994.

Sussman C, Bates-Jensen BM. Wound Care. *A Collaborative Practice Manual for Physical Therapists and Nurses.* Gaithersburg, Md: Aspen Publishers;1998.

Sussman C, Swanson G. Utility of the Sussman Wound Healing Tool in predicting wound healing outcomes in physical therapy. *Adv Wound Care.* 1997;10:74–77.

Chapter 15

Women's Health Disorders

Dysmenorrhea

Also known as *primary dysmenorrhea* or *functional dysmenorrhea*.

DESCRIPTION

Dysmenorrhea is painful menstruation. Primary dysmenorrhea is defined as pain that accompanies the menstrual cycle. The pain is typically felt in the lower abdomen and lower back during the early stages of a cycle. Pain usually decreases with an increase in blood flow. Secondary dysmenorrhea is painful menstruation caused by pathology.

CAUSE

Primary dysmenorrhea is thought to be caused by ischemia from uterine contractions and the release of the hormone prostaglandin. It may also be caused by hypertonicity in the uterine isthmus, leading to increased pressure and pain. Anxiety, lack of exercise, extrusion of tissue through the cervix, especially with a narrow cervical opening, or a malpositioned uterus can exacerbate the pain.

Secondary dysmenorrhea is caused by an abnormality or pathology such as endometriosis, adenomyosis, fibroids, pelvic cysts or tumors, and pelvic inflammatory disease.

ASSESSMENT

Note: See APTA's Guide to Physical Therapist Practice. 2nd ed. *Physical Therapy.* 2001;81.

AREAS
- History, including general health
- Pain
- Posture, including the effect of position on pain
- Strength, including pelvic floor muscle strength, if indicated

INSTRUMENTS/PROCEDURES

See References for sources.

Pain
- body diagram
- Numeric Pain Rating Scale
- visual analog scale

Special Tests to Which the Physical Therapist May or May Not Have Access
- breast exam
- examination of perineum, vagina, and cervix
- cervical cytology
- bimanual pelvic exam
- urinalysis

PROBLEMS
- The client often has cramping in the abdominal region.
- The client may have low back pain and pain may refer down the leg.
- The client often reports premenstrual tension.
- The client may also experience nausea, vomiting, or fainting.

TREATMENT/MANAGEMENT
- Consider use of modalities for pain such as transcutaneous electrical nerve stimulation (TENS) or interferential current.

- Try TENS with a conventional mode first, and then adjust parameters as indicated. Electrode placement effectiveness varies. One regimen suggests placement posteriorly at the level of uterine innervation, T10-L1, or anterolaterally, in suprapubic region of abdomen, between umbilicus and anterosuperior iliac spine. An additional option for electrode placement is at accupressure point spleen 6 and spleen 10. Over large areas of pain, additional electrodes have been used.
- With interferential current, the use of 2 electrodes of 100 cm2 placed anteriorly and 2 electrodes of 200 cm2 placed posteriorly is suggested. Intensity varies with client tolerance, with treatment duration of 15 to 20 minutes daily or on alternate days. Rhythmical frequency at 90 to 100 Hz has been suggested.
- Consider use of shortwave diathermy or superficial heat.
- Teach relaxation techniques or distraction techniques.
- Encourage vigorous exercise.
- Recommend specific exercises. The pelvic tilt may offer some relief, especially for a woman who has a retroverted uterus.
- Positioning and stretching should also be addressed; a supine position with knees flexed against the chest with a 10-second hold can offer relief. Leaning forward toward a wall can assist a stretch of the abdominal area that some women find beneficial.
- Soft tissue mobilization techniques, such as myofascial release, can also be used for dysmenorrhea and endometriosis.

PRECAUTIONS/CONTRAINDICATIONS

- Pain due to secondary dysmenorrhea may increase with activity.

DESIRED OUTCOME/PROGNOSIS

- The client will experience a reduction in pain and tension.
- There will be increased circulation to the abdominal region.
- The pain can diminish with age and after pregnancy.

Note: Dysmenorrhea is one of the of the main reasons given for a hysterectomy. The physical therapist can offer a woman the option of conservative treatment, thus possibly avoiding surgery.

REFERENCES

Assessment

American Physical Therapy Association. Guide to physical therapist practice. 2nd ed. *Phys Ther.* 2001;81.

King PM, Ling FW, Myers CA. Screening for female urogenital system disease. In: Boissonnault WG, ed. *Examination in Physical Therapy Practice—Screening for Medical Disease.* 2nd ed. New York, NY; 1995.

Treatment

Adams C, Frahm J. Genitourinary System. In: Myers RS, ed. *Saunders Manual of Physical Therapy Practice.* Philadelphia, Pa: WB Saunders Co; 1995:459–504.

Anonymous. Considering DM for women's health? Dysfunctional uterine bleeding a good place to start. *Healthcare Demand and Disease Management.* 1999;5:170–173.

Beal MW. Acupuncture and acupressure. Application to women's reproductive health care. *J Nurse Midwifery.* 1999;44:217–230.

Headley BJ. Chronic pain management. In: O'Sullivan SB, Schmitz TJ. *Phys Rehabil.* 3rd ed. Philadelphia, Pa: FA Davis Co; 1994:577–602.

Kaplan B, Peled Y, Pardo, et al. Transcutaneous electrical nerve stimulation (TENS) as a relief for dysmenorrhea. *Clin Exp Obstet Gynecol.* 1994;21:87–90.

Kokjohn K, Schmid DM, Triano JJ, et al. The effect of spinal manipulation on pain and prostaglandin levels in women with primary dysmenorrhea. *J Manipulative Physiol Ther.* 1992;15:279–285.

LeRida Ortega MA, Platero RD, Pone Castro J, et al. Rehabilitation of primary dysmenorrhea. *Rehabil.* 1999;33:335–338.

Mathias SD, Kuppermann M, Liberman RF, et al. Chronic pelvic pain: prevalence, health-related quality of life and economic correlates. *Obstet Gynecol.* 1996;87:321–327.

Milsom I, Hedner M, Mannheimer C. A comparative study of the effect of high-intensity transcutaneous nerve stimulation and oral naproxen on intrauterine pressure and menstrual pain in patients with primary dysmenorrhea. *Am J Obstet Gynecol.* 1994; 170:123–129.

Pauls J. Hysterectomy. In: Pauls J, *Therapeutic Approaches to Women's Health: A Program of Exercise and Education.* Gaithersburg, Md: Aspen Publishers; 1995:7–2:1–7.

Sapsford R, Bullock-Saxton J, Markwell S. *Women's Health: A Textbook for Physiotherapists.* Philadelphia, Pa: WB Saunders Co; 1999.

Stephenson RG, O'Connor LJ. *Obstetric and Gynecologic Care in Physical Therapy.* 2nd ed. Thorofare, NJ: Slack Inc; 2000.

Ushokova OE, Davydova PB, Iarustovskaia PV, et al. The effect of contrast baths on central nervous system function in patients with a disordered menstrual function. *Vopr Kurotol Fizioter Lech Fiz Kult.* 1997; Jul–Aug:25–27.

Vance AR, Hayes SH, Spielhlz NI. Microwave diathermy treatment for primary dysmenorrhea. *Phys Ther.* 1996;76:1003–1008.

Wilder E, ed. *The Gynecological Manual.* Section on Women's Health. Alexandra, Va: American Physical Therapy Association; 1997.

High-Risk Pregnancy

DESCRIPTION

In a high-risk pregnancy, there is an increased chance of morbidity or mortality for either the mother or the baby. Reportedly, as many as 25% of pregnant women can be included in the category of high-risk pregnancy.

CAUSE

Inherent risk factors include maternal age of 16 or below or maternal age of above 35, prepregnancy weight below 100 pounds, inadequate weight gain, maternal obesity, and height below 5 feet.

Risk factors related to obstetrical history or medical conditions are numerous and carry differing levels of risk. Some of the more frequently encountered problems are disseminated intravascular coagulation, gestational diabetes, hydraminos, hypertensive disorders, intrauterine growth retardation, incompetent cervix, multifetal gestation, oligohydramnios, placenta abruptio or placenta previa, preterm labor, and premature rupture of membranes.

Preexisting medical problems such as cardiac or respiratory abnormalities or diabetes can make an otherwise normal pregnancy complicated.

ASSESSMENT

Note: See APTA's Guide to Physical Therapist Practice. 2nd ed. *Physical Therapy.* 2001;81.

Cardiovascular/Pulmonary Preferred Practice Pattern: B

AREAS
- History, including detailed obstetrical and medical history
- Vital signs at rest and with activity
- Skin and soft tissue, including edema, if indicated, using volumetrics and girth
- Strength, including voluntary movement; do not perform resistive testing
- Cardiovascular, including endurance
- Mobility, including range of motion (ROM)
- Gait, if ambulatory
- Functional level; including activities of daily living (ADLs), bed mobility, and transfers

INSTRUMENTS/PROCEDURES

See References for sources.
- Algorithm for physical therapy decisions for high-risk pregnancy

PROBLEMS
- The client is often on restricted activity level; often on bed rest.
- Bed rest may lead to depression about being confined.
- Deconditioning occurs secondary to bed rest.
- The client may have blood pressure irregularities.
- The client may have premature contractions in excessive numbers.
- The client often has musculoskeletal problems.
- The client often has decreased independence in ADLs.
- The client may have increased intra-abdominal pressure during ADLs.

TREATMENT/MANAGEMENT

GENERAL GUIDELINES

When individualizing the treatment plan, include the following:
- Consider the primary diagnosis and secondary diagnoses and preexisting conditions of the patient which might lead to contraindications.
- Avoid any increased intra-abdominal pressure through straining or Valsalva maneuver.
- Teach the client relaxation techniques.
- Instruct the client in proper positioning and body mechanics for comfort and to enhance circulation.
- Consider the use of aquatic therapy for the benefit that hydrostatic pressure brings to a pregnant woman.
- Provide a list of resources and literature for the client.

UPPER EXTREMITIES
- Establish an exercise program for the upper extremities.
- Upper extremity exercises may include biceps, triceps, deltoids, and rotator cuff musculature.
- Consider use of devices such as Theraband or Theratubing. Use light weights as tolerated if no complications arise.
- Monitor for signs to stop exercise, such as dizziness, overfatigue, dyspnea, or increase in contractions.

LOWER EXTREMITIES
- Assess the client's response to exercise carefully.
- Instruct the client in circulatory exercises that include leg exercises (to be done every hour, when awake) to avoid deep-vein thrombosis.
- Consider the use of the following exercises:
  1. ankle circles for circulation
  2. active-assistive, passive, or active exercise as tolerated, without weights or manual resistance
- Consider the use of an aquatic program.

PRECAUTIONS/CONTRAINDICATIONS
- Avoid resistance when testing strength.
- Avoid the Valsalva maneuver and inadvertent breath holding during exercises, especially isometric exercise.
- Avoid stress on the abdominal or pelvic floor muscles.
- Monitor medical status to check for any changes such as an increase in blood pressure, any bleeding or leaking of fluid, and any increase in contractions, especially during or within 30 minutes of the exercise session.
- Avoid the plantar-flexed position at the ankle to avoid a calf cramp.

DESIRED OUTCOME/PROGNOSIS
- The woman will maintain or increase strength while on a restricted activity level.
- The woman will avoid an increase in intra-abdominal pressure or increased strain during ADLs.
- The woman will minimize the physiological effects of bed rest.
- The woman will maintain optimal uterine blood flow.
- There will be increased venous return to prevent thrombosis.
- There will be diminished stress and an increased sense of control.
- The woman will reduce musculoskeletal problems associated with pregnancy.
- The woman will prepare for optimal postpartum recovery.

REFERENCES

Assessment

American Physical Therapy Association. Guide to physical therapist practice. 2nd ed. *Phys Ther.* 2001;81.

Appel C. Obstetrical considerations. In: Myers RS, ed. *Saunders Manual of Physical Therapy Practice.* Philadelphia, Pa: WB Saunders Co; 1995:522.

Pauls J. *Therapeutic Approaches to Women's Health: A Program of Exercise and Education.* Gaithersburg, Md: Aspen Publishers; 1995.

Sapsford R, Bullock-Saxton J, Markwell S. *Women's Health: A Textbook for Physiotherapists.* Philadelphia, Pa: WB Saunders Co; 1999.

Treatment

Appel C. Obstetrical considerations. In: Myers RS, ed. *Saunders Manual of Physical Therapy Practice.* Philadelphia, Pa: WB Saunders Co; 1995:505–541.

Fitzpatrick M, O'Herlihy C. The effects of labour and delivery on the pelvic floor. *Best Pract Res Clin Obstet Gynaecol.* 2001;15:63–79.

Larson AI. Congenital malformations and exposure to high-frequency electromagnetic radiation among Danish physiotherapists. *Scand J Work, Environ Health.* 1991;17:318–323.

Larson AI, Olsen J, Svane O. Gender-specific reproductive outcome and exposure to high-frequency electromagnetic radiation among physiotherapists. *Scand J Work, Environ Health.* 1991;17:324–329.

Mayberry LJ, Smith M, Gill P. Effect of exercise on uterine activity in the patient in preterm labour. *J Perinatol.* 1992;12:354–358.

Onyeije CI, Sherer DM, Ham L, et al. Transient marked atelectasis: an unusual complication of asthma in pregnancy. *Am J Perinatol.* 1999;16:521–524.

Ouellet-Hellstrom R, Stewart WF. Miscarriages among female physical therapists who report using radio and microwave-frequency electromagnetic radiation. *Am J Epidemiol.* 1993;138:775–786.

Pauls J. *Therapeutic Approaches to Women's Health: A Program of Exercise and Education.* Gaithersburg, Md: Aspen Publishers; 1995.

Rasmussen B. Reimbursement for obstetric and gynecologic physical therapy. *J Obstetr Gynecol Phys Ther.* 1994;18:2:10–12.

Sapsford R, Bullock-Saxton J, Markwell S. *Women's Health: A Textbook for Physiotherapists.* Philadelphia, Pa: WB Saunders Co; 1999.

Taskinen H, Kyyronen P, Hemminki K. Effects of ultrasound, shortwaves, and physical exertion on pregnancy outcome in physiotherapists. *J Epidemiol Community Health.* 1990; 44:196–201.

Incontinence

DESCRIPTION

Urinary incontinence is the involuntary loss of urine. Incontinence can occur at any age, but it is common during pregnancy, affecting around 40% to 85% of pregnant women. There are several forms of incontinence, including:

- *Stress incontinence:* the loss of urine during increases in intra-abdominal pressures produced by stresses such as coughing, sneezing, and lifting or straining. Stress incontinence is the most common cause of incontinence in women.
- *Urge incontinence:* named for an urgent need to urinate combined with the involuntary loss of urine.
- *Overflow incontinence:* continuous or intermittent loss of urine in small amounts due to bladder overdistention.
- *Mixed incontinence:* combination of both urge and stress incontinence.
- *Transient incontinence:* temporary incontinence.

CAUSE

Incontinence in women is affected in part by diminished levels of estrogen during menopause. Childbirth and pelvic trauma can lead to weakness of pelvic floor muscles due to damage of the pudendal nerve, resulting in loss of urine. Chronic constipation can also lead to pelvic floor muscle damage.

Increased weight gain can increase intra-abdominal pressure, and chronic cough, usually due to smoking, can lead to urine leakage. Side effects of some medications, surgical procedures, infection in the urinary tract (UTI), diseases of the neurological system, and thyroid disorder can also trigger incontinence.

Causes of the specific types of incontinence:

- *Stress incontinence* can be caused by weakness of the urinary sphincter with relaxation of the pelvic floor muscles and downward displacement of the urethra during increases in intra-abdominal pressure. Stress incontinence may also be caused by perineal nerve damage secondary to childbirth (stretching of the perineal nerve or tearing of the perineum), excessive straining during defecation, trauma from childbirth or sexual abuse, or other trauma. In men, it can follow prostatectomy or trauma and intrinsic or neurogenic sphincter defect. In women, it can also be caused by cystocele (pelvic relaxation that allows the bladder to protrude into the vagina).
- *Urge incontinence* is usually idiopathic, but it may be caused by UTI, uninhibited neurogenic bladder dysfunction, multiple sclerosis, obstructive neuropathy, bladder calculi, tuberculosis, interstitial cystitis, or neoplasms.
- In *overflow incontinence,* bladder overdistention is due to a defect in the detruser muscle caused by sensory neuropathy, a stricture in the urethra, or lesion. In men, overflow incontinence is caused by disease of the prostate gland. In women, it is caused by incontinence surgery or pelvic prolapse (severe).
- *Mixed incontinence* has the same causes as those listed for components of stress and urge incontinence.
- *Transient incontinence* may be caused by delirium, infection, atrophy associated with menopause, medication side effects, depression, endocrine imbalance, impacted stool, or functional incontinence associated with restricted mobility.

ASSESSMENT

Note: See APTA's Guide to Physical Therapist Practice. 2nd ed. *Physical Therapy.* 2001;81.

Integumentary Preferred Practice Patterns: A, C, D

Musculoskeletal Preferred Practice Patterns: A, B, C, D, E, F, G, H

AREAS
- History, including occupation, surgery, menopausal state, medications, and medical conditions that may affect incontinence, such as allergy, diabetes, heart disease, neurological disease, and respiratory disorders
- Social/psychological, including emotional reaction to incontinence
- Bowel habits, including any constipation
- Functional level, including activity level
- Urogenital: perineal area, pelvic floor muscle strength, urinary frequency, urgency, stress, and nocturia

INSTRUMENTS/PROCEDURES

See References for sources. Table 15.1 compares various methods of recording pelvic muscle strength.

Special Tests to Which the Physical Therapist May or May Not Have Access
- urodynamic studies
- cystourethrography
- videourodynamics
- electromyography

Urogenital
- stop test or urine stream interruption test
- 1-hour office pad test

TABLE 15.1

Comparison of Four Methods to Record Pelvic Muscle Strength

Number	Grade (Modified Oxford Grading Scale)	Traditional Rating	Description
0	Nil	Nothing	No contraction
1	Flicker	Rapid fatigue	Just a bit
2	Weak	Not full range, not against gravity	Slight bulge in posterior wall as pelvic floor moves forward
3	Moderate	Full range in gravity eliminated position	Feel some lift
4	Good	Full range against gravity	Feels like "baby sucking on your finger"
5	Strong	Full range against resistance	Strong squeezing in with a strong lift

Source: Reprinted from Pauls J. *Therapeutic Approaches to Women's Health: A Program of Exercise and Education.* Aspen Publishers; 1995:5-1:16.

- internal evaluation of pelvic floor muscle strength
- daily intake and output diary
- urinary stress test

PROBLEMS

INCONTINENCE
- The client has involuntary loss of urine with exertion or sudden increase in intra-abdominal pressure.
- There is often an increased frequency and/or urgency to urinate.
- The client may also have chronic constipation.
- The incontinence may be accompanied by backache or lower abdominal pain.
- Incontinence may lead to extreme changes in a client's activities of daily living (ADLs).

PROLAPSE, CYSTOCELE, RECTOCELE
- The client may report a feeling of heaviness in the vulvar area.
- The client may complain of backache.
- The client often has increased frequency in urination and/or incontinence, especially stress incontinence. The client may also report pain or burning with urination.

TREATMENT/MANAGEMENT

Physical therapy for incontinence usually involves behavioral therapy. For rehabilitation purposes, the term behavioral therapy is used for an array of techniques, including pelvic muscle exercise, biofeedback, weight training with vaginal cones, electrical stimulation, and bladder retraining, habit (or timed) voiding, and prompted voiding.

PELVIC MUSCLE EXERCISE

Pelvic floor muscle exercise means increasing awareness and use of these muscles.

- For increasing awareness, have the client feel the muscle working and make sure she is not substituting or bearing down.
- For increasing actual strength, after the woman knows how to do a contraction, have her hold for a few seconds and relax for twice as long as the hold. See how many times she can do this. This is her baseline number. Continue to increase from the baseline number to stress the muscle. Be careful not to overfatigue, or the woman may end up more discouraged. Chart her progress. One regimen suggests a goal of 20 contractions at least 6 times a day. Another suggested schedule is a 10-10-10 schedule: 10 repetitions 10 times a day with a 10-second hold. Consider the use of very brief contractions, or flicks, to stimulate the phasic component of the pelvic floor muscles.
- For some women, being in a gravity-upright position may be too stressful at first. You can incorporate a progressive sequence for learning, going from a supine position to side-lying and then standing.

BIOFEEDBACK

Consider biofeedback using a perineometer or electronic biofeedback equipment. Auditory and/or visual feedback of information from surface or internal electrodes facilitates pelvic floor control. Follow instructions from the manufacturer or the references to this chapter for detailed instruction. A perineometer is a pneumatic device that uses pressure to measure effort. Visual feedback can be provided by simply giving the client a mirror to watch the external effects of a pelvic floor muscle contraction.

WEIGHT TRAINING WITH VAGINAL CONES

Vaginal cones usually come in a set of 5 cone-shaped weights, numbered from 1 (20 g) to 5 (70 g). Follow instructions from the manufacturer or the references to this chapter for detailed instruction. Select the appropriate cone. Insert the lightest cone with the pointed end and string downward. The cone should be able to stand vertically above the level of the pelvic floor. Once it is in place, the client walks around. If it can be held and retained for 1 minute, the client progresses on to the next cone, which is heavier, and so on until she is unable to retain for at least 1 minute. The heaviest cone that can be retained for 1 minute is used for exercise. The client should insert the cone twice a day and walk around for 15 minutes. If it slips, it should be pushed back up. If it can be retained, the next cone can be used, or the client can try the same cone with more challenging activities, such as jumping.

ELECTRICAL STIMULATION

For electrical stimulation, choose from faradic current or interferential current as indicated. Follow instructions from the manufacturer or the references to this chapter for a detailed protocol. One regimen suggests that the parameters be varied with the stimulation as follows:

- *Intensity:* per patient tolerance.
- *Frequency:* measured in Hz (hertz), pps (pulses per second), or cycles; 5 to 10 Hz is suggested for urgency and detrusor instability.
  35 Hz is used to increase muscle awareness and elicit a cortical response.
  50–60 Hz may fatigue the muscle.
- *Rest:* a weak muscle needs more rest than a trained muscle; the rest period should at least be equal to length of stimulation or greater (slow-twitch fiber, or

slow oxidative, needs stimulation of 10 to 20 seconds, fast-twitch fibers, or fast glycolytic, needs 30 to 60 seconds).
- *Pulse width:* 200 to 400 microseconds ideal.

BLADDER TRAINING

Educate the client about incontinence and set up a schedule of voiding that allows for increasing longer intervals between voiding. Habit training or timed voiding is especially helpful or useful for the client needing dependent care. (See Table 15.2.)

PRECAUTIONS/CONTRAINDICATIONS
- Bladder retraining is not indicated for clients with stress or overflow incontinence.
- Electrical stimulation (ES) is contraindicated during menstruation or pregnancy. ES is not to be used if the client has malignancy, metal implants, or a pacemaker.
- The following information should be given to the client who uses weighted cones:
    1. Excess lubrication, as at ovulation or other times, may affect cone retention.
    2. Vaginal cones are not used during the client's menstrual cycle.
    3. A wide introitus may make retention impossible. Permanent damage of innervation to pelvic floor may leave the woman a poor candidate for cones.
    4. A woman may be challenged by as little as 10 seconds, and the times listed may be unrealistic or fatigue inducing. Concentrate on increasing duration as opposed to resistance. A woman should not view reaching the No. 5 cone as the final goal. Adjust schedule to tailor the program to the client's individual needs.
    5. For infection control purposes, cones should be for one client's use only.

TABLE 15.2
Summary of Appropriate Activities Based on Muscle Grade

Strength	Activity
Weak muscles: Grade 1 or 2	
	Use gravity-eliminated position.
	Facilitate muscle with quick stretch.
	Use proprioceptive neuromuscular facilitation with patterns and over-flow activity from gluteal and adductor muscles.
	Use sensory stimulation with electrical stimulation.
	Repetitions should be fewer but more frequent to avoid overfatigue and promote myelin sheath development.
Stronger muscles: Grade 3, 4, or 5	
	Progress with full range of motion, increasing the hold time or number of repetitions.
	Add resistance with cones.
	Vary positions with weight bearing.
	Try with full bladder and quick contractions; quick ones are especially important to splint with contraction prior to a stress such as a cough.

TABLE 15.3
Successful Pelvic Floor Rehabilitation

Components of Successful Pelvic Floor Exercise Program
The client has an understanding of the anatomical aspects affecting the exercise program.
The therapist obtains an accurate baseline of the initial degree of incontinence.
The client is highly motivated.
The client receives feedback for her efforts.
The exercise program is customized and regularly supervised.
Supervision includes ongoing re-evaluation for assessment and treatment purposes.

Source: Reprinted with permission from Adams C, Frahm J. Genitourinary System. In: Myers RS, *Saunders Manual of Physical Therapy Practice.* WB Saunders Co; 1995:459–504.

DESIRED OUTCOME/PROGNOSIS
- The client will experience a reduction or stop in urine leaking.
- Therapy will normalize reflex activity for proper bladder functioning.
- The client will increase the strength of her pelvic floor and abdominal region.
- Therapy will stimulate proprioceptive feedback to the client, increase awareness of pelvic floor muscle function, and increase ability to differentiate and control pelvic floor contractions as opposed to contractions in regions such as adductor and abdominal musculature.
- Improved support of pelvic organs may preclude the need for surgery or enhance surgical outcomes.
- The overall outcome for client will be the restoration and increase in voluntary control of pelvic floor (see Table 15.3).

REFERENCES

Assessment

Adams C, Frahm J. Genitourinary system. In: Myers RS, ed. *Saunders Manual of Physical Therapy Practice.* Philadelphia, Pa: WB Saunders Co; 1995:459–504.

American Physical Therapy Association. *Guide to physical therapist practice.* 2nd ed. *Phys Ther.* 2001;81.

Jeyaseelan SM, Haslam J, Winstanley J, Roe BH. Digital vaginal assessment: An inter-tester reliability study. *Physiotherapy.* 2001;87:243–251.

Pauls J. *Therapeutic Approaches to Women's Health: A Program of Exercise and Education.* Gaithersburg, Md: Aspen Publishers; 1995.

Sapsford R, Bullock-Saxton J, Markwell S. *Women's Health: A Textbook for Physiotherapists.* Philadelphia, Pa: WB Saunders Co; 1999.

Treatment

American Physical Therapy Association. Taking back control. *PT-Magazine Phys Ther.* 1999; 7:44–45.

Ashworth PD, Hagan MT. Some social consequences of non-compliance with pelvic floor exercises. *Physiotherapy.* 1993;79:465–471.

Berghmans LC, Frederiks, CM, deBie RA, et al. Efficacy of biofeedback, when included with pelvic floor muscle exercise treatment, for genuine stress incontinence. *Neurol Urodynamics*. 1996;37–52.

Berghmans LC, Hendriks HJ, Bo K, et al. Conservative treatment of stress urinary incontinence in women: a systematic review of randomized clinical trials. *Br J Urology*. 1998; 82:181–191.

Berghmans LC, Hendriks HJ, DeBie RA, et al. Conservative treatment of urge urinary incontinence in women: a systematic review of randomized clinical trials. *Br J Urology Int*. 2000;85:254–263.

Bo K. Pelvic floor exercise for the treatment of stress urinary incontinence: an exercise physiology perspective. *Int Urogynecology J*. 1995;6:282–291.

Bo K. Effect of electrical stimulation on stress and urge urinary incontinence. Clinical outcome and practical recommendations based on randomized controlled trials. *Acta Obstetricia Gynecologica Scandinavica*. 1998;168:3–11.

Bo K, Stien R. Needle EMG registration of striated urethral wall and pelvic floor muscle activity patterns during cough, valsalva, abdominal, hip adductor and gluteal muscle contractions in nulliparous healthy females. *Neurol Urodynamics*. 1994;13:35–41.

Bo K, Stien R, Kulseng-Hanssen S, et al. Clinical and urodynamic assessment of nulliparous young women with and without stress incontinence symptoms—a case control study. *Obstetr Gynecol*. 1994;84:1028–1032.

Bo K, Talseth T. Long term effect of pelvic floor muscle exercise 5 years after cessation of organized training. *Obstetr Gynecol*. 1996;87:261–265.

Bo K, Talseth T, Holme I. Single blind, randomized controlled trial of pelvic floor exercises, electrical stimulation, vaginal cones, and no treatment in management of genuine stress incontinence in women. *BMJ*. 1999;318:487–493.

Broome BA. Development and testing of a scale to measure self-efficacy for pelvic muscle exercises in women with urinary incontinence. *Urologic Nurs*. 1999;19:258–268.

Brubaker L, Kotarinos R. Kegel or cut? Variations on this theme. *J Reprod Med*. 1993; 38:672–678.

Cammu H, Van Nylen M. Pelvic floor muscle exercises in genuine urinary stress incontinence. *Int. Urogynecology J Pelvic Floor Dysfunction*. 1997;8:297–300.

Cammu H, Van Nylen M, Amy JJ. A 10-year follow-up after Kegel pelvic floor muscle exercises for genuine stress incontinence. *Br J Urology Int*. 2000;85:655–658.

Cardozo L, Kelleher C. Sex hormones and the female lower urinary tract. *Physiotherapy*. 1994;80:135–138.

Chiarelli PE. *Women's Waterworks: Curing Incontinence*. Rushcutters Bay, NSW, Australia: Gore and Osment; 1992.

Chiarelli PE. *Let's Get Things Moving*. Sydney, Australia: Gore and Osment; 1992.

Clark GL. Innovations. Commercial vaginal weights for treatment of women with urinary incontinence. *Phys Ther Case Rep*. 1998;1:311–312.

Clarke SS. Pelvic floor intervention with a work conditioning patient. *J Section Women's Health*. 1997;21:15–17.

Cook T. Group treatment of female urinary incontinence: literature review. *Physiotherapy*. 2001;87:226–234.

Demain S, Smith F, Hiller L, et al. Comparison of group and individual physiotherapy for female urinary incontinence in primary care: pilot study. *Physiotherapy*. 2001;87:235–242.

Dumoulin C, Seabourne DE, Quirion-DeGirardi C, et al. Pelvic-floor rehabilitation, part 1: comparison of two surface electrode placements during stimulation of the pelvic-floor musculature in women who are continent using bipolar interferential currents. *Phys Ther*. 1995;75:1067–1074.

Dumoulin C, Seabourne DE, Quirion-DeGirardi C, et al. Pelvic-floor rehabilitation, part 2: pelvic-floor reeducation with interferential currents and exercise in the treatment of genuine stress incontinence in postpartum women-a cohort study. *Physical Therapy.* 1995;75:1075–1081.

Farragher DJ. The assessment and treatment of anorectal incontinence, a pudendal neuropathy. *J Assoc Chartered Physiotherapists Obstetr Gynecol.* 1993;72:7–9.

Farragher DJ. Evaluation of neuromuscular electrical stimulation in the treatment of genuine stress incontinence. *Physiotherapy.* 1998;84:199.

Fischer W, Linde A. Pelvic floor findings in urinary incontinence- results of conditioning using vaginal cones. *Acta Obstetricia et Gynecologica Scandinavica.* 1997;76:455–460.

Frahm J. The role of the PT in incontinence: innovation and communication to improve patient care. *Ostomy Wound Manage.* 1997;42:42–50.

Glazer H, MacConkey D. Functional rehabilitation of pelvic floor muscles; a challenge to tradition. *Urologic Nursing.* 1996;16:68–69.

Haslam J. Promotion of continence and management of incontinence. *Physiotherapy.* 1992;78:667–672.

Hulme JA, Wallace K, Kotarinos R, Huge BS. AHCPR Clinical Practice Guideline no. 2, update. Urinary incontinence in adults: acute and chronic management. *PT-Magazine Phys Ther.* 1997;5:56–63.

Jackson A, Irion J. Urinary incontinence in primiparous and multiparous. *J Section Women's Health.* 1998;22:9–14

Johnson JL. Biofeedback versus verbal instruction for pelvic floor training in the treatment of urinary incontinence. *J Section Women's Health.* 2000;24:7–13.

Kahn J. Electrodes and procedures for treatment of stress incontinence. *J Obstetr Gynecol Phys Ther.* 1993;17:1:7.

Kato K, Kondo A. Clinical value of vaginal cones for the management of female stress incontinence. *Int Urogynecology J Pelvic Floor Dysfunction.* 1997;8:314–317.

Knight SJ, Laycock J. The role of biofeedback in pelvic floor re-education. *Physiotherapy.* 1994;80:145–148.

Laycock J. Female pelvic floor assessment: the Laycock ring of continence. *Aust Physiotherapy Assoc women's Health J.* 1994;13;40–44.

Laycock J. Pelvic muscle exercises: physiotherapy for the pelvic floor. *Urologic Nurs.* 1994; 14:136–140.

Laycock J. Continence. Must do better. *Nurs Times.* 1995;91:64.

Laycock J, Green GR. Interferential therapy in the treatment of incontinence. *Physiotherapy.* 1988;74:161–168.

Laycock J, Jerwood D. Does pre-modulated interferential therapy cure genuine stress incontinence? *Physiotherapy.* 1993;79:553–560.

Laycock J, Jerwood D. Development of the Bradford Perineometer. *Physiotherapy.* 1994; 80:3:139–143.

Laycock J, Knight S, Naylor D. Prospective, randomized, controlled clinical trial to compare acute and chronic electrical stimulation in combination therapy for GSI. *Neurol Urodynamics.* 1995;14:425–426.

Ling FW, King PM, Myers CA. Screening for female urogenital system disease. In: Boissonnault WG, ed. *Examination in Physical Therapy Practice.* 2nd ed. New York, NY: Churchill Livingstone; 1995.

Malone-Lee J. Recent developments in urinary incontinence in late life. *Physiotherapy.* 1994; 80:133–134.

Mantle J. Focus on continence. *Physiotherapy.* 1994;80:126–131.

Markwell SJ, Sapsford RR. Physiotherapy management of obstructed defaecation. *Aust J Physiotherapy*. 1995;41:279–283.

McCandless S, Mason G. Physical therapy as an effective change agent in the treatment of patients with urinary incontinence. *J Mississippi Med Assoc*. 1995;271–274.

McIntosh LJ, Frahm JE, Mallett VT, Richardson DA. Pelvic floor rehabilitation in the treatment of incontinence. *J Reprod Med*. 1993;38:662–666.

McIntosh LJ, Mallett VT, Frahm JD, et al. Gynecologic disorders in women with Ehlers-Danlos syndrome. *J Soc Gynecol Invest*. 1995;2:559–564.

Noble E. The female pelvic floor: review and commentary. *J Obstetr Gynecol Phys Ther*. 1993;17:3:12–15.

Nygaard IE. Nonoperative management of urinary incontinence. *Curr Opinion Obstetr Gynecol*. 1996;8:347–350.

Pages IH, Jahr S, Schaufele MK. Comparative analysis of biofeedback and physical therapy for treatment of urinary stress incontinence in women. *Am J Phys Med Rehabil*. 2001;80:494–502.

Paterson J, Pinnock CB, Marshall VR. Pelvic floor exercises as a treatment for post-micturition dribble. *Br J Urology*. 1997;79:892–297.

Pauls J. Female urinary incontinence. In: *Therapeutic Approaches to Women's Health: A Program of Exercise and Education*. Gaithersburg, Md: Aspen Publishers; 1995:5–1:16.

Pauls S, Shelly E. The guide to physical therapist practice to women's health physical therapy. *J Section Women's Health*. 1999;23:8–12.

Rieger NA, Wattchow DA, Sarre RG, et al. Prospective trial of pelvic floor retraining in patients with fecal incontinence. *Dis Colon Rectum*. 1997;821–826.

Salamey J, Nof L. Physical therapists' practice patterns and perceptions related to urinary incontinence. *J Section Women's Health*. 1999;23:8–14.

Santiesteban AJ. Electromyographic and dynamometric characteristics of female pelvic floor musculature. *Phys Ther*. 1988;68:344–351.

Sapsford R, Bullock-Saxton J, Markwell S. *Women's Health: A Textbook for Physiotherapists*. Philadelphia, Pa: WB Saunders Co; 1999.

Sayer TR. Stress incontinence of urine: a connective tissue problem? *Physiotherapy*. 1994; 80:143–144.

Schussler B, Laycock J, Norton P, Stanton S, eds. *Pelvic Floor Rehabilitation*. London, England: Springer-Verlag; 1994.

Seim A, Sivertsen B, Eriksen BC, et al. Treatment of urinary incontinence in women in general practice: observational study. *Br Med J*. 1996;312:1459–1462.

Tries J, Eisman E. The use of biofeedback in the treatment of urinary incontinence. *Phys Ther Pract*. 1993;2:2:49–56.

Van Der Spuy A, Papadopoulis M. A 72 year-old lady with urinary incontinence: a case study. *S Afr J Physiotherapy*. 1999;55:21–23.

Walker JM. Curricular content on urinary incontinence in entry-level physical therapy programmes in three countries. *Physiotherapy Res Int*. 1998;3:123–134.

Wall LL, Davidson TG. The role of muscular re-education by physical therapy in the treatment of genuine stress urinary incontinence. *Obstetr Gynecol Survey*. 1992;47:322–331.

Wallace K. Female pelvic floor functions, dysfunctions, and behavioural approaches to treatment. *Clin Sports Med*. 1994;13:459.

Webb RJ, Powell PH. Transcutaneous electrical nerve stimulation in patients with idiopathic detrusor instability. *Neurol Urodynamics*. 1992;11:40.

White D, Stiller K, Roney F. The prevalence and severity of symptoms of incontinence in adult cystic fibrosis patients. *Physiotherapy Theory Pract.* 2000;16:35–42.

Wilder E, ed. *The Gynecological Manual.* Section on Women's Health. Alexandria, Va: American Physical Therapy Association; 1997.

Incontinence in Men and Children

DeJong TP, Van Gool JD, Dik P, et al. The treatment of post-urethrotomy incontinence in pediatric and adolescent females. *J Urology.* 2001;165:929–933.

Don't put up with it, incontinence experts tell men [editorial] *Physiotherapy Moves.* 2000; 14:13.

Dorey G. Physiotherapy for male continence problems. *Physiotherapy.* 1998;84:556–563.

Van Kampen M, De Weerdt W, Van Poppel H. Urinary incontinence following transurethral, transvesical and radical prostatectomy. *Acta Urologica Belgica.* 1997;65:1–7.

Wiener JS, Scales MT, Hampton J, et al. Long-term efficacy of simple behavioural therapy for daytime wetting in children. *J Urology.* 2000;164:785–790.

Zermann DH, Wunderlich H, Reichelt O, et al. Early post-prostatectomy pelvic floor biofeedback. *J Urology.* 2000;164:783–784.

Interstitial Cystitis

Also known as *Hunner's ulcer.*

DESCRIPTION

Interstitial cystitis (IC) is characterized by inflammation and irritation of the bladder but is not thought to be an infectious disorder.

CAUSE

The cause of IC is unknown, but IC can be a disorder of the autoimmune system, an allergic reaction, or a type of collagen disease. It may be manifested secondary to an infectious agent that is, as yet, unidentified.

ASSESSMENT

Note: See APTA's Guide to Physical Therapist Practice. 2nd ed. *Physical Therapy.* 2001;81.

Musculoskeletal Preferred Practice Patterns: C, D

AREAS
- History, including any medical conditions or symptoms such as bleeding or discharge, occupation, surgery, menopausal state, and medications
- Social/psychological
- Urinary symptoms: frequency, urgency, stress, and nocturia
- Bowel habits, including any constipation
- Pain, including any dyspareunia (painful intercourse)
- Functional level, including activities of daily living (ADLs)
- Perineal examination: observation and strength, if indicated

INSTRUMENTS/PROCEDURES

See References for sources.

No specific evaluation was identified for IC. Consider use of elements from evaluations for incontinence.

Urinary Symptoms
- daily intake and output diary

PROBLEMS
- The client often has severe pelvic pain which can become chronic.
- There is often painful urination with increased frequency.
- There can be increased pain after consumption of acidic or carbonated drinks, alcohol, or drinks with caffeine.

TREATMENT/MANAGEMENT
- Instruct the client in bladder training. Educate the client about incontinence, and establish a schedule of voiding that allows for increasing longer intervals between voiding.
- Teach habit training or timed voiding, especially for the client needing dependent care.
- Consider use of transcutaneous electrical nerve stimulation (TENS). One regimen suggests electrode placement using 2 sets of electrodes, 1 at the suprapubic area and another on paraspinal musculature at the T-10 level, with intensity as tolerated and frequency at BID for 2 hours.
- Consider use of interferential current; see manufacturer's suggestion for protocol and electrode placement.

PRECAUTIONS/CONTRAINDICATIONS

None indicated.

DESIRED OUTCOME/PROGNOSIS
- The client will experience a decrease in symptoms.

REFERENCES

Assessment

Adams C, Frahm J. Genitourinary system. In: Myers RS, ed. *Saunders Manual of Physical Therapy Practice*. Philadelphia, Pa: WB Saunders Co; 1995:477–483.

American Physical Therapy Association. Guide to physical therapist practice. 2nd ed. *Phys Ther*. 2001;81.

King PM, Ling FW, Myers CA. Screening for female urogenital system disease. In Boissonnault WG, ed. *Examination in Physical Therapy Practice—Screening for Medical Disease*. 2nd ed. New York, NY; 1995.

Sapsford R, Bullock-Saxton J, Markwell S. *Women's Health: A Textbook for Physiotherapists*. Philadelphia, Pa: WB Saunders Co; 1999.

Treatment

Adams C, Frahm J. Genitourinary system. In: Myers RS, ed. *Saunders Manual of Physical Therapy Practice*. Philadelphia, Pa: WB Saunders Co; 1995:459–504.

Kotarinos RK. Interstitial cystitis. *J Obstetr Gynecol Phys Ther*. 1994;18:4:5–7.

Meadows E, Taylor L. Treatment of interstitial cystitis using intra-anal biofeedback and electrical stimulation: a case study. *J Section Women's Health*. 1999;23:8–10.

Sapsford R, Bullock-Saxton J, Markwell S. *Women's Health: A Textbook for Physiotherapists*. Philadelphia, Pa: WB Saunders Co; 1999.

Wilder E, ed. *The Gynecological Manual. Section on Women's Health*. Alexandra, Va: American Physical Therapy Association; 1997.

Labor and Birth

DESCRIPTION

Labor involves contractions of the uterus that usually progress by getting longer, stronger, and more frequent. These contractions lead to dilation and effacement of the cervix. For descriptive purposes, labor is divided into 4 stages:

- The first stage covers the onset of labor until the cervix is completely dilated (about 10 cm).
- The second stage, or the pushing stage, begins at full cervical dilation and ends with the birth of the baby.
- The third stage begins after the baby is born and is complete when the placenta is delivered.
- The fourth stage is an observation time lasting from the placental delivery until 4 hours postpartum.

Note: Labor typically lasts between 12 and 14 hours in a first pregnancy and lasts 6 to 8 hours in subsequent pregnancies.

CAUSE

The stimulus that triggers the beginning of labor has not been established. One theory suggests that the hormone oxytocin, which is released from the pituitary gland, begins the process.

ASSESSMENT

AREAS
- History
- Respiration: rate and rhythm of breathing pattern
- Areas of tension/pain
- Uterine contractions
- Progress of labor: dilation and effacement from primary caregiver
- Pain
- Posture: positions of comfort/effect of posture on circulation and pain

INSTRUMENTS/PROCEDURES
- Palpation of areas of tension/pain
- External palpation of uterine contractions

PROBLEMS
- The client often has gradually increasing pain with contractions.
- Approximately 25% of women feel contractions primarily in the back; this is known as back labor.
- The client may have difficulty relaxing.
- The client may have anxiety and fear about labor.

TREATMENT/MANAGEMENT

- Educate the client about pregnancy, labor, birth, and the postpartum period prior to labor with childbirth education instruction. The physical therapist can also be a childbirth educator or can refer the client to a childbirth educator. Organizations that certify educators have varied philosophies. Three of the largest organizations include Lamaze/ASPO (American Society for Psychoprophylaxis in Obstetrics, Inc), ICEA (International Childbirth Education Association), and the Bradley method (American Academy of Husband-Coached Childbirth).
- A physical therapist may also assume the role of professional labor support and lactation consultant.

LABOR SUPPORT

- Provide encouragement and emotional support.
- Provide information about the labor and birth process and the comfort measures available.
- Provide advocacy of the client's choices regarding the birth experience.
- Instruct in stress management techniques to calm the parasympathetic nervous system, including:
  1. massage, especially slow, rhythmical strokes
  2. slow-paced abdominal breathing
  3. soothing surroundings
  4. warmth from water, moist heat packs, or compresses
  5. avoiding worry
  6. meditation on calming thoughts
  7. muscular release through relaxation techniques
- Relaxation techniques include the Mitchell method of reciprocal relaxation, Benson's relaxation response, progressive relaxation, modified progressive relaxation, selective dissociative relaxation, and differential relaxation.
- Consider use of ice for labor pain.
- Consider use of transcutaneous electrical nerve stimulation (TENS) for labor pain, especially for pain in low back. Electrode placement may vary. One suggested option is to place one set of electrodes paraspinally at level T-10 to L-1 (level of uterine innervation) and another set paraspinally at S-2 to S-4. (An additional option includes anterior placement of the electrodes in a V shape in the suprapubic area.) Parameters may vary. One option includes a pulse rate at 80 to 120 Hz, pulse width at 150 Ês, and intensity as desired by client.

POSITIONING DURING LABOR

During labor, positions for pushing can be modified.

- A side-lying or partially reclined position is recommended for many disabled women, especially if they cannot use a position in which the legs are widely spread. Side-lying is also useful for a patient with the diagnosis of herniated nucleus pulposus or spinal stenosis.
- Avoid standing for women with spondylolisthesis. Avoid the lithotomy position with sacroiliac dysfunction if standing is uncomfortable. Avoid hip abduction with pubic symphysis dysfunction.
- Women with a spinal cord injury may need extra padding to avoid pressure sores when assuming positions for prolonged periods. (See Table 15.4.)

BACK LABOR

Approximately 25% of women experience some or all of their labor contractions in the lower back area. Back labor is often caused by a baby in an occiput-posterior position.

TABLE 15.4

Selected Labor Considerations for Pregnant Women with Disabilities

Disability	Considerations During Labor
Arthritis	Side-lying may be the least stressful position for second-stage labor; epidural may not be an option.
Amputation with use of prosthesis	Avoid prolonged positions, which may lead to skin breakdown under prosthesis.
Asthma	Extra cortisone and adrenaline released naturally during labor provide increased protection against an asthma attack.
Cerebral Palsy	Cesarean is often recommended; there is no research to support this assumption; more research is needed.
Diabetes	Blood sugar levels will be closely monitored.
Epilepsy	Avoid any medications that might trigger convulsion; breathing techniques might trigger an attack in some women; avoid overbreathing.
Heart disease	Close monitoring during labor is warranted; interventions may be used during second-stage labor to diminish the stress of expulsive efforts.
Multiple Sclerosis	Epidural may not be an option due to concerns of exacerbating disorder; no research to confirm this assumption.
Scoliosis	Epidural may not be an option; pelvic size is usually unaffected by this disorder.
Spina Bifida	Abdominal muscle strength is usually sufficient for second-stage labor; careful positioning is indicated.
Spinal cord injury	Instruction in manual palpation of contractions is indicated to determine when labor is beginning; contractions of uterus are usually sufficient to expel baby during second-stage; positioning is important; degree of intervention needed during second-stage depends on level of lesion; spasm in pelvic floor muscle may be present during delivery.

Source: Reprinted from Pauls J. *Therapeutic Approaches to Women's Health: A Program of Exercise and Education.* Aspen Publishers; 1995:3–1:10.

Comfort measures for back labor include:
- changing positions—all-fours, sitting, side-lying (avoid supine)
- firm counterpressure on the back (muscular area) with the heel of partner's hand, tennis ball, or rolling pin
- passive pelvic tilt by partner with woman in side-lying position
- active pelvic tilt—any position
- massage
- heat or cold compresses—whichever works most effectively
- TENS

PRECAUTIONS/CONTRAINDICATIONS
- Occasionally, TENS may interfere with equipment such as a fetal monitor, if in use (see Table 15.5).

DESIRED OUTCOME/PROGNOSIS
- The client will be informed about the process of labor and options for birth.
- The client will have coping measures for labor.
- The client will have a positive birth experience.

TABLE 15.5
Cautions Concerning TENS Usage

Contraindications: TENS Units
Any electrode placement that applies current to the carotid sinus (neck) region
Presence of a demand-type cardiac pacemaker
Any electrode placement that causes current to flow transcerebrally (through the head)
Presence of undiagnosed pain syndromes until etiology is established
The safety of TENS devices for use during pregnancy or delivery has not been established
Not effective for pain of central origin (includes headache)
Should only be used under the continued supervision of a physician
Have no curative value
A symptomatic treatment and suppresses the sensation of pain that would otherwise serve as a protective mechanism
User must keep the device out of the reach of children
Electronic monitoring equipment (eg, ECG monitors and alarms) may not operate properly when TENS stimulation is in use
If the device is capable of delivering a charge per pulse of 25 microcoulombs or greater, there should be a prominently placed statement warning that stimulus delivered by this device may be sufficient to cause electrocution; electrical current of this magnitude must not flow through the thorax as it may cause cardiac arrythmia

Source: Reprinted with permission from Pomerantz E. TENS and Pregnancy: Rules for Safe Practice In: *J Obstetr Gynecol Phys Ther.* American Physical Therapy Association; 1988:12;3:5.

REFERENCES

Assessment

Pauls J. *Therapeutic Approaches to Women's Health: A Program of Exercise and Education.* Gaithersburg, Md: Aspen Publishers; 1995.

Sapsford R, Bullock-Saxton J, Markwell S. *Women's Health: A Textbook for Physiotherapists.* Philadelphia, Pa: WB Saunders Co; 1999.

Stephenson RG, O'Connor LJ. *Obstetric and Gynecologic Care in Physical Therapy.* 2nd ed. Thorofare, NJ: Slack Inc; 2000.

Treatment

Appel C. Continuing education: positioning for labor and delivery for women with spinal dysfunction by J. Boissonnault. *J Obstetr Gynecol Phys Ther.* 1992;16:3:6.

Bell JA, Saltikov JB. Mitchell's relaxation technique: is it effective? *Physiotherapy.* 2000;86:473–478.

Carroll D, Tramer M, McQuay H, et al. Transcutaneous electrical nerve stimulation in labour pain: a systematic review. *Br J Obstetr Gynaecol.* 1997;104:169–175.

Checca JB, Appel C, Frahm J. The challenge of labor and birth in the woman with a spinal cord injury. *J Section Women's Health.* 1998;22:9–17.

Crouthers E. Labour pains: a study of pain control mechanisms during labour. *J Assoc Chartered Physiotherapists Obstetr Gynaecol.* 1994;74:4–9.

Dunbar A. Relief of back labor pain by transcutaneous electrical nerve stimulation. *J Section Women's Health.* 1998;22:18–20.

Kaplan B, Rabinerson D, Lurie S, et al. Transcutaneous electrical nerve stimulation (TENS) for adjuvant pain-relief during labor and delivery. *Int J Obstetr Gynecol.* 1998;60:251–255.

Li A, Yoshida K. Women with physical disabilities and their health: implications for health promotion and physical therapy. *Physiotherapy Can.* 1998;50:309–315.

McMillan CM. Transcutaneous electrical stimulation of Neiguan anti-emetic acupuncture point in controlling sickness following opioid analgesia in major orthopaedic surgery. *Physiotherapy.* 1994;80:5–9.

Nolan MF, Wilson MB. Patient-controlled analgesia: a method for the controlled self-administration of opioid pain medications. *Phys Ther.* 1995;75:374–379.

Pauls J. *Therapeutic Approaches to Women's Health: A Program of Exercise and Education.* Gaithersburg, Md: Aspen Publishers; 1995.

Pauls J. Cesarean birth and vaginal birth after cesarean: an update for physical therapists. *J Section Women's Health.* 1998;22:15–21.

Pipp LM. Compendium of selected TENS literature. *J Obstetr Gynecol Phys Ther.* 1993; 17:12.

Rogers J. Perinatal education for women with physical disabilities. *AWHONNS.* 1993;4:141–146.

Roubal PJ, Chavinson AH, LaGrandeur RM. Bilateral radial nerve palsies form use of the standard birthing bar. *Obstetr Gynecol.* 1996;87:820–821.

Sapsford R, Bullock-Saxton J, Markwell S. *Women's Health: A Textbook for Physiotherapists.* Philadelphia, Pa: WB Saunders Co; 1999.

Simkin P. The labor support person: latest addition to the maternity care team. *Int J Childbirth Educ.* 1992;7:1:19–27.

Simkin P. Overcoming the legacy of childhood sexual abuse: the role of caregivers and childbirth educators. *Birth: Issues in Perinatal Care and Education.* 1992;4:224–225.

Simkin P. When should a child attend a sibling's birth? A guideline for parents. *Midwifery Today Childbirth Educ.* 1993;28:37.

Simkin P. Epidural epidemic. *Birth Gazette.* 1994;10:4:28–34.

Simkin P. Potential risks of epidural anesthesia. *Midwifery Today Childbirth Educ.* 1994; 31:27.

Simkin P. What you should know about active management of labor. *Childbirth Instructor Magazine.* 1995;5:1:8–10.

Stephenson RG, O'Connor LJ. *Obstetric and Gynecologic Care in Physical Therapy.* 2nd ed. Thorofare, NJ: Slack Inc; 2000.

Thornton SI, Thornton SJ. Management of gross devarication of the recti abdominis in pregnancy and labour. *Physiotherapy.* 1993;79:457–458.

Osteoporosis

DESCRIPTION

Osteoporosis is a progressive reduction in bone tissue mass per unit volume. This decrease in bone mass leads to skeletal weakness characterized by bone fractures. The most common adult metabolic bone disease, osteoporosis leads to between 1 and 1.5 million fractures in the United States annually. Colles fracture and vertebral crush fractures, as well as fractures in the hip and pelvic region, are often the result of osteoporosis.

CAUSE

Research suggests that diminished weight bearing leads to less stress on bones, which triggers calcium resorption, resulting in bone loss. Increased risk factors for primary osteoporosis include female gender, never having been pregnant, early menopause, white or oriental race, thinness, aging, family history, and inactivity.

There are Three Types of Primary Osteoporosis:

- idiopathic osteoporosis
- Type I or postmenopausal osteoporosis, which occurs around age 51 to 75 in women due to endocrinologic changes but can also occur in men.
- Type II or involutional osteoporosis, which occurs in clients over age 70, although it actually begins in the third decade. Women are 2 times as likely as men to be affected. This type is possibly related to a decrease in vitamin D synthesis.

ASSESSMENT

Note: See APTA's Guide to Physical Therapist Practice. 2nd ed. *Physical Therapy.* 2001;81.

Musculoskeletal Preferred Practice Patterns: A, B, C, G, H

AREAS

- History, including previous fractures, symptoms of dysmenorrhea or menopause, use of hormones, and any medications that may affect skeletal health
- Posture
- Pain
- Balance
- Gait
- Mobility, including active range of motion (ROM)
- Strength, especially trunk strength
- Neurological, including coordination and balance, in static and dynamic state
- Cardiovascular, including endurance level
- Functional level, including activities of daily living (ADLs) and leisure activities
- Equipment, including home environment

INSTRUMENTS/PROCEDURES

See References for sources.

Balance
- One-Legged Stance Test (OLST)
- Sharpened Rhomberg test (SR)
- step-width measurements
- Quantitative Muscle Tester (QMT)
- Get Up and Go Test
- Sensory Organization Test (SOT) for standing balance

Functional Level
- PULSES profile

Mobility
- Timed Up and Go Test

Posture
- postural stress test
- posturography
- Reedco Posture Score Sheet

Special Tests to Which the Physical Therapist May or May Not Have Access
- bone mineral density measurement
- trunk muscle strength testing

- isometric and isokinetic torque evaluation
- work measurements
- electromyography (EMG)

PROBLEMS

- The client often has extreme pain.
- The pain is often chronic.
- The pain is often in thoracic region, especially if the client shows signs of kyphosis and is a postmenopausal woman.

TREATMENT/MANAGEMENT

GENERAL

- Provide education, including fall prevention information (see Table 15.6).
- Increase functional activity level.
- Encourage weight-bearing exercise or exercise that stresses bone. Ideally, an exercise program should be started premenopausally, but even after an osteoporosis fracture, exercise such as walking, jogging, or stair climbing can be safe.
- Increase activity level and postural alignment with various activities, including calisthenics, weight lifting, swimming, cycling, walking, running, golfing, tennis, gardening, and dancing. Almost all have been more or less successful in either preventing age-related bone loss in the postmenopausal woman or actually increasing bone density, especially in the extremely sedentary woman. Stress as many parts of the skeleton (safely) as possible (see Table 15.7).
- Progress by adding light weights, Theraband, etc., for resistance. Areas for stretching including pectoral and shoulders. Areas for strengthening include back extension, abdominal upper extremity and lower extremity. Balance, coordination, and function can be facilitated by combining many of the exercises, along the order of dynamic stabilization routines.
- Every day, try to walk briskly, keeping an erect posture and swinging arms freely.
- Excessive flexion and rotation activities should be avoided.
- Consider use of back supports and bracing but avoid overuse and include the posture training support system.

TABLE 15.6
Education Topics for Osteoporosis

Topics for Client Education
Unavoidable versus avoidable risk factors
Do's and don'ts of exercise and activities
Proper body mechanics, perhaps including a "back school," and work simplification
Proper posture
Consultation with nutritionist regarding diet, calcium supplements, and so on
Individualized instruction in an exercise program to address identified dysfunction and needs
Supportive or orthotic devices where needed
Review of home environment and activities to minimize the risk of falls and fractures (eg, installing handrails, eliminating slippery throw rugs, refraining from climbing on ladders)
Work consolidation
Possible modification of diet and/or lifestyle to help minimize those risk factors that are avoidable

TABLE 15.7
Tips for Avoiding Injuries

Tips for Client Safety Education
Remove all loose or slippery area rugs.
Keep electrical cords well out of the way.
Keep walkways and porches clear.
Be especially careful around pets; man's best friend may inadvertently cause a fall both in the home and when out for a walk.
Monitor medications—both prescription and over-the-counter—drug interactions can account for dizziness, loss of balance, sedation, and so on.
Avoid situations where you are vulnerable to falling; let someone else climb up on the ladder.
Be extra careful during winter when sidewalks, porches, and driveways may be icy.
Be sure to have a clear path from your bed to the bathroom in case the need arises in the middle of the night.
Use ample lighting; use plenty of nightlights.

Source: Reprinted from Gleeson PB. Osteoporosis. In: Pauls J. *Therapeutic Approaches to Women's Health; A Program of Exercise and Education.* Aspen Publishers; 1995:5:6-1:1–6-1:27.

PAIN REDUCTION MEASURES
- For fracture pain, provide heat to areas of muscle spasm.
- Instruct the client in extension exercise following vertebral fracture.
- Post hip fracture, provide gait training, usually with partial weight bearing with internal fixation for 6 weeks. Consult with the surgeon on weight-bearing status.
- Any appropriate modalities may be used during the pain management aspect of treatment. Heat and/or cold and massage as well as transcutaneous electrical nerve stimulation (TENS) may provide temporary pain relief. Positioning for relaxation and proper alignment should always be emphasized. Splints, corsets, or other orthotic devices may be indicated.

PRECAUTIONS/CONTRAINDICATIONS
- Women with a significant amount of bone loss should consult their physicians before the physical therapist designs an individualized exercise program for each client.
- Avoid flexion exercises if the client has suffered vertebral fracture.
- After internal fixation, the client should avoid hip flexion (keeping the angle no less than 90 degrees), adduction past midline, and internal rotation.
- An added caution before prescribing an exercise program for the elderly population: cervical vertebrae may collapse with osteoporosis, resulting in a disruption of the vertebral artery flow. Vertebral artery syndrome may be present, with symptoms including dizziness, blurred vision, or blackouts with extension, lateral flexion, or rotation of their cervical spine. The physical therapist should determine if there is any compromise of the vertebral artery prior to prescribing neck exercises and should educate clients concerning this possibility. (See Table 15.8.)

DESIRED OUTCOME/PROGNOSIS
- The client will increase soft tissue flexibility.
- The client will increase muscular strength.
- The client will increase muscular endurance.
- The client will improve balance (both static and dynamic).

TABLE 15.8
Exercise and Leisure Time Do's and Don'ts

Tips for Client Well-being Education
Do make an appointment with a physical therapist to discuss work consolidation, safe body mechanics, and ways of making your environment more "user-friendly."
Do follow a regular exercise program that includes a variety of different activities; although weight-bearing activities such as walking have been shown to be the most effective in preventing bone loss, all forms of activity—including swimming—are beneficial.
Do be sure that your exercise program includes plenty of gentle, controlled movements emphasizing extension, especially of the shoulders, trunk, and legs.
Don't perform unnecessary flexion activities, especially those that also involve rotation movements; exercises such as sit-ups, toe touches from a standing position, and other form of purposeful flexion should be avoided; discuss the safest methods for making beds, weeding gardens, and so on, to minimize flexion forces on the spine.
Don't engage in ballistic types of exercise routines, such as high-impact aerobics and rope jumping.

Source: Reprinted from Gleeson PB. Osteoporosis. In: Pauls J. *Therapeutic Approaches to Women's Health; A Program of Exercise and Education.* Aspen Publishers; 1995:5:6-1:1-6-1:27.

- The client will improve coordination.
- The client will correct any asymmetry.
- The client will increase joint ROM.
- The client will improve function.

Notes: Exercise is only one component in the efforts to prevent the complications associated with osteoporosis. Estrogen replacement therapy, as well as nutritional considerations, must be addressed for optimum skeletal health. Exercise alone is not the complete answer to replacing bone mass in the aging skeleton.

REFERENCES

Assessment

American Physical Therapy Association. Guide to physical therapist practice. 2nd ed. *Phys Ther.* 2001;81.

Arnold CM, Beatty B, Harrison EL, et al. The reliability of five clinical postural alignment measures for women with osteoporosis. *Physiotherapy Can.* 2000;52:279–285.

Gleeson PB. Osteoporosis. In: Pauls J, *Therapeutic Approaches to Women's Health: A Program of Exercise and Education.* Gaithersburg, Md: Aspen Publishers; 1995:6–1:1–6–1:27.

Goodman C, Snyder TE. *Differential Diagnosis in Physical Therapy.* 2nd ed. Philadelphia, Pa: WB Saunders Co; 2000.

Lydick E, Zimmerman SI, Yawn B, et al. Development and validation of a discriminative quality of life questionnaire for osteoporosis (the OPTQoL). *J Bone Mineral Res.* 1997;12:456–463.

Murray C, O'Brien K. Osteoporosis workup: evaluation bone loss and risk of fracture. *Geriatrics.* 1995;50:9:41–53.

Sapsford R, Bullock-Saxton J, Markwell S. *Women's Health: A Textbook for Physiotherapists.* Philadelphia, Pa: WB Saunders Co; 1999.

Balance/Fall Prevention

Anacker SL, DiFabio RP. Influence of sensory inputs on standing balance in community-dwelling elders with a recent history of falling. *Phys Ther.* 1992;72:575–581.

Dean E, Ross J. Relationships among cane fitting, function, and falls. *Phys Ther.* 1993;73:494–500.

Duncan PW, Chandler J, Studenski S, et al. How do physiological components of balance affect mobility in elderly men? *Arch Phys Med Rehabil.* 1993;74:1343–1349.

Judge JO, Lindsey C, Underwood M, Winsemius D. Balance improvements in older women: effects of exercise training. *Phys Ther.* 1993;73:254–262.

Lord SR, Sambrook PN, Gilbert C, et al. Postural stability, falls and fractures in the elderly: results from Dubbo Osteoporosis Epidemiology Study. *Med J Aust.* 1994;160:684–691.

Meldrum D, Funn AM. An investigation of balance function in elderly subjects who have and have not fallen. *Physiotherapy.* 1993;79:339–342.

Simpson JM. Elderly people at risk of falling: the role of muscle weakness. *Physiotherapy.* 1993;79:831–835.

Steinmetz HM, Hobson JG. Prevention of falls among the community-dwelling elderly: an overview. *Phys Occup Ther Geriatr.* 1994;12:13–29.

Therapy Management Innovations, Inc. *Falls Assessment for the Physical Therapist.* USA, Therapy Management Innovations; 1992.

Vandervoort AA, Chesworth BM, Cunningham DA, Rechnitzer PA, Paterson DH, Koval JJ. An outcome measure to quantify passive stiffness of the ankle. *Can J Public Health.* 1992;83(suppl 2):S19–S23.

Vandervoort A, Hill K, Sandrin M, et al. Mobility impairment and falling in the elderly. *Physiotherapy Can.* 1990;42:99–107.

Special Tests to Which the Physical Therapist May or May Not Have Access

BONE MINERAL DENSITY AND STRENGTH

Sinaki M, Itoi E, Roger J, et al. Correlation of back extensor strength with thoracic kyphosis and lumbar lordosis in estrogen deficient women. *Am J Phys Med Rehabil.* 1996;75:370–374.

Smidt GL, Lin SY, O'Dwyer KD, Blanpied PR. The effect of high-intensity trunk exercise on bone mineral density of postmenopausal women. *Spine.* 1992;17:280–285.

Treatment

American Association of Clinical Endocrinologists. AACE Clinical Practice Guidelines for the Prevention and Treatment of Postmenopausal Osteoporosis. *J Fla Med Assoc.* 1996;83:552–566.

ACSM Position Stand on Osteoporosis and Exercise. *Med Science Sports Exerc.* 1995;27:1–7.

Act-Fliedner R, Mink D, Schneider G, et al. Transient bilateral osteoporosis of the hip in pregnancy. A case report and review of the literature. *Gynecol Obstet Invest.* 2001;51:138–140.

American Physical Therapy Association. Walking tall. *PT-Magazine Phys Ther.* 1999;7:36–37.

Anderson FH. Osteoporosis in men. *Int J Clin Pract.* 1998;52:176–180.

Barber BH. Niche practices in geriatrics. *PT—Magazine of Physical Therapy*. 2000;8:36–42.

Berard A, Bravo G, Gauthier P. Meta-analysis of the effectiveness of physical activity for the prevention of bone loss in postmenopausal women. *Osteoporosis Int*. 1997;7:331–337.

Brown AM. The effects of exercise on bone mass; implications for manipulative therapy. *J Manual Manipulative Ther*. 1995;3:3–8.

Broy SB. A "whole patient" approach to managing osteoporosis. *J Musculoskeletal Med*. 1996; 13:15–28.

Culham EG. Osteoporosis and osteoporotic fractures. In: Pickles B, Compton A, Simpson JM et al., eds. *Physiotherapy with Older People*. London, England: WB Saunders Co; 1995: 213–230.

Cumming SR, Nevitt MC, Browner WS, Stone K, et al. Risk factors for hip fracture in white women. *N Engl J Med*. 1995;332:767–773.

Dowd R, Cavalieri RJ. Help your patient live with osteoporosis. *Am J Nurs*. 1999;99:55–60.

Ernst E. Exercise for female osteoporosis. A systematic review of randomized clinical trials. *Sports Med*. 1998;25:359–368.

Fries JF. Prevention of osteoporotic fractures: possibilities, the role of exercise, and limitation. *Scand J Rheumatol*. 1996;25(suppl 103):6–10.

Gleeson PB. Osteoporosis. In: Pauls J, *Therapeutic Approaches to Women's Health: A Program of Exercise and Education*. Gaithersburg, Md: Aspen Publishers; 1995:6–1:1–6–1:27.

Gleeson PB. Osteoporosis prevention: rational and target population. *J Section Women's Health*. 1997;21:6–16.

Gleeson PB, Protas EJ, LeBlanc AD, Schneider VS, Evans HJ. Effects of weight lifting on bone mineral density in premenopausal women. *J Bone Miner Res*. 1990;5:153–158.

Grabois M, Garrison SJ, Hart KA, Lehmkuhl LD. *Physical Medicine and Rehabilitation: The Complete Approach*. Malden, Mass: Blackwell Science; 2000.

Gregg EW, Cauley JA, Seely DG, et al. Physical activity and osteoporotic fracture risk in older women. *Annals of Intern Med*. 1998;129:81–88.

Harrington S, Smith J, Thompson J, et al. Idiopathic transient osteoporosis: a hidden cause of hip pain. *Physician and Sportsmedicine*. 2000;28:82–96.

Hertel KI, Trahiotis MG. Exercise in the prevention and treatment of osteoporosis: the role of physical therapy and nursing. *Nurs Clin North Am*. 2001;36:441–453.

Hertling D, Kessler RM, eds. *Management of Common Musculoskeletal Disorders*. 3rd ed. Philadelphia, Pa: JB Lippincott Co; 1996:32, 456, 559, 562.

Hizmetli S, Elden H, Kaptanoglu E, et al. The effect of different doses of calcitonin on bone mineral density and fracture risk in postmenopausal osteoporosis. *Int J Clin Pract*. 1998;52:453–455.

Itoi E, Sinaki M. Effect of back-strengthening exercise on posture in healthy women 49 to 65 years of age. *Mayo Clin Proc*. 1994;69:1054–1059.

Johnston CC Jr. Development of clinical practice guidelines for prevention and treatment of oteoporosis. *Calcified Tissue Int*. 1996;59(suppl 1):S30–33.

Kanis JA, Delmas P, Burckhardt P, et al. Guidelines for diagnosis and management of osteoporosis. *Osteoporosis Int*. 1997;7:390–406.

Koval KJ, Zuckerman JD, eds. *Fractures in the Elderly*. Philadelphia, Pa: Lippincott-Revenn; 1998.

Lewis CB. The relationship between posture and psychological variables in students aged 18–25. In: Lewis CB, Lundon KM, Li AM, Bibershtein S, eds. Interrater and intrarater reliability in the measurement of kyphosis in postmenopausal women with osteoporosis. *Spine.* 1998;23:1978–1985.

Malmros B, Mortensen L, Jensen MB, et al. Positive effects of physiotherapy on chronic pain and performance in osteoporosis. *Osteoporosis Int.* 1998;8:215–221.

McGilvray L, Cott CA. A key informant survey of osteoporosis exercise programs in Ontario. *Physiotherapy Can.* 2000;52:146–152.

McNearney T. *The Functional Tool Box: Clinical Measures of Functional Outcomes.* Washington, DC: Learn Publications; 1994.

Moore S, Woollacott MH. The use of biofeedback devices to improve postural stability. *Phys Ther Pract.* 1993;2:2:1–10.

Murray C, O'Brien K. Osteoporosis workup: evaluating bone loss and risk of fractures. *Geriatr.* 1995;50:41–55.

Nelson ME, Fiatrone MA, Morganti CM. Effects of high-intensity strength training on multiple risk factors for osteoporotic fractures: A randomized controlled trial. *JAMA.* 1994; 272:1909–1914.

Rizzo A. Insights. Before the fractures. *PT—Magazine Phys Ther.* 1996;4:128.

Rizzo A. Building better bones: reaching out to the community. *PT—Magazine Phys Ther.* 1996;4:46–48.

Sapsford R, Bullock-Saxton J, Markwell S. *Women's Health: A Textbook for Physiotherapists.* Philadelphia, Pa: WB Saunders Co;1999.

Saunders CS. The active woman: special health concerns. *Patient Care.* 1998;184–195.

Shipp KM. Osteoporosis: to manage fragility. *PT—Magazine Phys Ther.* 1993;1:70–75.

Tamayo-Orozco J, Arzac-Palumbro P, Peon-Vidales H, et al. *Am J Med.* 1997;103:44S–48S.

Turner PA. Osteoporosis—its causes and prevention: an update. *Physiotherapy Theory Pract.* 2000;16:135–149.

Vandervoort AA. Effects of aging on human neuromuscular function: implications for exercise. *Can J Sport Sci.* 1992;17:178–184.

Varenna M, Binelli Zucchi F, et al. Is the metatarsal fracture in postmenopausal women an osteoporotiac fracture? A cross-sectional study on 113 cases. *Osteoporosis Int.* 1997; 7:558–563.

Woods EN. Building better bones: managing and preventing osteoporosis. *PT—Magazine Phys Ther.* 1996;4:40–42.

Pelvic Floor Tension Myalgia

Also known as *coccygodynia, levator ani spasm, pyriformis syndrome,* and *spastica pelvic diaphragm.*

DESCRIPTION

Pelvic floor tension myalgia is pain in the pelvic floor muscles and surrounding area.

CAUSE

Pelvic floor tension myalgia can be caused by muscular imbalances of the abdominal and back musculature or habitual muscular contraction due to pain. Spasm in the levator ani muscle can be caused by trauma, surgery, pathology, or excessive anxiety.

ASSESSMENT

Note: See APTA's Guide to Physical Therapist Practice. 2nd ed. *Physical Therapy.* 2001;81.

Musculoskeletal Preferred Practice Pattern: C

AREAS

- History, including occupation, surgery, menopausal state, medical conditions, medications
- Psychological/social
- Urinary symptoms
- Bowel habits, including any constipation
- Pain
- Perineal examination, including strength of pelvic floor musculature

INSTRUMENTS/PROCEDURES

See References for sources.

- Female Urogenital System Checklist

Special Tests to Which the Physical Therapist May or May Not Have Access
- perineometer
- urodynamic assessment

PROBLEMS

- There is pain in the rectum, pelvis, or back.
- There may be leg pain.
- There may be pain with bowel movement.
- There may be constipation.
- There is often dyspareunia.

TREATMENT/MANAGEMENT

- Consider rectal diathermy or high-voltage pulsed current stimulation as per the manufacturer's instructions.
- Consider Thieles massage.
- Instruct in relaxation exercises.
- Encourage daily warm soaks or baths.

EXPECTED OUTCOME/PROGNOSIS

- The client will experience relaxation of the pelvic floor muscles.

REFERENCES

Assessment

Adams C, Frahm J. Genitourinary system. In: Myers RS, ed. *Saunders Manual of Physical Therapy Practice.* Philadelphia, Pa: WB Saunders Co; 1995:494.

American Physical Therapy Association. Guide to physical therapist practice. 2nd ed. *Phys Ther.* 2001;81.

King PM, Ling FW, Myers CA. Screening for female urogenital system disease. In: Boissonnault WG, ed. *Examination in Physical Therapy Practice—Screening for Medical Disease.* 2nd ed. New York, NY; 1995.

Treatment

Adams C, Frahm J. Genitourinary system. In: Myers RS, ed. *Saunders Manual of Physical Therapy Practice*. Philadelphia, Pa: WB Saunders Co; 1995:459–504.

American Physical Therapy Association. *Guidelines for Recognizing and Providing Care for Victims of Domestic Violence*. Alexandria, Va; 1997; P-138.

Bo K, Stien R. Needle EMG registration of striated urethral wall and pelvic floor muscle activity patterns during cough, Valsalva, abdominal, hip adductor and gluteal contractions in nulliparous healthy females. *Neurol Urodynamics*. 1994;13:35–41.

Chiarelli P. *Women's Waterworks—Curing Incontinence*. Snohomish, WA: Khera Publications; 1995.

Costello K. Myofascial syndromes. In: Steege JF, Metzger DA, Levy BS, eds. *Chronic Pelvic Pain*. Philadelphia, Pa: WB Saunders Co; 1998:251–266.

Hay-Smith. Therapeutic ultrasound for postpartum perineal pain and dyspareunia. *Cochrane Database System Review*. 2000;CD 000495.

Kegel A. Progressive resistance exercises in the functional restoration of the perineal muscles. *Am J Obstetr Gynecol*. 1948;56:238.

Kegel A. Sexual function of the pubococcygeus muscle. *West J Surg Obstetr Gynecol*. 1952; 10:521.

King-Baker P. Musculoskeletal origins of chronic pelvic pain. *Obstetr Gynecol Clin North Am*. 1993;20:719.

King PB. Musculoskeletal problems. In: Steege JF, Metzger DA, Levy BS, eds. *Chronic Pelvic Pain*. Philadelphia, Pa: WB Saunders Co; 1998:215–240.

King PM, Ling FW, Myers CA. Screening for female urogenital system disease. In: Boissonnault WG, ed. *Examination in Physical Therapy Practice—Screening for Medical Disease*. 2nd ed. New York, NY: Churchill Livingstone; 1995.

Markswell SJ, Mumme GA. A role for physiotherapy in perianal and perineal pain syndromes. In: Shacklock MO, ed. *Moving in on Pain*. Australia: Butterworth Heinemann; 1995:145–152.

Mathias SD, Kuppermann M, Liberman RF, et al. Chronic pelvic pain: prevalence, health-related quality of life ad economic correlates. *Obstetr Gynecol*. 1996;87:321–327.

Sapsford R, Bullock-Saxton J, Markwell S. *Women's Health: A Textbook for Physiotherapists*. Philadelphia, Pa: WB Saunders Co; 1999.

Schachter CL, Stalker CA, Teram E. Toward sensitive practice: issues for physical therapists working with survivors of childhood sexual abuse. *Phys Ther*. 1999;79:248–261.

Schussler B, Laycock J, Norton P, Stanton S, eds. *Pelvic Floor Re-education Principles and Practice*. New York, NY: Springer-Verlag; 1994.

Theve-Gibbons S. Women and chronic pelvic pain: stigma, invisibility and sexuality. *J Section Women's Health*. 2000;24:7–12.

Wallace K. Female pelvic floor functions, dysfunctions, and behavioural approaches to treatment. *Clin Sports Med*. 1994;13:459–481.

Wilder E, ed. *The Gynecological Manual. Section on Women's Health*. Alexandria, Va: American Physical Therapy Association; 1997.

Pelvic Inflammatory Disease

Also known as *salpingitis*.

DESCRIPTION

Pelvic inflammatory disease (PID) is an infection of the fallopian tubes, and possibly the cervix, uterus, and ovaries as well.

CAUSE

Infection usually begins intravaginally, spreading upward due to microorganisms transmitted during intercourse. Women using an intrauterine device (IUD) are particularly vulnerable because the IUD device allows transmission of pathogens. Childbirth, ruptured ectopic pregnancy, or surgical procedures such as an abortion may also, although less commonly, allow transmission of an infecting organism.

ASSESSMENT

Note: See APTA's Guide to Physical Therapist Practice. 2nd ed. *Physical Therapy.* 2001;81.

Musculoskeletal Preferred Practice Patterns: C, D

AREAS
- History, including any medical conditions or symptoms such as bleeding or discharge, occupation, surgery, menopausal state, and medications
- Psychosocial
- Urinary symptoms: frequency, urgency, stress, and nocturia
- Bowel habits, including any constipation
- Pain, including any dyspareunia (painful intercourse)
- Activities of daily living (ADLs)
- Perineal examination, including pelvic floor strength

INSTRUMENTS/PROCEDURES

See References for sources.

No specific evaluation for PID was identified. Consider use of elements from evaluation for incontinence.

Urinary Symptoms
- daily intake and output diary

PROBLEMS
- The woman will often have extreme pain in lower abdominal region, which can become chronic.
- The woman may have swelling and tenderness accompanying the pain.
- The woman may have backache.
- The woman may have dysmenorrhea and may have increased menstrual flow.
- The woman may feel generally lethargic.
- The woman may have dyspareunia.
- The woman may have infertility.
- The women may have ectopic pregnancy.

TREATMENT/MANAGEMENT
- In the acute phase of infection, the client should be receiving medical attention.
- In the chronic phase, perform gentle mobilization exercises, instruct the client in relaxation exercises, and try shortwave or microwave diathermy at daily frequency or on alternate days for a duration of 20 minutes.

DESIRED OUTCOME/PROGNOSIS
- The client will have a decrease in pain.
- There will be a reduction in infection.

REFERENCES

Assessment

Adams C, Frahm J. Genitourinary system. In: Myers RS, ed. *Saunders Manual of Physical Therapy Practice*. Philadelphia, Pa: WB Saunders Co; 1995:494.

American Physical Therapy Association. Guide to physical therapist practice. 2nd ed. *Phys Ther*. 2001;81.

Goodman C, Snyder TE. *Differential Diagnosis in Physical Therapy*. 2nd ed. Philadelphia, PA; WB Saunders Co; 2000.

King PM, Ling FW, Myers CA. Screening for female urogenital system disease. In: Boissonnault WG, ed. *Examination in Physical Therapy Practice—Screening for Medical Disease*. 2nd ed. New York, NY: Churchill Livingstone; 1995.

Treatment

Adams C, Frahm J. Genitourinary system. In: Myers RS, ed. *Saunders Manual of Physical Therapy Practice*. Philadelphia, Pa: WB Saunders Co; 1995:459–504.

Markswell SJ, Mumme GA. A role for physiotherapy in perianal and perineal pain syndromes. In: Shacklock MO, ed. *Moving in on Pain*. Australia: Butterworth Heinemann; 1995:145–152.

Mathias SD, Kuppermann M, Liberman RF, et al. Chronic pelvic pain: prevalence, health-related quality of life and economic correlates. *Obstetr Gynecol*. 1996;87:321–327.

Polden M, Mantle J. *Physiotherapy in Obstetrics and Gynecology*. London, England: Butterworth Heinemann; 1990.

Sapsford R, Bullock-Saxton J, Markwell S. *Women's Health: A Textbook for Physiotherapists*. Philadelphia, Pa: WB Saunders Co; 1999.

Wilder E, ed. *The Gynecological Manual. Section on Women's Health*. Alexandria, Va: American Physical Therapy Association; 1997.

Postpartum Period

Also known as the *puerperium*.

DESCRIPTION

The postpartum period describes the time following birth. The uterus undergoes a process of involution, or returning to near prepregnant size, usually 5 to 6 weeks after birth. Most describe the period as lasting 6 to 12 weeks; each woman's adjustment period is different.

CAUSE

During the time following birth, the mother's body undergoes a physiological adjustment to the changes from pregnancy and delivery.

ASSESSMENT

Note: See APTA's Guide to Physical Therapist Practice. 2nd ed. *Physical Therapy.* 2001;81.

Musculoskeletal Preferred Practice Pattern: D

AREAS

- History, including type of delivery, complications, medical history
- Activity level
- Mobility, including transfers, bed, and gait
- Pain
- Strength, if indicated
- Range of motion (ROM)
- Posture
- Musculoskeletal, including joints, presence of diastasis recti after third postpartum day
- Functional level

INSTRUMENTS/PROCEDURES

See References for sources.

Strength
- manual muscle testing

PROBLEMS

- The woman often feels physically exhausted.
- There are often contractions, called afterpains, after birth and during nursing, which may be painful. They are usually stronger with second or subsequent deliveries.
- There may be breast discomfort.
- The abdominal muscles are often very lax.
- There may be bladder distention.
- The client may be constipated. Hemorrhoids can be present.
- The client often has perineal pain if she sustained a laceration or if an episiotomy was performed.
- The woman may have had perineal trauma, such as hematoma, edema, ecchymosis, or erythema.
- The woman often has "postpartum blues" characterized by crying spells, anxiety, worry, loneliness, and mood swings.
- The woman may have postpartum depression, usually beginning as soon as 24 hours after delivery, but possibly beginning several weeks later. Symptoms of depression include feeling hopeless, being overly concerned or underconcerned about baby, losing appetite, having a fear of touching the baby, being unable to sleep, and having little concern about appearance.

Note: Postpartum psychosis is a more extreme reaction to birth and is rare.

TREATMENT/MANAGEMENT

GENERAL

- Referral to a support group is almost always welcome for new mothers, especially those with postpartum depression.

- Instruct in postural correction as needed. During the postpartum period, there is a tendency for a forward head and rounded shoulder posture due to holding and feeding the baby.
- Instruct in proper body mechanics. Proper instruction in activities of daily living (ADLs) for child care includes topics such as lifting, feeding, changing, and use of equipment.

EXERCISE

After checking for diastasis of the abdominal muscles, the therapist can teach exercises, stressing the importance of the restoration of the abdominal and the pelvic floor muscles. The synergistic nature of the pelvic floor with the abdominal muscles can also be taught. Provide the woman with guidance for general and specific exercises after birth. These exercises can include the following:

- First 2 to 3 days after an uncomplicated delivery
  1. gentle abdominal exercise coordinated with breathing
  2. ROM exercises for the feet and ankles
  3. pelvic tilt
  4. pelvic floor toning
  5. heel slides and gluteal toning
- After first 2 to 3 days
  1. abdominal exercise as indicated by state of abdominal wall: begin with head lifts if diastasis is larger than 2 cm; if less than 2 cm, curl-ups are indicated; progress as indicated to bridging and curl-ups with diagonal or reverse components added
  2. upper back release and upper extremity exercises
  3. leg toning

EPISIOTOMY HEALING

- Ice packs can be used during the first 48 hours; then switch to mild heat, sitz baths, Kegel exercises, and a pericare bottle. Follow up with a pelvic floor rehabilitation program.

BREAST-FEEDING

Tips to New Mothers About How to Get Started with Breast-Feeding

- Stroke nipple near the infant's mouth to encourage reflexive rooting response and to facilitate sucking.
- Let the infant breast-feed on demand and not on a fixed schedule. It is normal for newborns to nurse 10 to 12 times in a 24-hour period.
- Refer to books, nurses, lactation consultants, hospital classes, or a support group such as La Leche League International as indicated.
- Discuss inverted nipples during pregnancy so intervention can begin before the baby arrives.

Common Problems Encountered in Breast-Feeding

- Engorgement—fullness as milk production begins
  1. Breast-feed as soon as possible after birth.
  2. Feed frequently.
  3. Use both breasts at each feeding.
  4. Apply warmth before feeding (use warm cloth or take shower).
  5. Apply cold after feeding.
- Sore nipples
  1. Use the less sore nipple first.
  2. Let air get to breasts.
  3. Coat nipples and aureola with breast milk.

4. Make the feedings shorter and more frequent.
5. Position the infant's chest to the mother's chest, with the infant and breast well supported under and on top.
6. Vary nursing positions.
- Mastitis—reddened, lump in breast, painful, may begin with flulike symptoms
  1. Rest with the infant, and feed the infant every 2 to 2-1/2 hours.
  2. Use medication for fever as prescribed by physician.
  3. Generally, it is advisable to continue to breast-feed.
- Musculoskeletal conditions affecting breast-feeding mothers
  1. Discuss proper body mechanics postpartum.
  2. Recommend supports such as nursing pillows and stools for arm and foot support.

AFTER A CESAREAN DELIVERY
- Instruct the woman in abdominal breathing and huffing techniques with incisional support via a pillow.
- Consider transcutaneous electrical nerve stimulation (TENS) for post-cesarean delivery pain control. Electrode placement may vary depending on the type of incision. For horizontal incisions possible locations include above and below the incision, parallel at each end of the incision, or in an inverted V shape at each end of the incision.
- Beginning exercises for after cesarean delivery, as indicated by recovery, are breathing exercises, ankle ROM, isometric leg exercises. Gradually add, as recovery allows, pelvic tilt, bridging, modified curl-ups, and leg sliding exercises.

PRECAUTIONS/CONTRAINDICATIONS
- The new mother can resume aerobic activity at the 60% level after clearance from her physician and when her body feels ready.
- Referral is indicated if the pathological condition of postpartum psychosis appears. It is manifested by symptoms of persistent depression, lack of interest in the baby, thoughts of harming the baby or self, hallucinations, and/or other psychotic behavior.
- The mother should notify the primary caregiver if she experiences any of the following symptoms:
  1. The entire breast is hot and hard, and there is also fever, chills, nausea, or aching; the woman may have mastitis.
  2. The leg has an area that is hot, swollen, and red; the woman may have thrombophlebitis.
  3. There is a frequent urge to urinate, but little or no urine is passed, and there is pain in the lower abdomen or back; the woman may have cystitis.
  4. Lochia, vaginal discharge, changes back to a bright red color; there may be some placental retention.
  5. Vaginal discharge is foul smelling, accompanied by pain and itching; there may be infection.
  6. There is a fever higher than 100.4 degrees F for more than 1 day, with persistent, intense pain from the vaginal area.

DESIRED OUTCOME/PROGNOSIS
- Pain will be diminished.
- The client will increase strength and endurance.
- The client will be independent in mobility and ADLs.
- The client will be educated about body mechanics for child care with the infant.
- The client will be continent in bladder and bowel.
- Musculoskeletal dysfunction will be corrected.

REFERENCES

Assessment

American Physical Therapy Association. Guide to physical therapist practice. 2nd ed. *Phys Ther.* 2001;81.

Appel C. Obstetrical considerations. In: Myers RS, ed. *Saunders Manual of Physical Therapy Practice.* Philadelphia, Pa: WB Saunders Co; 1995:522.

Pauls J, ed. *Therapeutic Approaches to Women's Health: A Program of Exercise and Education.* Gaithersburg, Md: Aspen Publishers; 1995.

Sapsford R, Bullock-Saxton J, Markwell S. *Women's Health: A Textbook for Physiotherapists.* Philadelphia, Pa: WB Saunders Co; 1999.

Treatment

Appel C. Obstetrical considerations. In: Myers RS, ed. *Saunders Manual of Physical Therapy Practice.* Philadelphia, Pa: WB Saunders Co; 1995:522.

Daniels L, Worthingham C. *Muscle Testing: Techniques of Manual Examination.* 6th ed. Philadelphia, Pa: WB Saunders Co; 1995.

Duffy-Rath J, Rath W, Mielcarski E, et al. Low back pain during pregnancy: helping patients take control: movements, postures that ease symptoms are basis of physical therapy. *J Musculoskeletal Med.* 2000;17:223–232.

Everett T, Macintosh J, Grant A. Ultrasound therapy for persistent postnatal perineal pain and dyspaerunia. *Physiotherapy.* 1992;78:263–267.

Gilleard WL, Brown JM. Structure and function of the abdominal muscles in primigravid subjects during pregnancy and the immediate postbirth period. *Phys Ther.* 1996;76:750–762.

Goldman L, Ishigami S, Raynovich, et al. A comparison of back pain characteristics of pregnant, postpartum, and not pregnant women. *J Section Women's Health.* 2000;24:14.

Hay-Smith EJ. Therapeutic ultrasound for postpartum perineal pain and dyspareunia. *Cochrane Database Systematic Review.* 2000;2:CD000495.

Hay-Smith J, Mantle J. Surveys of the experience and perceptions of post-natal superficial dyspareunia of post-natal women, general practitioners and physiotherapists. *Physiotherapy.* 1996;82:91–97.

Kendall FP, McCreary EK, Provance PG. *Muscles: Testing and Function.* 4th ed. Baltimore, Md: Williams and Wilkins; 1993.

Luscombe D, Jones S, Cox D, et al. The effects of therapeutic ultrasound on breast milk composition: a single case experimental study. *Aust Physiotherapy Assoc Natl Women's Health J.* 1995;14:48.

Markswell SJ, Mumme GA. A role for physiotherapy in perianal and perineal pain syndromes. In: Shacklock MO, ed. *Moving in on Pain.* Australia: Butterworth Heinemann; 1995:145–152.

Nicholson W. Mastitis and ultrasound. *Aust J Phys Ther.* 1994;40:49.

Nilsson-Wikmar L, Harms-Ringdahl K, Pilo C. Back pain in women post-partum is not a unitary concept. *Physiotherapy Res Int.* 1999;4:201–213.

Pauls J, ed. *Therapeutic Approaches to Women's Health: A Program of Exercise and Education.* Gaithersburg, Md: Aspen Publishers; 1995.

Pauls J. Cesarean birth and vaginal birth after cesarean: an update for physical therapists. *J Section Women's Health.* 1998;22:15–21.

Pipp LM. Compendium of selected TENS literature. *J Obstetr Gynecol Phys Ther*. 1993; 17:12.

Pirie A, Herman H. *How to Raise Children Without Breaking Your Back*. West Somerville, Mass: IBIS Publications; 1995.

Riddoch S, Grimmer K. Developing a clinical indicator for obstructive mastitis. *Aust J Phys Ther*. 1993;39:321–322.

Sapsford R, Bullock-Saxton J, Markwell S. *Women's Health: A Textbook for Physiotherapists*. Philadelphia, Pa: WB Saunders Co; 1999.

Sheppard S. Management of postpartum gross divarication recti. *Midwifery Digest*. 1997; 7:84–86.

Pregnancy—Musculoskeletal Conditions

DESCRIPTION

Pregnancy changes can lead to or aggravate musculoskeletal conditions. About half of all pregnant women experience back pain. Some common musculoskeletal conditions during pregnancy:

- back pain, including postural pain, sacroiliac dysfunction, disk derangement, and sciatica
- diastasis abdominis recti
- pubic symphysis pain
- coccydynia
- calf cramps
- costal margin pain
- transient osteoporosis of pregnancy
- thoracic outlet pain
- carpal tunnel syndrome

CAUSE

Low back pain has many causes, but two of the most common are faulty posture combined with poor body mechanics. During pregnancy, factors contributing to musculoskeletal dysfunction include increased weight gain, hormonal relaxation of tissues, stretching of abdominal muscle, increase in lumbar lordosis and thoracic kyphosis, genu recurvatum, and forward head posture.

ASSESSMENT

Note: See APTA's Guide to Physical Therapist Practice. 2nd ed. *Physical Therapy*. 2001;81.

Musculoskeletal Preferred Practice Pattern: D

AREAS
- History
- Edema
- Posture
- Range of motion (ROM)
- Gait
- Joint integrity and structural deviations/neurological involvement
- Strength
- Pain
- Functional level

INSTRUMENTS/PROCEDURES

See References for sources.

Edema
- volumetrics
- girth measurements

Joint Integrity and Structural Deviations/Neurological Involvement
- carpal tunnel syndrome tests
  1. Phalen's test
  2. Tinel's sign
- diastasis recti abdominis test (see Table 15.9)
- lumbar lordosis measurement
- orthopedic tests for sacroiliac joint
  1. limb-length test
  2. Gillet test: palpation of anterior and posterior superior iliac spines (patient standing, then sitting), palpation of iliac crests (patient standing, then sitting)
  3. side-lying iliac compression test
  4. sitting flexion text
  5. standing flexion test
  6. standing Gillet test
  7. supine iliac gapping test
- standing march test for irritated symphysis
- thoracic outlet syndrome tests
  1. Adson's test
  2. hyperabduction test
  3. Wright's test

Special Tests to Which the Physical Therapist May or May Not Have Access
- nerve conduction studies (see Carpal Tunnel Syndrome Tests in references)

PROBLEMS

LOW BACK PAIN

Muscle Strain
- The woman may have localized swelling.
- The woman often has pain with movement.
- The woman often has decreased and painful ROM.
- Passive movement is often within normal limits.
- The woman may show painful recovery from movement.
- The woman may have unilateral pain.
- The woman may have pain radiate distally.

TABLE 15.9
Test for Diastasis Recti Abdominals

Diastasis Recti Abdominals Test for the Female Client

The therapist has the woman in the supine position with no pillow under her head. The woman lifts her chin and shoulders forward to bring the rectus muscle belly forward. The therapist palpates the gap between the rectus abdominis muscle at the level of the umbilicus and also 4.5 cm (approximately 2 fingers) above and 4.5 cm below this level. A gap equal to the width of 2 or more fingers (ie, 4.5 cm) is considered positive. Below the umbilical line, a separation of 1 finger may be significant.

Source: Reprinted from Pauls J. *Therapeutic Approaches to Women's Health; A Program of Exercise and Education.* Aspen Publishers; 1995:2-1:4.

Muscle Spasm
- The woman often has decreased ROM, pain, and tenderness over a muscle.
- There is often increased tone in the muscles.
- The woman may find that continued spasm becomes a source of additional pain due to a self-perpetuating cycle.

Postural Syndrome
- The woman often finds that pain eases with activity.
- Often, standing or sitting posture is beyond normal limits.
- The woman may find pain only during sustained supine positions.

Sacroiliac Joint Dysfunction

In general sacroiliac joint dysfunction:

- The woman often complains of pain with sitting.
- The woman often has pain on leaning forward.
- The woman may have pain with an increase in intra-abdominal pressure.
- The woman may have a sudden onset of unilateral sacroiliac pain.
- The woman may have a sharp pain or catching sensation during rolling from side to side.
- The woman may feel pain in the posterior thigh.
- The woman may have anterior hip pain.
- The woman may report paresthesia in the absence of neurological signs.
- The woman may find ipsilateral sacroiliac dysfunction present with L 3–4 or L 4–5 lesions.
- A pattern of right sacroiliac dysfunction has been described as causing associated discomfort at left T-12, right T-8, left T-2, and right C2-3.

Notes: In the case of anterior rotation of the ilium on the sacrum, the long-sitting versus supine leg-length test makes the leg appear longer when the client is in a supine position and shorter when she is in a sitting position.

In the case of posterior rotation of the ilium on the sacrum, the long-sitting versus supine leg-length test makes the leg appear shorter when the client is in a supine position and longer when she is in a sitting position.

Pubic Symphysis Pain
- The woman may have pain over the area of the symphysis pubis and sacroiliac joints, groin, and adductor muscles.
- There may be palpable separation of the joint, especially during weight shifting.
- The woman may have pain with forward bending.
- The woman may not be able to move in bed.
- The woman may not be able to walk.
- The woman may not be able to move her legs.

Pregnancy-Associated Osteoporosis
- The woman often has a back pain that is unexplained by another diagnosis.
- The woman may have hip fracture.

Disk Derangement

In the case of acute posterolateral disk prolapse:

- The woman may have a sudden onset of unilateral lumbosacral pain.
- Often, the pain is severe or knifelike, but it may be dull and aching.
- The woman may have aching into the leg, usually unilateral.
- Often the pain is worse with sitting or sudden straining, and it may be hard to stand up.
- The woman may have lumbar deformity with loss of lordosis.
- The woman often has lumbar scoliosis (convexity on involved side).

- Often, there is marked, painful restriction of spinal movement, with a decrease of extension mobility.
- Often, the pain increases with repeated flexion and/or sustained flexion.
- Often, the mechanism of onset involves flexion.

In the case of disk herniation:

- The woman may have neurological involvement (reflexes, myotome and/or dermatome).
- The woman may have pain and/or paresthesia distal to knee.
- The mechanism of onset typically involves lumbar flexion.
- The woman may have pain aggravated by sitting.

In the case of lower lumbar disc herniation (extrusion) with nerve root impingement:

- The woman may have unilateral leg pain, but bilateral is possible.
- The woman often feels leg pain in the posterolateral thigh and the anterior lateral or posterior aspect of the lower leg.
- The woman may have back pain alone; the combination of back and leg pain is less common.
- Often, lumbar extension will peripheralize pain. Extremity pain is usually worse than back pain.
- The woman often has mild segmental neurologic deficit, indicated by the presence of a specific dermatome sensory loss or specific motor weakness.
- Rarely, rupture leads to decreased pain but increased neurological signs.

Sciatica
- The woman often has pain following the course of the sciatic nerve, with radiating pain into the buttocks.

DIASTASIS ABDOMINIS RECTI
- This condition often goes undetected by the pregnant woman.

PIRIFORMIS SYNDROME
- The woman often has persistent, severe, radiating low back pain that extends from the sacrum to the hip joint over the gluteal region and posterior portion of the upper leg (sciatic distribution).
- The hip on the involved side may demonstrate an increase in external rotation secondary to a shortened piriformis muscle.
- Often, on palpation, the buttock on the involved side is very tender. The leg on the involved side may appear shorter from contracture.

COCCYDYNIA
- The woman is often unable to sit directly on the coccyx because of localized tenderness.

CALF CRAMPS
- The woman often has pain in the calf triggered by pointing the toes.

COSTAL MARGIN PAIN
- The woman may often have pain on the anterior aspect of the lower ribs secondary to the changes in abdominal muscle alignment and the flaring of the ribs.

THORACIC OUTLET SYNDROME
- The woman often has parethesia in the upper extremity.
- The woman may complain of fatigue with arm use.
- Often, upper extremity stretching leads to pain.

CARPAL TUNNEL SYNDROME

- The woman often has weakness in the hands.
- The woman may have thenar atrophy.
- The woman often has paresthesia, especially at night.
- The woman may have diminished median nerve conduction velocity.
- The woman may have swelling over the volar aspect of the wrist.
- Pitting edema may be present.

TREATMENT/MANAGEMENT

LOW BACK PAIN

Muscle Strain
In acute cases:

- Try ice (except over the kidney area), any modalities not contraindicated during pregnancy, and relaxation techniques, as tolerated.
- The client should be advised to rest.

In subacute cases:

- Begin with gentle movement, and progress to full movement.
- Superficial heat and massage can be added, along with gentle stretching techniques, graded isometric exercise, and resistive dynamic exercise.
- Use the side-lying position if needed. Usually the left side-lying position is the most comfortable, and a client can perform these exercises from this position: gluteal set, pelvic tilt, and adductor set.
- Correct posture abnormalities with kinesthetic training, and correct flexibility and strength imbalances. Posture exercises include axial extension, stretching the pectoralis major muscle, strengthening the midthoracic area muscles, and toning abdominal shortening contractions of the external obliques along with the rectus abdominis.
- Stabilization exercises to promote isolation and cocontraction of muscle groups should be considered.

Muscle Spasm
In acute cases:

- Ice or cold packs and passive support can be helpful. Avoid ice over the kidney region.
- The following techniques are indicated: elongation of muscle to tolerance via positioning, reverse muscle action techniques, and passive to active ROM in a pain-free range.

In subacute and chronic cases:

- Moist heat and/or ice, cold packs, and massage are indicated.
- Progress the exercise program as tolerated.
- Consider using postural retraining with kinesthetic awareness and relaxation exercises. Education should be emphasized, along with a search for the underlying cause of the pain.

Postural Syndrome
Posturally related back pain is especially suited to the self-treatment principles learned in a back school.
Possible topics for back school include the following:

- Basic information: anatomy, biomechanics, pain, drugs, sex, stress, physical fitness, health, resources
- Rehabilitation/prevention: posture, awareness, movement, body/mind relationship, self-help techniques, physical interventions
- Ergonomic principles: human considerations, environmental conditions, work dynamics, relevance of person to equipment

- Basic rules of working and lifting
- Supplement education with appropriate strengthening and stretching exercises.
- Treatment sessions in the water can be helpful. Immersion is an effective treatment for edema, significantly decreasing swelling in the lower extremities.

Sacroiliac Joint Dysfunction
In general:

- Instruct the client in how to stretch shortened muscles and strengthen weakened muscles. Treatment aims to decrease pain and improve joint mobility and mechanics.
- The area is supported with an orthosis if it is acute and inflamed or in need of increased stability. A support with a special pad for the sacroiliac region is especially helpful. The client should be cautioned, however, that an orthosis does not substitute for strengthening exercises and can actually weaken muscles if overused. A heel lift may be indicated if leg-length difference is demonstrated. The client should avoid any painful activities or vigorous exercise, such as jogging, until the pelvis is level and she is symptom-free.
- For acute pain, the client rests with legs adducted and flexed. She may get some relief by applying pressure around the hips with an orthosis.
- Ice packs and supported weight bearing with crutches or a walker may be needed.
- The typical treatment of ultrasound or electrical stimulation over the sacral sulci is contraindicated during pregnancy (see Precautions following).
- Provide education about the vulnerability of this joint. Teach posture awareness and body mechanics. Avoid high heels and prolonged standing.
- Use gentle mobilization or muscle energy techniques. Strengthen pelvic floor muscles and abdominal musculature.
- Teach proper relaxation positions (avoid the supine position after the first trimester if the client experiences symptoms of supine hypotension).
- Avoid unilateral weight bearing.

In cases of anterior rotation of the ilium on the sacrum:

- Consider eccentric contraction of hamstrings on the involved side, isometric or resisted hip extension, and knee extension to the gluteal and hamstring muscles on the involved side.
- Extreme abduction of lower extremities should be avoided.
- If tight, the hip piriformis muscle and iliotibial band should be stretched; weakened lower extremity muscles and abdominal musculature need to be strengthened.
- Progress can be facilitated with orthotic support, but the client can be weaned from the device if her pelvis can stay level on its own. If not, orthotic support will be needed during the remainder of her pregnancy and perhaps into the postpartum period.

In cases of posterior rotation of the ilium on the sacrum:

- Consider isometric contraction of the hip flexors, with the client in a position with 90-degree hip flexion and 90-degree knee flexion, squeezing the forearm between the knees during isometric hip adduction within a sitting position, and stretching and strengthening as before.

In cases of locking of the joint:

- The client lies on her back briefly, bends the knee of the involved side, and wraps her toes under the outer side of the straight leg. The therapist can gently place the client's bent knee across her body, while gently pressing the shoulder of the involved side in the opposite direction. This can be combined with a gentle rocking motion.

- A self-help position is similar. If the right side is involved, the client gently pulls her right flexed knee up and out with the right hand. With her left hand, she cups the right foot. She can also simply lie supine with the leg on the affected side crossed over the other leg with some rotation to get a traction effect to the sacroiliac joint through the weight of the leg. After staying in this position for 15 minutes or so, she cautiously resumes normal activity. The supine position should be avoided after the first trimester if the client is experiencing symptoms of supine hypotension. She follows with support and avoids overuse of any manipulation. The client rests in a side-lying position with pillows for support.
- Single weight-bearing exercises should be avoided.

Pubic Symphysis Pain

- Try moist heat or cold packs for pain relief.
- Positions in which the legs are widely separated should be avoided.
- Crutches or a walker may be needed for weight-bearing activities.
- The symphysis pubis joint can be immobilized with a binder around the hips at pubic level as tight as the client can tolerate after the joint is aligned.
- A depressed pubis can be raised by gentle pressure to the anterior ilium and ischial tuberosity.
- Having the client squeeze the forearm between the knees during isometric hip adduction in a sitting position is also helpful.
- Another self-correction technique involves the use of the abdominals to pull on the pubis.
- Resisted hip extension also utilizes the energy and movement from the muscle action to achieve the desired effect.

Pregnancy-Associated Osteoporosis

- If hip fracture is ruled out, treatment consists of rest, pain-reducing measures, and a gentle exercise routine that progresses to partial and then full weight bearing if well tolerated.

Disk Derangement
In cases of acute posterolateral disk prolapse:

- Reduce derangement with appropriate movement; the client may find pain reduced with repeated extension.
- Maintain reduction with posture correction and restore function. Avoid poor posture by providing education.
- Self-treatment with repeated movements can be tried first and may progress to mobilization if indicated (see Precautions following).
- Gentle traction can be tried with caution (see Precautions following).
- Use appropriate modalities for pain.
- Transcutaneous electrical nerve stimulation (TENS) should be considered as a last resort (see Precautions following).
- Treatments such as massage and localized moist heat packs can decrease disk pain by increasing the blood supply and facilitating relaxation.
- Massage can be done either in the water or on land, in a sitting or side-lying position. Massage can be performed prone during pregnancy if a special maternity support or table adaption is present and the client is comfortable.

In cases of disk herniation:

- For protrusion with neurological signs, use modalities and advise the client to rest. Avoid aggravation with postures that cause increased intradiscal pressure (especially sitting and flexion).
- Gentle traction can be considered (see Precautions following).
- Maintain correct posture and provide education.
- External support with a pregnancy back orthosis is indicated.

- Consider a trial of extension exercises, and extension in prone lying, if this is still a tolerable position, with gentle anterior-posterior glides.
- Contact the referring physician if neurological signs progress.

In cases of lower lumbar disc herniation (extrusion) with nerve root impingement:

- TENS for pain may be considered as a last resort (see Precautions following). Contact referring physician if neurological signs worsen.

Sciatica

- Reduction in activity may help in the acute stage.

DIASTASIS ABDOMINIS RECTI

- Treatment consists of splinting the two sides of the rectus abdominis toward midline while doing any stressful activity or during abdominal exercises. Splinting can be accomplished using the hands or with a wrap.
- An attempt should be made to approximate the rib with the pubic symphysis without bulging the abdominal wall.
- Teach the client shortening active contractions of the transversus and the internus and externus obliquus abdominal muscle in combination with breath exhalation.
- The client might consider using a maternity binder, reducing intra-abdominal stress with proper body mechanics, and avoiding a Valsalva maneuver.

PIRIFORMIS SYNDROME

- Moist heat is applied, with the client in the side-lying position (affected side up) and support at the waist, abdomen, and knees.
- Tightness is treated with pressure to insertion while adducting and internally rotating hip of the affected side.
- Gentle stretching is added. With the client in a sitting position, stretching is performed with hip flexion, adduction, and internal rotation. Equal weight bearing while standing should be stressed.
- Contract/relax, proprioceptive neuromuscular facilitation techniques, friction massage, and myofascial release techniques can also be used.
- Rule out any sacroiliac dysfunction.

COCCYDYNIA

- Treatment includes gentle mobilization when necessary.
- Myofascial techniques, examination and treatment of trigger points, and strain–counterstrain techniques can be considered.
- The use of specially designed ischial support cushions or 2 cushions with a gap in the middle to avoid pressure on coccyx while sitting and the application of ice or heat are helpful.
- Encourage proper sitting posture.

CALF CRAMPS

- "Runner's" stretch with dorsiflexion of the ankle can provide relief. Lock the foot up into supination before stretching.
- Stretching can also be performed by the therapist using a contract/relax technique on the gastrocnemius muscle tendon.
- Increase strength in the dorsiflexor muscles to counteract the strength of the cramp.
- Consider massage if no contraindications.

COSTAL MARGIN PAIN

- Raising the arms and flexing the trunk to the side away from the pain often gives relief.

- A posterior stretch can be accomplished by wrapping the arms around a chair while straddling it backwards.
- Teach proper posture, with emphasis on avoiding slumped sitting.
- Prescribe exercise for upper back strengthening.
- Consider muscle energy techniques for rib region.

THORACIC OUTLET SYNDROME

- General treatment consists of gentle mobilization of the clavicle at either joint and posture exercises to elevate the shoulder girdle.
- More specific treatments for the 3 types of thoracic outlet syndrome are described below.

Scalenus Anticus and Cervical Rib Syndrome

- Treatment consists of local heat, massage, ultrasound (away from the area near the baby in utero), traction, stretching of scalenus muscles, and active strengthening of upper trapezius and levator scapular muscles.

Costoclavicular Syndrome

- Treatment consists of exercise, posture training, and mobilization of the clavicle.

Hyperabduction Syndrome

- Treatment consists of stretching pectoral muscle and postural training.

CARPAL TUNNEL SYNDROME (CTS)

- Treatment for CTS varies and usually aims at symptomatic relief. Treatment consists of resting splints unilaterally or bilaterally, as needed.
- Splints are useful in decreasing wrist pressure.
- Splints can also be alternated during the day if both hands are involved. A splint on the wrist in a neutral position can be used as frequently as needed, perhaps even through the remainder of the pregnancy.
- Other therapists use a splint that "cocks" up the wrist into an extended position or keeps the wrist in a neutral position. The patient is told to avoid vigorous flexion and extension.
- Night splints, which may fit into a patient's lifestyle better, can also counteract the pain caused by increased heat, with subsequent increased metabolism, that occurs at night.
- Ice packs can be applied for pain relief.
- Postural exercises, such as thoracic outlet exercise, may help to alleviate brachial plexus pressure.
- Ergonomic considerations, such as maintaining 90 degrees' flexion of the elbow when working at a desk, can prevent repetitive motion strain.
- Ultrasound is sometimes helpful. Avoid sonating the abdomen, pelvis, and lumbar-sacral area (see Precautions).
- For posturally related pain, exercises, posture re-education, and conservative physical therapy may alleviate symptoms.
- Isometric and stretching exercises to consider include wrist circles, thumb and finger stretches, finger-thumb squeeze, wrist curls with the palm up and with the palm down, arm curls, and shoulder shrugs.

PRECAUTIONS/CONTRAINDICATIONS

The following precautions should be observed during the examination and treatment of a pregnant woman:

- The therapist should avoid testing that leaves the client excessively uncomfortable or that she is unable to tolerate.

- Having the woman's buttocks higher than the level of her chest could possibly, in rare instances, cause an air embolism infarct; this position has been associated with introduction of air into the vaginal canal in a forced manner.
- The woman should change positions slowly to allow time for postural and circulatory changes.
- The therapist should use caution with any maneuvers that could lead to shearing forces on a joint, secondary to laxity, or transient osteoporosis. Some therapists consider manipulation contraindicated during pregnancy, but, if indicated, and if special precautions are taken, the benefits may outweigh any risk. Most pregnant clients can be treated with an appropriate mobilizing technique without any undue complication (see Maitland and Corrigan, *Practical Orthopaedic Medicine*, in References). Adequate posturing of clients needs to be considered. Mobilization grades 1 and 2 are the most commonly used techniques in the lumbar spine during pregnancy. Muscle energy techniques are also used to affect joint alignment. Vigorous thrusting techniques are contraindicated.
- Avoiding the supine position for periods longer than 3 minutes is important to prevent supine hypotension syndrome.
- The physical therapist must be careful not to let pregnancy mask causes unrelated to the baby, such as a herniated disk, fibromyalgia, or ankylosing spondylosis.
- Correction of a lateral shift may cause increased back pain (a centralization effect) but should not cause increased leg pain. Discontinue the extension exercise if this happens. Extension of the spine is contraindicated if it does not decrease or centralize the pain, if bladder weakness or paresthesia in the saddle region is present, or if the patient is unable to assume a position due to pain or stage of pregnancy. Avoid flexion if it increases pain or peripheralizes the symptoms. Flexion positions and exercises may harm patients with herniated nucleus pulposus with protrusion. If any increase in mobility increases pain or an inflammatory response, try another approach.
- Clients with pain and stiffness usually progress in improvement. If a client is not following patterns of improvement, this may be a warning to consider an organic disease or psychogenic disorder.
- Special caution should be taken when using physical agents and modalities with a pregnant woman:
  1. Modalities such as deep heat (ultrasound or diathermy) or electrical stimulation are contraindicated over areas near the baby, especially the sacral sulci.
  2. Some therapists consider mechanical traction to be contraindicated during pregnancy. Traction has, however, been used successfully in the first 2 trimesters, provided it is with small poundage. Check with the equipment manufacturer for guidelines.
  3. TENS for pain relief in pregnancy has not been approved by the FDA and should be considered only as a last resort and only in the last 2 trimesters. Because TENS and other forms of electromagnetic and ultrasonic therapy have not been proved safe for use during pregnancy, they must be used with caution until the short-term and long-term effects on the fetus have been documented sufficiently. Some authors consider its use contraindicated in pregnancy (see Pipp, "TENS Update," in References). But TENS has been used during pregnancy in areas other than over the uterus. In special circumstances, under the consultation of the physician, the benefit may outweigh any potential risk. It may also carry less risk than pharmaceutical and surgical alternatives. The conventional mode has been used.
  4. Modalities can be overused, particularly with musculoskeletal strain or sprain and inflammation. Pain relief through modalities should not cause you to ignore loss of motion and strength.

    5. Whirlpools with very hot water and saunas should be used with caution, and water temperature should be monitored carefully. If body temperature rises more than 1 degree, it is time to get out. Raised internal temperature can interfere with fetal cell division.

- Discuss the following symptoms with primary caregiver:
  1. swelling in feet and ankles not better after 30 minutes of elevation
  2. swelling in both hands
  3. eyes and/or face are puffy
  4. leg has painful, hot, red, or swollen area
  5. bloody vaginal discharge
  6. thin, watery discharge
  7. abdominal pain accompanied by nausea or vomiting, or dizziness or pain lasting longer than 2 minutes
  8. frequent contraction prematurely more than 6 times in an hour
  9. major decrease in fetal movement
  10. visual disturbances
  11. significant decrease in urine production
- Contraindications associated with aquatic exercise and pregnancy are toxemia, cerclage secondary to a dilated cervix, antepartum bleeding, and fetal hypotrophy. General contraindications include heart insufficiency, uncontrolled hypertension, respiratory insufficiency, tuberculosis, infections, incontinence, epilepsy, and diabetes.

DESIRED OUTCOME/PROGNOSIS

The goals of treatment will vary depending upon clinical findings but in general:

- The client will experience a decrease in pain and a relief of symptoms.
- The client will have an increase in movement and restore function or stabilize excessive movement.
- Therapy will prevent the progression and recurrence of the disorder.

Note: Early intervention is important to decrease the severity of pain and disability.

REFERENCES

Assessment

American Physical Therapy Association. Guide to physical therapist practice. 2nd ed. *Phys Ther.* 2001;81.

Feldt CM. Applying the Guide to Physical Therapist Practice to Women's Health Physical Therapy: Part II. *J Section Women's Health.* 2000;24:7–14.

Noble E. *Essential Exercises for the Childbearing Years.* 4th ed. Boston, Mass: Houghton Mifflin; 1995.

Pauls J, ed. *Therapeutic Approaches to Women's Health: A Program of Exercise and Education.* Gaithersburg, Md: Aspen Publishers; 1995.

Stephenson RG, O'Connor LJ. *Obstetric and Gynecologic Care in Physical Therapy.* 2nd ed. Thorofare, NJ: Slack Inc; 2000.

Treatment

American College of Obstetricians and Gynecologists. Exercise during pregnancy and the postpartum period. Technical Bulletin 189. *Int J Gynaecol Obstetr.* 1994;45:65–70.

Association of Chartered Physiotherapists in Women's Health. *Physiotherapy.* 1997;83:41–42.

Ashworth PD, Hagan MT. Some social consequences of non-compliance with pelvic floor exercises. *Physiotherapy.* 1993;79:465–471.

Bernstein S. Components and approaches of current perinatal exercise classes: part 1, a literature review. *J Obstetr Gynecol Phys Ther.* 1994;18:4:10–14.

Boissonnault WG, Boissonnault JS. Transient osteoporosis of the hip associated with pregnancy. *J Orthop Sports Phys Ther.* 2001;31:359–367.

Boxer SE, Jones S. Intra-rater reliability of rectus abdominis diastasis measurement using dial calipers. *Aust J Physiotherapy.* 1997;43:109–114.

Clark TJ, McKenna LS Jewell MJ, Callinan-Moore K. Managing diastasis recti. *Aus Physiotherapy Assoc J Natl Women's Health Group.* 1993;12:15–19.

Dinniny P. Women's health issues: coming of age. *PT-Magazine Phys Ther.* 1995;3:9:46–55.

Duffy-Rath J, Rath W, Mielcarski E, et al. Low back pain during pregnancy: helping patients take control: movements, postures that ease symptoms are basis of physical therapy. *J Musculoskeletal Med.* 2000;17:223–232.

Editorial. Physio helps new mums to stay dry. *Physiotherapy Moves.* 1999;10:20.

Feldt CM. Applying the Guide to Physical Therapist Practice to Women's Health Physical Therapy: Part II. *J Section Women's Health.* 2000;24:7–14.

Franklin ME, Conner-Kerr T. An analysis of posture and back pain in the first and third trimesters of pregnancy. *J Orthop Sports Phys Ther.* 1998;28:133–138.

Friend B. PT: proving positive in women's health. *Physiotherapy Frontline.* 1998;4:8–9.

Gilleard WL, Brown JM. Structure and function of the abdominal muscles in primigravid subjects during pregnancy and the immediate postbirth period. *Phys Ther.* 1996;76:750–762.

Gleeson PB, Pauls JA. Obstetrical physical therapy: review of the literature. *Phys Ther.* 1988;68:1699–1702.

Hainline B. Low back pain in pregnancy. In: Devinsky O, Feldman E, Hainline B, eds. *Nerological Complications of Pregnancy.* New York, NY: Raven Press; 1994:65–76.

Hakeem F. Baby, what a difference a decade can make. *PT—Magazine Phys Ther.* 1995;3:46–48.

Harris SR, Osborn JA, Weinberg J, Loock C, Junaid K. Effects of prenatal alcohol exposure on neuromotor and cognitive development during early childhood: a series of case reports. *Phys Ther.* 1993;73:608–617.

Hertling D, Kessler RM. *Management of Common Musculoskeletal Disorders.* 3rd ed. Philadelphia, Pa: JB Lippincott Co; 1996.

Hsia M, Jones S. Natural resolution of rectus abdominis diastasis. Two single case studies. *Aust J Physiotherapy.* 2000;46:301–307.

Johnstone J. Exercise in pregnancy. *J Obstetr Gynecol Neonatal Nurs.* 1997;26:143.

Kelderman C, Johnsen L. Exercise and pregnancy: a review of literature. *J Section Women's Health.* 1998;22:3–8.

Kisner C, Colby LA. *Therapeutic Exercise: Foundations and Techniques.* 3rd ed. Philadelphia, Pa: FA Davis Co; 1996.

Levangie PK. Association of low back pain with self-reported risk factors among patients seeking physical therapy services. 1999;79:757–766.

Li A, Yoshida K. Women with physical disabilities and their health: implications for health promotion and physical therapy. *Physiotherapy Can.* 1998;50:309–315.

Lo T, Candido G, Janssen P. Diastasis of the Recti abdominis in pregnancy: risk factors and treatment. *Physiotherapy Can.* 1999;51:32–37.

Maitland GD, Corrigan B. *Practical Orthopaedic Medicine*. London, England: Butterworth and Co Ltd; 1983.

Mantle J. Back pain in the childbearing year. In: Boyling JD, Palastanga N, eds. *Grieve's Modern Manual Therapy*. 2nd ed. New York, NY: Churchill Livingstone; 1994:799–808.

Marcus DA, Scharff L, Turk DC. Nonpharmacological management of headaches during pregnancy. *Psychosomatic Med*. 1995;57:527–535.

Nilsson-Wikmar L, Harms-Ringdahl K, Nygren A. Back pain in women post-partum is not a unitary concept. *Physiotherapy Research International*. 1999;4:201–213.

Noble E. *Essential Exercises for the Childbearing Year*. 4th ed. Boston, Mass: Houghton Mifflin; 1995.

Noren L, Ostgaard S, Nielsen TF, et al. Reduction of sick leave for lumbar back and posterior pelvic pain in pregnancy. *Spine*. 1997;22:2157–2160.

O'Connor G. My pelvis and I-symphysis pubic dysfunction. *Midwifery Matters*. 2000;84:8–9.

O'Connor LJ. Exercising more ways, enjoying it less. *J Obstetr Gynecol Phys Ther*. 1989;13:8–9.

Olney E. Spotlight on women's health. *Physiotherapy Moves*. 1999;10:19.

Onyeije CI, Sherer DM, Ham L. Transient marked atelectasis; an unusual complication of asthma in pregnancy. *Am J Perinatology*. 1999;16:521–524.

Ostgaard HC, Zetherstrom G, Roos-Hansson E. Back pain in relation to pregnancy: a 6 year follow-up. *Spine*. 1997;22:2945–2950.

Otman AS, Beksac MS, Bagoze O. The importance of lumbar lordosis measurement device application during pregnancy, and post-partum isometric exercise. *Eur J Obstetr Gynecol Reprod Biol*. 1989;31:155–162.

Ouellet-Hellstrom R, Stewart WF. Miscarriages among female physical therapists who report using radio and microwave-frequency electromagnetic radiation. *Am J Epidemiol*. 1993;138:775–786.

Osborn JA, Harris SR, Weinberg J. Fetal alcohol syndrome: review of the literature with implications for physical therapists. *Phys Ther*. 1993;73:599–607.

Paul JA, Frings-Drsen MHW, Sale HJA, et al. Pregnant women and working surface height and working surface areas for standing manual work. *Appl Ergonomics*. 1995;26:129–133.

Pauls J, ed. *Therapeutic Approaches to Women's Health: A Program of Exercise and Education*. Gaithersburg, Md: Aspen Publishers; 1995.

Pipp LM. TENS update: compendium of selected TENS literature. *J Obstetr Gynecol Phys Ther*. 1993;17:1:12.

Polden M. Health after childbirth: are we neglecting women's problems? *Professional Care of Mother and Child*. 1993;3:121–122.

Poncelet C, Perdu M, Levy-Weil F. Reflex sympathetic dystrophy in pregnancy: nine cases and a review of the literature. *Eur J Obstetr Gynecol Reprod Biol*. 1999;86:55–63.

Potter P, Horne R, Le May K, et al. The sensitivity of thermography to temperature changes in breast tissue. 1997;43:205–210.

Rasmussen B. Reimbursement for obstetric and gynecologic physical therapy. *J Obstetr Gynecol Phys Ther*. 1994;18:2:10–12.

Roubal PJ, Chavinson AH, LaGrandeur RM. Bilateral radial nerve palsies from use of the standard birthing bar. *Obstetr Gynecol*. 1996;87:820–821.

Samsford R, Bullock-Saxton J, Markwell S. *Women's Health: A Textbook for Physiotherapists*. Philadelphia, Pa: WB Saunders Co; 1999.

Scharff L, Marcus Da, Turk DC. Maintenance of effects in the nonmedical treatment of headaches during pregnancy. *Headache*. 1996;36;285–290.

Simkin P, Whalley J, Keppler A. Gracefully pregnant. *Am Baby.* 1992;54:76–80.

Sittler K. Effects of exercise and exercise combined with electrical stimulation on diastasis recti: a single-subject design. *J Section Women's Health.* 1997;21:5.

Stephenson RG, O'Connor LJ. *Obstetric and Gynecologic Care in Physical Therapy.* 2nd ed. Thorofare, NJ: Slack Inc; 2000.

Thornton SI, Thornton SJ. Management of gross devarication of the recti abdominis in pregnancy and labour. *Physiotherapy.* 1993;79:457–458.

Tomberlin JP, Saunders HD. *Evaluation, Treatment and Prevention of Musculoskeletal Disorders. Vol 2: Extremities.* Chaska, Minn: The Saunders Group; 1994.

Wedenberg K, Moen B, Norling A. A prospective randomized study comparing acupuncture with physiotherapy for low-back and pelvic pain in pregnancy. *Acta Obstetricia et Gynecologica Scandinavica.* 2000;79:331–335.

Vulvar Vestibulitis

DESCRIPTION

Vulvar vestibulitis is inflammation and pain in the area of the vaginal vestibule and vulva.

CAUSE

No specific cause has been identified.

ASSESSMENT

No specific evaluation has been identified. Consider use of elements from the evaluation for incontinence.

Note: See APTA's Guide to Physical Therapist Practice. 2nd ed. *Physical Therapy.* 2001;81.

Musculoskeletal Preferred Practice Patterns: C, D

AREAS
- History, including any medical conditions or symptoms such as bleeding or discharge, occupation, surgery, menopausal state, and medications
- Psychological/social
- Urinary symptoms: frequency, urgency, stress, and nocturia
- Bowel habits, including any constipation
- Pain, including any dyspareunia (painful intercourse)
- Activities of daily living (ADLs)
- Musculoskeletal evaluation, including any contributing postural problems and adductor muscle spasm, hip, or pelvic floor muscle imbalance
- Perineal examination: strength or spasm, if indicated

INSTRUMENTS/PROCEDURES

See References for sources.
- Female Urogenital System Checklist

PROBLEMS
- The client often has severe pain localized at the vestibule of the vagina and vulvar area.
- The pain may be described as burning.
- The client is hypersensitive in the labia minora area, especially if clothing is tight.

- There is often dyspareunia.
- The condition may be accompanied by urgency in urination, cystitis, or interstitial cystitis.

TREATMENT/MANAGEMENT
- Consider use of acupressure, joint mobilization, soft tissue work, trigger point therapy, or myofascial release.
- Modalities can include electrotherapy, ultrasound or diathermy, superficial heat, ice, or transcutaneous electrical nerve stimulation (TENS).
- Encourage a fitness program with a stretching component.
- Instruct in relaxation techniques.

DESIRED OUTCOME/PROGNOSIS
- The client will experience symptom relief.

REFERENCES

Assessment

Adams C, Frahm J. Genitourinary system. In: Myers RS, ed. *Saunders Manual of Physical Therapy Practice*. Philadelphia, Pa: WB Saunders Co; 1995:459–504.

American Physical Therapy Association. Guide to physical therapist practice. 2nd ed. *Phys Ther.* 2001;81.

Glazer H, Jantos M, Hartmann EH, et al. Electromyographic comparisons of the pelvic floor in women with dyesthetic vulvodynia and asymptomatic women. *J Reprod Med.* 1998;43:959–962.

Samsford R, Bullock-Saxton J, Markwell S. *Women's Health: A Textbook for Physiotherapists.* Philadelphia, Pa: WB Saunders Co; 1999.

Wilder E, ed. *The Gynecological Manual. Section on Women's Health.* Alexandria, Va: American Physical Therapy Association; 1997.

Treatment

Becka EG, Hahn S, Hunter D, et al. Reducing pelvic floor hypertonicity in patients with vulvodynia. *Phys Ther Case Reports.* 2000;3:247–257.

Glazer HI, Rodke G, Swencionis C. Treatment of vulvar vestibulitis syndrome with electromyographic biofeedback of pelvic floor musculature. *J Reprod Med.* 1995;40:283–290.

Markswell SJ, Mumme GA. A role for physiotherapy in perianal and perineal pain syndromes. In: Shacklock MO, ed. *Moving in on Pain*. Australia: Butterworth Heinemann; 1995:145–152.

Mathias SD, Kuppermann M, Liberman RF, et al. Chronic pelvic pain: prevalence, health-related quality of life and economic correlates. *Obstetr Gynecol.* 1996;87:321–327.

Pomerantz E. Vulvodynia: Etiology and treatment strategies. *J Obstetr Gynecol Phys Ther.* 1994;18:10.

Samsford R, Bullock-Saxton J, Markwell S. *Women's Health: A Textbook for Physiotherapists.* Philadelphia, Pa: WB Saunders Co; 1999.

Wilder E, ed. *The Gynecological Manual. Section on Women's Health.* Alexandria, Va: American Physical Therapy Association; 1997.

Appendix

Pediatric Assessments

AAMR Adaptive Behavior Scales
> Nihira K, Leland H, Lambert N. *AAMR Adaptive Behavior Scale.* Austin, Tex: PRO-ED; 1974.

Alberta Infant Motor Scale (AIMS)
> Piper M, Darrrah J. *Motor Assessment of the Developing Infant.* Philadelphia, Pa: WB Saunders Co; 1994.

Assessment, Evaluation, and Programming System for Infants and Children (AEPS)
> Bricker D. *Assessment, Evaluation, and Programming System for Infants and Children. Volume 1. Measurement for Birth to Three Years.* Baltimore, Md: Paul H Brookes; 1993.
> Bricker D. *Assessment, Evaluation, and Programming System for Infants and Children. Volume 3. Measurement for Three to Six Years.* Baltimore, Md: Paul H Brookes; 1996.

Assessment of Muscle Tone
> Howle JMW. Assessment of muscle tone. In: Campbell SK ed. *Decision Making in Pediatric Neurologic Physical Therapy.* New York, NY: Churchill Livingstone; 1999:37.

Assessment of Preterm Infant Behavior (APIB)
> Als H, Lester B, Tronick EZ, Brazelton TB. *Assessment of Preterm Infant Behavior.* Boston, Mass: Children's Hospital; 1982.

Battelle Developmental Inventory Screening Test (BDIST)
> Newborg J, Stock JR, Wnek L. *Battelle Developmental Inventory Screening Test.* Chicago: Riverside Publishing Co; 1988.

Bayley Infant Neurodevelopmental Screener (BINS)
> Aylward GP. *Bayley Infant Neurodevelopmental Screener Manual.* San Antonio, Tex: The Psychological Corporation; 1995.

Bayley Scales of Infant Development–II (BSID–II)
> Bayley N. *Bayley Scales of Infant Development–II.* San Antonio, Tex: The Psychological Corporation; 1993.

Beery-Buktenica Developmental Test of Visual-Motor Integration, 4th ed, rev. (VMI-4)
> Beery KE, Buktenica NA. *Beery-Buktenica Developmental Test of Visual-Motor Integration.* 4th ed. Parsippany, NJ: Modern Curriculum Press; 1997.

Borg's Scale of Ratings of Perceived Exertion
> Borg GAV. Psychophysical bases of perceived exertion. *Medicine and Science in Sports and Exercise.* 1982;14:377–381.

Brief Functional Evaluation of Muscle Strength
> Kuchta G, Davidson I, Petty RE. Connective tissue diseases in children. In: Melvin JL, Wright FB, eds. *Pediatric Rheumatic Diseases.* (Rheumatologic rehabilitation

services, v. 3). Bethesda, Md: American Occupational Therapy Association; 2000: 80.

Brigance Diagnostic Inventory of Early Development–Revised
Brigance A. *Brigance Diagnostic Inventory of Early Development–Revised*. North Billerica, Mass: Curriculum Associates; 1991.

Bruininks-Oseretsky Test of Motor Proficiency (BOTMP)
Bruninks RH. *Bruininks-Oseretsky Test of Motor Proficiency*. Circle Pines, Minn: American Guidance Service; 1978.

Canadian Occupational Performance Measure (COPM)
Law M, Baptiste S, Carswell A, McColl MA, Polatajko H, Pollock N. *Canadian Occupational Performance Measure*. 3rd ed. Ottawa, Ontario: Canadian Association of Occupational Therapists; 1998.

Carolina Curriculum for Handicapped Infants at Risk
Johnson-Martin N, Jens KG, Attermeier SM, Hacker BJ. *Carolina Curriculum for Handicapped Infants at Risk*. Baltimore, Md: Paul H. Brookes; 1986.

Carolina Curriculum for Preschoolers with Special Needs
Johnson-Martin N, Attermeier SM, Hacker BJ. *Carolina Curriculum for Preschoolers with Special Needs*. Baltimore, Md: Paul H. Brookes; 1990.

Chandler Movement Assessment of Infants Screening Test (CMAI-ST)
Chandler L. Neuromotor assessment. In: Gibbs Ed, Teti DM, eds. *Interdisciplinary Assessment of Infants: A Guide for Early Intervention*. Baltimore, Md: Paul H. Brookes; 1990.

Childhood Health Assessment Questionnaire
Singh G, Arthreya B, Fries JF, Goldsmith DP. Measurement of health status in children with JFA. *Arthritis and Rheumatism*; 1994;37:1761–1769. Scale is provided in Campbell, Vander Linden, Palisano, *Physical Therapy for Children*. 2nd ed. 2000: 236–237.

Clinical Assessment of Gestational Age in the Newborn Infant
Dubowitz L, Dubowitz V, Goldberg C. Clinical assessment of gestational age in the newborn infant. *Journal of Pediatrics*. 1970;77:1–10.

Clinical Observation of Motor and Postural Skills (COMPS)
Wilson BN, Pollock N, Kaplan BJ, Law M. *Clinical Observations of Motor and Postural Skills*. 2nd ed. Farmingham, Mass: Therapro; 2000.

Coma/Near Coma
Rappaport M, Doughery AM, Kelting DL. Evaluation of coma and vegetative states. *Archives of Physical Medicine and Rehabilitation*. 1992;73:628–634.

DeGangi-Berk Test of Sensory Integration
Berk RA, DeGangi GA. *DeGangi-Berk Test of Sensory Integration*. Los Angles: Western Psychological Services;1987.

Denver II
Frankenburg WK, Dodds J, Archer P. *Denver II Technical Manual*. Denver, Colo: Denver Developmental Materials Inc; 1990.

Duncan Reach Tests
See Functional Reach Test.

Early Intervention Developmental Profile (EIDP)
Rogers SJ, D'Eugenio DB. Assessment and application. In: Schafer DS & Moersch MS, eds. *Developmental Programming for Infants and Young Children*. Vol. 3. Ann Arbor: The University of Michigan Press; 1977.

Developmental Test of Visual Perception–2 (DTVP–2)
Hammill DD, Pearson NA, Voress JK. *Developmental Test of Visual Perception*. Austin, Tex: PRO-ED; 1993.

Early Learning Accomplishment Profile for Young Children (Early LAP)
>Glover ME, Preminger JL. *Early LAP–The Early Learning Accomplishment Profile for Young Children Birth to 36 Months.* Lewisville, NC: Kaplan Press; 1995.

First STEP: Screening Test for Evaluating Preschoolers
>Miller LJ. *First STEP.* San Antonio, Tex: The Psychological Corporation; 1992.

Functional Independence Measure
>Data Management Service of the Uniform Data System for Medical Rehabilitation and the Center for Functional Assessment Research. *Guide for the Use of the Uniform Data Set for Medical Rehabilitation Including the Functional Independence Measure* (Version 3.1). Buffalo, NY: State University of New York at Buffalo; 1990.

Functional Independence Measure for Children (WeeFIM)
>Granger CV, Hamilton BB, Kayton R. *Guide for the Use of the Functional Independence Measure for Children (WeeFIM) of the Uniform Data Set for Medical Rehabilitation.* Buffalo, NY: State University of New York at Buffalo; 1989.

Functional Reach Test (FRT)
>Duncan PW, Weiner DK, Chadler J, Studenske S. Functional reach. A new clinical measure of balance. *Journal of Gerontology.* 1990;45(6):M192–M197.

Functional Standing Test
>Triolo RJ, Reilley B, Freedman W, Betz RR. The functional standing test. *IEEE Engineering and Medical Biology.* 1992;11(4):32–34.

Gesell Developmental Schedules
>Knobloch H, Parsamanick B. *Gesell and Amatruda's Developmental Diagnosis.* 3rd ed. Philadelphia, Pa: JB Lippincott; 1974.

Gesell & Amatruda Developmental and Neurological Examination, Revised
>Knobloch H, Stevens F, Malone AT. *Manual of Developmental Diagnosis: The Administration and Interpretation of the Revised Gesell & Armatruda Developmental and Neurological Examination.* New York, NY: Harper & Row; 1980.

Glasgow Coma Scale
>Teasdale G, Jennett B. Assessment of coma and impaired consciousness. *Lancet.* 1974; 2:81–83.

Glasgow Outcome Scale
>Jennett B, Snoek J, Bond MR, Brooks N. Disability after severe head injury: Observations on the use of Glasgow Outcome Scale. *Journal of Neurology, Neurosurgery and Psychiatry.* 1981;44:285–287.

Gross Motor Function Measure (GMFM)
>Russell D, Rosenbaum P, Gowland C, Hardy S, Lane M, Plews N, McGavin H, Cadman D, Jarvis S. *Gross Motor Function Measure Manual.* 2nd ed. Hamilton, Ontario: MacMaster University; 1993.

Gross Motor Performance Measure (GMPM)
>Boyce W, Gowland C, Rosenbaum P, Hardy L, Lane C, Plews N, Goldsmith C, Russell D, Wright V, Potter S, Harding D. *Gross Motor Performance Measure.* Kingston, Ontario: Queen's University, School of Rehabilitation Therapy; 1998.

Gubbay Tests of Motor Proficiency
>Gubbay SS. *The Clumsy Child: A Study of Developmental Apraxic and Agnostic Ataxia.* London: WB Saunders; 1975:155–156. Also see Campbell SK, Vander Linden DW, Palisano RJ. *Physical Therapy for Children.* 2nd ed; 2000:500–501.

Harris Infant Neuromotor Test (HINT)
>Harris SR, Daniels LE. Content validity of the Harris Infant Neuromotor Test. *Physical Therapy.* 1996;76:727–737.

Hawaii Early Learning Profile (HELP)
>Parks S. *Inside HELP–Administration and Reference Manual for the Hawaii Early Learning Profile.* Palo Alto, Calif: VORT Corp; 1999.

Health-Related Physical Fitness Test
> American Alliance for Health Physical Education Recreation and Dance. *Lifetime: Health-Related Physical Fitness Test.* Reston, Va: AAHPERD; 1980.

Helping Babies Learn
> Furuno S, O'Reilly KA, Hosaka CM, Inatsuka TT, Falbey BZ. *Helping Babies Learn. Developmental Profiles and Activities for Infants and Toddlers.* San Antonio, Tex: The Psychological Corporation/Communication Therapy Skill Builders; 2000.

INFANIB: Infant Neurological International Battery
> Andre-Thomas C, Chesni Y, Dargassies SS. *Neurological Examination of the Infant.* London: National Spastics Society; 1950:11–50.

Infant Motor Screen (IMC)
> Nickel RE. *The Manual for the Infant Motor Screen.* Eugene, Ore: Child Development and Rehabilitation Center, The Oregon Health Sciences Center; 1987.

Infant Neuromotor Assessment (INA)
> Magasiner VA, Molteno CD, Lachman P, Thompson C, Buccimazza SS, Burger EJ. A neuromotor screening test for high-risk infants in a hospital or community setting. *Pediatric Physical Therapy.* 1997;9(4):166–172.

Joint Alignment and Motion (JAM) Scale
> Speigel TM, Speigel JS, Paulus HE. The joint alignment and motion scale: a simple measure of joint deformity in patients with rheumatoid arthritis. *Journal of Rheumatology.* 1987;14:887–892.

Juvenile Arthritis Functional Assessment Scale (JAFAS)
> Lovell DJ, Howe S, Shear E, Hartner S, McGirr G, Schulte M, Levinson J. Development of a disability measurement tool for juvenile rheumatoid arthritis: The Juvenile Arthritis Functional Assessment Scale. *Arthritis and Rheumatism.* 1989;21:1390–1395.
> Scale provided in Scull, In: Campbell SK, ed. *Physical Therapy for Children.* 2nd ed. Philadelphia, Pa: WB Saunders Co; 2000:234.

Juvenile Arthritis Status Index (JASI)
> Wright FV, Longo-Kimber J, Law M, Goldsmith CJ, Dent P. Validation of a functional status index for juvenile arthritis. *Physiotherapy Canada.* 1992;44:S6 (abstract).

Manual Muscle Testing
> Hislop HJ, Montgomery J, eds. *Daniels' and Worthingham's Muscle Testing: Techniques of Manual Examination.* 6th ed. Philadelphia, Pa: WB Saunders; 1995.

Manual Muscle Testing
> MacDonald CM, Jaffe KM, Shurles DB. Assessment of muscle strength in children with meningomyelocele: Accuracy and stability of measurements over time. *Archives of Physical Medicine and Rehabilitation.* 1986;67:855–861.

Milani-Comparetti Motor Development Screening Test (MCMDST)
> Stuberg WA, Dehne P, Miedaner J, White P. *The Milani-Comparetti Motor Developmental Screening Test.* 3rd ed rev. Omaha, Neb: University of Nebraska Medical Center; 1992.

Miller Assessment of Preschoolers (MAP)
> Miller LJ. *Miller Assessment for Preschoolers.* San Antonio, Tex: The Psychological Corporation; 1988.

Modified Ashworth Scale
> Bohannon RW, Smith MB. Interrater reliability of a Modified Ashworth Scale of muscle spasticity. *Physical Therapy.* 1987;67:206–7.

Morgan Neonatal Neurobehavioral Examination
> Sheahan MC, Brockway NF, Tecklin JS. The high-risk infant. In: Tecklin JS, ed. *Pediatric physical therapy.* 3rd ed. Philadelphia, Pa: Lippincott Williams and Wilkins; 1999: 88–91.

Motor-Free Visual Perception Test–Revised (MVPT-R)
Colarusso R, Hammill D. *Motor-Free Visual Perception Test–Revised*. Novato, Calif: Academic Therapy Publications; 1996.

Motor Assessment of the Development Infant
See Alberta Infant Motor Scale.

Movement Assessment Battery for Children (Movement ABC)
Henderson SE, Sugden D. *Movement Assessment Battery for Children*. San Antonio, Tex: The Psychological Corporation; 1992.

Movement Assessment of Infants (MAI)
Chandler LS, Andrews MS, Swanson MW. *Movement Assessment of Infants–A Manual*. Rolling Bay, Wash: Rolling Bay Press; 1980.

Naturalistic Observation of Newborn Activity
Als H. *Naturalistic Observation of Newborn Activity*. Neonatal Individualized Development Care and Assessment Program (NIDCAP). Boston, Mass: Childrens' Hospital; 1984.

NCAST Feeding Scale
See Nursing Child Assessment Feeding Scale.

Neonatal Behavioral Assessment Scale (NBAS)
Brazelton TB. *Neonatal Behavioral Assessment Scale*. 3rd ed. Clinics in Developmental Medicine No. 137. London, England: Mac Keith Press; 1995.

Neonatal Oral-Motor Assessment Scale (NOMAS)
Braum MA, Palmer MM. A pilot study of oral-motor dysfunction in "at-risk" infants. *Physical and Occupational Therapy in Pediatrics*. 1985;5:13–25.

Neurobehavioral Assessment for Preterm Infants (NAPI)
Korner AF, Constantinou J, Dimiceli S, Brown BW Jr, Thom VA. Establishing the reliability and developmental validity of neurobehavioral assessment for preterm infants: A methodological process. *Child Development*. 1991;62:1200–1208.

Neurologic Assessment of the Preterm and Full-Term Newborn Infant
Dubowitz L, Dubowitz V. *The Neurological Assessment of the Preterm and Full-Term Newborn Infant*. London: Heinemann; 1981.

Nicholas Manual Muscle Tester
Horvat M, Croce R, Roswal G. Intratester reliability of the Nicholas Manual Muscle Tester on individuals with intellectual disabilities by a tester having minimal experience. *Archives of Physical Medicine and Rehabilitation*. 1994;76:808–811.

Nine Hole Peg Test
Kellor M, Frost J, Silverberg N, Iversen I, Cummings R. Hand strength and dexterity. Norms for clinical use. *American Journal of Occupational Therapy*. 1971;25(1): 77–83.

Nursing Child Assessment Feeding Scale (NCAFS)
Barnard KE, Eyres SJ. Feeding scale. In: *Child Health Assessment* (DHEW publication no. HRA 78–25). Hyattsville, Md: U.S. Department of Health, Education and Welfare, Health Resources Administration, Bureau of Health Manpower, Division of Nursing; 1979.

Peabody Developmental Motor Scales–2 (PDMS-2)
Folio MR, Fewell RR. *Peabody Developmental Motor Scales–2*. Austin, Tex: PRO-ED; 1999.

Pediatric Clinical Test of Sensory Interaction for Balance (P-CTSIB)
Crowe TK, Deitz JC, Richardson PK, Atwater SW. Interrater reliability of the Pediatric Clinical Test of Sensory Interaction for Balance. *Physical and Occupational Therapy in Pediatrics*. 1990;10(4):1–27.

Pediatric Evaluation of Disability Inventory (PEDI)
> Haley SM, Coster WJ, Ludlow LH, Haltiwanger JT, Andrellos PJ. *The Pediatric Evaluation of Disability Inventory.* San Antonio, Tex: Therapy Skills Builders; 1992.

Perceived Competence Scale for Children
> Harter S. The perceived competence scale for children. *Child Development.* 1982;53: 87–97.

Quick Neurological Screening Test-II (QNST)
> Mutti M, Sterling HM, Spalding NV, Crawford CS. *Quick Neurological Screening Test–II.* Novato, Calif: Academic Therapy; 1988.

School Function Assessment (SFA)
> Coster W, Deeney T, Haltiwanger J, Haley S. *School Function Assessment.* San Antonio, Tex: The Psychological Corporation/Therapy Skill Builders; 1998.

Seated Postural Control Measure
> Story M, Fife S. *Seated Postural Control Measure.* Vancouver, BC: Sunny Hill Hospital for Children; 1992.

Sensory Integration and Praxis Tests (SIPT)
> Ayres AJ. *Sensory Integration and Praxis Tests.* Los Angeles, Calif: Western Psychological Corporation; 1991.

Sitting Assessment for Children with Neuromotor Dysfunction (SACND)
> Reid DT. *Sitting Assessment for Children with Neuromotor Dysfunction.* San Antonio, Tex: The Psychological Corporation/Therapy Skill Builders; 1997.

Sitting Assessment Scale
> Myhr U, von Wendt L. Improvement of functional sitting position for children with cerebral palsy. *Developmental Medicine and Child Neurology.* 1991;33:236–256.

Southern California Postrotary Nystagmus Test (PRNT)
> Ayres AJ. *Southern California Postrotary Nystagmus Test.* Los Angeles, Calif: Western Psychological Corporation; 1975.

Supported Walker Ambulation Performance Scale (SWAPS)
> Malouin F, Richards CL, Menier C, Dumas F, Marcoux S. Supported Walker Ambulation Performance Scale (SWAPS): Development of an outcome measure of locomotor status in children with cerebral palsy. *Pediatric Physical Therapy.* 1997;9(2): 48–53.

Test of Infant Motor Performance (TIMP)
> Campbell SK, Osten ET, Kolobe THA, Fisher AG. *Development of the Test of Infant Motor Performance.* In: Granger CV & Gresham GE, eds. *New Developments in Functional Assessment. [Physical Medicine and Rehabilitation Clinics of North America]* Philadelphia, Pa: WB Saunders Co; 1993:541–550.
> Campbell DK, Kolobe THA, Osten E, Lemke M, Girolami GL. Construct validity of the Test of Infant Motor Performance. *Physical Therapy.* 1995;74:585–596.

Test of Sensory Function in Infants
> DeGangi GA, Greenspan SI. *Test of Sensory Function in Infants.* Los Angles, Calif: Western Psychological Services; 1988.

The T.I.M.E.: Toddler and Infant Motor Evaluation
> Miller LJ, Roid GH. *The TIME. Toddler and Infant Motor Evaluation: A Standardized Assessment.* San Antonio, Tex: Therapy Skills Builders; 1994.

Timed Get-Up-and-Go Test
> See Timed Up and Go.

Timed Up and Go (TUG)
> Podsciadlo D, Richardson S. The Timed "Up and Go": A test of basic functional mobility for frail elderly persons. *Journal of the American Geriatric Society.* 1991;39: 142–148.

Torticollis Evaluation Form
>Karmel-Ross K. Torticollis evaluation form. *Physical and Occupational Therapy in Pediatrics.* 1997;17(2):23–27.

Tufts Assessment of Motor Performance (TAMP)
>Gans BM, Saley SM, Hallenborg SC, Mann N, Inacio CA, Faas RM. Description and interobserver reliability of the Tufts Assessment of Motor Performance. *American Journal of Physical Medicine and Rehabilitation.* 1988;67:202–210.

Upright Motor Control Test
>Hislop HJ & Montgomery J. Upright motor control. In: *Daniels' and Worthingham's Muscle Testing: Techniques of Manual Examination.* 6th ed. Philadelphia, Pa: WB Saunders; 1995:320.

Vineland Adaptive Behavior Scales-Revised (VABS)
>Sparrow SS, Balla DA, & Cicchetti DV. *Vineland Adaptive Behavior Scales, Revised.* Circle Pines, Minn: American Guidance Service; 1984.

Vulpe Assessment Battery, 2nd ed. (VAB)
>Vulpe S. *Vulpe Assessment Battery: Developmental Assessment, Performance Analysis, Individualized Programming for the Atypical Child.* 2nd ed. East Aurora, NY: Slosson Educational Publications; 1994.

WeeFIM
>See Functional Independence Measure for Children.

Western Neuro Sensory Stimulation Profile
>Ansell BJ, Keenan JE. The Western Neuro Sensory Stimulation Profile: A tool for assessing slow-to-recover head-injured patients. *Archives of Physical Medicine and Rehabilitation.* 1989;70:104–108.

Index

About the Authors

Julie A. Pauls, PhD, PT, ICCE, is an associate professor at Montgomery College and president of PhysiCare for Women, P.C., a consultative practice. She is the author of *Therapeutic Approaches to Women's Health*. She lives in The Woodlands, Texas, with her husband and children.

Kathlyn L. Reed, PhD, OTR, FAOTA, MLIS, AHIP, is visiting professor, School of Occupational Therapy, at Texas Woman's University–Houston Center. She is the author of *Quick Reference to Occupational Therapy* and co-author of *Quick Reference to Speech Language Pathology*.